ORAL TOLERANCE:
MECHANISMS AND APPLICATIONS

ANNALS OF THE NEW YORK ACADEMY OF SCIENCES
Volume 778

ORAL TOLERANCE: MECHANISMS AND APPLICATIONS

Edited by Howard L. Weiner and Lloyd F. Mayer

The New York Academy of Sciences
New York, New York
1996

Library of Congress Cataloging-in-Publication Data

Oral tolerance : mechanisms and applications / edited by Howard L. Weiner and Lloyd F. Mayer.
    p.   cm. — (Annals of the New York Academy of Sciences, ISSN 00778923 : v. 778)
    Includes bibliographical references and index.
    ISBN 0-89766-995-9 (cloth : alk. paper). — ISBN 0-89766-996-7 (pbk. : alk. paper)
    1. Immunological tolerance—Congresses.   2. Oral mucosa—Immunology—Congresses.   3. Gastrointestinal mucosa—Immunology—Congresses.   4. Autoimmune diseases—Congresses.   I. Weiner, Howard L.   II. Mayer, Lloyd F.   III. Series.
    [DNLM: 1. Immune Tolerance—physiology. 2. Administration, Oral. W1 AN626YL v. 778 1996 / QW 504 O63 1996]
Q11.N5   vol. 778
[QR188.4]
500 s—dc20
[616.07′9]
DNLM/DLC
    for Library of Congress

95-48330
CIP

PCP
Printed in the United States of America
ISBN 0-89766-995-9 (cloth)
ISBN 0-89766-996-7 (paper)
ISSN 0077-8923

ANNALS OF THE NEW YORK ACADEMY OF SCIENCES

Volume 778
February 13, 1996

ORAL TOLERANCE:
MECHANISMS AND APPLICATIONS [a]

Editors and Conference Organizers
HOWARD L. WEINER and LLOYD F. MAYER

CONTENTS

[a] This volume is the result of a conference, entitled **Oral Tolerance: Mechanisms and Applications,** held in New York City on March 30–April 2, 1995, by the New York Academy of Sciences.

Financial assistance was received from:

Major Funders

- AUTOIMMUNE INC.
- FOUNDATION FOR NEUROLOGIC DISEASES

Supporters

- BERLEX LABORATORIES

Contributors

- ELI LILLY AND COMPANY
- GLAXO INC.
- GLAXO RESEARCH INSTITUTE
- HOFFMANN-LA ROCHE INC.
- MERCK RESEARCH LABORATORIES
- NATIONAL INSTITUTE OF ALLERGY AND INFECTIOUS DISEASES—NATIONAL INSTITUTES OF HEALTH
- NATIONAL INSTITUTE OF ARTHRITIS AND MUSCULOSKELETAL AND SKIN DISEASES—NATIONAL INSTITUTES OF HEALTH
- NATIONAL INSTITUTE OF DIABETES AND DIGESTIVE AND KIDNEY DISEASES—NATIONAL INSTITUTES OF HEALTH
- NATIONAL MULTIPLE SCLEROSIS SOCIETY
- PFIZER INC., CENTRAL RESEARCH DIVISION
- SOLVAY PHARMACEUTICALS

Introduction

HOWARD L. WEINER [a] AND LLOYD F. MAYER [b]

[a]Center for Neurologic Diseases
Brigham and Women's Hospital and
Harvard Medical School
221 Longwood Avenue
Boston, Massachusetts 02115

[b]Mount Sinai Medical Center
Division of Clinical Immunology and
Department of Cell Biology
Box 1089, One Gustave L. Levy Place
New York, New York 10029

Oral tolerance is a long recognized method of inducing immune tolerance. It refers to the observation that if one feeds a protein and then immunizes with the fed protein, a state of systemic hyporesponsiveness to the fed protein exists. In recent years, as more has been learned about the general mechanisms of immune tolerance, investigators have begun to apply oral tolerance as a method to manipulate injurious immune responses, primarily in the area of autoimmune diseases, although its applications appear broader and have included transplantation as well. The conference entitled Oral Tolerance: Mechanisms and Applications was organized to bring together investigators who are studying both basic mechanisms of oral tolerance and its application to pathologic immune states. This is an area that has become of intense interest and one that is likely to grow inasmuch as manipulation of systemic immune responses through the mucosal immune system has major practical and theoretical advantages. TABLE 1 lists the wide range of topics discussed at the conference and contained in this volume.

Oral tolerance was first described in 1911 when Wells fed hen's egg proteins to guinea pigs and found them resistant to anaphylaxis when challenged.[1] In 1946, Chase fed guinea pigs the contact-sensitizing agent, DCNB, and observed that animals had decreased skin reactivity to DCNB.[2] Subsequently, numerous investigators have found that animals fed proteins such as ovalbumin or sheep red blood cells do not respond as well to these antigens when subsequently immunized but do respond normally to other antigens.[3] The phenomenon of oral tolerance has also been observed in humans fed and immunized with keyhole-limpet hemocyanin.[4]

Immunologic tolerance is a basic property of the immune system that provides for self/nonself-discrimination so that the immune system can protect the host from external pathogens without reacting against self. When the immune system reacts against itself, autoimmune disease results. For a time it was thought that self/nonself-discrimination was a simple matter of deleting autoreactive cells in the thymus, but it is now clear that the maintenance of immunologic tolerance is a much more complicated process. Autoreactive cells, such as those reacting with the brain, are not deleted and can be found in normal individuals.[5,6] Why these cells become activated and cause disease in some individuals, whereas in others they remain harmless, is a major question in basic immunology. How to control the autoimmune process once it has been initiated is the major problem in clinical medicine.

These two areas have come together in recent years, as oral tolerance has been successfully used to treat autoimmune diseases in animal models (reviewed in ref. 7),

TABLE 1. Oral Tolerance

A. Mechanisms
    Deletion
    Anergy
    Active suppression
    (Regulation)
B. Types of Immune Responses Affected
    Cellular Responses
        Th1
        Th2
    Humoral Responses
        IgG1
        IgG2a
        IgA
        IgE
C. Regulating Factors
    Dose of antigen
    Form/nature of antigen
    Antigen-presenting cells
    Cytokine mileu
    Adjuvants
    Luminal factors
    Age

and is now being applied for the treatment of human disease states.[8,9] Furthermore, an understanding of the basic mechanisms by which orally administered antigens induce immune tolerance is beginning to emerge. As with immunologic tolerance in general, oral tolerance involves multiple mechanisms.[10-13] Thus the term, oral tolerance, is in some ways misleading, as it implies that there is one unique mechanism of tolerance induction when antigens are administered orally. This is not the case. Although the gut clearly has unique properties that favor tolerance induction, the type of tolerance induced must now be defined when factors that influence oral tolerance are investigated.

Orally administered antigen encounters the gut-associated lymphoid tissue or GALT, a very well-developed immune network that evolved not only to protect the host from ingested pathogens, but also developed the inherent property of preventing the host from reacting to ingested proteins. The GALT consists of epithelial cells capable of antigen presentation, specialized epithelium or M cells capable of transporting certain antigens across the mucosal barrier, intraepithelial lymphocytes, and lamina propria lymphocytes.[14] In addition, there are Peyer's patches, lymphoid nodules underlying the dome epithelium among the villi, which are one of the primary areas in the GALT where specific immune responses are generated. Investigators have attempted to stimulate the GALT in the development of oral vaccines but have been hampered by the systemic hyporesponsiveness or oral tolerance that is naturally generated. Nonetheless, as described below, active induction of selected immune responses in the GALT is one of the primary mechanisms by which oral antigen suppresses systemic immunity.

In addition to stimulating the GALT, some oral antigen is absorbed. Although dietary antigens are degraded by the time they reach the small intestine, studies in humans and rodents have indicated that the degradation is partial and that some intact antigen is absorbed.[15,16] Absorbed antigen, either undegraded or partially degraded, appears to have an important role in the generation of certain types of oral tolerance.

MECHANISMS OF ORAL TOLERANCE

It is now known that the mechanisms by which oral tolerance is mediated include the generation of active cellular suppression (regulatory cells), clonal energy, or clonal deletion; the determining factor is the dose of antigen fed.[10-13] Low doses favor active suppression, whereas higher doses favor anergy and deletion. Active suppression is mediated by the induction of regulatory T cells in the GALT, such as Peyer's patches. These cells then migrate to the systemic immune system. When higher doses of antigen are fed, clonal anergy results and can be demonstrated by reversal of systemic hyporesponsiveness by culturing with recombinant IL-2.[10,12] Anergy may be favored by the passage of antigen into the systemic circulation. When large doses of antigen are fed, clonal deletion occurs.[13] Thus, oral tolerance is not a single immunologic event.

Active cellular suppression of immune responses has been studied extensively over the years and has remained ill-defined, due to difficulties in cloning suppressor cells and defining their mechanism of action. More recently, it appears that one of the primary mechanisms of active cellular suppression is through the secretion of suppressive cytokines, such as TGF-β, IL-4, and IL-10 after antigen-specific triggering.[17] In this sense, the GALT is unique, as it favors the induction of cells that secrete these cytokines, Th2 as opposed to Th1 cells, and T cells that secrete TGF-β, a potent immunosuppressive cytokine. T cells in lymphoid organs drained by mucosal sites secrete IL-4 as a primary T-cell growth factor, whereas those drained by nonmucosal sites secrete IL-2.[18] Oral tolerance has often been demonstrated by a decreased delayed-type hypersensitivity (DTH) response to the fed antigen,[2,3,7] and it is known that DTH is a Th1 response inhibited by IL-4-producing Th2 cells. TGF-β plays an important role in local function of the gut, as it serves as a switch factor for IgA production in the mucosa[19] and may also be involved in the homing mechanism of the cells to high-endothelial venules and into the epithelium.[20] TGF-β is produced by both CD4+ and CD8+ GALT-derived T cells[17,21] and is an important mediator of the active component of oral tolerance. TGF-β secreting MBP-specific CD4+ cells have recently been cloned from the mesenteric lymph nodes of orally tolerized SJL mice.[17] These clones were structurally identical to Th1 disease-inducing clones in T-cell receptor usage, MHC restriction, and epitope recognition, but these clones suppressed rather than induced disease. Thus, mucosally derived CD4+ cells that primarily produce TGF-β may be a unique T-cell subset with both mucosal T-helper function and down-regulatory properties for Th1 and other immune cells.

BYSTANDER SUPPRESSION AND ORAL TOLERANCE

Bystander suppression was discovered during the investigation of regulatory cells induced by oral administration of low doses of myelin-basic protein.[22] It solves a major conceptual problem related to designing antigen or T-cell specific therapy of inflammatory autoimmune diseases, such as multiple sclerosis, type-1 diabetes, and rheumatoid arthritis in which the autoantigen is unknown or where there are reactivities to multiple autoantigens in the target tissue. In animal models of autoimmunity, during the course of the chronic inflammatory autoimmune process, there is an intra- and interantigenic spread of autoreactivity at the target organ.[23-27] Similar findings have been observed in human autoimmune disease in which there are reactivities to multiple autoantigens from the target tissue. For

TABLE 2. Suppression of Autoimmunity by Oral Tolerance

A. Animal Models	Protein Fed
EAE	MBP, PLP
Arthritis (CII[a], AA[b], Ag[c], Pris[d])	Type II collagen
Uveitis	S-antigen, IRBP[e]
Diabetes (NOD mouse)	Insulin, glutamate decarboxylase
Myasthenia gravis	AChR
Thyroiditis	Thyroglobulin
Transplantation	Alloantigen, MHC peptide
B. Human Disease Trials	Protein
Multiple sclerosis	Bovine myelin
Rheumatoid arthritis	Chicken type II collagen
Uveoretinitis	Bovine S-antigen
Type I diabetes	Human insulin

[a] Collagen.
[b] Adjuvant arthritis.
[c] Antigen.
[d] Pristane.
[e] Interphotoreceptor retinoid-binding protein.

example, in multiple sclerosis there is immune reactivity to three myelin antigens, MBP, proteolipid protein (PLP), and myelin-oligodendrocyte glycoprotein.[5,6] In type-1 diabetes, there are multiple islet-cell antigens that could be the target of autoreactivity, including glutamate decarboxylase, insulin, and heat-shock proteins.[28] Because regulatory cells induced by oral antigen secrete antigen nonspecific cytokines after being triggered by the fed antigen, they suppress inflammation in the microenvironment where the fed antigen is localized. Thus, for an organ-specific inflammatory disease, one need not know the specific antigen that is the target of an autoimmune response but only feed an antigen capable of reducing regulatory cells that then migrate to the target tissue and suppress inflammation. Bystander suppression was demonstrated *in vitro* when it was shown that cells from MBP-fed animals suppressed proliferation of an ovalbumin line across a transwell, but only when triggered by the fed antigen.[22] The soluble factor was identified as TGF-β. Bystander suppression has also been demonstrated in autoimmune disease models. One can suppress PLP peptide-induced experimental autoimmune encephalomyelitis (EAE) by feeding MBP,[29] and MBP-specific T-cells clones from orally tolerized animals that secrete TGF-β also suppress PLP-induced disease. Other examples include the suppression of adjuvant-[30] and antigen-[31] induced arthritis by feeding type II collagen, the suppression of insulitis in the nonobese diabetic (NOD) mouse by feeding glucagon,[7] and the suppression of lymphocytic choriomeningitis virus (LCMV)-induced diabetes in mice that have had LCMV proteins expressed by way of the insulin promoter on the pancreatic islets by feeding insulin.[32]

TREATMENT OF AUTOIMMUNE DISEASES IN ANIMALS

A large series of studies has demonstrated that orally administered autoantigens can suppress several experimental models of autoimmunity and transplantation (TABLE 2, reviewed in ref. 7). The mechanism of suppression in these models depends on dosage administered; in some instances active suppression has been shown, whereas in other instances, clonal anergy. Immunohistochemical studies have demonstrated the up-regulation of antiinflammatory cytokines, such as TGF-β and IL-4 in the target organ of animals fed low doses of autoantigens.[33-35] Importantly, for human trials, feeding after immunization[30] and feeding in chronic disease models, such as chronic EAE, have been successful.[36] Thus, it does not appear that feeding an autoantigen to an already sensitized animal necessarily results in further priming. Suppression of disease, however, may be most effective when homologous protein is administered,[37] which has important implications for treatment of human autoimmune diseases for which recombinant human proteins would be required. Although one can suppress the generation of antibodies by oral feeding, much larger doses are required, and because the gut preferentially induces Th2 responses, the degree to which oral tolerance will be successful in suppressing antibody-mediated diseases is unclear.

TREATMENT OF AUTOIMMUNE DISEASES IN HUMANS

Investigators have shown that exposure of a contact sensitizing agent by way of the mucosa prior to subsequent skin challenge led to unresponsiveness in a portion of patients studied.[39] Orally administered KLH, 50 mg given daily for 10 days over a two- to three-week period to human subjects, has been reported to decrease subsequent cell-mediated immune responses, although antibody responses were not affected.[4]

Based on the long history of oral tolerance and the apparent safety of the approach, human trials have been initiated in multiple sclerosis,[8] rheumatoid arthritis,[9] and uveitis.[40] These initial phase I/II trials have involved a relatively small number of patients, and the clinical efficacy of oral antigen in these diseases must await the results of large-scale trials that are currently in progress (TABLE 2). What can be said from the initial trials is that there was no apparent toxicity or exacerbation of disease. In MS patients, a decrease in MBP-reactive cells was observed in the peripheral blood, and in rheumatoid arthritis, joint swelling was decreased. In multiple sclerosis, there is presently a 500-patient double-blind phase III trial in which patients are randomized by sex and DR haplotype, which may be linked to the response. In rheumatoid arthritis, a 280-patient double-blind phase II dosing trial has just been completed in which doses ranging from 20 μg to 2500 μg were tested. Preliminary analysis of the data demonstrates a positive effect in patients fed 20 μg. In uveitis, a double-masked trial of S-antigen and an S-antigen mixture is currently in progress. In addition, trials are being planned both in juvenile and new-onset diabetes in which oral recombinant human insulin will be administered. Thus, we have evolved from a phenomenon known over the past century as "oral tolerance" to a potential therapeutic modality that is now understood in modern immunologic terms.

REFERENCES

1. WELLS, H. G. 1911. J. Infect. Dis. **8:** 147-171.
2. CHASE, M. 1946. Proc. Soc. Exp. Biol. Med. **61:** 257-259.
3. MOWAT, A. M. 1987. Immunol. Today **8:** 93-98.
4. HUSBY, S., J. MESTECKY, Z. MOLDOVEANU, S. HOLLAND & C. O. ELSON. 1994. J. Immunol. **152:** 4663.
5. KERLERO, DE ROSBO, N., R. MILO, M. B. LEES, D. BURGER, C. C. A. BERNARD & A. BEN-NUN. 1993. J. Clin. Invest. **92:** 2602-2608.
6. ZHANG, J., S. MARKOVIC, J. RAUS, B. LACET, H. L. WEINER & D. A. HAFLER. 1993. J. Exp. Med. **179:** 973-984.

7. WEINER, H. L., A. FRIEDMAN, A. MILLER, S. J. KHOURY, A. AL-SABBAGH, L. M. B. SANTOS, M. SAYEGH, R. B. NUSSENBLATT, D. E. TRENTHAM & D. A. HAFLER. 1994. Annu. Rev. Immunol. **12**: 809-837.
8. WEINER, H. L., G. A. MACKIN, M. MATSUI, E. J. ORAV, S. J. KHOURY, D. M. DAWSON & D. A. HAFLER. 1993. Science **259**: 1321-1324.
9. TRENTHAM, D. E., R. A. DYNESIUS-TRENTHAM, E. J. ORAV, D. COMBITCHI, C. LORENZO, K. L. SEWELL, D. A. HAFLER & H. L. WEINER. 1993. Science **261**: 1727-1730.
10. WHITACRE, C. C., I. E. GIENAPP, C. G. OROSZ & D. BITAR. 1991. J. Immunol. **147**: 2155-2163.
11. GREGERSON, D. S., W. F. OBRITSCH & L. A. DONOSO. 1993. J. Immunol. **151**: 5751-5761.
12. FRIEDMAN, A. & H. L. WEINER. 1994. Proc. Natl. Acad. Sci. USA **91**: 6688-6692.
13. CHEN, Y., J. INOBE, R. MARKS, P. GONELLA, V. J. KUCHROO & H. L. WEINER. 1995. Nature **376**: 177-180.
14. BRANDTZAEG, P. 1989. Curr. Top. Microbiol. Immunol. **146**: 13-28.
15. HUSBY, S., J. C. JENSENIUS & S.-E. SVEHAG. 1986. Scand. J. Immunol. **24**: 447-452.
16. BRUCE, M. G. & A. FERGUSON. 1986. Immunology **59**(2): 295-300.
17. CHEN, Y., V. K. KUCHROO, J.-I. INOBE, D. A. HAFLER & H. L. WEINER. 1994. Science **265**: 1237-1240.
18. DAYNES, R., B. ARANEO, T. DOWELL, K. HUANG & D. DUDLEY. 1990. J. Exp. Med. **171**(April): 979-996.
19. KIM, P.-H. & M. F. KAGNOFF. 1990. J. Immunol. **144**: 3411-3416.
20. CHIN, Y. H., J. P. CAI & X. M. XU. 1992. J. Immunol. **148**(4): 1106-1112.
21. SANTOS, L. M. B., A. AL-SABBAGH, A. LONDONO & H. L. WEINER. 1994. Cell. Immunol. **157**: 439-447.
22. MILLER, A., O. LIDER & H. L. WEINER. 1991. J. Exp. Med. **174**: 791-798.
23. MCCARRON, R., R. FALLIS & D. MCFARLIN. 1990. J. Neuroimmunol. **29**: 73-79.
24. LEHMANN, P., T. FORSTHUBER, A. MILLER & E. SERCARZ. 1992. Nature **358**: 155.
25. CROSS, A. H., V. K. TUOHY & C. S. RAINE. 1993. Cell. Immunol. **146**: 261-270.
26. KAUFMAN, D. L., M. CLARE-SALZIER, J. TIAN, T. FORSTHUBER, G. S. P. TING, P. ROBINSON, M. A. ATKINSON, E. E. SERCARZ, A. J. TOBIN & P. V. LEHMANN. 1993. Nature **366**: 72-75.
27. TISCH, R., X.-D. YANG, S. M. SINGER, R. S. LIBLAU, L. FUGGER & H. O. MCDEVITT. 1993. Nature **366**: 72-75.
28. HARRISON, L. C. 1992. Immunol. Today **13**: 348-352.
29. AL-SABBAGH, A., A. MILLER, L. M. B. SANTOS & H. L. WEINER. 1994. Eur. J. Immunol. **24**: 2104-2109.
30. ZHANG, J. Z., C. S. Y. LEE, O. LIDER & H. L. WEINER. 1990. J. Immunol. **145**: 2489-2493.
31. YOSHINO, S., E. WUATTROCCHI & H. L. WEINER. 1995. Arthritis Rheum. **38**: 1092-1096.
32. HERRATH, M., T. DYRBERG, M. B. A. OLDSTONE. 1995. Int. Congr. Immunol. Abstr. **5018**: 846.
33. KHOURY, S. J., W. W. HANCOCK & H. L. WEINER. 1992. J. Exp. Med. **176**: 1355.
34. HANCOCK, W., M. SAYEGH, C. KWOK, H. L. WEINER & C. CARPENTER. 1993. Transplantation **55**(5): 1112-1118.
35. HANCOCK, W., M. POLANSKI, J. ZHANG, N. BLOGG & H. L. WEINER. 1995. Am. J. Pathol. **147**: 1193-1199.
36. BROD, S. A., A. AL-SABBGH, R. A. SOBEL, D. A. HAFLER & H. L. WEINER. 1991. Ann. Neurol. **29**: 615-622.
37. MILLER, A., O. LIDER, A. AL-SABBAGH & H. L. WEINER. 1992. J. Neuroimmunol. **39**: 243-250.
38. DAKIN, R. 1829. Am. J. Med. Sci. **4**: 98-100.
39. LOWNEY, E. D. 1968. J. Invest. Dermatol. **51**(6): 411-417.
40. NUSSENBLATT, R. B., M. D. DE SMET, H. L. WEINER & I. GERY. 1993. The treatment of the ocular complications of Behcet's disease with oral tolerization. Sixth International Conference on Behcet's disease. Elsevier Press. Amsterdam.

History of Oral Tolerance and Mucosal Immunity[a]

PER BRANDTZAEG

Laboratory for Immunohistochemistry and Immunopathology (LIIPAT)
Institute of Pathology
University of Oslo
The National Hospital
Rikshospitalet, N-0027 Oslo, Norway

INTRODUCTION

The true history of the immune system is written in our genes. Much of this instrumental information was established several million years before our ancestors (*Homo sapiens*) started the migration throughout Africa and to other continents some 100,000 years ago. Evolutionary gene modifications took place as an adaptation to the environmental microbial pressure and the dietary impact influenced by various ways of living, such as hunting, fishing, and farming. In this manner the mucosal immune system has over time apparently generated two arms to defend the body: an immune exclusion system for protection against epithelial penetration of noxious antigens and colonization of pathogens, and hyporesponsiveness to innocuous antigens bombarding the extensive mucosal surfaces (FIG. 1). The latter phenomenon is called ''oral tolerance'' when it is induced in the gut by dietary antigens, and similar down-regulation of immune responsiveness can be generated through the airway mucosae. Parallel protective and suppressive mechanisms have developed in other mammalian species but with considerable variations as to details of expression.

In the face of the immense perspective of the genetic instruction that guides our immune system, a historical overview of mucosal immunity and oral tolerance based on available scientific information will appear to be less than the tip of an iceberg. Solid facts about oral tolerance mechanisms are scant, although this arm of the mucosal immune system seems to have developed rather successfully; more than a ton of nutrients passes through the gastrointestinal tract of an adult every year, but the antigenic challenge this variety of peptides represents causes no hypersensitivity in most individuals. Conversely, mucosal defence against infections is by no means patent, as highlighted in a regrettable manner in the developing countries, although this situation could have been significantly improved by reimplementation of traditional breast feeding.[1] Mucosal infections are now the major killer below the age of five years, being responsible for more than 14 million deaths of children annually. Diarrheal disease alone claims a toll of five million children per year or about 500 deaths per hour. These unfortunate figures document the need for mucosal vaccines to enhance surface defence against common infectious diseases in addition to advocating breast feeding. Moreover, there is hope that the obscure mechanisms of mucosal tolerance induction to soluble protein antigens in the future may be exploited for therapeutic immunosuppression in certain T cell–mediated autoimmune diseases as

[a] Studies in the author's laboratory are supported by the Norwegian Cancer Society, the Research Council of Norway, and Anders Jahre's Fund.

1

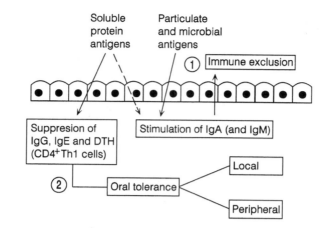

FIGURE 1. Schematic depiction of two major defense mechanisms induced in the gut. Immune exclusion limits epithelial colonization of microorganisms and inhibits penetration of foreign material. This first-line defense is principally mediated by secretory antibodies of the IgA (and IgM) class in cooperation with various nonspecific innate protective factors. Secretory immunity is stimulated mainly by particulate and live microbial antigens. Soluble protein antigens, on the other hand, primarily induce suppression of proinflammatory humoral immune responses (IgG and IgE antibodies) as well as delayed-type hypersensitivity (DTH) mediated by activated helper T cells (CD4⁺) of the Th1 subset. This poorly defined phenomenon induced by dietary antigens, which may operate both locally and in the periphery, is called oral tolerance.

well as for modulation of immunity in infancy to avoid atopic allergy against inhalant allergens.

Although mucosal immunology has suffered from slow recognition as a scientific discipline, work in this field is now moving faster and faster; a final goal of these extensive efforts is the development of rational protocols for mucosal stimulatory or down-regulating antigen application that are efficient, safe, practical, and inexpensive. However, the complexity of the local immune system is an obstacle to rapid success with regard to efficient manipulation. It is therefore essential to join forces in terms of basic and practical research. An international Society for Mucosal Immunology (SMI) has been organized to promote this important branch of biological science.[2] In 1994, SMI sponsored a major publishing project: a Handbook of Mucosal Immunology. This 766-page multiauthor text will be referred to several times below; it gives an excellent update of the remarkable advances recently made in this field, both with regard to immunity against infections and oral tolerance mechanisms.

The following overview will attempt to place some of the advances in mucosal immunology in a historical perspective. Both the early and recent history of this field has been previously discussed, and the readers are referred to two interesting reviews for a more detailed historical account.[3,4]

INDUCTIVE SITES OF THE MUCOSAL IMMUNE SYSTEM

Role of Lymphoepithelial Structures

In view of the slow recognition of the importance of mucosal immunity, it is a paradox that the organized gut-associated lymphoid tissue (GALT), which now is considered to

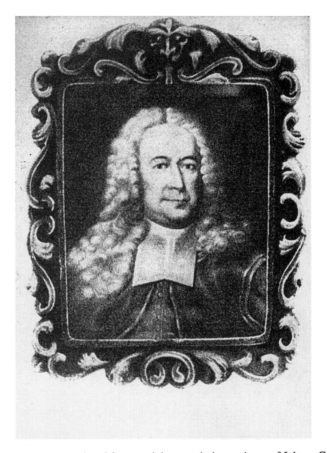

FIGURE 2A. Portrait reproduced from a miniature painting on ivory of Johann Conrad Peyer (1653-1712).

be the major inductive site of the mucosal immune system, was discovered more than 300 years ago. The Swiss physician and professor of medicine, Johann Conrad Peyer (FIG. 2A), first described the Peyer's patches in 1677; he claimed that these lymphoid structures were intestinal glands,[5] although this was strongly disputed by his friend and colleague at the Schaffenhauser Ärzteschule, Johann Conrad Brünner, who earlier had discovered the duodenal submucosal glands (Jan-Olaf Gebbers, personal communication).

GALT was later shown to be composed of subcompartments designed for sampling, processing, and presentation of luminal antigens to the local immune system. It is composed of approximately 30,000 scattered solitary lymphoid follicles, which are particularly frequent in the large bowel, but a major part consists of the Peyer's patches. These lymphoid aggregates can be up to 25 cm long and appear at the antimesenteric location in the small intestine as whitish, oval, slightly raised structures composed of at least five lymphoid follicles (FIG. 2B). The human Peyer's patches are usually largest and most abundant in

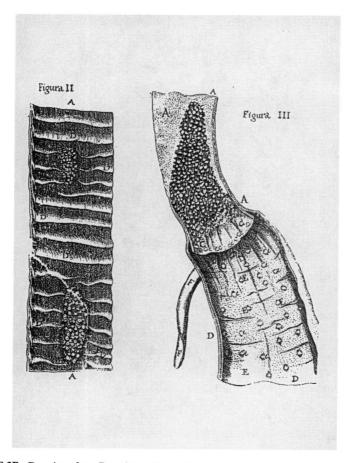

FIGURE 2B. Drawings from Peyer's treatise (1677) depicting a segment of the small intestine (left) and the distal ileum with connected appendix and cecum (right). Peyer's patches and solitary lymphoid follicles are nicely indicated by raised areas. Illustrations kindly provided by Dr. Jan-Olaf Gebbers, Luzern, Switzerland.

the distal ileum but they may also occur more proximally. Their numbers change with age, increasing from approximately 50 at the beginning of the last trimester to some 250 around puberty and then decreasing again to around 100 in individuals over 70 years.[6]

An important component of GALT is the follicle-associated epithelium (FAE), which is fit for antigen sampling; in addition, it contains phenotypically and functionally distinct B-, T-, and accessory-cell populations. GALT exerts mucosal selectivity in the potential for extravasation and dissemination of lymphoid cells.[7,8] Through such restrictions of its afferent and efferent limbs, GALT is at least partially independent of the systemic immune apparatus.

Although mainly being involved in immune protection of the gut, GALT also contributes to dissemination of primed B cells, and probably T cells, to other secretory tissues

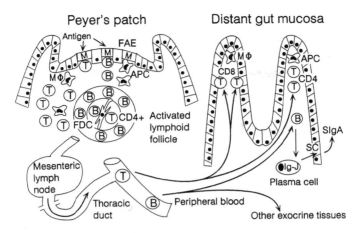

FIGURE 3. Scheme for induction of intestinal immune responses and cell traffic in the integrated mucosal immune system. Luminal antigens are mainly transported into Peyer's patch through M cells (M) of follicle-associated epithelium (FAE) and are presented to T cells (T) by macrophages (MØ), dendritic types of antigen-presenting cells (APC), and probably by B cells. Lymphoid follicles become activated and generate high-affinity memory B cells by retaining and presenting antigen on the follicular dendritic cell (FDC) under the influence of CD4+ regulatory T cells. Primed T and B cells migrate through lymph to the peripheral blood circulation and extravasate mainly in the intestinal lamina propria but also to some extent in other exocrine tissues. Intestinal B cells differentiate in the lamina propria under the influence of MØ, APC, and CD4+ T cells mainly to plasma cells producing polymeric immunoglobulin with J chain (Ig-J), which is transported to the lumen by epithelial transmembrane secretory component (SC), the chief product being secretory IgA (SIgA). Most CD8+ T cells migrate into the villus epithelium, perhaps to mediate oral tolerance to food antigens.

(FIG. 3), including the mucosae of the upper respiratory tract as well as the lacrimal, salivary, and lactating mammary glands. There is evidence for such an integrated mucosal immune system both in experimental animals and in humans. This is the cellular basis for the current interest in exploitation of GALT for oral vaccination against a variety of infectious diseases.

GALT is the best defined of all lymphoepithelial structures collectively called mucosa-associated lymphoid tissue (MALT). These inductive sites include, in addition to GALT, the bronchus-associated lymphoid tissue (BALT) and the tonsils, as well as other organized lymphoid tissue of the Waldeyer's pharyngeal ring.[9,10] It was suggested by John Bienenstock and his co-workers in the mid-1970s that the dissemination of primed lymphoid cells from MALT takes place in an integrated manner to exocrine tissues all over the body, and this observation gave rise to the term a "common mucosal immune system."[11] Paul Ehrlich exploited this functional feature of MALT as early as 1891 by inducing conjunctival resistance against abrin and ricin in guinea pigs after oral immunization with the same plant poisons.[3] However, recent studies have revealed more clearly than previously assumed that the mucosal immune system is not completely integrated;[12] accumulating evidence suggests a certain regionalization or subcompartmentalization both in humans and animals, especially a dichotomy between the gut and the upper aerodigestive tract with regard to homing properties and terminal differentiation of B cells.[13,14] Such a disparity may be explained by microenvironmental differences in the local antigenic repertoire as well as

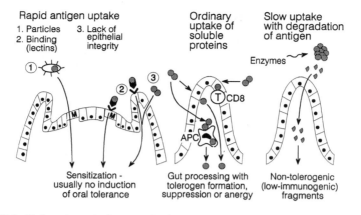

FIGURE 4. Various theoretical routes of antigen uptake in the gut and putative immunological consequences. Live microorganisms and dead particles (1) as well as proteins with special lectin-like properties (2) are rapidly transported through M cells (M) of follicle-associated epithelium (to the left). Breaching of the gut epithelium (3) also allows rapid antigen uptake. Soluble proteins may be taken up by the paracellular route through villus epithelium and then become processed by subepithelial antigen-presenting cells (APC), or they are transported and presented by enterocytes to intraepithelial (CD8) or subepithelial T cells (T). The transcellular route through the enterocyte is presumably speeded up by lectin-like properties of the antigen (2). If the antigen is aggregated, luminal enzymes may degrade it extensively (to the right).

in the expression of lymphoid and endothelial adhesion molecules involved in the regional B-cell extravasation (see below).

The notion that antigen priming of naive B and T cells belonging to the mucosal immune system primarily takes place in MALT is mainly based on studies of the inductive mechanisms operating in Peyer's patches of experimental animals.[12,15] Proliferating and dead particulate antigens are preferentially taken up from the lumen through specialized areas of the dome epithelium or FAE, so-called M ("membrane") cells, and are then transported into the underlying lymphoid tissue.[15,16] B and T cells as well as macrophages and other antigen-presenting cells (APC) of the dendritic variety are present immediately underneath the FAE (FIG. 3). The M cell-associated activated B lymphocytes may function as efficient APC even for naive T cells and facilitate the diversification of secretory IgA (SIgA) antibody responses;[17] this may be an important mechanism to cope with the continuous antigenic drift of the mucosal microbiota.

Much less is known about the preferential portal of entry and handling of soluble luminal protein antigens; most likely such molecules are taken up also through the extensive epithelial surfaces covering the diffuse lymphoid tissue of the mucosae—that is, directly into effector sites. This aspect is particularly unclear for soluble antigens with no affinity to the epithelium (FIG. 4), whereas proteins with lectin-like properties have been shown to be taken up as efficiently by villus epithelium as by FAE.[18]

Dissemination of Memory Cells to Mucosal Effector Sites

As late as 1958, it was stated in a large review that "although lymphocytes have been studied for over a hundred years, not a single function can yet be ascribed to them with any confidence, and their role in the body remains both an enigma and a challenge."[19] In the mid-1960s their immunological role had started to become unraveled, and their recirculation became a field of great interest.[20] The classical work from James Gowans' laboratory published in 1964 showed that thoracic duct lymphocytes after entering into the blood could give rise to plasma cells in the intestinal mucosa.[21] This observation initiated a series of important animal experiments in many laboratories on mucosal homing of MALT-derived lymphoid cells.[15] In 1971 it was directly documented by Susan W. Craig and John J. Cebra that the rabbit Peyer's patches are a major precursor source for IgA-producing plasma cells terminating in the gut lamina propria after allogeneic transfer to irradiated recipients.[22]

It is now well established that after antigen-induced activation, proliferation, and partial differentiation in MALT, B cells (and to some extent probably also T cells) migrate rapidly to regional lymph nodes where they may differentiate further and then exit through efferent lymphatics into the peripheral blood circulation (FIG. 3). These memory cells express adhesion molecules or "homing receptors" specific for corresponding determinants ("addressins") on endothelial cells in mucosal and glandular tissues; they will therefore extravasate preferentially at such exocrine effector sites.[23,24]

Most of the lymphoid cells stimulated in GALT migrate to distant intestinal lamina propria, and an important "traffic signal," and perhaps "retention signal," appears to be their prominent expression of the $\alpha 4\beta 7$ integrin.[25,26] Certain T-cell subsets, particularly those bearing CD8 and the $\alpha E\beta 7$ integrin, for unclear reasons selectively enter the intestinal epithelium; in this compartment they are retained apparently by binding of their $\alpha E\beta 7$ to epithelial E-cadherin.[27] As mentioned previously, an undefined fraction of GALT-derived B cells (and perhaps T cells) end up in mucosal effector sites and exocrine glands outside the gut (FIG. 3), notably also in lactating mammary glands.[12,15]

This integrated dissemination of memory cells from GALT to all exocrine tissues is the functional basis for oral vaccines.[12] Conversely, migration to the gut lamina propria of B cells induced in the lymphoid tissue of Waldeyer's ring (and in BALT, if such organized structures normally occur in humans)[28] appears to be negligible.[10,13,14] This dichotomy may to some extent be explained by disparity in relevant homing molecules as mentioned above. There is good evidence that endothelial determinants with affinity for GALT-derived lymphoid cells are shared among Peyer's patches, mesenteric lymph nodes, and the intestinal lamina propria;[23–25] one may postulate that another set of slightly different homing molecules is shared among the inductive sites and exocrine tissues of the upper aerodigestive tract.[9,13] Such putative heterogeneity or subcompartmentalization must be better defined and eventually exploited in the development of effective versatile mucosal vaccines.[29]

THE SECRETORY IMMUNE SYSTEM

Antibodies in Exocrine Fluids

Mucosal immunology has a history dating back to anecdotes more than two thousand years old; such early observations, as well as several important milestones on the long way to scientific recognition of this field, have been reviewed previously.[3,4] Induction of adaptive resistance by planned ingestion of foreign substances was exploited by Mithridates VI-Eupator (132-63 B.C.), King of Pontus (Northern shores of present Turkey), to defend himself against being poisoned by enemies. He made a sophisticated mixture containing the blood of ducks habitually fed poisonous weeds; this antidote was taken every morning on an empty stomach. After an unsuccessful battle with the Roman army and the subsequent revolt of his own soldiers, Mithridates tried in vain to poison himself, thereby apparently proving the efficacy of oral immunization. As a "negative control" his two daughters successfully committed suicide by means of the same poison, whereas the desperate king had to ask his devoted Gallic mercenary to stab him to death.[3]

According to old myths most ancient people recognized the natural antimicrobial properties of external secretions; local application of colostrum, saliva, or urine was commonly employed both as a cure and as a prophylactic.[30] This medical use of external body fluids might have originated from primitive man's observation that animals lick their wounds, but a therapeutic effect of secretions should not necessarily be ascribed to SIgA antibodies alone. Many innate defence factors have been identified in such fluids, exhibiting more or less broad antimicrobial activities, which obviously is important for the barrier function of mucous membranes in addition to the physical protective aid by the ciliary activity in the airways and the peristalsis of the gut. These natural cleansing mechanisms cooperate intimately with the specific mucosal humoral immune system whose major mediator substances are the noninflammatory SIgA antibodies[7,8] that perform immune exclusion (Fig. 1). The cellular basis for this quantitatively dominating and highly adaptive "first line" defence system is the fact that exocrine glands and secretory mucosae contain the majority of activated B cells, particularly the gut lamina propria, where at least 80% of all Ig-producing immunocytes (B-cell blasts and plasma cells) occur—almost 90% normally being accounted for by the IgA class.[31]

The concept of mucosal humoral immunity was developed by the Russian scientist, Alexandre Besredka, who in 1893 settled in Paris to become Chief of the Pasteur Institute in 1918. He showed the existence of an adaptive defence system, functioning in the gut lumen rather independently of systemic immunity, by demonstrating that rabbits, after oral immunization with *Shigella dysenteriae,* were protected against fatal dysentery, irrespective of their serum antibody titer.[32] He further elaborated on the principle of oral vaccination in his interesting treatise on local immunity published in 1927 by Williams & Wilkins, Baltimore. In the meantime, the British military doctor Arthur Davies had reported supporting evidence in humans for an operative intestinal immune system; he was able to detect antibodies against the dysentery bacillus in the stools from infected soldiers several days before similar antibodies appeared in their serum.[33] Nevertheless, research on local immunity was not significantly revived until the early 1960s when it became evident in several independent studies, shortly after Joseph F. Hereman's discovery of IgA, that this antibody class is generally dominating in human external secretions.[4,34]

External Transfer of Immunoglobulins

The interest in secretory immunity was particularly boosted in 1965 when Thomas B. Tomasi documented that SIgA has unique physicochemical properties;[35] it consists of IgA dimers (and a variable proportion of larger polymers), which contain an epithelial glycoprotein of approximately 80 kDa, now called bound secretory component (SC). A comprehensive literature has accumulated about SIgA, and its function as a highly stabilized antibody performing immune exclusion is well established (Fig. 1). The small amounts of IgM and IgG that normally occur in external secretions may likewise participate in immunological exclusion of luminal antigens, although these antibody classes are less stable than SIgA.[7,8,15] In a pure glandular secretion, with minimum contamination by paracellular epithelial leakage of tissue fluid, the concentration ratio of IgG : IgA is reduced to about 0.2% of that in serum, and the IgG:IgM ratio is reduced to 2% or less.[36] When this was first recognized by our laboratory in 1970, it was taken to signify preferential external translocation of IgM as well as of IgA.[37]

Around 1970 several authors speculated that SC might facilitate the entry of IgA into secretory epithelial cells. SC was therefore originally called "transport piece" by Mary

Ann South, but there was no obvious explanation for such a putative function.[36] Our laboratory proposed initially that the external preferential transport of dimeric IgA and pentameric IgM takes place independently of SC, perhaps as a result of affinity between "transfer sites" in their heavy chains and an unknown epithelial receptor.[37] This view originated from our initial failure to demonstrate a regular association between SC and purified exocrine IgM;[38] but in 1975 we showed that secretory IgM (SIgM) in parotid secretion contains noncovalently bound SC.[39] Altogether, various studies in the early 1970s made it increasing likely that transmembrane SC acts as a selective polymeric Ig (pIg) receptor basolaterally on secretory epithelia. In 1973-74 our laboratory, therefore, proposed a common receptor-mediated transport mechanism for dimeric IgA and pentameric IgM.[40,41]

Transport Models for Secretory Immunoglobulins

The first models proposed for external IgA transport suggested that SC-producing epithelial cells facilitate uptake of serum-derived or locally produced IgA monomers, which subsequently are dimerized intracellularly by complexing with SC. As previously reviewed in detail,[36] various modifications of this model were published, each with particular features (FIG. 5) that often have been neglected in the subsequent literature. The model proposed by our laboratory in 1973-74 differed from the others by implying that the pIg molecules are subjected to SC-mediated transcytosis.[40,41] An important basis for this formulation was the independent discovery by two American laboratories in 1970-71 of the J ("joining") chain, which is a 15-kDa polypeptide common to all varieties of pIg molecules.[42,43] We subsequently obtained evidence suggesting that the presence of J chain in the pIg molecules is decisive for their specific SC binding site (see below). It was also a prerequisite for the proposal of our pIg transport model that Singer and Nicolson[44] in 1972 had described the fluid mosaic structure of the cell membrane. In our model, ligand-receptor complexes were suggested to form at the basolateral epithelial cell membrane, thereby being subjected to endocytosis followed by vesicular transport through the cytoplasm outside the Golgi complex. However, it was not possible to understand how SC could first reach the basolateral cell faces and then the apical surface, although our model implied that SC was expressed as a transmembrane protein when it functioned as a pIg receptor.[41]

In 1970-71, Mach[45] and Radl et al.[46] independently proposed that the polymer configuration of IgA is important for its ability to complex with purified free SC in vitro. Complexing with IgM was also noted in one of these studies, but only polymers larger than pentamers were thought to be active.[46] Subsequently, however, we showed that SC was able to complex with pentameric IgM in vitro even more efficiently than with polymeric IgA and that the initial interactions depended on noncovalent forces rather than on the formation of disulphide bonds. These observations were important for the proposed pIg receptor function of transmembrane SC and have been confirmed by other laboratories as reviewed elsewhere.[36]

In the early 1970s, our laboratory succeeded in providing the first direct evidence for preferential synthesis of J chain-containing polymeric IgA by immunocytes present at exocrine sites such as the gut lamina propria;[40,47] this finding provided additional and necessary support for the proposed pIg transport mechanism. When Mach[45] published his SC-binding results, the J chain had just been detected in polymeric IgA;[42] in an addendum to his paper, he therefore postulated a role for this polypeptide in the SC-binding process. The first direct evidence for such a J-chain dependency was obtained in our laboratory with a monoclonal IgM protein lacking J chain;[48] this polymer failed to complex with free SC, but we were unable to show convincingly that the J chain alone constitutes the

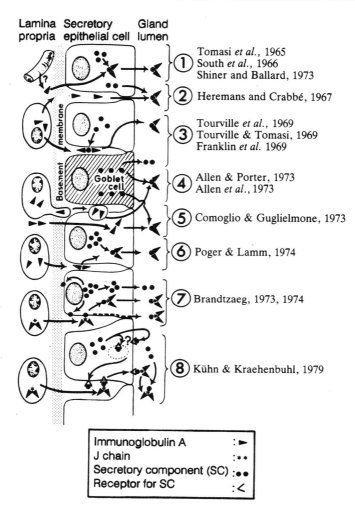

Lamina   Secretory   Gland
propria   epithelial cell   lumen

① Tomasi *et al.*, 1965
   South *et al.*, 1966
   Shiner and Ballard, 1973

② Heremans and Crabbé, 1967

③ Tourville *et al.*, 1969
   Tourville & Tomasi, 1969
   Franklin *et al.* 1969

④ Allen & Porter, 1973
   Allen *et al.*, 1973

⑤ Comoglio & Guglielmone, 1973

⑥ Poger & Lamm, 1974

⑦ Brandtzaeg, 1973, 1974

⑧ Kühn & Kraehenbuhl, 1979

Immunoglobulin A	: ►
J chain	: **
Secretory component (SC)	: ••
Receptor for SC	: <

FIGURE 5. Schematic representation of the formation and epithelial transport of SIgA as proposed by various research groups, each of the eight models presenting particular features. Model 7 was the first one proposing that SC acts as a transmembrane receptor for J chain-containing dimeric IgA (and pentameric IgM), as detailed in Fig. 6. Model 8 was an extension of model 7; it included steps by which SC finally reached the basolateral surface after initial secretion and binding to a receptor at the luminal face (or in cytoplasmic vesicles?). Model 8 also suggested that luminal release of dimeric IgA takes place because of displacement by free SC. (Adapted from Ref. 36, where the citations included in the Figure are listed.)

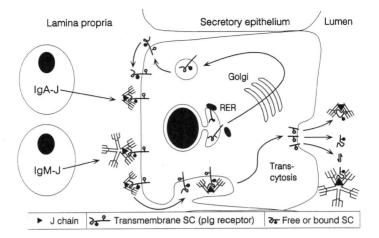

FIGURE 6. Schematic representation of various steps involved in the production of human secretory IgA (right, top) and secretory IgM (right, bottom) by way of SC-mediated epithelial transport of J chain–containing polymeric IgA (IgA-J) and pentameric IgM (IgM-J) secreted by local plasma cells (left). Transmembrane SC is synthesized in the rough endoplasmic reticulum (RER) of secretory epithelial cells and matures by terminal glycosylation (●) in the Golgi complex. After sorting through the trans-Golgi network, SC is phosphorylated (o) and expressed as a polymeric Ig (pIg) receptor at the basolateral plasma membrane. Endocytosis of noncovalently ligand-complexed and unoccupied pIg receptor is followed by transcytosis and finally by cleavage and release of secretory Ig molecules with bound SC, as well as an excess of free SC at the luminal cell face. During the external translocation, covalent stabilization of the IgA-SC complexes regularly occurs (two disulphide bridges indicated secretory IgA), whereas free SC in the secretion apparently serves to stabilize the noncovalent IgM-SC complexes (dynamic equilibrium indicated for secretory IgM).

SC-binding site.[36] Recent studies have suggested that the first ligand-receptor binding step depends on a conserved 23-amino-acid-long sequence in the N-terminal domain of SC, followed by noncovalent interactions extending beyond this domain.[49,50] Although the $C\alpha2$ domain and particularly the $C\alpha3$ domain of polymeric IgA are involved in these interactions, the exact part of the pIg molecules initially contacting SC remains undefined.[7,51] However, the presence of J chain in the pIg molecules is crucial for specific stabilization of their noncovalent interactions with transmembrane SC,[52] because the first step in the ligand binding is promiscuous in terms of Ig class.[49] The final covalent stabilization of SIgA apparently takes place between the membrane-proximal domain of SC and one $C\alpha2$ domain by means of disulphide exchange reactions; such bonding is not facilitated in SIgM, which therefore remains a noncovalent complex.[36]

Molecular Biology of SC-dependent pIg Transport

Epithelial transport of pIg is undoubtedly the best defined aspect of mucosal immunity (FIG. 6); this position has been fortified by recent studies based on molecular and cellular biology as reviewed in detail elsewhere.[51,53] An exciting phase of penetrating experimentation started in 1980 with the documentation by Keith E. Mostov and Jean-Pierre Kraehenbuhl that rabbit SC, which is structurally more heterogeneous than the human counterpart, is produced as a transmembrane protein family 25-30 kDa larger than the secreted free or bound form of SC.[54] The authors proposed that the relatively large cytoplasmic tail of transmembrane SC functions as an effector domain that contains guiding information for its complex migration through the epithelial cell. This has been confirmed by subsequent extensive *in vitro* studies with different mutants of rabbit transmembrane SC.[53]

When Mostov and his colleagues in 1984 cloned cDNA for rabbit transmembrane SC,[55] this receptor protein was found to contain five extracellular domains that showed remarkable homology to each other and to Ig variable regions, as previously reported by Eiffert *et al.*[56] for free SC purified from human colostrum. Both cDNA and the gene for human transmembrane SC were subsequently cloned by our laboratory;[57,58] it has become clear that SC is a remarkably conserved protein in keeping with its important immunological function.[7,51] SC cDNA has now been cloned not only in rabbits and humans, but also in the rat,[59] the mouse,[60] and the cow.[61]

Although transmembrane SC is constitutively expressed by secretory epithelia even before birth,[6] its production can be up-regulated by various cytokines derived from activated T cells and macrophages,[7,51] particularly in combination with metabolites of the normal gut flora, that is, the short fatty acid butyrate.[62] The SC-dependent external translocation of pIg antibodies can in this way be adapted to the degree of local immunostimulation, for which there is supporting *in vivo* evidence in active mucosal lesions such as untreated celiac disease.[63]

INTRAEPITHELIAL LYMPHOCYTES

The early history of intraepithelial lymphocytes (IEL) of the gut has been reviewed by Anne Ferguson.[64] Small round cells within the epithelium of the upper small intestine were described in 1847 by E. H. Weber who thought they were involved in nutrient absorption. In 1864 C. F. Eberth first recognized that these cells were leukocytes, but their function was unclear and, as will become apparent below, still is. In 1912 A. Guieysse-Pellissier proposed that IEL rejuvenate aging nuclei of enterocytes; another hypothesis was that the gut was the graveyard of lymphocytes.[64] Today it is believed that IEL may perform a variety of protective immunological functions, but direct supporting evidence is scarce.

In humans, IEL occur mainly in the villi of the small intestine and are mostly positive for the pan-T-cell marker CD3, about 75% expressing the T-cell receptor (TCR) α/β with a limited (oligoclonal) repertoire and generally being of the CD45R0/RB memory phenotype.[31,65–67] Human IEL further show a striking predominance (80%-90%) of the CD8 (mostly α/β heterodimeric) phenotype, whereas the lamina propria mainly contains the CD4 subset (FIG. 3). Some evidence for an epithelium-directed cytolytic activity of human CD8+ IEL has been presented, and their possible contribution to local oral tolerance is also of interest (see later). Their oligoclonality, as deemed from restricted TCR usage in each individual, suggests specificity for a limited number of antigens that may be presented by MHC class I or class I-like (class Ib or CD1) molecules expressed by the gut epithelium (FIG. 7). Thus, there is some evidence that nonpolymorphic CD1d molecules act as a recognition element for human IEL.[67] Interestingly, CD1d occurs on the surface of human intestinal epithelial cells without associated β2-microglobulin.[68] Although enterocytes in the small intestine express MHC class II both apically and basolaterally,[63] these molecules show, at least in the mouse, an unusual confirmation that may be inadequate for efficient antigen presentation.[69] This may contribute to a preferential engagement of CD8+ T cells by the gut epithleium.

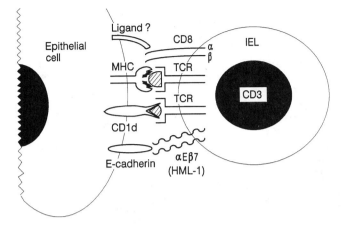

FIGURE 7. Molecules involved in putative interactions between human intestinal epithelial cells and intraepithelial (IEL) or subepithelial T lymphocytes (CD3). The epithelial cell may present processed antigen (hatched fragments) to the T-cell receptor (TCR) by polymorphic MHC molecules or by nonpolymorphic CD1d molecules. Accessory molecules may be integrin αEβ7, which binds to E-cadherin, and CD8, which binds to MHC class I and/or a putative ligand (?) with affinity for the α chain of CD8. Costimulation through the latter ligand activates rapidly the tyrosine kinase p56[lck]. Neither CD1d nor the latter ligand seems to be expressed by the airway epithelium; this difference may explain preferential induction of CD8+ T cells with suppressor function by the gut epithelium.

Human T cells bearing the TCRγ/δ, which are poorly represented (approximately 5%) in peripheral blood, often lack CD4 and CD8, thus being "double negative." Normal human small intestinal epithelium usually contains only a minor fraction (on average <8%) of TCRγ/δ+ cells; most of these IEL (50%-75%) are double negative[65,66] and show, in contrast to circulating γ/δ cells, a preferential usage of the Vδ1/Jδ1-encoded receptor (60%-70%); this may reflect some specificity in their local expansion or accumulation, but molecular TCR analysis has nevertheless revealed considerable diversity.[65,66]

It has been speculated that γ/δ T cells have a special role in the immunological surveillance of mucosal surfaces, perhaps to some extent by eliminating infected or damaged epithelial cells through interaction with heat-shock proteins.[70] At the same time, this particular IEL subset may contribute to maintaining epithelial integrity by secreting keratinocyte growth factor, which may promote the proliferation of enterocytes.[71] However, the antigenic repertoire and putative restriction element of TCRγ/δ+ cells are still obscure, although T-cell clones of this subset have variably been reported to recognize allospecific MHC class I, class II, and class I-like molecules. It has recently been suggested that γ/δ IEL may recognize unprocessed luminal antigens presented to them on the surface of bacteria or viruses without any restriction element being involved;[72] such a direct antigen-presenting mechanism could endow these cells with unique defense properties in the gut (FIG. 8). As mentioned earlier, the intraepithelial retention of TCRα/β+CD8+ IEL may be explained by their abundant expression of αEβ7 that binds to E-cadherin (FIG. 7); this integrin is also present on the intraepithelial γ/δ T cells (I.N. Farstad, personal communication) and may in fact function as a costimulatory molecule for T-cell activation.[71]

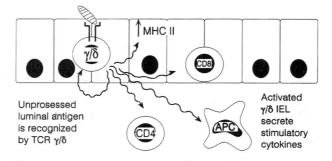

FIGURE 8. Putative local immunoregulatory consequences of direct activation of TCRγ/δ⁺ IEL by unprocessed antigen (hatched) at the epithelial cell surface. Rapid release of cytokines (wavy arrows) may enhance protective immune functions in the microenvironment and perhaps abrogate oral tolerance by stimulating CD4⁺ lamina propria T cells, antigen-presenting cells (APC), and epithelial cells to secretion of mediator substances and enhanced expression (↑) of MHC class II and accessory molecules.

Direct microbial activation of γ/δ T cells might induce local secretion of cytokines that enhance other protective mucosal immune functions or perhaps abrogate oral tolerance (Fig. 8), in keeping with the contrasuppressor activity suggested for this subset of murine IEL.[73] If the latter is true in humans, the expansion of TCRγ/δ⁺ IEL noted in celiac disease could contribute to the striking increase of Ig-producing immunocytes with a proinflammatory potential, as well as to the activated lamina propria T-helper cells (CD4⁺CD25⁺) seen in the untreated lesion, apparently reflecting a break of oral tolerance to gluten peptides.[66,74] Conversely, experimental induction of tolerance in the respiratory tract of rats has suggested an important role of γ/δ T cells in suppressing CD4⁺ T-cell (Th2)-dependent IgE production directly by way of their own cytokine profile or indirectly through TCRα/β⁺CD8⁺ cells triggered by them.[75] It has to be admitted that the function of both TCRα/β⁺CD8⁺ and TCRγ/δ⁺ T cells in mucosal immunity remains more elusive than that of the lamina propria CD4⁺ subset.

ORAL TOLERANCE

A Long History of Experimentation

A peripheral immunosuppressive effect of oral immunization was apparently exploited by ancient people. It has been claimed in several articles about oral tolerance that ingestion of shrub (*Rhus*) leaves was practiced among American Indians for centuries to dampen the severity of delayed-type hypersensitivity reactions upon subsequent contact with poison ivy plants. This anecdotal information is often documented by a reference to R. Dakin, who in 1829 published a report on the clinical appearance of this type of skin sensitization.[76] However, as pointed out by Jiri Mestecky and Jerry R. McGhee,[3] there is no mention of Indians in his paper. He states that "Some good meaning, mystical, marvelous physicians, or favoured ladies with knowledge inherent, say the bane will prove the best antidote, and hence advise the forbidden leaves to be eaten, both as a preventive and cure to the external disease. I have known the experiment tried, which resulted in an eruption, swelling, redness, and intolerable itching, around the verge of the anus."

Altogether, Dakin's paper reflected a rather pessimistic view of oral tolerance induction. Nevertheless, the phenomenon has since 1910 been subjected to numerous feeding experiments in rodents, as recently reviewed by Allan Mcl. Mowat.[77] The American scientist Harry Gideon Wells (1875-1943) conducted a large series of experiments in guinea pigs and showed that anaphylactic reactions to proteins could be inhibited by prior feeding of the same soluble antigens. The immunological nature of oral tolerance was established in 1946 by another American scientist, Merrill Chase, who applied contact-sensitizing agents. By exploiting the increasing knowledge on cellular immunity and on the induction of tolerance in other test systems, Chase demonstrated how readily the immune system could be down-regulated in an antigen-specific manner. This phenomenon came to be known by his name and by that of his contemporary, Marion Baldur Sulzberger.

A variety of immune mechanisms appears to operate in the Chase-Sulzberger phenomenon depending on the species, genetic background, oral antigen dose, timing of antigen exposure, nature and activation state of antigen-presenting cells, generation of tolerogenic peptides, and polarization or deviation of cytokine profiles (Th1 or Th2) in activated T cells. The phenomenon is significantly influenced by the nature of the actual dietary antigen, as recently shown in mice with various cereal proteins.[78] Soluble proteins with lectin-like properties do not induce tolerance in the humoral immune system (FIG. 4) but, instead, elicit good systemic antibody responses.[79] Likewise, a dietary antigen incorporated into a live vector (*Escherichia coli*) induces a strong immune response.[80] On the contrary, aggregated protein antigens (FIG. 4) may be degraded in the gut lumen to an extent that they become nontolerogenic and of low immunogenicity.[81]

Recent experiments in CD8 knock-out mice suggested that there may be separate mechanisms operating in the oral induction of local tolerance and peripheral tolerance (FIG. 1); thus, CD8[+] T cells were crucial for the down-regulaiton of mucosal immunity but not for suppression of systemic antibody responses.[82] Moreover, the read-out system will have a marked impact on the interpretation of the result—that is, whether only humoral immunity or only cell-mediated immunity is examined.[83] Although similar possibilities of inducing local and peripheral hyporesponsiveness by the mucosal route seem to exist in the upper respiratory tract, the mechanisms may be quite different from those operating in the gut, as discussed below. The lack of precise knowledge in this field is reflected by theories suggesting that the primary driving force of the immune system is the ability to tell the difference between dangerous antigens that should be eliminated (stimulatory immunity) and others that should be left alone (tolerance induction).[84]

Putative Mechanisms of Oral Tolerance

The information obtained from animal experiments discussed above shows that oral tolerance must be a very complex immunological phenomenon.[77] Although there is little direct evidence that such down-regulating mechanisms operate in human mucosae, it seems justified to believe so. This possibility is supported by the fact that small amounts of intact dietary antigens are taken up after meals, even in the healthy state;[15] and the vulnerable intestinal mucosa, which is exposed to at least 1000 kg of nutrients per year in adult life, normally exhibits no substantial IgG response[31] and contains very few T cells with markers of recent activation, such as the IL-2 receptor or CD25.[66] Moreover, the systemic IgG response to dietary antigens tends to decrease in humans with increasing age,[85,86] and direct evidence for a hyporesponsive state to bovine serum albumin was indeed obtained as early as 1968 by intradermal testing of this antigen in adults.[87] Quite recently experimental feeding in healthy adults with keyhole-limpet hemocyanin (KLH) resulted in down-regulation of the peripheral T-cell response but stimulation of local as well as systemic humoral immunity.[88] Conversely, intranasal application of KLH tended to suppress both cell-mediated and humoral peripheral immunity to this antigen.[89] The mechanisms remain unclear, and sequestration of specific immune cells into the mucosae or regional lymph nodes is one possible pitfall that is difficult to refute because local immunity was enhanced in both studies.

With regard to down-regulating immunoregulatory mechanisms operating in the gut, it is tempting to speculate how the prominent TCRα/β⁺CD8⁺ human IEL population might contribute to oral tolerance. There is some supporting evidence to this end,[90] and one possibility is that luminal peptides are inadequately presented to the IEL by the entero-cytes.[91] According to the model formulated by Peter Bretscher and Melvin Cohn in 1970, complete T-cell activation with cytokine production and proliferation requires two signaling events, one through the TCR and another through a receptor for some costimula-tory molecule.[92] Without the latter signal the T cells mount only a partial response and, more importantly, are subjected to tolerance induction. In this anergic state they do not produce their own growth factor IL-2 on restimulation.[93] The required costimulation might be provided by soluble mediators such as IL-1 or through cellular interactions,[94] particularly ligation of B7 (CD80/CD86) on antigen-presenting cells (APC) with CD28 on T cells (FIG. 9).

A central role of the gut epithelium in the induction of oral tolerance is supported by the observation that this phenomenon depends on a preserved integrity of the mucosal barrier.[95,96] Moreover, recent studies have provided considerable information about the immunoregulatory function of nonprofessional APC, such as keratinocytes.[83] As reviewed elsewhere,[31] the chief effect obtained when enterocytes have been used as APC in various test systems has been stimulation of CD8⁺ T cells with suppressor function. Although

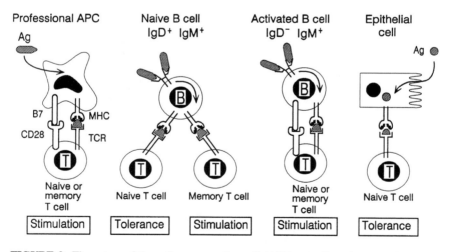

FIGURE 9. The nature of the antigen-presenting cell (APC) as well as the properties of the responding T cell (naive or memory) influence the outcome of encounter with antigen (Ag). Professional APC and activated B cells carry costimulatory molecules, such as B7, whereas naive B cells and intestinal epithelial cells normally lack such molecules. The M-cell pockets of Peyer's patches contain both naive and activated B cells, and the availability of antigen may determine whether stimulation or tolerance induction is favored by the local immune response. Uptake of soluble antigen by enterocytes and subsequent presentation through their MHC (or MHC-like) molecules may normally result in tolerance.

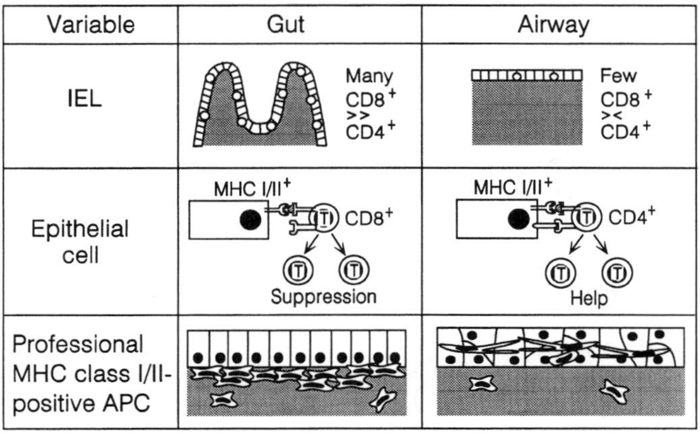

Variable	Gut	Airway
IEL	Many CD8⁺ >> CD4⁺	Few CD8⁺ >< CD4⁺
Epithelial cell	MHC I/II⁺ ● CD8⁺ Ⓣ Ⓣ Suppression	MHC I/II⁺ ● CD4⁺ Ⓣ Ⓣ Help
Professional MHC class I/II-positive APC		

FIGURE 10. Schematic depiction of three biological variables that may contribute to the apparent disparity in immunoresponsiveness between the gut and the airways. Upper panel: numbers and phenotypic distribution of intraepithelial lymphocytes (IEL). Middle panel: capacity for antigen presentation as well as expression of costimulatory signals to T cells by epithelial cells leading to preferential suppression or help. Bottom panel: distribution of subepithelial and intraepithelial professional antigen-presenting cells (APC).

human enterocytes express MHC class II apically as well as basolaterally,[63] recent evidence suggests that the interaction with CD8⁺ T cells is rather mediated by the nonclassical class I molecule CD1d (FIG. 7).[97] In addition, human enterocytes apparently express an additional ligand (gp180) that by interaction with the α chain of CD8 may rapidly activate the tyrosine kinase p56^{lck} (FIG. 7) and thereby trigger preferentially CD8⁺ T cells.[98] IEL to which antigen is presented by enterocytes in this context could theoretically be left in a state of anergy. Such unresponsive cells might inhibit the IL-2 receptor on mucosal CD4⁺ helper cells, a possibility suggested by the effect of CD8⁺ suppressor cell lines.[99] Perhaps CD8 molecules released from stimulated IEL function as inhibitory ligands, affecting naive T cells during immunological priming.[100]

Immunosuppressive mechanisms similar to those in the gut, appear to operate in the upper respiratory tract, particularly in relation to IgE responses.[101,102] However, hypersensitivity reactions to allergens and microbial antigens are much more frequent and persistent in the airways than in the gut.[103] It is possible that this disparity to some extent is explained by the relative scarcity of CD8⁺ T cells in the airway epithelium.[104] There are also other putative immunoregulatory differences between the airways and the gut (FIG. 10). Numerous MHC class I⁺ and class II⁺ dendritic cells are located within the airway epithelium and may be involved in antigen uptake and mediate down-regulation or up-regulation of immunity depending on their state of activation.[101,102,105] Interestingly, CD1d, that apparently participates in the interaction between the gut enterocytes and CD8⁺ IEL (FIG. 7), does not seem to be expressed by airway epithelium.[97] It is not surprising, therefore, that MHC class II⁺ respiratory epithelium may stimulate CD4⁺ helper T cells rather than CD8⁺ suppressor T cells.[106] Moreover, the intercellular adhesion molecule-1 (ICAM-1 or CD54) is readily induced basally on airway epithelium but not on gut epithelium *in vivo*.[104] Because ICAM-1 may provide a costimulatory signal for T-cell activation, it seems justified to conclude that the epithelium of the respiratory tract, in contrast to that of the normal intestine, appears to possess properties favoring immunological help instead of

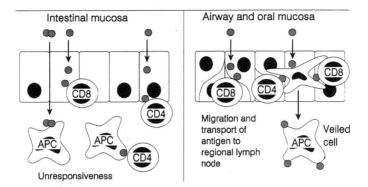

FIGURE 11. Antigen unresponsiveness may be induced differently by soluble antigen (hatched) in the gut and in the airway or oral mucosa. Lack of costimulatory signal on epithelial cells and on subepithelial antigen-presenting cells (APC) in normal intestinal mucosa will presumably favor tolerance induction. In airway mucosa, stimulation of CD4+ helper T cells may be favored unless antigen is rapidly transported away by intraepithelial APC with low levels of MHC class II molecules.

suppression (FIG. 10). This difference could be conducive to the preferential development of airway allergy through break of immunological tolerance.

Patrick G. Holt has focused on the role of the dendritic cells in the airway epithelium as a central immunoregulatory element both in the normal state and in immunopathological reactions.[103,107] The subepithelial band of APC in the gut lamina propria may have a similar function and, after mobilization, migrate with antigen to regional lymph nodes.[108] Also intestinal APC normally express quite low levels of costimulatory molecules, such as B7 (J. Rugtveit, personal communication), and may therefore be involved in tolerance induction (FIG. 11).[94] However, an increasing functional complexity of dendritic cells is emerging.[109] In the normal state of the respiratory tract, Holt and co-workers postulate that such cells are locally inert but transport allergens to regional lymph nodes where leakage of processed peptides from the MHC class II to the MHC class I pathway may provide stimulation of CD8+ regulatory T cells (FIG. 12). The cytokine pattern resulting from this immune deviation causes down-regulation of the Th2 helper cells that are necessary for IgE responses.[75,103] However, other types of immune modulation may make Th2 cells tolerant as well.[110] Perhaps vaccines may be designed in the future for down-regulation or deviation of immune responses in the airway to avoid the development of allergy in genetically predisposed individuals.[110,111] Likewise, a central role of dendritic cells and CD8+ T cells has been suggested in both humans and mice for down-regulation of delayed-type hypersensitivity to nickel, presumably penetrating by way of the oral epithelium.[112,113]

The immunoregulatory phenomena discussed above seem to be mainly antigen-specific, whereas recent efforts to induce therapeutic tolerance through the gut in various autoimmune disease models rely on a bystander effect of T cells secreting down-regulating cytokines, such as TGF-β.[114] In these models it is thought that the beneficial effect of TGF-β is exerted directly in the peripheral lesions. However, this cytokine may also be involved in oral tolerance by preserving the epithelial barrier function in the gut.[115] The immunosuppressive cells operating in the periphery are apparently in the main derived from organized GALT rather than from the intestinal lamina propria. It is interesting in this context that naive B cells may act as potent APC for the induction of tolerance (FIG.

9).[94] Because of their surface Ig, B cells can specifically take up antigen perhaps 10,000 times more efficiently than professional APC; if little antigen is available, competition between the two cell types may skew the immune response towards suppression. It is quite possible that such an interplay takes place in the M-cell pockets of Peyer's patches where B cells of different phenotypes are present.[17]

The exciting recent information that the recombinant B subunit of cholera toxin enhances tolerance induction in mice is quite intriguing.[29] At present it is only possible to speculate about the mechanism (FIG. 13). Concomitantly the B subunit may enhance an intestinal IgA response to luminal protein antigens, even in its pure (recombinant) form.[116] However, locally produced IgA *per se* probably plays no role in oral tolerance, although in early studies such antibodies, or IgA-containing immune complexes, were considered important. Hervé Bazin has reviewed this initial phase of animal experimentation when he and his colleagues presented the thesis of antigenic filtration through the gut mucosa with emerging tolerogenic molecules.[117] Intestinal tolerogen formation (FIG. 4) indeed remains an actual possibility under continuing investigation.[118]

Additional uncertainties are related to the role of the liver that in several studies has been shown to be involved in the induction of oral tolerance.[119] This organ may sequester immunoregulatory cells and immunogenic components of antigen-antibody complexes and allow tolerogenic fragments to exert their effect. Access of antigens from the gut directly to the liver through the portal blood circulation may in fact enhance the induction of T cells with immunosuppressive properties.[120] Finally, an interesting role has been suggested for the normal microbial gut flora in recovery of suppressive mechanisms after toxin-mediated abrogation of oral tolerance as well as in prolongation of a hyporesponsive state in terms of systemic humoral immunity (IgG and IgE) in mice.[121] Such observations add to the extreme complexity of oral tolerance.

SUMMARY

Mucosal immunity depends on antigen stimulation in specialized lymphoepithelial structures such as the Peyer's patches. Although these inductive compartments were discovered more than 300 years ago, their functional role has become clear only over the

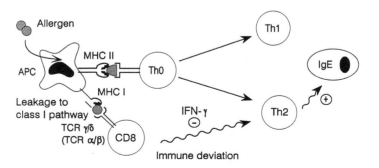

FIGURE 12. Putative immune deviation induced in the upper respiratory tract leading to down-regulation of IgE response. Allergen is transported to regional lymph node by antigen-presenting cells (APC) in which immunogenic peptides leak from the MHC class II pathway to the class I pathway. Subsequent stimulation of CD8+ cells results in production of interferon-γ (IFN-γ) that suppresses CD4+ Th2 helper cells, which are necessary for IgE synthesis.

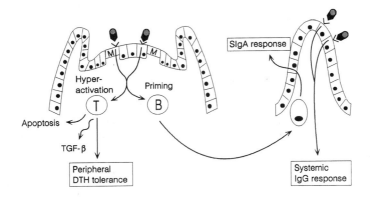

FIGURE 13. Soluble antigen (hatched) conjugated to cholera toxin B subunit (black) is efficiently taken up through both M cells (M) of Peyer's patches (left) and through enterocytes of villi (right). In Peyer's patch such a conjugate may produce hyperactivation with apoptosis and dissemination of T cells, which by secretion of transforming growth factor-β (TGF-β) may cause systemic bystander suppression. This may be one mechanism of tolerance induction to down-regulate delayed-type hypersensitivity (DTH) in peripheral lesions. Priming of B cells also occurs in Peyer's patch, thereby giving rise to an enhanced secretory IgA (SIgA) response in the distant mucosa; at the same time, a systemic IgG response is elicited by excessive antigen uptake.

last few decades. Research on homing of primed lymphoid cells to the intestinal mucosa began with animal experimentation in the 1960s and 1970s and has recently been brought to the molecular level. The major effector substance of mucosal immunity is secretory IgA (SIgA). The first evidence for its local antibody activity was obtained in humans in 1922, but its unique properties were not defined until in the mid-1960s. Several models were subsequently proposed for selective external transport of IgA involving the secretory component (SC). In the early 1970s SC was suggested to act as a transmembrane polymeric Ig receptor common for dimeric IgA and pentameric IgM; this transport mechanism has now been confirmed by detailed studies at the level of cellular/molecular biology. Although SIgA antibodies performing immune exclusion are the main goal for exploitation of the mucosal immune system by oral vaccination, little is known about the precise mechanisms for induction of mucosal immunity against soluble proteins and chemicals. A peripheral immunosuppressive effect of oral immunization with such substances was apparently exploited by ancient people, and "oral tolerance" has since 1910 been subjected to numerous feeding experiments in rodents. The basis for the whole phenomenon appears to be an intact epithelial barrier. Mucosal induction of suppression may in the future be exploited not only to modulate autoimmune diseases through the gut but also to prevent the development of IgE-mediated allergy and other untoward immune reactions by way of the respiratory tract.

ACKNOWLEDGMENTS

Dr. J.-O. Gebbers (Luzern, Switzerland) is gratefully acknowledged for providing the information and illustrations related to the work of J. C. Peyer. I thank Hege E. Svendsen for excellent secretarial assistance, and Espen Baekkevold for the drawings.

REFERENCES

1. HANSON, L. Å., R. ASHRAF, B. CARLSSON, F. JALIL, J. KARLBERG, B. S. LINDBLAD, S. R. KHAN & S. ZAMAN. 1993. Child health and the population increase. *In* Peace, Health and Development. L. Å. Hanson & L. Köhler, Eds. **4:** 31-38.

2. BRANDTZAEG, P. 1995. The SMI—an international society for mucosal immunology. Immunologist **3:** 67-69.

3. MESTECKY, J. & J. R. MCGHEE. 1989. Oral immunization: past and present. Curr. Top. Microbiol. Immunol. **146:** 3-11.

4. BIENENSTOCK, J. 1991. A non-historical overview of mucosal immunology. *In* Frontiers of Mucosal Immunology. Proc. Sixth Int. Congr. Mucosal Immunology. M. Tsuchiya, H. Nagura, T. Hibi & I. Moro, Eds.: XV-XViii. Excerpta Medica, Elsevier (Biomed. Div.). Amsterdam.

5. PEYER, J. C. 1677. Exercitatio anatomico-medica de glandulis intestinorum. Schaffhausen. Switzerland.

6. BRANDTZAEG, P., D. E. NILSSEN, T. O. ROGNUM & P. S. THRANE. 1991. Ontogeny of the mucosal immune system and IgA deficiency. Gastroenterol. Clin. North Am. **20:** 397-439.

7. BRANDTZAEG, P. 1995. Molecular and cellular aspects of the secretory immunoglobulin system. APMIS **103:** 1-19.

8. BRANDTZAEG, P. 1995. Basic mechanisms of mucosal immunity—a major adaptive defense system. Immunologist **3:** 89-96.

9. KUPER, C. F., P. J. KOORNSTRA, D. M. HAMELEERS, J. BJEWENGA, B. J. SPIT, A. M. DUIJVESTIJN, P. J. VAN BREDA VRIESMAN & T. SMINIA. 1992. The role of nasopharyngeal lymphoid tissue. Immunol. Today **13:** 219-224.

10. BRANDTZAEG, P. & T. S. HALSTENSEN. 1992. Immunology and immunopathology of tonsils. Adv. Oto-rhino-laryngol. **7:** 64-75.

11. MCDERMOTT, M. R. & J. BIENENSTOCK. 1979. Evidence for a common mucosal immunologic system. I. Migration of B immunoblasts into intestinal, respiratory, and genital tissues. J. Immunol. **122:** 1892-1898.

12. MESTECKY, J., R. ABRAHAM & P. L. OGRA. 1994. Common mucosal immune system and strategies for the development of vaccines effective at the mucosal surfaces. *In* Handbook of Mucosal Immunology. P. L. Ogra, J. Mestecky, M. E. Lamm, W. Strober, J. R. McGhee & J. Bienenstock, Eds.: 357-372. Academic Press. Orlando, Florida.

13. BRANDTZAEG, P. 1992. Humoral immune response patterns of human mucosae: induction and relation to bacterial respiratory tract infections. J. Infect. Dis. **165:** Suppl. 1: S167-176.

14. VANCOTT, J. L., T. A. BRIM, J. K. LUNNEY & L. J. SAIF. 1994. Contribution of antibody-secreting cells induced in mucosal lymphoid tissues of pigs inoculated with respiratory or enteric strains of coronavirus to immunity against enteric coronavirus challenge. J. Immunol. **152:** 3980-3990.

15. BRANDTZAEG, P., K. BAKLIEN, K. BJERKE, T. O. ROGNUM, H. SCOTT & K. VALNES. 1987. Nature and properties of the human gastrointestinal immune system. *In* Immunology of the Gastrointestinal Tract. K. Miller & S. Nicklin, Eds.: 1-86. CRC Press. Boca Raton, Florida.

16. KATO, T. & R. L. OWEN. 1994. Structure and function of intestinal mucosal epithelium. *In* Handbook of Mucosal Immunology. P. L. Ogra, J. Mestecky, M. E. Lamm, W. Strober, J. R. McGhee & J. Bienenstock, Eds.: 11-26. Academic Press. Orlando, Florida.

17. FARSTAD, I. N., T. S. HALSTENSEN, O. FAUSA & P. BRANDTZAEG. 1994. Heterogeneity of M-cell-associated B and T cells in human Peyer's patches. Immunology **83:** 457-464.

18. LINDNER, J., A. F. GECZY & G. J. RUSSELL-JONES. 1994. Identification of the site of uptake of the *E. coli* heat-labile enterotoxin, LTB. Scand. J. Immunol. **40:** 564-572.

19. TROWELL, O. A. 1958. The lymphocyte. Int. Rev. Cytol. **7:** 235-293.

20. YOFFEY, J. M. 1966. Lymphocytes—the fourth circulation. Discovery **27:** 24-29.

21. GOWANS, J. L. & E. J. KNIGHT. 1964. The route of re-circulation of lymphocytes in the rat. Proc. R. Soc. (Lond.) **B159:** 257-282.
22. CRAIG, S. W. & J. J. CEBRA. 1971. Peyer's patches: an enriched source of precursors for IgA-producing immunocytes in the rabbit. J. Exp. Med. **134:** 188-200.
23. DUIJVESTIJN, A. & A. HAMANN. 1989. Mechanisms and regulation of lymphocyte migration. Immunol. Today **10:** 23-28.
24. SALMI, M. & S. JALKANEN. 1991. Regulation of lymphocyte traffic to mucosa-associated lymphatic tissues. Gastroenterol. Clin. North Am. **20:** 495-510.
25. PICKER, L. J. 1994. Control of lymphocyte homing. Curr. Opinion Immunol. **6:** 394-406.
26. FARSTAD, I. N., T. S. HALSTENSEN, A. I. LAZAROVITS, J. NORSTEIN, O. FAUSA & P. BRANDTZAEG. 1995. Human intestinal B-cell blasts and plasma cells express the mucosal homing receptor integrin α4β7. Scand. J. Immunol. In press.
27. CEPEK, K. L., S. K. SHAW, C. M. PARKER, G. J. RUSSELL, J. S. MORROW, D. L. RIMM & M. B. BRENNER. 1994. Adhesion between epithelial cells and T lymphocytes mediated by E-cadherin and the α4β7 integrin. Nature **372:** 190-193.
28. PABST, R. & I. GEHRKE. 1990. Is the bronchus-associated lymphoid tissue (BALT) an integral structure of the lung in normal mammals, including humans? Am. J. Respir. Cell. Mol. Biol. **3:** 131-135.
29. CZERKINSKY, C. & J. HOLMGREN. 1995. The mucosal immune system and prospects for anti-infectious and anti-inflammatory vaccines. Immunologist **3:** 97-103.
30. GORDON, B. L. 1945. The Romance of Medicine. The Story of the Evolution of Medicine from Occult Practices and Primitive Times. *In* Anonymous pp. 395-398. Davis Co. Philadelphia.
31. BRANDTZAEG, P., T. S. HALSTENSEN, K. KETT, P. KRAJČI, D. KVALE, T. O. ROGNUM, H. SCOTT & L. M. SOLLID. 1989. Immunobiology and immunopathology of human gut mucosa: humoral immunity and intraepithelial lymphocytes. Gastroenterology **97:** 1562-1584.
32. BESREDKA, A. 1919. De la vaccination contre les états typhoides par la voie buccale. Ann. Inst. Pasteur **33:** 882-903.
33. DAVIES, A. 1922. An investigation into the serological properties of dysentery stools. Lancet **ii:** 1009-1012.
34. HANSON, L. A. & P. BRANDTZAEG. 1993. The discovery of secretory IgA and the mucosal immune system. Immunol. Today **14:** 416-417.
35. TOMASI, T. B., E. M. TAN, A. SOLOMON & R. A. PRENDERGAST. 1965. Characteristics of an immune system common to certain external secretions. J. Exp. Med. **121:** 101-124.
36. BRANDTZAEG, P. 1985. Role of J chain and secretory component in receptor-mediated glandular and hepatic transport of immunoglobulins in man. Scand. J. Immunol. **22:** 111-146.
37. BRANDTZAEG, P., I. FJELLANGER & S. T. GJERULDSEN. 1970. Human secretory immunoglobulins. I. Salivary secretions from individuals with normal or low levels of serum immunoglobulins. Scand. J. Haematol. Suppl. **12:** 3-83.
38. BRANDTZAEG, P., I. FJELLANGER & S. T. GJERULDSEN. 1968. Immunoglobulin M: local synthesis and selective secretion in patients with immunoglobulin A deficiency. Science **160:** 789-791.
39. BRANDTZAEG, P. 1975. Human secretory immunoglobulin M. An immunochemical and immunohistochemical study. Immunology **29:** 559-570.
40. BRANDTZAEG, P. 1973. Two types of IgA immunocytes in man. Nature New Biol. **243:** 142-143.
41. BRANDTZAEG, P. 1974. Mucosal and glandular distribution of immunoglobulin components: differential localization of free and bound SC in secretory epithelial cells. J. Immunol. **112:** 1553-1559.
42. HALPERN, M. S. & M. E. KOSHLAND. 1970. Novel subunit in secretory IgA. Nature **228:** 1276-1278.

43. MESTECKY, J., J. ZIKAN & W. T. BUTLER. 1971. Immunoglobulin M and secretory immunoglobulin A: presence of a common polypeptide chain different from light chains. Science **171:** 1163-1165.
44. SINGER, S. J. & G. L. NICHOLSON. 1972. The fluid mosaic model of the structure of cell membranes. Science **175:** 720-731.
45. MACH, J. P. 1970. *In vitro* combination of human and bovine free secretory component with IgA of various species. Nature **228:** 1278-1282.
46. RADL, J., F. KLEIN, P. VAN DEN BERG, A. M. DE BRUYN & W. HIJMANS. 1971. Binding of secretory piece to polymeric IgA and IgM paraproteins *in vitro*. Immunology **20:** 843-852.
47. BRANDTZAEG, P. 1974. Presence of J chain in human immunocytes containing various immunoglobulin classes. Nature **252:** 418-420.
48. ESKELAND, T. & P. BRANDTZAEG. 1974. Does J Chain mediate the combination of 19S IgM and dimeric IgA with the secretory component rather than being necessary for their polymerization? Immunochemistry **11:** 161-163.
49. BAKOS, M. A., A. KUROSKY & R. M. GOLDBLUM. 1991. Characterization of a critical binding site for human polymeric Ig on secretory component. J. Immunol. **151:** 3419-3426.
50. COYNE, R. S., M. SIEBRECHT, M. C. PEITSCH & J. E. CASANOVA. 1994. Mutational analysis of polymeric immunoglobulin receptor/ligand interactions. Evidence for the involvement of multiple complementarity determining region (CDR)-like loops in receptor domain I. J. Biol. Chem. **269:** 31620-31625.
51. BRANDTZAEG, P., P. KRAJČI, M. E. LAMM & C. S. KAETZEL. 1994. Epithelial and hepatobiliary transport of polymeric immunoglobulins. *In* Handbook of Mucosal Immunology. P. L. Ogra, J. Mestecky, M. E. Lamm, W. Strober, J. R. McGhee & J. Bienenstock, Eds.: 113-126. Academic Press. Orlando, Florida.
52. BRANDTZAEG, P. & H. PRYDZ. 1984. Direct evidence for an integrated function of J chain and secretory component in epithelial transport of immunoglobulins. Nature **311:** 71-73.
53. MOSTOV, K. E. 1994. Transepithelial transport of immunoglobulins. Annu. Rev. Immunol. **12:** 63-84.
54. MOSTOV, K. E., J. P. KRAEHENBUHL & G. BLOBEL. 1980. Receptor-mediated transcellular transport of immunoglobulin: synthesis of secretory component as multiple and larger transmembrane forms. Proc. Natl. Acad. Sci. USA **77:** 7257-7261.
55. MOSTOV, K. E., M. FRIEDLANDER & G. BLOBEL. 1984. The receptor for transepithelial transport of IgA and IgM contains multiple immunoglobulin-like domains. Nature **308:** 37-43.
56. EIFFERT, H., E. QUENTIN, J. DECKER, S. HILLEMEIR, M. HUFSCHMIDT, D. KLINGMÜLLER, M. H. WEBER & N. HILSCHMANN. 1984. Die Primärstruktur der menschlichen freien Sekretkomponente und die Anordnung der Disulfidbrücken. Hoppe-Seyler's Z. Physiol. Chem. **365:** 1489-1495.
57. KRAJČI, P., K. H. GRZESCHIK, A. H. GEURTS VAN KESSEL, B. OLAISEN & P. BRANDTZAEG. 1991. The human transmembrane secretory component (poly-Ig receptor): molecular cloning, restriction fragment length polymorphism and chromosomal sublocalization. Hum. Genet. **87:** 642-648.
58. KRAJČI, P., D. KVALE, K. TASKEN & P. BRANDTZAEG. 1992. Molecular cloning and exon-intron mapping of the gene encoding human transmembrane secretory component (the poly-Ig receptor). Eur. J. Immunol. **22:** 2309-2315.
59. BANTING, G., B. BRAKE, P. BRAGHETTA, J. P. LUZIO & K. K. STANLEY. 1989. Intracellular targeting signals of polymeric immunoglobulin receptors are highly conserved between species. FEBS Lett. **254:** 177-183.
60. PISKURICH, J. F., M. H. BLANCHARD, K. R. YOUNGMAN, J. A. FRANCE & C. S. KAETZEL. 1995. Molecular cloning of the mouse polymeric Ig receptor. Functional regions

of the molecule are conserved among five mammalian species. J. Immunol. **154:** 1735-1747.

61. KULSETH, M. A., P. KRAJČI, O. MYKLEBOST & S. ROGNE. 1995. Cloning and characterization of two forms of bovine polymeric immunoglobulin receptor cDNA. DNA Cell Biol. **14:** 251-256.

62. KVALE, D. & P. BRANDTZAEG. 1995. Constitutive and cytokine induced expression of HLA molecules, secretory component, and intercellular adhesion molecule-1 is modulated by butyrate in the colonic epithelial cell line HT-29. Gut **36:** 737-742.

63. BRANDTZAEG, P., T. S. HALSTENSEN, H. S. HUITFELDT, P. KRAJČI, D. KVALE, H. SCOTT & P. S. THRANE. 1992. Epithelial expression of HLA, secretory component (poly-Ig receptor), and adhesion molecules in the human alimentary tract. Ann. N.Y. Acad. Sci. **664:** 157-179.

64. FERGUSON, A. 1977. Intraepithelial lymphocytes of the small intestine. Gut **18:** 921-937.

65. CERF-BENSUSSAN, N., M. CERF & D. GUY-GRAND. 1993. Gut intraepithelial lymphocytes and gastrointestinal diseases. Curr. Opinion Gastroenterol. **9:** 953-961.

66. HALSTENSEN, T. S. & P. BRANDTZAEG. 1994. Phenotypic characteristics of human intraepithelial lymphocytes. *In* Mucosal Immunology: Intraepithelial Lymphocytes. Advances in Host Defense Mechanisms. H. Kiyono & J. R. McGhee, Eds.: 147-161. Raven Press. New York.

67. BLUMBERG, R. S. & S. P. BALK. 1994. Intraepithelial lymphocytes and their recognition of non-classical MHC molecules. Int. Rev. Immunol. **11:** 15-30.

68. BALK, S. P., S. BURKE, J. E. POLISCHUK, M. E. FRANTZ, L. YANG, S. PORCELLI, S. P. COLGAN & R. S. BLUMBERG. 1994. β_2-microglobulin-independent MHC class Ib molecule expressed by human intestinal epithelium. Science **265:** 259-262.

69. VIDAL, K., C. SAMARUT, J.-P. MAGAUD, J.-P. REVILLARD & D. KAISERLIAN. 1993. Unexpected lack of reactivity of allogeneic anti-Ia monoclonal antibodies with MHC class II molecules expressed by mouse intestinal epithelial cells. J. Immunol. **151:** 4642-4650.

70. BORN, W., M. P. HAPP, A. DALLAS, C. REARDON, R. KUBO, T. SHINNICK, P. BRENNAN & R. O'BRIEN. 1990. Recognition of heat shock proteins and $\gamma\delta$ cell function. Immunol. Today **11:** 40-43.

71. ERLE, D. J. 1995. Scratching the surface. Curr. Biol. **5:** 252-254.

72. KLEIN, J. R. & M. HAMAD. 1995. $\gamma\delta$ T cells, antigen recognition and intestinal immunity. Immunol. Today **16:** 108-109.

73. KIYONO, H. & J. R. McGHEE. 1994. T helper cells for mucosal immune responses. *In* Handbook of Mucosal Immunology. P. L. Ogra, J. Mestecky, M. E. Lamm, W. Strober, J. R. McGhee & J. Bienenstock, Eds.: 263-274. Academic Press. Orlando, Florida.

74. BRANDTZAEG, P., T. S. HALSTENSEN, M. HVATUM, D. KVALE & H. SCOTT. 1993. The serologic and mucosal immunologic basis of celiac disease. *In* Immunophysiology of the Gut. Bristol-Myers Squibb/Mead Johnson Nutrition Symposia. W. A. Walker, P. R. Harmatz & B. K. Wershil, Eds.: 295-333. Academic Press. London.

75. McMENAMIN, C., C. PIMM, M. McKERSEY & P. G. HOLT. 1994. Regulation of IgE responses to inhaled antigen in mice by antigen-specific $\gamma\delta$ T cells. Science **265:** 1869-1871.

76. DAKIN, R. 1829. Remarks on a cutaneous affection, produced by certain poisonous vegetables. Am. J. Med. Sci. **4:** 98-100.

77. MOWAT, A. M. 1994. Oral tolerance and regulation of immunity to dietary antigens. *In* Handbook of Mucosal Immunology. P. L. Ogra, J. Mestecky, M. E. Lamm, W. Strober, J. R. McGhee & J. Bienenstock, Eds.: 185-201. Academic Press. Orlando, Florida.

78. JOHNSON, R. B., J. T. LABROOY & J. H. SKERRITT. 1990. Antibody responses reveal differences in oral tolerance to wheat and maize grain protein fractions. Clin. Exp. Immunol. **79:** 135-140.

79. DE AIZPURUA, H. J. & G. J. RUSSELL-JONES. 1988. Oral vaccination. Identification of classes of proteins that provoke an immune response upon oral feeding. J. Exp. Med. **167:** 440-451.

80. DAHLGREN, U. I. H., A. E. WOLD, L. Å. HANSON & T. MIDTVEDT. 1991. Expression of a dietary protein in *E. coli* renders it strongly antigenic to gut lymphoid tissue. Immunology **73**: 394-397.

81. PENG, H.-J., Z.-N. CHANG, S.-H. HAN, M.-H. WON & B.-T. HUANG. 1995. Chemical denaturation of ovalbumin abrogates the induction of oral tolerance of specific IgG antibody and DTH responses in mice. Scand. J. Immunol. **42**: 297-304.

82. HÖRNQUIST, C. E., K. D. GRDIC, T. W. MAY & N. LYCKE. 1994. Augmented mucosal immune responses and intact adjuvant effects of cholera toxin in CD8- but not in CD4-deficient mice. Immunology. In press.

83. NICKOLOFF, B. J. & L. A. TURKA. 1994. Immunological functions of non-professional antigen-presenting cells: new insights from studies of T-cell interactions with keratinocytes. Immunol. Today **15**: 464-469.

84. MATZINGER, P. 1994. Tolerance, danger, and the extended family. Annu. Rev. Immunol. **12**: 991-1045.

85. ROTHBERG, R. M. & R. S. FARR. 1965. Anti-bovine serum albumin and anti-alpha lactalbumin in the serum of children and adults. Pediatrics **35**: 571-588.

86. SCOTT, H., T. O. ROGNUM, T. MIDTVEDT & P. BRANDTZAEG. 1985. Age-related changes of human serum antibodies to dietary and colonic bacterial antigens measured by an enzyme-linked immunosorbent assay. Acta Pathol. Microbiol. Immunol. Scand. [C] **93**: 65-70.

87. KORENBLAT, P. E., R. M. ROTHBERG, P. MINDEN & R. S. FARR. 1968. Immune responses of human adults after oral and parenteral exposure to bovine serum albumin. J. Allergy **41**: 226-235.

88. HUSBY, S., J. MESTECKY, Z. MOLDOVEANU, S. HOLLAND & C. O. ELSON. 1994. Oral tolerance in humans. T cell but not B cell tolerance after antigen feeding. J. Immunol. **152**: 4663-4670.

89. WALDO, F. B., A. W. VAN DEN WALL BAKE, J. MESTECKY & S. HUSBY. 1994. Suppression of the immune response by nasal immunization. Clin. Immunol. Immunopathol. **72**: 30-34.

90. SACHDEV, G. K., H. R. DALTON, P. HOANG, M.-C. DIPAOLO, B. CROTTY & D. P. JEWELL. 1993. Human colonic intraepithelial lymphocytes suppress in vitro immunoglobulin synthesis by autologous peripheral blood lymphocytes and lamina propria lymphocytes. Gut **34**: 257-263.

91. HOYNE, G. F., M. G. CALLOW, M. C. KUO & W. R. THOMAS. 1993. Presentation of peptides and proteins by intestinal epithelial cells. Immunology **80**: 204-208.

92. JENKINS, M. K. 1992. The role of cell division in the induction of clonal anergy. Immunol. Today **13**: 69-73.

93. SCHWARTZ, R. H. 1990. A cell culture model for T lymphocyte clonal anergy. Science **248**: 1349-1356.

94. DURIE, F. H., T. M. FOY, S. R. MASTERS, J. D. LAMAN & R. J. NOELLE. 1994. The role of CD40 in the regulation of humoral and cell-mediated immunity. Immunol. Today **15**: 406-411.

95. NICKLIN, S. & K. MILLER. 1983. Local and systemic immune responses to intestinally presented antigen. Int. Arch. Allergy Appl. Immunol. **72**: 87-90.

96. STROBEL, S., A. M. MOWAT, H. E. DRUMMOND, M. G. PICKERING & A. FERGUSON. 1983. Immunological responses to fed protein antigens in mice. II. Oral tolerance for CMI is due to activation of cyclophosphamide-sensitive cells by gut-processed antigen. Immunology **49**: 451-456.

97. PANJA, A., R. S. BLUMBERG, S. P. BALK & L. MAYER. 1993. CD1d is involved in T cell-intestinal epithelial cell interactions. J. Exp. Med. **178**: 1115-1119.

98. LI, Y., X. Y. YIO & L. MAYER. 1995. Human intestinal epithelial cell-induced CD8+ T cell activation is mediated through CD8 and the activation of CD8-associated p56^{lck}. J. Exp. Med. **182**: 1079-1088.

99. Aune, T. M. & S. L. Pogue. 1989. Generation and characterization of continuous lines of CD8⁺ suppressor T lymphocytes. J. Immunol. **142**: 3731-3739.

100. Hambor, J. E., D. R. Kaplan & M. L. Tykocinski. 1990. CD8 functions as an inhibitory ligand in mediating the immunoregulatory activity of CD8⁺ cells. J. Immunol. **145**: 1646-1652.

101. Holt, P. G. & C. McMenamin. 1989. Defence against allergic sensitization in the healthy lung: the role of inhalation tolerance. Clin. Exp. Allergy **19**: 255-262.

102. McMenamin, C. & P. G. Holt. 1993. The natural immune response to inhaled soluble protein antigens involves major histocompatibility complex (MHC) class I-restricted CD8⁺ T cell-mediated but MHC class II-restricted CD4⁺ T cell-dependent immune deviation resulting in selective suppression of immunoglobulin E production. J. Exp. Med. **178**: 889-899.

103. Holt, P. G. 1994. Immunoprophylaxis of atopy: light at the end of the tunnel? Immunol. Today **15**: 484-489.

104. Brandtzaeg, P. 1995. Immunocompetent cells of the upper airway: functions in normal and diseased mucosa. Eur. Oto-rhino-laryngol. **252**(Suppl. 1): S8-S21.

105. Grabbe, S., S. Beissert, T. Schwarz & R. D. Granstein. 1995. Dendritic cells as initiators of tumor immune responses: a possible strategy for tumor immunotherapy? Immunol. Today **16**: 117-121.

106. Kalb, T. H., M. T. Chuang, Z. Marom & L. Mayer. 1991. Evidence for accessory cell function by class II MHC antigen-expressing airway epithelial cells. Am. J. Respir. Cell. Mol. Biol. **4**: 320-329.

107. McWilliam, A. S., D. Nelson, J. A. Thomas & P. G. Holt. 1994. Rapid dendritic cell recruitment is a hallmark of the acute inflammatory response at mucosal surfaces. J. Exp. Med. **179**: 1331-1336.

108. MacPherson, G. G., C. D. Jenkins, M. J. Stein & C. Edwards. 1995. Endotoxin-mediated dendritic cell release from the intestine. Characterization of released dendritic cells and TNF dependence. J. Immunol. **154**: 1317-1322.

109. Stingl, G. & P. R. Bergstresser. 1995. Dendritic cells: a major story unfolds. Immunol. Today **16**: 330-333.

110. Yssel, H., S. Fasler, J. Lamb & J. E. De Vries. 1994. Induction of non-responsiveness in human allergen-specific type 2 T helper cells. Curr. Opinion Immunol. **6**: 847-852.

111. Holt, P. G. 1994. A potential vaccine strategy for asthma and allied atopic diseases during early childhood. Lancet **344**: 456-458.

112. Van Hoogstraten, I. M. W., K. E. Andersen, B. M. E. Von Blomberg, D. Boden, D. P. Bruynzeel, D. Burrows, J. G. Camarasa, A. Dooms-Goossens, G. Kraal, A. Lahti et al. 1991. Reduced frequency of nickel allergy upon oral nickel contact at an early age. Clin. Exp. Immunol. **85**: 441-445.

113. Van Hoogstraten, I. M. W., C. Boos, D. Boden, M. E. Von Blomberg, R. J. Scheper & G. Kraal. 1993. Oral induction of tolerance to nickel sensitization in mice. J. Invest. Dermatol. **101**: 26-31.

114. Weiner, H. L., A. Friedman, A. Miller, S. J. Khoury, A. Al-Sabbagh, L. Santos, M. Sayegh, R. B. Nussenblatt, D. E. Trentham & D. A. Hafler. 1994. Oral tolerance: immunologic mechanisms and treatment of animal and human organ-specific autoimmune diseases by oral administration of autoantigens. Annu. Rev. Immunol. **12**: 809-837.

115. Planchon, S. M., C. A. P. Martins, R. L. Guerrant & J. K. Roche. 1994. Regulation of intestinal epithelial barrier function by TGF-β1: Evidence for its role in abrogating the effect of a T cell cytokine. J. Immunol. **153**: 5730-5739.

116. Stok, W., P. J. Van Der Heijden & A. T. J. Bianchi. 1994. Conversion of orally induced suppression of the mucosal immune response to ovalbumin into stimulation by conjugating ovalbumin to cholera toxin or its B subunit. Vaccine **12**: 521-526.

117. BAZIN, H. 1976. The secretory antibody system. *In* Immunological Aspects of the Liver and Gastrointestinal Tract. A. Ferguson & R. N. M. MacSween, Eds.: 33-82. MTP Press Ltd. Lancaster, England.
118. STROBEL, S. 1995. Development of oral tolerance. *In* Intestinal Immunology and Food Allergy. A. de Weck & H. A. Sampson, Eds.: Vol. 34. Nestlé Nutrition Workshop Series. 155-166. Nestec Ltd., Vevey/Raven Press, Ltd. New York.
119. ROGOFF, T. M. & P. E. LIPSKY. 1981. Role of the Kupffer cells in local and systemic immune responses. Gastroenterology **80:** 854-860.
120. DUMONT, A. E. 1979. Orally induced tolerance. J. Immunol. **122:** 2134-2135.
121. GABORIAU-ROUTHIAU, V. & M.-C. MOREAU. 1996. The gut flora allows recovery of oral tolerance to ovalbumin after a transient breakdown mediated by cholera toxin or *Escherichia coli* heat-labile enterotoxin in mice. Pediatr. Res. In press.

Antigen Trafficking in the Intestine[a]

L. MAYER, L. P. SO, X. Y. YIO, AND G. SMALL

Mount Sinai Medical Center
Division of Clinical Immunology and Department of Cell Biology
Box 1089
One Gustave L. Levy Place
New York, New York 10029

It is generally recognized that the intestine is the largest lymphoid organ in the body, encompassing the greatest number of lymphocytes and generating significant amounts of antibody. Although much of this antibody is directed against luminal antigens, the majority of luminal contents do not generate active immunologic responses. This may result from two processes: physical barriers present along the epithelial border (mucus barrier, tight junctions) prevent access of antigens (Ags) to lymphoid tissues, or, as is the theme of this volume, many such Ags induce an active immunologic nonresponse, that is, oral tolerance. The dilemma here is to determine why, in a similar environment, some Ags induce active immunity while others induce suppression or anergy. The key then is to determine how Ags are handled in the gut. Clearly this is quite different from Ags administered systemically. Antigen in the gut lumen is subject to a variety of agents that can alter it prior to uptake (Table 1). Peptides are affected by gastric acid, pancreatic proteases, bacterial products, as well as other compounds. A result of this "luminal processing" may be a decrease in the requirements for processing by antigen-presenting cells (APCs) in the gut and differences in T-cell responses, inasmuch as different epitopes may be displayed. As a consequence of the luminal effects on antigen, there are many novel types of cells involved in antigen trafficking, either as APCs or as conduits to lymphoid aggregates. Specialized epithelium or M cells overlying Peyer's patches have been shown to transfer particulate Ags from the lumen to the patch.[1-3] As will be discussed

TABLE 1. Nonimmunologic Factors Regulating Mucosal Immune Responses

Chemical barriers
  Salivary secretions
    amylase, lysozyme

  Gastric secretions
    acid, pepsin

  Intestinal/pancreatic secretions
    proteases, trypsin, chymotrypsin, bile salts
    lipase, amylase

Physical barriers
  Epithelial tight junctions
  Mucus barrier

[a]This work was supported by PHS Grants AI 23504, AI 24671, and DK 44156.

28

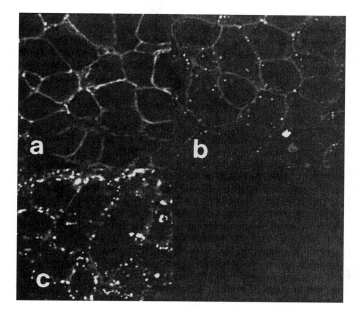

FIGURE 1. HT29 cells were grown on cover slips and incubated for varying periods with FITC-tetanus toxoid (60 μg). At each point, cells were washed, fixed with PBS-buffered formalin, and analyzed by fluorescence microscopy. a, time 0; b, 30 minutes; c, 5 hours.

later, several viruses and bacteria specifically bind to M cells by way of expressed receptors, allowing for the directed transport of certain microorganisms. Such a pathway typically results in the induction of an active IgA immune response. Although M cells can clearly transport antigen, data supporting their ability to act as APCs are less compelling.[4] However, within the GI tract, several conventional APCs exist and appear to be functional (macrophages, dendritic cells), but these cannot explain the immunologically suppressed tone of the gut.[5,6] Therefore, several groups have recently focused on nonprofessional APCs as potential regulators of mucosal immune responses. Intestinal epithelial cells (IEC) have been shown to process and present soluble Ags to immunocompetent T cells *in vitro*.[7-9] The unique feature here is that T cells proliferating in such co-cultures express CD8 and are functional suppressor cells.[7,8] Thus a scenario can be developed that not only is the form of Ag important in gut responses but that the route of Ag trafficking (M cells vs. IEC) also plays a major role.

We initiated studies to define the types of Ag capable of trafficking within the IEC and followed their routes intracellularly. Human adenocarcinoma cell lines were used as model systems either grown as monolayer cultures or polarized on collagen-coated filters. Fluorescein-coupled tetanus toxoid (FITC-TT) was added (60 μg), and intracellular trafficking was assessed by fluorescence; and confocal and electron microscopy. As seen in FIGURE 1, soluble FITC-TT is taken up by HT29 after 30 min of culture, and intracellular fluorescence within vesicles persists for 5 hours. No uptake was detected if cells were maintained at 4° C or if cells were pretreated with 1% PBS-buffered formalin. Furthermore this uptake appeared to be cell specific. That is, when pulsing T cells with the same concentration of FITC-TT, no uptake was detected. When comparing the kinetics of Ag

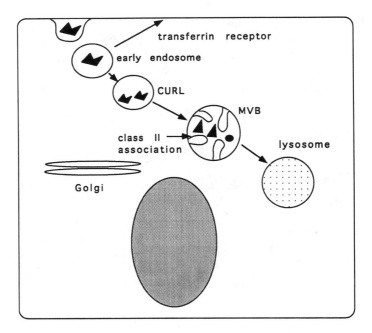

FIGURE 2. Schematic representation of studies monitoring the traffic of tetanus toxoid by confocal and electron microscopy. Antigen enters into early endosomes, into the compartment of uncoupling ligand and receptor (CURL), subsequently to multivesicular bodies (MVB) where class II/peptide association is reported to occur, and finally to the lysosomal compartment. Receptor-mediated uptake, such as that seen for transferrin, results in recycling to the cell surface after early endosome or CURL compartments. No transport of antigen into the cytoplasm, ER, or Golgi is noted.

uptake with conventional APCs, IEC were considerably slower. In monocytes, intracellular fluorescence signals were detected at 5 min, peaked at 60 min, and were markedly decreased by 2 H (data not shown). These kinetics were consistent with Ag processing and reexpression of processed peptides in association with products of the major histocompatibility complex (MHC) on the cell surface. As described above, uptake was slower in IEC, and fluorescence signals persisted. This, coupled with data from Bland in a rat model,[10] suggest that IEC are inefficient antigen-processing cells.

We have previously shown that Ags presented by IEC selectively activate CD8+ T cells.[8] It was therefore of interest to determine whether Ag trafficking within the IEC after exogenous uptake followed an endolysosomal pathway consistent with a classical class II-presentation pathway or whether Ags gained access to the cytoplasm, where they might be transported to the endoplasmic reticulum and allowed to associate with class I molecules, more consistent with CD8+ T cell-activation pathways. As seen in FIGURE 2 (schematic), exogenously administered Ag followed an endolysosomal route within IEC, being taken up initially in early endosomes and subsequently in late endosomes and lysosomes. This schematic represents the cumulative findings of confocal and electron microscopy and were confirmed using dual-labeling fluorescence microscopy (using antibodies against endolysosomal compartments along with FITC-TT).

Thus Ag processing and presentation by IEC does not appear to be classical in any sense and raises the concept that nonclassical restriction elements may play a role here. This concept is supported by the finding that blocking monoclonal antibodies (mAbs) to class I and class II fail to inhibit CD8+ T-cell activation induced by normal IEC.[11] By contrast, antibodies to the class Ib molecule CD1d are capable of inhibiting proliferation in these co-cultures.[12] Thus, not only may the APC be different in the gut but also the restriction element governing IEC:T-cell interactions may be distinct from those regulating common systemic immune responses. However, CD1d is not alone in this process. CD1d is not polymorphic and by itself does not bind to CD8. Furthermore CD1d transfectants fail to activate CD8-associated $p56^{lck}$, a src-like tyrosine kinase whose activity appears to be necessary for T-cell activation by IEC.[11] Thus other surface molecules may be involved. Therefore one scenario might be that CD1d associates with a CD8 ligand, allowing for engagement of the T-cell receptor and formation of a coreceptor complex with CD8 (FIG. 3). Because CD1d has an endosomal localization motif and can bind peptides larger than those associated with class I (8-10mers) or class II (10-14mers), it is plausible that the limited endosomal processing occurring in IEC[13] may favor peptide (or other compounds) binding to CD1d. This model needs to be formally proven, but the currently available data fit with this scenario and support the concept that Ags sampled from the lumen by IEC would favor the activation of CD8+ suppressor T cells.

Other factors may aid in dictating the site of Ag sampling. Our data reported above describe the uptake of soluble protein Ags. Regardless of size, soluble Ags were taken up by IEC with similar kinetics (data not shown). However, if Ag is aggregated or expressed in the form of an insoluble immune complex, the IEC is no longer capable of taking up these Ags (FIG. 4). Insolubility or globular Ags may favor uptake by cells in the dome epithelium or M cells. As stated earlier, numerous studies have reported that M-cell uptake is associated with an active IgA response. In addition, several bacteria and/ or viruses for whom a receptor is expressed on the M cell will induce a protective IgA response,[14] as is the case with polio virus, the first protective oral vaccine. An interesting series of experiments reported by Rubin *et al.*[15] in 1982 underscores this concept. Reovirus type I and III evoke distinct immune responses in the mouse. Reovirus III passes through M cells and elicits a protective IgA response, whereas reovirus I infects surface epithelium and induces tolerance. From these data as well as our own, one can develop the following model: Ags that exist in an insoluble form or that have receptors for their surface coats expressed on M cells will be selectively taken up by M cells and elicit an active immune response. Soluble protein Ags as well as luminally processed peptides may be taken up by IEC, resulting in the induction of anergy or tolerance, depending upon the presence or absence of costimulatory signals (FIG. 5). If this scenario is valid, then tolerogens might be turned into immunogens by altering the form of the Ag, therefore focusing it onto the M cell (FIG. 6).

There are refinements to this model as well. Invasive bacteria (invading IEC) can evoke an active immune response without passing through the M cell. If one analyzes invasive *Salmonella,* the intracellular trafficking pattern is quite distinct from that of soluble protein Ags, where there is endolysosomal localization. Rather, bacteria are transported in separate vesicles from the apical to the basolateral surface, without the interaction of potential suppressor-inducing mechanisms in the IEC. It appears then that IEC may contribute to both tolerance and active immunity, depending upon the Ag-trafficking pathway within the cell. A similar scenario may exist for M cells.

There are some inconsistencies with this model, however. Several groups have documented that Peyer's patches T cells can promote tolerance as well as an active IgA response.[16] This may be due to the production of TGF_B within the patch. However, the secretion of this cytokine may be Ag dose dependent and not a generalizable event.

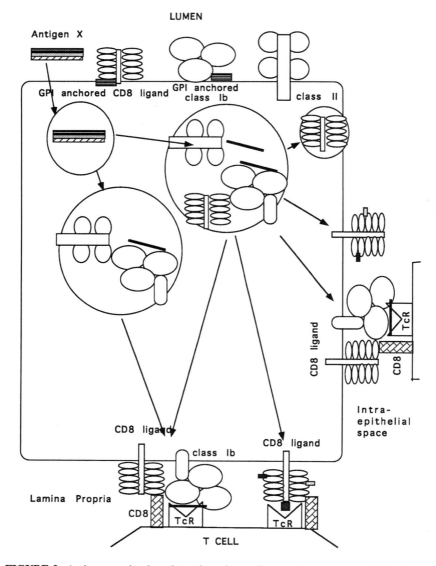

FIGURE 3. Antigen entering into the early endosomal compartment, as described in FIGURE 2, is subject to proteolysis and association with either class II or class Ib molecules, such as CD1d. Because CD1d is incapable of binding to CD8, one must invoke a novel CD8 ligand, allowing for the formation of a coreceptor complex when the MHC/peptide complex is re-expressed either on the lateral aspect of the cell (allowing for interaction with intraepithelial lymphocytes) or basally (allowing for interaction with lamina propria lymphocytes).

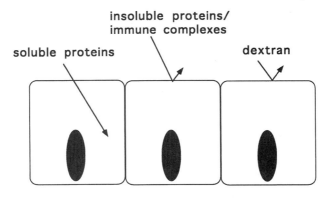

FIGURE 4. As shown in FIGURE 1, soluble antigens are capable of being taken up by IEC (intestinal epithelial cells). Neither immune complexes nor aggregated insoluble proteins are taken up, despite similarity in molecular weight. Similarly, soluble dextran is not taken up by IEC, demonstrating selectivity in this process.

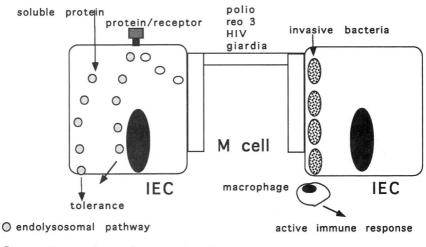

FIGURE 5. The outcome of distinct routes of antigen trafficking in the gut. Soluble protein antigens taken up by IEC will process these antigens and invoke a suppressor T cell response or anergy, depending upon the presence or absence of costimulatory molecules. Specific viruses and bacteria selectively enter M cells by virtue of expressed receptors for these microorganisms. Invasive bacteria appear to bypass the IEC tolerogenic pathway by trafficking in a distinct set of vacuoles. Bacteria that translocate can be taken up by subepithelial macrophages and stimulate an active immune response.

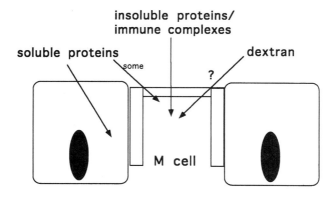

FIGURE 6. Alteration of the form of antigen can alter the trafficking pattern and potentially the type of immune response generated. As depicted here, aggregation of soluble antigen can inhibit its uptake by IEC and focus the same antigen onto the M cell, where an active immune response will be generated.

In summary, it is recognized that administration of soluble proteins by way of an oral route can result in the induction of tolerance. Some forms of oral tolerance appear to be mediated by suppressor T cells. These cells may be generated in the intestine by the interaction of novel APCs with CD8[+] T cells. However, the ability to generate suppression may also relate to various exogenous factors affecting orally administered antigen. The degree of processing, the site of entry, and the intracellular pathways may dictate the type of response generated.

REFERENCES

1. WOLF, J. L. & W. A. BYE. 1984. The membranous epithelial (M) cell and the mucosal immune system. Annu. Rev. Med. **35:** 95–112.
2. OWEN, R. L. & A. L. JONES. 1974. Epithelial cell specialization within human Peyer's patches: An ultrastructural study of intestinal lymphoid follicles. Gastroenterology **66:** 189.
3. OWEN, R. L., N. F. PIERCE, R. T. APPLE & W. C. CRAY, JR. 1986. M cell transport of *Vibrio cholerae* from the intestinal lumen into Peyer's patches: A mechanism for antigen sampling and for microbial transepithelial migration. J. Infect. Dis. **153:** 1108–1118.
4. ALLAN, C. H., D. L. MENDRICK & J. S. TRIER. 1993. Rat intestinal M cells contain acidic endosomal-lysosomal compartments and express class II major histocompatibility complex determinants. Gastroenterology **104:** 698–708.
5. BLAND, P. W. & D. M. KAMBARAGE. 1991. Antigen handling by the epithelium and lamina propria macrophages. Gastroenterol. Clin. North Am. **20:** 3.
6. PANJA, A. & L. MAYER. 1994. Diversity and function of antigen presenting cells in mucosal tissues. *In* Handbook of Mucosal Immunology. P. L. Ogra, M. E. Lamm, J. R. McGhee, J. Mestecky, W. Strober & J. Bienenstock, Eds.: 177–181. Academic Press. San Diego, CA.
7. BLAND, P. W. & L. G. WARREN. 1986. Antigen presentation by epithelial cells of the rat small intestine. II. Selective induction of suppressor T cells. Immunology **58:** 9–14.
8. MAYER, L. & R. SHLIEN. 1987. Evidence for function of a Ia molecule on gut epithelial cells in man. J. Exp. Med. **166:** 1471.

9. KAISERLIAN, D., K. VIDAL & J. P. REVILLARD. 1989. Murine enterocytes can present soluble antigen to specific class II restricted CD4⁺ T cells. Eur. J. Immunol. **19:** 1513.

10. BLAND, P. W. & C. V. WHITING. 1989. Antigen processing by isolated rat intestinal villus enterocytes. Immunology **68**(4): 497-502.

11. LI, Y., X. Y. YIO & L. MAYER. 1995. Human intestinal epithelial cell-induced CD8⁺ T cell activation is mediated through CD8 and the activation of CD8-associated p56^{lck}. J. Exp. Med. **182:** 1079-1088.

12. PANJA, A., R. S. BLUMBERG, S. P. BALK & L. MAYER. 1993. CD1d is involved in T cell:epithelial cell interactions. J. Exp. Med. **178:** 1115-1120.

13. CASTANO, A. R., S. TANGRI, J. E. MILLER, H. R. HOLCOMBE et al. 1995. Peptide binding and presentation by mouse CD1. Science **269**(5221): 223-6.

14. SICINKI, P. J., J. B. ROWINSKI, A. WARCHOL et al. 1990. Poliovirus type I enters the human host through intestinal M cells. Gastroenterology **98:** 56-58.

15. RUBIN, D., H. L. WEINER, B. N. FIELDS & M. I. GREENE. 1981. Immunologic tolerance after oral administration of reovirus: Requirement for two viral gene products for tolerance induction. J. Immunol. **127**(4): 1697-701.

16. MILLER, A., A. AL-SABBAGH, L. M. SANTOS, M. P. DAS & H. L. WEINER. 1993. Epitopes of myelin basic protein that trigger TGF-beta release after oral tolerization are distinct from encephalitogenic epitopes and mediate epitope-driven bystander suppression. J. Immunol. **151**(12): 7307-15.

The Role of the Thymus in Intestinal Intraepithelial T-cell Development

LEO LEFRANÇOIS AND LYNN PUDDINGTON

Department of Medicine, MC1310
University of Connecticut Health Center
263 Farmington Avenue
Farmington, Connecticut 06030

INTRODUCTION

The intestinal immune system, although integrated with the peripheral immune system, is made up of lymphocyte populations that are functionally and phenotypically distinguishable from other lymphocytes. Lamina propria T and B cells are categorized by a predominance of "memory" phenotype cells in the former case and the production of IgA for the latter. The Peyer's patches are specialized structures geared toward uptake of luminal antigen and subsequent antigen presentation of these antigens to T and B cells. In keeping with this compartmentalized specialization of the intestinal immune response, intraepithelial lymphocytes (IEL) of the small intestine develop along a pathway quite different from that followed by other T cells.[1] Whereas the vast majority of non-IEL T cells are derived from precursors that have matured and been selected in the thymus, IEL have unique requirements for the thymus in completing their developmental program.[2-4] However, whether there is an absolute necessity for the thymus in IEL maturation has been questioned. Thus, thymectomized irradiated bone-marrow or fetal liver reconstituted (ATXBM) mice contain IEL.[2,5,6] In the mouse, TCRαβ and TCRγδ cells each comprise roughly 50% of IEL, and both of these subsets are present in ATXBM mice.[7,8] Moreover, CD8αα IEL, which contain TCRγδ and TCRαβ IEL and have been touted as the extrathymic IEL component,[9] are produced in ATXBM mice, but CD8αβ TCRαβ IEL are also generated.[6] More recently, Rocha *et al.* showed that reconstitution of RAG2$^{-/-}$ mice with nude mouse bone marrow resulted in production of only CD8αα IEL expressing either TCR type but in significantly lower numbers than found in euthymic mice.[10] It should be noted that congenitally athymic nude mice contain approximately 5-fold fewer TCRγδ IEL and few TCRαβ IEL.[11-13] Taken together, these results would suggest that the thymus is required for CD8αβ IEL production and that it is involved in efficient production of all IEL. The reasons why ATXBM mice produce all IEL subsets is unclear but could be due to influence of the thymus on the intestine prior to thymectomy or due to effects of radiation on T-cell development.

We have now used neonatal thymectomy and thymus grafting as a means of studying the role of the thymus in IEL development.[3] In the case of thymus grafting, we asked whether the thymus is capable of producing IEL, rather than asking whether removal of the thymus affects IEL maturation. Overall, the results demonstrate that the thymus plays a dual role in IEL development: as a source of IEL precursors and as a source of as yet unidentified factors that aid IEL maturation.

MATERIAL AND METHODS

Mice

C57BL/6J, Balb/cJ, and CB6F$_1$ nude mice were obtained from the Jackson Laboratory, Bar Harbor, ME. B6-Ly5.2 mice were obtained from Harlan.

Monoclonal Antibodies

The following monoclonal antibodies (mAbs) were used in this study: GL3, anti-TCRγδ;[8] H57.597, anti-TCRαβ;[14] 3.168, anti-CD8;[15] anti-CD4-PE (Becton-Dickinson, San Jose, CA); and H35-17-2, anti-CD8β,[16] anti-Ly5.1, and anti-Ly5.2.[17]

Neonatal Thymectomy

Within 24 hours of birth, mice were thymectomized using suction according to the protocol of Sjokin et al.[18]

Grafting and Reconstitution Studies

Fetal and neonatal thymus lobes were grafted subcutaneously to adult neonatally thymectomized (nTx) or SCID mice. Either B6-Ly5.2 or C57BL/6J (Ly5.1) mice were used as graft donor or recipient, which allowed distinction between host and graft-derived cells. IEL and lymph node (LN) cells were isolated 4-8 weeks after grafting and examined by fluorescence flow cytometry. Day-19 fetal intestine or fetal thymus (from B6-Ly5.1 mice) was grafted subcutaneously into thymectomized, irradiated (1100 rad) (BALB/c × B6-Ly5.2)F$_1$ mice that had been reconstituted with T-cell depleted bone marrow from B6-Ly5.2 mice. Grafting was performed three weeks after reconstitution. For reconstitution of nude mice, (BALB/c × B6-Ly5.2)F$_1$ day-13 fetal liver was injected intravenously into irradiated (1100 rad) (BALB/c × C57BL/6)F$_1$ nude mice.

Isolation of IEL

IEL were isolated essentially as described previously.[19] Briefly, the small intestines of individual mice were cut into 5 mm pieces and washed twice with medium. The washed intestinal pieces were then stirred at 37°C for 20 min in medium with the addition of 1 mM dithioerythritol. This step was repeated, and the resultant supernatants were rapidly filtered through nylon wool and the filtrate centrifuged through a 44%/67.5% Percoll gradient. The cells at the interface of the Percoll gradient were collected and prepared for flow cytometry.

Isolation of LN Subsets

Inguinal, brachial, cervical, and mesenteric lymph nodes were removed and pooled, and single cell suspensions were prepared using a tissue homogenizer. The preparation was filtered through Nytex, and the filtrate centrifuged to pellet the cells.

Immunofluorescence Analysis

Lymphocytes were resuspended in PBS-0.2% BSA-0.1% NaN_3 (PBS/BSA/NaN_3) at a concentration of 1×10^6-1×10^7 cells/mL followed by incubation at 4 °C for 30 min with 100 μL of properly diluted mAb. The mAbs were either directly labeled with fluorescein isothiocyanate (FITC), phycoerythrin (PE), or were biotinylated. For the latter, avidin-phycoerythrin (Av-PE) or avidin-Red 613 (Av-R613; BRL Life Technologies, Gaithersburg, MD) were used as secondary reagents for detection. After staining, the cells were washed twice with PBS/BSA/NaN_3, and relative fluorescence intensities were measured with a FACScan (Becton-Dickinson, San Jose, CA).

RESULTS AND DISCUSSION

In order to determine whether the thymus was necessary during early life for generation of IEL, mice were neonatally thymectomized (nTx). IEL and LN T cells were isolated eight weeks later and analyzed for T-cell receptor (TCR) and coreceptor expression. Strikingly, TCRγδ IEL were greatly reduced in nTx mice (FIG. 1). As expected, few mature T cells were present in lymph nodes of nTx mice. In addition to γδ IEL depletion, interesting effects on the TCRαβ IEL population were noted. Specifically, the levels of TCR and of CD8 (not shown) were lower than normal in some animals (FIG. 2). Moreover, a population of CD8⁺ TCR⁻ IEL was greatly increased in some nTx mice as compared to controls (FIG. 3). These results suggest that the thymus was providing signals to IEL or to the epithelium that were essential for normal γδ and αβ IEL maturation. The presence of putative immature IEL (TCR^low, CD8⁺TCR⁻), which are also present in nude mice, further implies that the later developmental stages of IEL were occurring in the intestine.

One interpretation of the result of nTx on the IEL compartment, particularly with regard to γδ IEL, is simply that the thymus is the source of mature or immature IEL precursors (IELp). In order to test whether the thymus can produce IEL, we grafted fetal or neonatal thymus to immunodeficient hosts. B6-Ly5 congenic mice were used to allow tracking of graft and host-derived cells. Grafting of B6-Ly5.1 neonatal thymus to B6-Ly5.2 mice resulted in production of a significant population of thymus-derived IEL (FIG. 4), as well as LN cells (data not shown). All TCRαβ IEL subsets, including the so-called extrathymic subsets lacking Thy1 and CD8β, were generated from the thymus (FIG. 4 and ref. 3). In addition, TCRγδ IEL could also be produced by the thymus. Although our original observations suggested that the early thymus could not produce γδ IEL,[3] the large number of grafted animals that we have now examined suggests that γδ IEL can be produced by the thymus from early fetal to neonatal periods. However, the production of TCRαβ IEL by thymus grafts always outweighs γδ IEL production, sometimes exclusively.

Taken at face value, the results from nude mice would suggest that all TCRαβ IEL and 80% of TCRγδ IEL are thymus dependent. However, there has been some discussion of whether the nude mouse is a good model of extrathymic development. This is due in part to the possibility that an early thymic rudiment may influence limited T-cell development. Additionally, with regard to IEL development, it is possible that the nude epithelial defect extends to the intestine. It is also possible that the absence of a thymus throughout life, as opposed to adult thymectomy, results in a long-term defect in nude mouse intestine that will not allow IEL development. In order to test this possibility we lethally irradiated and reconstituted nude mice with day-13 fetal liver. Again, only donor fetal liver-derived cells were analyzed (FIG. 5). Small numbers of CD4⁻8⁻ and CD4⁻8⁺ IEL were produced as well as a population of CD4⁻8⁻ non-T cells. Thus, TCR analysis showed that ~45% of IEL expressed either TCRγδ or TCRαβ. The TCR⁻ population was not characterized further but contained ~15% sIg⁺ cells. Therefore, a significant population of non-T,

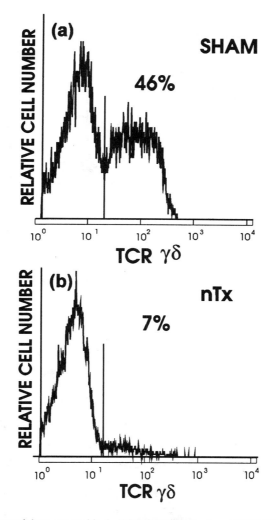

FIGURE 1. Neonatal thymectomy blocks TCRγδ IEL production. C57BL/6J mice were sham-operated (a) or thymectomized (b) within one day after birth. IEL were isolated 20 weeks later and reacted with phycoerythrin-coupled GL3 (anti-TCRγδ). Relative intensities of individual cells were measured with a Becton-Dickinson FACScan. Gating using forward and right angle light scatter was used to include only the lymphocyte population based on staining with an anti-CD45 mAb (not shown). The bold vertical line in the histograms represents the demarcation between positive and negative staining as determined using an appropriately labeled irrelevant mAb.

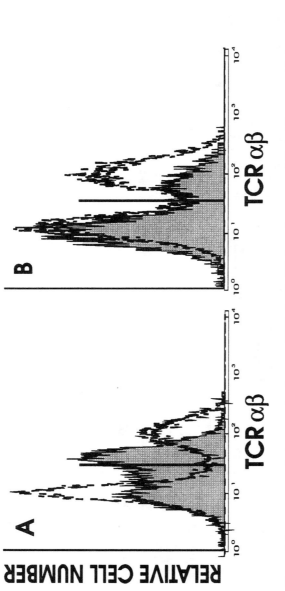

FIGURE 2. Neonatal thymectomy results in maturational arrest of TCRαβ IEL. IEL from sham-operated (dashed lines, open histograms) or nTx BALB/c mice (filled histograms) were analyzed for TCRαβ expression. Percoll-fractionated IEL were reacted with H57-PE (anti-TCRαβ) and analyzed by FACScan. The bold vertical line in the histograms represents the demarcation between positive and negative staining as determined using an appropriately labeled irrelevant mAb.

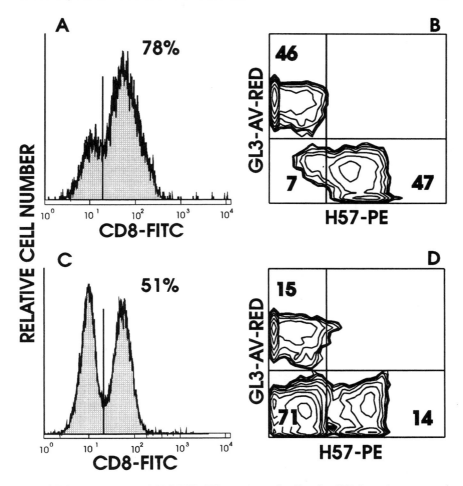

FIGURE 3. A population of CD8⁺TCR⁻ IEL are present in nTx mice. IEL from sham-operated (panels A and B) or nTx (panels C and D) C57BL/6J mice were analyzed by three-color fluorescence flow cytometry for CD8, TCRγδ, and TCRαβ expression. Cells were reacted with 3.168-FITC (anti-CD8), H57-PE (anti-TCRαβ), and with GL3-biotin. The latter was detected with avidin-Red 613 (BRL, Gaithersburg, MD). CD8⁺ cells to the right of the bold vertical line in panels A and C were analyzed for TCRγδ and TCRαβ expression as shown in panels B and D.

non-B cells were produced in these mice, which could represent IELp. These results indicate that the nude mouse intestine can support γδ and αβ IEL production, albeit limited. It should also be noted that in the absence of irradiation, no donor-derived IEL could be detected, despite the fact that few IEL are present in nude mice. This result indicated that IELp contained in fetal liver, and this is also true for adult bone marrow IELp, do not develop in the absence of irradiation in these experimental systems. This

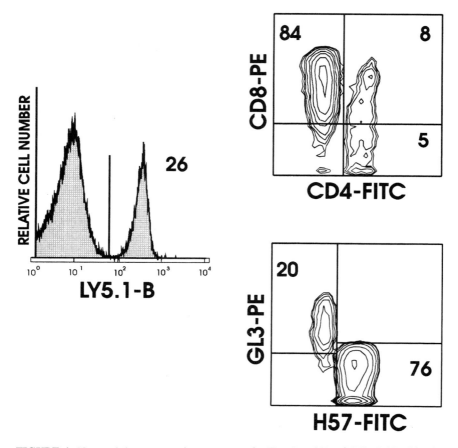

FIGURE 4. Neonatal thymus contains precursors for Tcrαβ and Tcrγδ IEL. B6-Ly5.2 mice that had been neonatally thymectomized six weeks earlier were grafted subcutaneously with neonatal (< 24 hours old) thymus lobes from C57BL/6 (Ly5.1) mice. Six weeks later IEL were isolated and reacted with mAbs specific for Ly5.1, CD8 and CD4, or Tcrγδ (GL3) and Tcrαβ (H57). The Ly5.1+ cells were analyzed for either CD4 and CD8 (upper right panel) or Tcrγδ and Tcrαβ (lower right panel) by fluorescence flow cytometry.

may be due either to an inability to home to the gut in the absence of intestinal damage by irradiation or could be the result of the production of radiation-induced factors that impinge on T-cell production. In regard to the latter, irradiation can induce immature thymocytes to differentiate to the CD4+8+ stage and can also induce TCRβ rearrangement in SCID mice.[20,21] The potential untoward effects of radiation should be considered when discussing T-cell development in these model systems.

The ability of the intestine to act as a surrogate thymus has been suggested by experiments using ectopic intestinal grafts.[22] In that system, fetal intestine was grafted to irradiated, thymectomized, bone-marrow reconstituted mice. Curiously, three weeks after grafting with fetal intestine under the kidney capsule or subcutaneously, an apparently

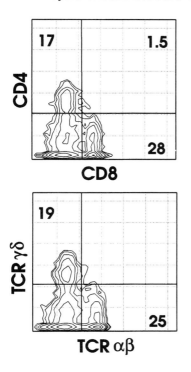

FIGURE 5. Reconstitution of IEL in nude mice. (BALB/c × C57BL/6)F$_1$ nude mice were irradiated (1100 rad) and reconstituted with 1×10^7 day-13 (BALB/c × B6-Ly5.2)F$_1$ fetal liver cells. Twelve weeks later IEL were isolated, and fetal liver-derived cells (Ly5.2$^+$) were examined for CD4, CD8, and TCR expression by fluorescence flow cytometry.

normal complement of CD4 and CD8 LN T cells appeared in these animals. T cells persisted in these mice for at least eleven weeks. Because the IEL compartment was not examined in that study, we sought to determine whether intestinal grafts could generate IEL. Our system was devised such that the source of all cells could be determined.

Irradiated, thymectomized (BALB/c × B6-Ly5.2)F$_1$ mice were reconstituted with T-depleted bone marrow from B6-Ly5.2 mice. Three weeks later these mice received B6-Ly5.1 fetal intestine or fetal thymus grafts, and five weeks after grafting, IEL and LN cells were analyzed. Grafts were examined at the time of sacrifice, and only mice in which the thymus or intestine grafts had obviously thrived were included in the analysis. Examination of lymphocytes for Ly5.1 and Ly5.2 expression simultaneously allows assignation of each cell to host, graft, or bone marrow derivation, as shown in FIGURE 6A. When ATXBM mice were grafted with fetal thymus, graft- and bone marrow-derived LN and IEL populations were detected. In LN, 15% of the cells were graft derived, and all expressed TCRαβ (data not shown). Forty-five percent of IEL were graft derived, and the majority expressed TCRαβ, again demonstrating that the thymus can produce IEL. Neither LN or IEL from fetal-intestine-grafted mice contained graft-derived cells, indicating that the fetal gut was not a source of T-cell precursors. However, it is possible that gut-resident IELp were present in the graft but were unable to traffic out of the tissue following *in situ* development.

In order to determine whether the presence of thymus or intestine grafts directed T-cell development from bone-marrow precursors, we examined TCR expression of the bone-marrow-derived population (FIG. 6B). In fetal thymus-grafted mice, ~11% of bone-marrow-derived LN cells expressed TCRαβ. This is a reasonable percentage, given that

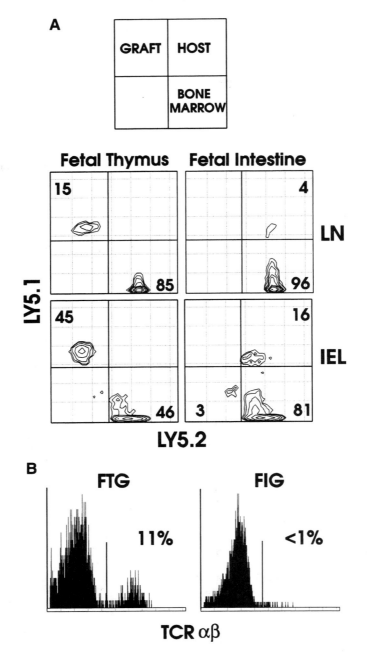

FIGURE 6. Fetal intestinal grafts do not support T-cell production. (BALB/c × B6-Ly5.2)F_1 mice were irradiated and reconstituted with 2×10^7 T-cell depleted B6-Ly5.2 bone marrow cells. Three weeks later, these mice received subcutaneous fetal thymus or fetal intestine grafts. Five weeks later IEL and LN cells were isolated and analyzed for Ly5.1, Ly5.2, and TCR expression by three-color fluorescence flow cytometry. Panel A shows the expression of Ly5.1 and Ly5.2 on LN cells and IEL. Panel B shows the expression of TCRαβ on Ly5.1⁻ Ly5.2⁺ LN cells from fetal thymus-grafted (FTG) or fetal intestine-grafted (FIG) mice.

complete reconstitution in a normal mouse generally requires at least 8 weeks. This analysis was performed 5 weeks after grafting, so the time until engraftment (*i.e.,* vascularization) should also be taken into account. In contrast to the results obtained with thymus-grafted animals, no T cells were present in LN cells from fetal intestine-grafted mice (FIG. 6B). Thus, we find no evidence that ectopic intestinal grafts can direct T-cell development in the peripheral or intestinal lymphoid tissues.

The data now available indicates clearly that the thymus plays a pivotal role in IEL development. Removal of the thymus early in life disrupts severely the maturation and/ or expansion of IEL subsets. This defect is long term, indicating that although bone marrow contains IELp, such cells are unable to generate IEL in the absence of a thymus. However, thymus-derived IELp can repopulate the intestine in this system. Nevertheless, our results suggest that IELp may leave the thymus prior to TCR rearrangement and undergo positive selection in the intestine.[23] Although arguments can be made against the use of the nude mouse as a model for athymic T-cell development, in the case of IEL, these mice may provide a valuable lesson. In the apparent complete absence of thymic influence due to a congenital defect, few TCRαβ IEL and low numbers of TCRγδ IEL can develop *in vivo*. In models in which the thymus is removed during adulthood and the animals are irradiated and reconstituted, TCRαβ and TCRγδ IEL can develop. Thus, taken in the extreme, either the thymus provides factors that induce competence in the intestinal epithelium (or elsewhere?), which subsequently allows IEL development, or the animal models employed are faulty. In any case, the main question that now confronts us is whether the unique developmental pathway of IEL provides the basis for specialized, organ-specific immunity.

REFERENCES

1. LEFRANÇOIS, L. & L. PUDDINGTON. 1995. Extrathymic intestinal T cell development: virtual reality? Immunol. Today **16:** 16-21.
2. LIN, T., G. MATSUZAKI, H. KENAI, T. NAKAMURA & K. NOMOTO. 1993. Thymus influences the development of extrathymically derived intestinal intraepithelial lymphocytes. Eur. J. Immunol. **23:** 1968-1974.
3. LEFRANÇOIS, L. & S. OLSON. 1994. A novel pathway of thymus-directed T lymphocyte maturation. J. Immunol. **153:** 987-995.
4. WANG, J. & J. R. KLEIN. 1994. Thymus-neuroendocrine interactions in extrathymic T cell development. Science **265:** 1860-1862.
5. MOSLEY, R. L., D. STYRE & J. R. KLEIN. 1990. Differentiation and functional maturation of bone marrow-derived intestinal epithelial T cells expressing membrane T cell receptor in athymic radiation chimeras. J. Immunol. **145:** 1369-1375.
6. POUSSIER, P., P. EDOUARD, C. LEE, M. BINNIE & M. JULIUS. 1992. Thymus-independent development and negative selection of T cells expressing T cell receptor α/β in the intestinal epithelium: evidence for distinct circulation patterns of gut and thymus-derived T lymphocytes. J. Exp. Med. **176:** 187-199.
7. LEFRANÇOIS, L. 1991. Phenotypic complexity of intraepithelial lymphocytes of the small intestine. J. Immunol. **147:** 1746-1751.
8. GOODMAN, T. & L. LEFRANÇOIS. 1989. Intraepithelial lymphocytes. Anatomical site, not T cell receptor form, dictates phenotype and function. J. Exp. Med. **170:** 1569-1581.
9. ROCHA, B., P. VASSALLI & D. GUY-GRAND. 1991. The Vβ repertoire of mouse gut homodimeric α CD8+ intraepithelial lymphocytes reveals a major extrathymic pathway of T cell differentiation. J. Exp. Med. **173:** 483-486.
10. ROCHA, B., P. VASSALLI & D. GUY-GRAND. 1994. Thymic and extrathymic origins of gut intraepithelial lymphocyte populations in mice. J. Exp. Med. **180:** 681-686.

11. BANDEIRA, A., S. ITOHARA, M. BONNEVILLE, O. BURLEN-DEFRANOUX, T. MOTA-SANTOS, A. COUTINHO & S. TONEGAWA. 1990. Extrathymic origin of intestinal intraepithelial lymphocytes bearing T-cell antigen receptor γδ. Proc. Natl. Acad. Sci. USA **88:** 43-47.

12. DEGEUS, B., M. VAN DEN ENDEN, C. COOLEN, L. NAGELKERKEN, P. VAN DER HEIJDEN & J. ROZING. 1990. Phenotype of intraepithelial lymphocytes in euthymic and athymic mice: implications for differentiation of cells bearing a CD3-associated γδ T cell receptor. Eur. J. Immunol. **20:** 291-298.

13. GUY-GRAND, D., N. CERF-BENSUSSAN, B. MALISSEN, M. MALASSIS-SERIS, C. BRIOTTET & P. VASSALLI. 1991. Two gut intraepithelial CD8+ lymphocyte populations with different T cell receptors: A role for the gut epithelium in T cell differentiation. J. Exp. Med. **173:** 471-481.

14. KUBO, R., W. BORN, J. W. KAPPLER, P. MARRACK & M. PIGEON. 1989. Characterization of a monoclonal antibody which detects all murine αβ T cell receptors. J. Immunol. **142:** 2736.

15. SARMIENTO, M., A. L. GLASEBROOK & F. W. FITCH. 1982. IgG or IgM monoclonal antibodies reactive with different determinants on the molecular complex bearing Lyt-2 antigen block T-cell mediated cytolysis in the absence of complement. J. Immunol. **125:** 2665.

16. GOLSTEIN, P., C. GORIDIS, A. M. SCHMITT-VERHULST, B. HAYOT, A. PIERRES, A. VAN AGTHOVEN, Y. KAUFMANN, Z. ESHAR & M. PIERRES. 1982. Lymphoid cell surface interaction structures detected using cytolysis-inhibiting monoclonal antibodies. Immunol. Rev. **68:** 5.

17. SHEN, F. W. 1991. Monoclonal antibodies to mouse lymphocyte differentiation alloantigens. *In* Monoclonal antibodies and T-cell hybridomas: Perspectives and technical advances. U. Hammerling & J. F. Kearney, Eds.: 25. Amsterdam: Elsevier/North Holland Inc.

18. SJOKIN, K., A. P. DALMASSO, J. M. SMITH & C. MARTINEZ. 1963. Thymectomy in newborn and adult mice. Transplantation **1:** 521-525.

19. GOODMAN, T. & L. LEFRANÇOIS. 1988. Expression of the γ-δ T-cell receptor on intestinal CD8+ intraepithelial lymphocytes. Nature **333:** 855-858.

20. DANSKA, J. S., F. PFLUMIO, C. J. WILLIAMS, O. HUNER, J. E. DICK & C. J. GUIDOS. 1994. Rescue of T cell-specific V(D)J recombination in SCID mice by DNA-damaging agents. Science **266:** 450-455.

21. ZUNIGA-PFLUCKER, J. C., D. JIANG, P. L. SCHWARTZBERG & M. J. LENARDO. 1994. Sublethal γ-radiation induces differentiation of CD4⁻/CD8⁻ into CD4+/CD8+ thymocytes without T cell receptor β rearrangement in recombinase activation gene 2⁻/⁻ mice. J. Exp. Med. **180:** 1517-1521.

22. MOSLEY, R. L. & J. R. KLEIN. 1992. Peripheral engraftment of fetal intestine into athymic mice sponsors T cell development: direct evidence for thymopoietic function of murine small intestine. J. Exp. Med. **176:** 1365-1373.

23. FULLER, B. & L. LEFRANÇOIS. 1995. Requirement for extrathymic class I histocompatibility antigens for positive selection of thymus-derived T lymphocytes. J. Immunol. **155:** 2808-2811.

The Role of Dendritic Cells in Antigen Processing in the Peyer's Patch

BRIAN L. KELSALL AND WARREN STROBER

Mucosal Immunity Section
Laboratory for Clinical Investigation
National Institute of Allergy and Infectious Diseases
National Institutes of Health
Building 10, Room 11N238
900 Rockville Pike
Bethesda, Maryland 22908

INTRODUCTION

Although it is clear that antigens and microorganisms from the intestinal lumen are transported into the Peyer's patch (PP) by microfold (M)-cells present in the follicle-associated epithelium (FAE), the details of antigen processing and presentation within the PP are poorly understood. Prior studies have suggested that dendritic cells (DCs) are a major antigen-presenting cell population in the subepithelial dome (SED) of the PP, the region just beneath the FAE.[1-3] In addition, isolated DCs from the PP have been shown to stimulate T cells in a mixed lymphocyte reaction (MLR),[4] and to support IgA B-cell development.[5-8] It was also demonstrated, using rats that had undergone mesenteric adenectomy, that DCs isolated from the thoracic duct lymph of animals fed OVA were capable, on adoptive transfer to an unimmunized animal, of inducing a primary T-cell response *in vivo,* suggesting that intestinal DCs carry antigens to the mesenteric lymph nodes or to other nonintestinal lymphoid sites.[9] These prior studies have provided important insight into the possible role of DCs in antigen presentation in the PP.

We have extended these findings by demonstrating the location of at least two different subsets of DCs in the mouse PP by performing immunohistochemistry with DC-reactive monoclonal antibodies (mAb), and by showing that PP DCs can efficiently process and present soluble antigens to T cells. We determined by immunoperoxidase staining that there is a striking concentration of cells lying just beneath the PP dome epithelium that stain with a mAb against murine CD11c (N418), an integrin, that in the mouse is present on nonfollicular dendritic cells.[10] These cells in the PP are poised to capture antigens transported from the intestinal lumen by overlying M cells. A separate population of dendritic cells was identified in the interfollicular T-cell regions (IFR) that stained with N418, but also with the DC-reactive mAbs NLDC-145, M342, and 2A1. The latter mAbs stain typical interdigitating DCs in the T-cell areas of peripheral lymphoid tissues. The expression of the intracellular antigens recognized by mAb M342 by the IFR DCs suggest that they are in a later stage of differentiation than the PP DCs in the SED.[11]

We went on to isolate PP and spleen DCs and analyze their surface phenotype by flow cytometry. We found that PP DCs expressed much higher levels of MHC class II molecules than similar cells from the spleen. In addition, we demonstrated using T cells from mice transgenic for a T-cell receptor (TCR) specific for either cytochrome C (CyC) or ovalbumin (OVA) that PP DCs are as effective as spleen DCs in processing CyC or

OVA for presentation to antigen-specific naive T cells. We were able to load PP DCs with antigens for presentation to T cells either *in vitro,* during the overnight culture required for their isolation, or *in vivo,* by feeding OVA to mice prior to PP DC isolation.[10] We concluded that the SED PP DCs are uniquely poised for the capture of antigens transported by overlying M cells; that the DCs in the IFRs appear to be in a more mature state, suggesting movement of DCs from the SED to the IFR; and that PP DCs are as efficient as spleen DCs for the processing and presentation of soluble antigen to naive T cells.

MATERIAL AND METHODS

Animals

Female B10.A and BALB/c mice 6-10 weeks of age were obtained from the Jackson Laboratory (Bar Harbor, ME). Mice transgenic for the Vα11/Vβ3 TCR that recognizes the 88-104 C-terminal peptide of pigeon cytochrome c and IE^k were originally provided by Ronald Schwartz (Laboratory of Cellular Immunology, NIAID, NIH, Bethesda, MD). The F-1 line used in these experiments was maintained by backcrossing B10.D2 (H-2^d) mice heterozygous for the TCR alpha and beta chains, with B10.A (H-2^k) mice (the Jackson Laboratory, Bar Harbor, ME). Mice homozygous for a TCR recognizing the 323-339 peptide of ovalbumin and IA^d were kindly provided by Dennis Loh (Howard Hughes Medical Institute, Washington University, St. Louis, MO).

Preparation of Dendritic Cells and Antigen-loading Protocols

DCs were prepared with a modification of established techniques.[12] Peyer's patches were digested with collagenase D (400 U/mL, Boeringher Mannheim, Germany) and DNAse (15 μg/mL, Boeringher Mannheim, Germany) in Iscove's modified Delbecco's media (IMDM), supplemented with 10% heat-inactivated fetal calf serum (FCS), penicillin/streptomycin, 2-mercaptoethanol (50 μM), L-glutamine (2 mM), and amphotericin B. Cells were plated on 15-cm plastic tissue culture dishes (#3025, Falcon Labware, Oxnard, CA), and nonadherent cells were washed free with warmed PBS. Adherent cells were cultured for 18 h with supplemented RPMI in the presence or absence of 100 μg/mL pigeon cytochrome c (Sigma, St. Louis, MO), or 1 mg/mL ovalbumin (Sigma, St. Louis, MO). DC-enriched, nonadherent cells were recovered by washing the plastic dishes with warmed PBS. By flow cytometry these cells were 75-90% N418$^+$, 10-25% B220$^+$, and 2-4% CD3$^+$. Spleen DCs were prepared in an identical fashion and by flow cytometry were 60-85% N418$^+$, 10-18$^+$ B220$^+$, and 1-3% CD3$^+$. Highly enriched N418$^+$ cell populations were prepared from nonadherent cell populations by flow cytometric sorting for N418$^+$ cells; the sorted cells were 98-99% N418$^+$. Whole PP populations yielded 0.1-0.5% DCs, whereas whole spleen populations yielded 0.5-1.2% DCs.

For studies with *in vivo* antigen loading, 3 doses of 250 mg of ovalbumin in 0.5 mL of PBS and 100 μL of a 2.5% solution of 0.5-0.75 μm latex beads was given by gavage to each of 15 BALB/c mice. The first two doses were separated by 15 hours, and the last dose was given after an additional 3 hours. In addition, the animals drinking water was supplemented with 5 mg/mL ovalbumin. Mice fed only microbeads served as controls. PP DCs were isolated 3 hours after the last feeding by transient plastic adherence and were used to stimulate transgenic T cells as indicated.

Preparation of T Cells

T cells were prepared by negative selection on immunoaffinity (anti-mouse Ig) columns from lymph nodes or spleens of 8- to 16-week-old TCR-transgenic mice. Briefly, single cell suspensions were made from peripheral lymph nodes (inguinal, popliteal, and axillary) or spleens by mechanical separation, and cells were passed over a T cell-enrichment column (Isocell® Mouse T cell Column, Pierce, Rockville, IL) according to the manufacturer's instructions. Resulting cell populations were 85-90% CD3$^+$ and 5-10% B220$^+$ as measured by flow cytometry; in addition, 70-90% of CD3$^+$ cells also expressed Vα11 or the KJ1-26 clonotype. CD4$^+$, LECAM-1^{hi} T cells were isolated by two-color flow cytometry sorting using FITC-labeled anti-CD4 and biotinylated-anti-LECAM-1, followed by streptavidin-PE.

Procedure for Immunoperoxidase Staining of Frozen Sections

PPs were dissected, placed in embedding medium for frozen sections (O.C.T. Compound, Miles, Elkhart, IN), and flash frozen. Immunoperoxidase staining of acetone-fixed 10 μm sections was carried out as follows: (1) Tissue sections were rehydrated in phosphate-buffered saline (PBS) containing 0.1% bovine serum albumin (fraction V, Sigma, St. Louis, MO, PBS/BSA) and then incubated for 30 minutes in PBS with 2% normal mouse serum and 3% normal goat or rabbit serum (same species as secondary antibody) to block nonspecific binding sites; (2) blocking solution was removed, and the tissue sections were incubated for 60 minutes with primary or control antibodies, prepared in PBS with 1% normal mouse serum and 2% goat or rabbit serum (PBS-serum); (3) sections were washed in PBS/BSA an then incubated for 30 minutes with biotinylated secondary antibody, prepared in PBS serum; (4) tissue sections were washed for 30 minutes in three changes of PBS/BSA and then incubated for 30 minutes with avidin-biotin-complex (ABC) linked to HRP (Vectastain Elite ABC Kit, Vector Labs, Burlingame, CA) prepared according to the manufacturer's instructions; (5) after washing for 30 minutes in six changes of PBS/BSA, tissue sections were incubated with 0.5% (wt/vol) 3,3 diaminobenzidine (Sigma, St. Louis, MO), 0.05% NiCl, and 0.03% H_2O_2; (6) sections were rinsed in PBS and counterstained with 5% methyl green (Fisher Scientific, Fair Lawn, NJ) in methanol; (7) finally, tissue sections were rinsed in distilled water, air dried, and permanently mounted with Permount (Fisher Scientific, Fair Lawn, NJ).

Antibodies

Monoclonal hamster anti-mouse CD11c (N418),[13] rat anti-Cd11b (MAC-1, M1/70),[14] rat anti-macrophage (F4/80),[15] and hamster anti-MHC II (M5) were obtained from American Type Culture Collection (Rockville, MD). Rat anti-mouse IDC (NLDC-145)[16] was kindly provided by George Kraal (Free University, Amsterdam, The Netherlands). Hamster (M342)[11] and rat (2A1)[17] DC-reactive mAbs were kindly provided by R. M. Steinman (Rockefeller University, New York, NY). The biotinylated monoclonals anti-B220 (RA3-6B2.1),[18] anti-CD4 (RM4-4), anti-CD8 (53-6.7), hamster anti-CD3ϵ (2C11),[19] anti-B7-1 (1G10),[20] anti-B7-2 (GL1),[21] and anti-LECAM-1 (Mel-14) were purchased from Pharmingen (San Diego, CA). Normal rat serum and normal hamster serum (1 : 1000 dilution) (Sigma, St. Louis, MO) served as control antibodies, along with 2C11, a hamster monoclonal that does not react with DCs. For flow cytometry, FITC-labeled goat F(ab')^2 anti-hamster IgG and PE-labeled goat anti-rat IgG were purchased from Caltag (South San Francisco, CA), and directly labeled FITC-anti-CD3 (2C11), FITC anti-B220 (RA3-

6B2.1), biotinylated anti-Vα11 TCR, and PE-streptavidin (PE-SA) were purchased from Pharmingen (San Diego, CA). KJ1-26[22] was kindly provided by K. Nakayama in Dennis Loh's laboratory.

Flow Cytometry and FACS Sorting

DC preparations were initially treated with anti-FcRγII mAb (2.4G2) to block nonspecific FcR binding of the primary antibody, followed by biotinylated anti-B7-1 or anti-B7-2 with PE-SA, FITC-labeled B220, or N418, NLDC-145, M5, or 2C11 mAbs, in the form of cell culture supernatants, and PE-labeled F(ab')^2 goat anti-hamster or anti-rat IgG (Caltag, South San Francisco, CA). Flow cytometric analysis was performed on a FACSCAN flow cytometer (Becton-Dickenson, Waltham, MA). FACS sorting for N418$^+$ cells was performed on a FACSTAR sorter (Becton-Dickenson, Waltham, MA). Sorted DCs were routinely 97–99% N418$^+$.

Proliferation Assay

5×10^4 purified cytochrome c or ovalbumin TCR T cells were cultured with purified DCs in round-bottom 96-well tissue culture plates (Nunc, Denmark) in RPMI 1640 media, supplemented as noted above for IMDM media for 48 hours. During the last 8 h of culture, 1 μCi/well of [^{3}H]thymidine (Amersham, Arlington Hts., IL) was added; cells were frozen and subsequently harvested (PHD Harvester, Cambridge Technologies, Watertown, MA) and counted in a beta emission scintillation counter. All cultures were set up in triplicate, with values expressed as mean values +/– standard deviation of the mean.

RESULTS AND DISCUSSION

We identified PP DC and macrophages (MP) *in situ* by immunoperoxidase staining of frozen sections of PPs from B10.A mice using the ABC technique. Cells typical of interdigitating DCs that stain with the mAb NLDC-145, M342, 2A1, and N418 (anti-CD11c) were located in the IFR (Fig. 1). Mac-1 (CD11b)^{hi} MPs were concentrated in the IFR, as well as the lamina propria of the overlying villi (not shown). Interestingly, we identified a population of N418$^+$, MHC II$^+$, MAC-1^{lo}, F4/80$^-$, B220$^-$, CD3$^-$, CD4$^-$, and CD8$^-$ cells with dendritic morphology that is concentrated just beneath the FAE (Fig. 1). The lack of MAC-1^{hi}, F4/80$^+$, or endogenous peroxidase positive cells beneath the FAE suggests there are few mature MPs at this site. In addition, the lack of staining for the intracellular DC antigen identified by M342 argues that the subepithelial DCs may be in an earlier state of differentiation than the DCs in the IFR. This suggestion is based on the finding that isolated spleen DCs express the M342-reactive antigen only after *in vitro* maturation in overnight culture.[11] The identification of two populations of PP DCs has implications for studies of antigen handling in the PP, and we believe the N418$^+$ cells in the subepithelial region are a population of DCs uniquely positioned to capture luminal antigens transported into the PP by overlying M cells.

In addition, we isolated DCs from the PPs of B10.A mice by transient plastic adherence and analyzed their surface phenotype by FACS analysis. After one day in culture, when compared to spleen DCs, PP DCs had the same surface expression of B7.1, B7.2, and antigens recognized by the DC-reactive antibodies NLDC-145 and N418. By contrast, a 5- to 10-fold higher level of MHC class II molecules (IE^k) was found on PP DCs (data not shown).

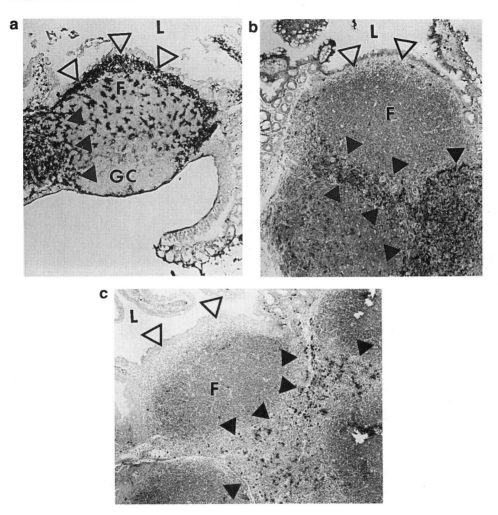

FIGURE 1. Immunoperoxidase staining of frozen sections of a mouse Peyer's patch. Positively stained cells appear dark. The subepithelial dome (SED) is indicated by the large open arrows, and the interfollicular T-cell region (IFR) is outlined by smaller filled arrows. The intestinal lumen (L), and the PP follicle (F) and germinal center (GC) are marked. **a:** DC-reactive mAb (anti-CD11c, N418). Note the intense staining of the SED and IFR, and of cells scattered throughout the follicle (F), but sparing of the germinal center (GC). **b:** Interdigitating DC-reactive mAb (NLDC-145). Note the positively stained cells in the IFR, but only occasional positive cells in the SED. **c:** DC-reactive mAb (M342). Note the positively stained cells in the IFR, but not in the SED.

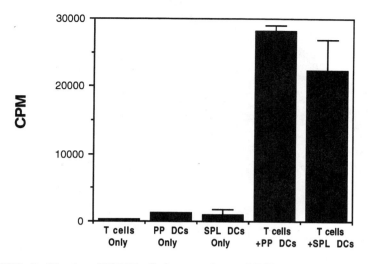

FIGURE 2. Proliferation of CD3[+] T cells from cytochrome C-TCR transgenic mice. Proliferation was measured by [^{3}H]thymidine uptake during the last 8 h of a 48-h culture. Results are presented as the mean counts per minute (CPM) of triplicate cultures ± standard error. 5 × 10^4 purified lymph node T cells were stimulated with 5 × 10^3 cytochrome C-pulsed DCs purified by FACS sorting for N418[+] cells from transiently adherent, DC-enriched populations. This graph shows results of a representative experiment. At least three separate experiments were conducted with similar results.

We went on to isolate DCs from the PP and spleen and compare their ability to stimulate T cells from TCR-transgenic mice. When T cells from CyC (shown) or OVA-TCR transgenic mice were stimulated with DCs from the PP or spleen pulsed *in vitro* with CyC or OVA, levels of proliferation (Fig. 2) and IL-2 production were equivalent. This was true for CyC and OVA-TCR transgenic T cells, and was true for T cells isolated by negative selection to yield CD3[+] enriched (85% CD3[+]) T cells, or by positive selection for CD4[+]/LECAM-1[hi] T "naive" T cells by FACS. These equivalent levels of T-cell proliferation were also found with DC populations enriched by transient plastic adherence (75-90% N418[+]), or purified by FACS sorting for N418[+] cells from the nonadherent fraction (98-99% N418[+]) (Fig. 2).

To demonstrate the importance of antigen presentation by PP DCs *in vivo,* we fed OVA to mice and demonstrated that DCs isolated from the PP after feeding were capable of stimulating proliferation in OVA-TCR T cells. Although the level of proliferation was modest (SI = 6, approximately 6000 cpm with 10^5 T cells and 10^4 DCs) when compared to proliferation induced by PP DCs from sham-fed mice, the findings were reproducible and statistically highly significant (p < 0.001) (data not shown). These data demonstrate that PP DCs process antigens transported into the PP from the gut lumen and can present these antigens to antigen-specific T cells.

CONCLUSION

In conclusion, we have found two separate populations of DCs present in the murine PP. The SED PP DCs are uniquely poised for the capture of antigens transported by overlying M cells, and the DCs in the IFR appear to be in a more mature state, suggesting movement of DCs from the SED to the IFR. We demonstrated that DCs can be isolated from the PP by transient plastic adherence and FACS sorting for N418$^+$ cells, and that when compared to spleen DCs, PP DCs express higher levels of MHC class II (IE^k), but process and present antigen to naive T cells from TCR-transgenic mice with similar efficiency. These findings have implications for how antigens are handled in the intestine and may be relevant to efforts to manipulate both positive (IgA responses) and negative (oral tolerance) immune responses to oral antigens.

REFERENCES

1. MAYRHOFER, G., C. W. PUGH & A. N. BARCLAY. 1983. The distribution, ontogeny and origin in the rat of Ia-positive cells with dendritic morphology and of Ia antigen in epithelia, with special reference to the intestine. Eur. J. Immunol. **13:** 112-122.

2. WITMER-PACK, M. D., D. A. HUGHES, G. SCHULER, L. LAWSON, A. McWILLIAM, K. INABA, R. M. STEINMAN & S. GORDON. 1993. Identification of macrophages and dendritic cells in the osteopetrotic (op/op) mouse. J. Cell Sci. **104:** 1021-1029.

3. SPENCER, J., T. FINN & P. G. ISAACSON. 1986. Human Peyer's patches: an immunohistochemical study. Gut **27:** 405-410.

4. PAVLI, P., C. E. WOODHAMS, W. F. DOE & D. A. HUME. 1990. Isolation and characterization of antigen-presenting dendritic cells from the mouse intestinal lamina propria. Immunology **70:** 40-47.

5. SPAULDING, D. M., W. J. KOOPMAN, J. R. McGHEE & R. M. STEINMAN. 1983. Accessory cells in murine Peyer's patches. I. Identification and enrichment of a functional dendritic cell. J. Exp. Med. **157:** 1646-1659.

6. SPAULDING, D. M., S. I. WILLIAMSON, W. J. KOOPMAN & J. R. McGHEE. 1984. Preferential induction of polyclonal IgA secretion by murine Peyer's patch dendritic cell-T cell mixtures. J. Exp. Med. **160:** 941-946.

7. SPAULDING, D. M. & J. A. GRIFFIN. 1986. Different pathways of differentiation of pre-B cell lines are induced by dendritic cells and T cells from different tissues. Cell **44:** 507-515.

8. GEORGE, A. & J. J. CEBRA. 1991. Responses of single germinal-center B cells in T-cell-dependent microculture. Proc. Natl. Acad. Sci. USA **88:** 11-15.

9. LIU, L. M. & G. G. PHERSON. 1993. Antigen acquisition by dendritic cells: intestinal dendritic cells acquire antigen administered orally and can prime naive T cells *in vivo*. J. Exp. Med. **177:** 1299-1307.

10. KELSALL, B. L. & W. STROBER. 1996. Distinct populations of dendritic cells are present in the subepithelial dome and T cell regions of the murine Peyer's patch. J. Exp. Med. In press.

11. AGGAR, R., N. WITMER-PACK, N. ROMANI, H. STOSSEL, W. J. SWIGGARD, J. P. METLAY, E. STOROZYNSKY, P. FREIMUTH & R. M. STEINMAN. 1992. Two populations of spleen dendritic cells detected with M342, a new monoclonal antibody to an intracellular antigen of interdigitating dendritic cells and some B lymphocytes. J. Leukocyte Biol. **52:** 34-42.

12. CROWLEY, M. K., M. INABA, M. WITMER-PACK & R. M. STEINMAN. 1989. The cell surface of mouse dendritic cells: FACS analyses of dendritic cells from different tissues including thymus. Cell. Immunol. **118:** 108-125.

13. METLAY, J. P., M. D. WITMER-PACK, R. AGGAR, M. T. CROWLEY & R. M. STEINMAN. 1990. The distinct leukocyte integrins of mouse spleen dendritic cells as identified with new hamster monoclonal antibodies. J. Exp. Med. **171:** 1753-1771.

14. SPRINGER, T. A., G. GALFRE, D. S. SECHER & C. MILSTEIN. 1979. Mac-1: A macrophage differentiation antigen identified by monoclonal antibody. Eur. J. Immunol. **9:** 301-306.

15. HUME, D. A., A. P. ROBINSON, G. G. MACPHERSON & S. GORDON. 1983. The mononuclear phagocyte system of the mouse defined by immunohistochemical localization of antigen F4/80. Relationship between macrophages, Langerhans' cells, reticulular cells, and dendritic cells in lymphoid and hematopoietic organs. J. Exp. Med. **158:** 1522-1536.

16. KRAAL, G. M., M. BREEL, M. JANSE & G. BRUIN. 1986. Langerhans' cells, veiled cells and interdigitating cells in the mouse recognized by a monoclonal antibody. J. Exp. Med. **163:** 981-997.

17. INABA, K., R. M. STEINMAN, M. WITMER-PACK, H. AYA, M. INABA, T. SUDO, S. WOLPE & G. SCHULER. 1992. Identification of proliferating dendritic cell precursors in mouse blood. J. Exp. Med. **175:** 1157-1167.

18. COFFMAN, R. L. 1982. Surface expression and immunoglobulin gene rearrangement during mouse pre-B cell development. Immunol. Rev. **69:** 5-23.

19. LEO, O., M. FOO, D. H. SACHS, L. E. SAMUELSON & J. A. BLUESTONE. 1987. Identification of a monoclonal antibody specific for a murine T3 polypeptide. Proc. Nat. Acad. Sci. USA **84:** 1374-1378.

20. NABAVI, N., G. L. FREEMAN, A. GAULT, D. GODFREY, L. M. NADLER & L. H. GLIMCHER. 1991. Signalling through the MHC class II cytoplasmic domain is required for antigen presentation and induces B7 expression. Nature **360:** 266-268.

21. HATHCOCK, K. S., G. LASZLO, H. B. DICKLER, P. BRADSHAW & R. J. HOADES. 1993. Identification of an alternative CTLA4 ligand costimulatory for T cell activation. Science **5:** 905-907.

22. HASKINS, K., R. KUBO, J. WHITE, M. PIGEON, J. KAPPLER & P. MARRACK. 1983. The major histocompatibility complex-restricted antigen receptor on T cells. I. Isolation with a monoclonal antibody. J. Exp. Med. **157:** 1149-1169.

Role of γδ T Cells in the Regulation of Mucosal IgA Response and Oral Tolerance[a]

KOHTARO FUJIHASHI, JERRY R. McGHEE, MASAFUMI YAMAMOTO, TAKACHIKA HIROI, AND HIROSHI KIYONO

The Immunobiology Vaccine Center
The Departments of Oral Biology and Microbiology
The University of Alabama at Birmingham, Medical Center
Birmingham, Alabama 35294
and
The Department of Mucosal Immunology
Research Institute for Microbial Diseases
Osaka University
Suita, Osaka 565, Japan

INTRODUCTION

Oral immunization has been shown to be a useful system to induce antigen-specific S-IgA and serum immune responses when certain adjuvants or vectors for delivery are used. However, oral immunization with large doses or multiple-spaced lower doses of free-protein antigen can also elicit distinct and opposite immune responses in mucosa-associated and systemic lymphoid tissues. For example, oral administration of large amounts of ragweed antigen or of *Streptococcus mutans* cell-wall antigen resulted in the induction of antigen-specific IgA responses in the mucosal compartment, whereas unresponsiveness to the same antigen was evident in the systemic immune system.[1,2] Further, soluble protein antigens, including ovalbumin (OVA), keyhole-limpet hemocyanin (KLH), gamma globulin, or casein, as well as heterologous erythrocytes, have all been shown to induce systemic unresponsiveness in both humoral as well as cell-mediated immune compartments when given by way of the oral route.[3-9] In this regard, our previous studies demonstrated that oral immunization of mice with sheep red blood cells (SRBC) for extended periods resulted in the induction of SRBC-specific unresponsiveness in the systemic immune compartment.[10-12] This study provided suggestive evidence that CD4+ and CD8+ T-cell subsets that reside in the mucosa-associated and systemic tissues are involved in the regulation of IgA responses and systemic unresponsiveness, respectively.[10] These immunologically unique responses, where systemic unresponsiveness to orally administered antigen was induced in the presence of mucosal IgA responses, have been termed oral tolerance.[2]

The most compelling evidence to date suggests that T lymphocytes are the major cell type involved in the induction of oral tolerance. For example, oral immunization with

[a] This work was supported by NIH Grants AI 35544, DE 09837, AI 18958, DK 44240, AI 35344, DE 08228, DE 04217, contract AI 15128, and a Grant from Asahi Chemical Co., Ltd.

SRBC resulted in the induction of CD4[+] T cells in mucosal inductive tissues (e.g., Peyer's patches (PP), which mediated antigen-specific IgA responses.[13,14] By contrast, Lyt-1[-], Lyt-2[+] (CD8[+]) T cells induced by oral antigen were responsible for the induction of systemic unresponsiveness.[10] These findings were also supported by other studies where oral immunization of rats with SRBC resulted in the induction of T cells that down-regulated antigen-specific responses initially in PP and later in the mesenteric lymph node and spleen (SP).[15] Further, feeding OVA to mice led to the generation of Th cells that supported IgA responses and suppressor T cells in SP that down-regulated antigen-specific IgM and IgG responses.[16]

Other studies in different systems have also shown that suppressor T-cell subsets are important in the induction of oral tolerance.[17–19] More recent studies have presented mechanisms for T cell-mediated suppression, and it was revealed that CD8[+] T cells, which produce TGF-β, are key cell types for the induction of oral tolerance.[20–22] Thus, oral administration of myelin basic protein (MBP) induced TGF-β-producing CD8[+] T cells, which were capable of inducing oral tolerance with resultant inhibition of experimental autoimmune encephalomyelitis.[20–22] By contrast, it was demonstrated that CD4[+] T cells anergized by high doses of oral feeding induced antigen-specific systemic unresponsiveness.[23]

In the context of T-cell subsets in oral tolerance, it is also important to consider roles for antigen-specific Th1 and Th2 cell responses for the development of oral tolerance, inasmuch as these two subsets of helper T cell can down-regulate each other through their derived specific cytokines, for example, IFN-γ, and IL-4 and IL-10, respectively.[24,25] Thus, both antigen-specific Th1 and Th2 cell responses could be inhibited by the influence of their derived respective cytokines (e.g., IFN-γ for Th2 or IL-4 and IL-10 for Th1 inhibition) in systemic lymphoid tissues, whereas polarized Th2 type responses might be maintained in the mucosal compartment for the induction of IgA responses. To this end, it was recently shown that both Th1- and Th2-type responses were susceptible to oral tolerance.[26] Further, systemic unresponsiveness was induced in IL-4 knockout (IL-4[-/-]) mice orally administered with a high dose of protein antigen, clearly suggesting that Th1-type cells were made tolerant.[26]

PROLONGED ORAL ADMINISTRATION OF PROTEIN VACCINE, DIPHTHERIA TOXOID RESULTS IN THE INDUCTION OF ORAL TOLERANCE

Our group has investigated the implications of oral tolerance for the development of mucosal vaccines. Thus, we have used diphtheria toxoid (DT) as an example of vaccine antigen for the development of systemic unresponsiveness (oral tolerance). BALB/c mice (8-12 weeks old) were immunized with 250 μg of DT by gastric intubation on either 6 or 12 occasions at 3- to 4-day intervals. Mice were then given 10 μg of antigen intravenously one week after the last oral dose of vaccine. Seven days later, serum and fecal extracts were obtained and assessed for isotype and levels of DT-specific antibodies (FIG. 1). Further, mononuclear cells were isolated from spleen and intestinal lamina propria of these orally immunized mice. These cells were then subjected to isotype and antigen-specific ELISPOT assays for the assessment of antibody-producing cells in both mucosal and systemic compartments (FIG. 1).

When DT-specific serum-antibody responses were compared between two groups of mice that received oral DT either 6 or 12 times, high levels of DT-specific serum IgM, IgG, and IgA responses were only seen in the former group following systemic challenge with DT (TABLE 1). By contrast, DT-specific systemic unresponsiveness was induced in mice given DT orally in 12 spaced doses. This result indicated that prolonged oral administration of protein-vaccine antigen induces systemic suppression, whereas a more

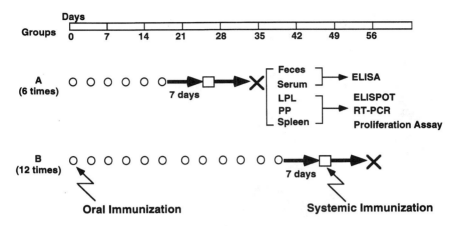

FIGURE 1. Immunization schedule for the induction of oral tolerance.

optimal regimen and dose of oral antigen application resulted in DT-specific serum antibody responses. When DT-specific serum IgG subclass responses were examined in the responsive mice, the main subclass of DT-specific IgG antibodies was IgG1, and no other subclass responses were noted in mice that received DT orally on 6 occasions (TABLE 1). Further, the levels of DT-specific IgG1 antibodies were comparable to antigen-specific total IgG responses. As one might expect, no IgG-subclass responses were seen in serum of orally tolerized mice (*e.g.*, given DT orally for 12 times). These findings showed that systemic unresponsiveness was induced following oral administration of DT for 12 times, whereas a more optimal schedule of 6 oral immunizations induced an appropriate systemic antibody response.

TABLE 1. Induction of Oral Tolerance or Mucosal and Systemic Immune Responses by Oral Vaccine

Characteristics of DT-specific Immune Responses		Oral Administration of DT for	
Site	Isotype and Subclasses	6 Times	12 Times
Systemic compartment	Serum IgG	↑↑↑	↓
	γ1	↑↑↑	—
	γ2a	—	—
	γ2b	—	—
	γ3	—	—
	Spleen IgG SFC	↑↑↑	↓
Mucosal compartment	Fecal IgA	↑↑	↑↑
	LPL IgA SFC	↑↑	↑↑

Inasmuch as antigen-specific unresponsiveness was induced in the blood circulation of mice orally immunized with DT 12 times, it was important to assess whether antigen-specific IgA responses were maintained in these mice. When fecal extracts from mice orally immunized with DT for 6 or 12 times were examined by ELISA, approximately the same levels of brisk DT-specific IgA responses were seen in both groups of mice (TABLE 1). These findings demonstrated that oral immunization with DT for 6 or 12 times induced antigen-specific IgA responses in the mucosal compartment. However, prolonged oral administration of DT resulted in the induction of systemic unresponsiveness in the presence of DT-specific mucosal IgA responses. In addition, our results further emphasize that mucosal immunization (*e.g.,* by way of the oral route) is an effective way to activate the mucosal immune system.

DT-SPECIFIC IgA B-CELL RESPONSES IN MUCOSA-ASSOCIATED TISSUES OF ORALLY TOLERIZED MICE

In order to ensure that DT-specific IgA responses were induced in mucosa-associated tissues of orally tolerized mice, DT-specific antibody-producing cells were enumerated by isotype- and antigen-specific ELISPOT assay. Single-cell suspensions were obtained from intestinal LP, PP and SP of mice orally immunized with 250 μg of DT for 12 times, as examples of mucosa-associated and systemic compartments, respectively. High numbers of DT-specific IgA spot-forming cells (SFC) were only found in LP of orally tolerized mice. By contrast, SP did not contain DT-specific SFC (TABLE 1). Because PP is an IgA-inductive tissue, elevated numbers of DT-specific antibody-producing cells were not detected in comparison to LPL. These findings provide additional supportive evidence that DT-specific unresponsiveness was only seen in the peripheral immune system of orally tolerized mice, whereas antigen-specific IgA responses were maintained in the mucosal compartment.

CHARACTERIZATION OF DT-SPECIFIC T-CELL RESPONSES IN SYSTEMIC COMPARTMENT OF ORALLY TOLERIZED MICE

In order to understand the contribution of DT-specific T-cell responses in oral tolerance, splenic lymphocytes were obtained from mice orally immunized with DT for 6 or 12 times prior to systemic challenge. These splenic cells were then incubated with DT for 3 to 7 days. When splenic lymphocytes from mice orally tolerized with DT were examined, DT did not induce any antigen-specific proliferative responses (TABLE 2). On the other hand, splenic lymphocytes isolated from mice orally immunized with DT for 6 times that harbor both mucosal and systemic antigen-specific immune responses induced high proliferative responses following 3–7 days of *in vitro* stimulation with antigen (TABLE 2). The highest proliferative response was noted in 7-day cultures. Similar findings were also obtained by purified T-cell cultures containing antigen-presenting cells and DT. These results suggest that T-cell unresponsiveness (anergy) was induced in the systemic compartment of orally tolerized mice.

We next compared DT-induced proliferative responses in lymphocytes isolated from mucosal-associated tissues of tolerized mice. When PP cells were incubated with DT for 7 days, no proliferative responses were seen in this culture. In contrast to PP, an example of a mucosal inductive site, lymphocytes from mucosal effector sites such as intraepithelial lymphocytes (IELs) from the same mice responded well to antigen stimulation (TABLE 2). These results suggested that lymphocytes that reside in mucosal effector tissues, for

TABLE 2. Characterization of DT-induced T-Cell Responses in Systemic and Mucosal Compartments of Orally Tolerized Mice

Source of Lymphocytes	Culture Stimulant	Oral Administration of DT for ([³H]thymidine incorporation)	
		6 Times	12 Times
Spleen	DT	50,000–55,000	2,000–3,000
	None	900–1,000	5,000–6,000
IELs	DT	12,000–13,000	10,000–12,000
	None	1,100–1,200	3,000–4,000

example, the intestinal IEL, may play an important role for the induction and maintenance of antigen-specific IgA responses in mucosal compartments in the presence of systemic unresponsiveness. To this end, our previous study has suggested that γδ T cells in IELs may play an important role for the maintenance of mucosal IgA responses in oral toler- ance.[27,28] We are currently testing Th1 and Th2 cytokine profiles of DT-stimulated mucosal and systemic T cells isolated from orally tolerized mice by using quantitative RT-PCR methods in order to elucidate the role of Th1- and Th2-type responses for the induction of systemic unresponsiveness and maintenance of mucosal IgA responses in a state of oral tolerance.

THE ROLE OF γδ T CELLS FOR MUCOSAL IgA RESPONSES

It is now established that the mucosal immune system is a separate entity from the systemic immune system and is regulated by different subsets of lymphoid cells. Mucosal sites such as the intestinal epithelium contain large numbers of γδ T cells in addition to αβ T cells that are referred to as IELs.[29,30] Further, the lamina propria of small intestine also contain a relatively higher frequency of γδ T cells when compared with systemic lymphoid tissues.[31] The mucosal γδ T cells have been shown to possess several unique features, which were extensively summarized in a recent review.[32] For example, the majority of γδ T cells that reside in the intestinal epithelium express CD8 molecules with αα homodimer chains.[33,34] Further, these γδ T cells may develop without thymus influence,[35–37] and usage of their Vγ gene is totally distinct from peripheral γδ T cells.[38,39] However, only limited information is currently available for their immunobiological func- tions.

Mutant mice lacking γδ T cells have been produced by introducing germ-line mutations in the TCR δ-chain gene.[40] This TCR-δ chain-deleted mouse could be a useful model to elucidate the exact role of γδ T cells for the induction and regulation of mucosal IgA immune response. Thus, we have taken advantage of these unique TCR-δ⁻/⁻ mice in order to determine the role of γδ T cells in mucosal immunity.

It was important to define the mucosal immune system in TCR-δ⁻/⁻ mice because the vast majority of γδ T cells are present in the epithelium of the small intestine.[29,30] The absence of this T-cell subset in this mucosal effector site may influence immunological homeostasis in the host; however, little attention has been given to mucosal γδ T cells for their contribution to IgA responses. Thus, we initially examined possible effects of TCR-δ gene disruption by characterizing total numbers of IgM-, IgG-, and IgA-producing cells in systemic and mucosa-associated tissues, and levels of IgM, IgG, and IgA titers in serum and fecal extracts obtained from TCR-δ$^{-/-}$ mice. When the frequency of Ig-producing cells were compared between SP of TCR-δ$^{-/-}$ mice and their background strains [(129 × B6)F$_2$], essentially identical numbers of IgM- and IgG-producing cells were seen. However, the numbers of IgA-secreting cells in mucosa-associated tissues, such as intestinal LP and PP of TCR-δ$^{-/-}$ mice, were significantly lower than in control background mice.

These observations were further confirmed by the assessment of serum and fecal extracts using isotype-specific ELISA. The level of IgA was reduced by approximately 40% in fecal extracts obtained from TCR-δ$^{-/-}$ mice when compared with normal background mice. In addition, serum IgA titers in TCR-δ$^{-/-}$ mice were also reduced. These results suggested that the depletion of γδ T cells resulted in the reduction of IgA synthesis but did not affect IgM and IgG isotypes. It has been shown that αβ T cells with CD4 phenotype are an essential T-cell subset for the induction and regulation of IgA responses. To this end, a significant reduction in IgA synthesis was noted in anti-L3T4-treated and athymic mice.[41,42] The CD4$^+$ T cell-depleted mice harbored PP, which were smaller with fewer germinal centers as well as low numbers of IgA-producing cells in the LPL.[41] Furthermore, our most recent and separate study showed that TCR-β$^{-/-}$mice contain almost no mucosal IgA-producing cells (Fujihashi *et al.*, manuscript in preparation). In addition to these previous observations, our present finding directly demonstrated that γδ T cells are also important regulatory T cells for IgA responses using TCR-δ knockout mice, despite the fact that TCR-δ$^{-/-}$ mice possess normal numbers of functional αβ T cells. We are currently using both TCR-δ$^{-/-}$ and TCR-β$^{-/-}$ mice in order to directly examine the contribution of γδ and αβ T cells for the induction and regulation of oral tolerance. Our preliminary results indicated that prolonged oral administration of protein antigen can lead to the induction of antigen-specific unresponsiveness in both systemic and mucosal compartments. These findings suggested that mucosal γδ T cells are essential regulatory T cells for the maintenance of IgA responses in the presence of systemic unresponsiveness.

SUMMARY

In this short review, we first described experiments that show that prolonged oral immunization with a protein vaccine, such as DT, induces systemic unresponsiveness in the presence of antigen-specific mucosal IgA responses. Mucosal T cells, such as IEL, may play an important role for the maintenance of antigen-specific IgA responses because these T cells are able to respond to stimulation signals provided by antigen even when T-cell unresponsiveness was induced in systemic tissue, such as spleen of mice orally tolerized with the protein DT. Inasmuch as IEL contain a high frequency of γδ T cells, it was logical to postulate that mucosal γδ T cells are essential regulatory T cells for the induction of IgA responses in oral tolerance. To this end, our previous studies showed that adoptive transfer of mucosal γδ T cells from IEL of mice orally tolerized with SRBC to the recipient mice with systemic unresponsiveness to the same antigen resulted in the abrogation of unresponsiveness to Ig synthesis, including those of IgA isotype.[27,28] In this regard, when the mucosal immune system of TCR-δ$^{-/-}$ and their control mice was examined, lower numbers of IgA antibody-producing cells were noted in TCR-δ$^{-/-}$ mice in comparison to control background mice. Further, the level of IgA in fecal extracts was also low in TCR-δ$^{-/-}$ mice. These findings suggested that loss of γδ T cells results in down-regulation of IgA B-cell responses.

REFERENCES

1. CHALLACOMBE, S. J. & T. B. TOMASI JR. 1980. Systemic tolerance and secretory immunity after oral immunization. J. Exp. Med. **152:** 1459–1472.
2. TOMASI, T. B., JR. 1980. Oral tolerance. Transplantation **29:** 353–356.
3. KAGNOFF, M. F. 1978. Effects of antigen-feeding on intestinal and systemic immune responses. III. Antigen-specific serum-mediated suppression of humoral antibody responses after antigen feeding. Cell. Immunol. **40:** 186–203.
4. VIVES, J., D. E. PARKS & W. O. WEIGLE. 1980. Immunologic unresponsiveness after gastric administration of human γ-globulin: antigen requirements and cellular parameters. J. Immunol. **125:** 1811–1816.
5. ELSON, C. O. & W. EALDING. 1984. Cholera toxin feeding did not induce oral tolerance in mice and abrogated oral tolerance to unrelated protein antigen. J. Immunol. **133:** 2892–2897.
6. CARR, R., S. FORSYTH & D. SADI. 1987. Abnormal responses to ingested substances in murine systemic lupus erythematosus: apparent effect of a casein-free diet on the development of systemic lupus erythematosus in NZB/W mice. J. Rheumatol. **14:** 158–165.
7. LAMONT, A. G., M. G. BRUCE, K. C. WATRET & A. FERGUSON. 1988. Suppression of an established DTH response to ovalbumin in mice by feeding antigen after immunization. Immunology **64:** 135–139.
8. PENG, H.-J., M. W. TURNER & S. STROBEL. 1990. The generation of a "tolerogen" after the ingestion of ovalbumin is time-dependent and unrelated to serum levels of immunoreactive antigen. Clin. Exp. Immunol. **81:** 510–515.
9. GESUALDO, L., M. E. LAMM & S. N. EMANCIPATOR. 1990. Defective oral tolerance promotes nephritogenesis in experimental IgA nephropathy induced by oral immunization. J. Immunol. **145:** 3684–3691.
10. KIYONO, H., J. R. McGHEE, M. J. WANNEMUEHLER & S. M. MICHALEK. 1982. Lack of oral tolerance in C3H/HeJ mice. J. Exp. Med. **155:** 605–610.
11. MICHALEK, S. M., H. KIYONO, M. J. WANNEMUEHLER, L. M. MOSTELLER & J. R. McGHEE. 1982. Lipopolysaccharide (LPS) regulation of the immune response: LPS influence on oral tolerance induction. J. Immunol. **128:** 1992–1998.
12. WANNEMUEHLER, M. J., H. KIYONO, J. L. BABB, S. M. MICHALEK & J. R. McGHEE. 1982. Lipopolysaccharide (LPS) regulation of the immune response: LPS converts germfree mice to sensitivity to oral tolerance induction. J. Immunol. **129:** 959–965.
13. KAGNOFF, M. F. 1980. Effects of antigen-feeding on intestinal and systemic immune responses. IV. Similarity between the suppressor factor in mice after erythrocyte-lysate injection and erythrocyte feeding. Gastroenterology **79:** 54–61.
14. KIYONO, H., J. L. BABB, S. M. MICHALEK & J. R. McGHEE. 1980. Cellular basis for elevated IgA response in C3H/HeJ mice. J. Immunol. **125:** 732–737.
15. MATTINGLY, J. A. & B. H. WAKSMAN. 1978. Immunologic suppression after oral administration of antigen. I. Specific suppressor cells formed in rat Peyer's patches after oral administration of sheep erythrocytes and their systemic migration. J. Immunol. **121:** 1878–1883.
16. RICHMAN, L. K., A. S. GRAEFF, R. YARCHOAN & W. STROBER. 1981. Simultaneous induction of antigen-specific IgA helper T cells and IgG suppressor T cells in the murine Peyer's patch after protein feeding. J. Immunol. **126:** 2079–2083.
17. NGAN, J. & L. S. KIND. 1978. Suppressor T cells for IgE and IgG in Peyer's patches of mice made tolerant by the oral administration of ovalbumin. J. Immunol. **120:** 861–865.
18. MOWAT, A. McI., A. G. LAMONT & D. M. W. PARROTT. 1988. Suppressor T cells, antigen presenting cells and the role of I-J restriction in oral tolerance to ovalbumin. Immunology **64:** 141–145.
19. KOSTER, F. T. & N. F. PIERCE. 1983. Parental immunization causes antigen specific cell mediated suppression of an intestinal IgA response. J. Immunol. **131:** 115–119.

20. LIDER, O., L. M. B. SANTOS, C. S. Y. LEE, P. J. HIGGINS & H. L. WEINER. 1989. Suppression of experimental autoimmune encephalomyelitis by oral administration of myelin basic protein. II. Suppression of disease and *in vitro* immune responses is mediated by antigen specific CD8⁺ T lymphocytes. J. Immunol. **142:** 748-752.

21. MILLER, A., O. LIDER & H. L. WEINER. 1991. Antigen-driven bystander suppression after oral administration of antigens. J. Exp. Med. **174:** 791-798.

22. MILLER, A., O. LIDER, A. B. ROBERTS, M. B. SPORN & H. L. WEINER. 1992. Suppressor T cells generated by oral tolerization to myelin basic protein suppress both *in vitro* and *in vivo* immune responses by the release of transforming growth factor-β after antigen-specific triggering. Proc. Natl. Acad. Sci. USA **89:** 421-425.

23. HIRAHARA, K., T. HISATSUNE, K. NISHIJIMA, H. KATO, O. SHIHO & S. KAMINOGAWA. 1995. CD4⁺ T cells anergized by high dose feeding establish oral tolerance to antibody responses when transferred in SCID and nude mice. J. Immunol. **154:** 6238-6245.

24. STREET, N. E. & T. R. MOSMANN. 1991. Functional diversity of T lymphocytes due to secretion of different cytokine patterns. FASEB J. **5:** 171-177.

25. MOORE, K. W., A. O'GARRA, R. W. MALEFYT, P. VIEIRA & T. R. MOSMANN. 1993. Interleukin-10. Annu. Rev. Immunol. **11:** 165-190.

26. GARSIDE, P., M. STEEL, E. A. WORTHEY, A. SATOSKAR, J. ALEXANDER, H. BLUETHMANN, F. Y. LIEW & A. MCL. MOWAT. 1995. T helper 2 cells are subject to high dose oral tolerance and are not essential for its induction. J. Immunol. **154:** 5649-5655.

27. FUJIHASHI, K., T. TAGUCHI, J. R. MCGHEE, J. H. ELDRIDGE, M. G. BRUCE, D. R. GREEN, B. SINGH & H. KIYONO. 1990. Regulatory function for murine intraepithelial lymphocytes: two subsets of CD3⁺, T cell receptor-1⁺ intraepithelial lymphocyte T cells abrogate oral tolerance. J. Immunol. **145:** 2010-2019.

28. FUJIHASHI, K., T. TAGUCHI, W. A. AICHER, J. R. MCGHEE, J. A. BLUESTONE, J. H. ELDRIDGE & H. KIYONO. 1992. Immunoregulatory functions for murine intraepithelial lymphocytes: γ/δ T cell receptor-positive (TCR⁺) T cells abrogate oral tolerance, while α/β TCR⁺ T cells provide B cell help. J. Exp. Med. **175:** 695-707.

29. GOODMAN, T. & L. LEFRANÇOIS. 1988. Expression of the γδ T cell receptor on intestinal CD8⁺ intraepithelial lymphocytes. Nature (Lond.) **333:** 855-858.

30. BONNEVILLE, M., C. A. JANEWAY, JR., K. ITO, W. HASER, I. ISHIDA, N. NAKANISHI & S. TONEGAWA. 1988. Intestinal intraepithelial lymphocytes are a distinct set of γδ T cells. Nature (Lond.) **336:** 479-481.

31. AICHER, W. K., K. FUJIHASHI, M. YAMAMOTO, H. KIYONO, A. M. PITTS & J. R. MCGHEE. 1992. Effects of the lpr/lpr mutation on T and B cell populations in the lamina propria of the small intestine, a mucosal effector site. Intern. Immunol. **4:** 959-968.

32. KIYONO, H. & J. R. MCGHEE, EDS. 1995. Mucosal immunology: Intraepithelial lympho-cytes. Adv. Host. Def. Melch. **9:** 1-194.

33. GUY-GRAND, D., N. CERF-BENSUSSAN, B. MALISSEN, M. MALASSIS-SERIS, C. BRIOTTET & P. VASSALLI. 1991. Two gut intraepithelial CD8⁺ lymphocyte populations with different T cell receptors: a role for the gut epithelium in T cell differentiation. J. Exp. Med. **173:** 471-481.

34. LEFRANÇOIS, L. 1991. Phenotypic complexity of intraepithelial lymphocytes of the small intestine. J. Immunol. **147:** 1746-1751.

35. LEFRANÇOIS, L., R. LECORRE, J. MAYO, J. A. BLUESTONE & T. GOODMAN. 1990. Extrathy-mic selection of TCR γδ⁺ T cells by class II major histocompatibility complex molecules. Cell **63:** 333-340.

36. MOSLEY, R. L., D. STYRE & J. R. KLEIN. 1990. Differentiation and functional maturation of bone marrow-derived intestinal epithelial T cells expressing membrane T cell receptor in athymic radiation chimeras. J. Immunol. **145:** 1369-1375.

37. BANDERIA, A., S. ITOHARA, M. BONNEVILLE, O. BURLEN-DEFRANOUX, T. MOTA-SANTOS, A. COUTINHO & S. TONEGAWA. 1991. Extrathymic origin of intestinal intraepithelial lymphocytes bearing T-cell antigen receptor γδ. Proc. Natl. Acad. Sci. USA **88:** 4347.

38. TAKAGAKI, Y., A. DeCLOUX, M. BONNEVILLE & S. TONEGAWA. 1989. Diversity of γδ T-cell receptors on murine intestinal intraepithelial lymphocytes. Nature (Lond.) **339:** 712–714.
39. ITOHARA, S., A. G. FARR, J. J. LAFAILLE, M. BONNEVILLE, Y. TAKAGAKI, W. HAAS & S. TONEGAWA. 1990. Homing of a γδ thymocyte subset with homogeneous T-cell receptors to mucosal epithelia. Nature (Lond.) **343:** 754–757.
40. ITOHARA, S., P. MOMBAERTS, J. LAFAILLE, J. IACOMINI, A. NELSON, A. FARR & S. TONEGAWA. 1993. T cell receptor δ gene mutant mice: independent generation of αβ T cells and programmed rearrangements of γδ TCR gene. Cell **72:** 337–348.
41. MEGA, J., M. G. BRUCE, K. W. BEAGLEY, J. R. McGHEE, T. TAGUCHI, A. M. PITTS, M. L. McGHEE, R. P. BUCY, J. H. ELDRIDGE, J. MESTECKY & H. KIYONO. 1991. Regulation of mucosal responses by CD4+ T lymphocytes: effects of anti-L3T4 treatment on the gastrointestinal immune system. Intern. Immunol. **3:** 793–805.
42. GUY-GRAND, D., C. GRISCELLI & P. VASSLLI. 1975. Peyer's patches, gut IgA plasma cells and thymic function: study in nude mice bearing thymic grafts. J. Immunol. **115:** 361–364.

The Role of Th1 and Th2 Cells for Mucosal IgA Responses[a]

MASAFUMI YAMAMOTO, JOHN L. VANCOTT,
NOBUO OKAHASHI,[b] MARIAROSARIA MARINARO,[b]
HIROSHI KIYONO, KOHTARO FUJIHASHI,
RAYMOND J. JACKSON, STEVEN N. CHATFIELD,[c]
HORST BLUETHMANN,[d] AND JERRY R. McGHEE

The Immunobiology Vaccine Center
The Departments of Microbiology and Oral Biology
University of Alabama at Birmingham
Medical Center
Birmingham, Alabama 35294

[b]*The Department of Mucosal Immunology*
Research Institute for Microbial Diseases
Osaka University
Suita, Osaka 565, Japan

[c]*Vaccine Research Unit*
Imperial College of Science
London, United Kingdom

[d]*Hoffmann-La Roche AG*
CH-4002, Basel, Switzerland

INTRODUCTION

The mucosal surface area where most pathogens enter the host are protected by antibodies of the secretory IgA (S-IgA) isotype. This isotype constitutes greater than 80% of all antibodies produced in mucosal-associated tissues of humans,[1,2] and S-IgA is induced, transported, and regulated by mechanisms that are completely different from those involved in systemic antibody responses.[1-3] Although the induction of S-IgA responses is known to be dependent on cognate help provided by CD4+ T-helper (Th) cells in mucosa-associated tissues, the regulatory cells and molecules important in the subsequent development of these S-IgA antibody responses are only partially understood.

Studies of cytokine production by murine Th-cell clones have provided direct evidence that effector CD4+ Th cells can be divided into two distinct classes, Th1 and Th2 cells, on the basis of the patterns of cytokines secreted.[4] For example, Th1 cells secrete IL-2, IFN-γ, and TNF-β, whereas Th2 cells secrete IL-4, IL-5, IL-6, and IL-10. The roles and potential interactions of these Th-cell subsets for the induction of specific immune responses are regulated in large part by the cytokines produced by Th1- and Th2-type cells. Further, the outcome of these distinct cytokine patterns are influenced by the unique

[a]This work was supported by NIH Contract AI 15128 and Grants AI 18958, DK 44240, DE 04217, AI 35544, DE 09837, AI 35344, and DE 08228.

microenvironment present in mucosa-associated tissues. Studies from our group[5-7] and by others[8-12] have shown that two Th2 cell-derived cytokines, for example, IL-5 and IL-6, are of particular importance for inducing surface IgA-positive (sIgA⁺) B cells to differentiate into IgA-plasma cells. In this regard, IL-6 induced high-rate IgA synthesis in cultures containing mucosal B cells from mice[5,6] and humans.[7] More recently, it was shown that mice with targeted disruption of the IL-6 gene resulted in a deficiency of IgA-plasma cells in mucosa-associated tissues.[13]

The development of effective mucosal vaccines will require the precise characterization of molecular mechanisms involved in the induction of antigen-specific immune responses in mucosal and systemic tissues. In this article, we will summarize our recent studies of the role of Th1 and Th2 cytokines for the induction and regulation of mucosal and systemic immune responses to well-defined oral vaccines. In particular, we will focus on two distinct mucosal vaccines, *Salmonella typhimurium*, expressing fragment C of tetanus toxin (Tox C), and soluble tetanus toxoid (TT) together with the mucosal adjuvant cholera toxin (CT) for the induction of antigen-specific immune responses in IL-4 (Th2) and IFN-γ (Th1) gene-disrupted (knockout) mice.

CT AS A MUCOSAL ADJUVANT

For the induction of Th1- and Th2-cell responses for provision of help for antigen-specific IgA responses, our recent studies have provided important evidence that the protein vaccine TT given orally with CT as adjuvant induced antigen-specific Th2-type immune responses. When fecal and serum samples from these orally immunized mice were analyzed for antigen-specific immune responses, the levels of TT-specific S-IgA and IgG antibodies were increased, respectively.[14,15] In these studies, both Peyer's patches (PP) and splenic (SP) CD4⁺ T cells were obtained during peak mucosal S-IgA and serum anti-TT and anti-CT-B responses,[14] and were restimulated *in vitro* with TT or CT-B conjugated to latex beads.[15,16] In all cases, high numbers of IL-4- and IL-5-producing cells were seen, whereas IFN-γ- and IL-2-secreting cells remained at levels seen in naive mice.[15] We thus concluded that CD4⁺ Th2-type cells, secreting IL-4 and IL-5, provide optimal help for mucosal S-IgA and serum IgG and IgA antibody responses.

More recently, it has been shown that mice orally immunized with TT and CT show marked increases in TT-specific mucosal IgA, and serum IgG and IgE responses, where IgG subclass-specific antibodies were mainly IgG1 followed by IgG2b. Further, CT as an adjuvant elicited identical antibody profiles to other protein antigens (*e.g.*, OVA and lysozyme) given by the oral route.[17] Analysis of cytokine-specific mRNA indicated that Th2-type cytokines (*e.g.*, IL-4, IL-5, and IL-6) were induced, and significant increases in IL-4 mRNA were revealed.[17] Taken together, these results suggest that CT acts as adjuvant through selective induction of Th2-type cytokines.

RECOMBINANT *SALMONELLA* VACCINE

Live attenuated *Salmonella* have been developed as mucosal vaccine delivery vectors for recombinant proteins associated with microbial virulence.[18-20] It has been shown that *Salmonella* vaccines elicit protective humoral and cellular immune responses in the host after either parenteral or oral immunization.[20,21] *Salmonella typhimurium*, like other intracellular microorganisms, that is, *Leishmania major, Listeria monocytogenes*, or *Mycobacterium tuberculosis*, have been shown to induce a Th1-dependent immune response.[22-26] Further, IFN-γ, a predominant Th1-type cytokine, is essential for clearing *S. typhimurium* infection *in vivo*, in part through the activation of macrophages for intracellular killing.[26-29]

In this study, we have used recombinant (r) *Salmonella typhimurium* BRD 847 (*aro A⁻, aro D⁻*), expressing the Tox C gene of TT under regulation of a *nir* B promoter. This delivery system has been shown to induce long-lasting immune responses and protection against systemic lethal tetanus toxin challenge in mice following a single oral dose of 10^{10} colony-forming units (CFU).[20,21] Our studies showed that oral administration of r*Salmonella*-Tox C to mice elicited mucosal S-IgA and serum IgG responses, largely of the IgG2a subclass. Further, supernatants from both SP and PP CD4⁺ T-cell cultures showed increases in Th1-type cytokines (*e.g.*, IFN-γ and IL-2) as well as a Th2 cytokine, IL-10, but not IL-4 or IL-5. To confirm these results, we assessed IFN-γ- and IL-2-specific T-cell responses by the ELISPOT assay. Significant numbers of IFN-γ and IL-2 spot-forming cells (SFCs) were noted in CD4⁺ T-cell cultures stimulated with TT. Analysis of cytokine-specific mRNA by RT-PCR using capillary electrophoresis also revealed predominant messages for Th1 (IL-2 and IFN-γ) and selective Th2 (IL-10) cytokines.[30] These results showed that TT-specific IgA responses were elevated in the gastrointestinal (GI) tract following induction of mainly Th1 cells producing IFN-γ, and Th2 cells producing IL-10, but not traditional Th2 cells producing IL-4 and IL-5 in GI tract inductive sites (*i.e.*, Peyer's patches).

Induction of TT-specific IgA responses in a Th1-dominant environment could be explained by the existence of alternate or compensatory Th1 and Th2 cell pathways. In the absence of traditional Th2-type cells producing IL-4 and IL-5, IL-10-secreting CD4⁺ Th cells along with Th1 cells may support both mucosal and systemic IgA responses. The inefficiency of Th1 cells for supporting mucosal IgA responses *in vivo* may be overcome by the production of Th2-type cytokines (*i.e.*, IL-6) by other cell types. In this regard, we found that Mac-1⁺ cells, which are enriched in macrophages, produced high levels of IL-6 in mice orally immunized with r*Salmonella*. IL-6 has been shown to be the most effective terminal differentiation factor for IgA-committed B cells to become IgA-producing cells in both human and mouse systems.[5,9,31,32] Further, it has been shown in humans that IL-10 plays an essential role in IgA B-cell differentiation.[33] These results suggested that Th2-derived IL-10, macrophage-derived IL-6 and antigen-specific Th1 cells may provide important signals for regulating mucosal IgA responses in the absence of traditional Th2 cells producing IL-4 and IL-5 in mice orally immunized with r*Salmonella* Tox C.

IMMUNE RESPONSES IN IL-4⁻/⁻ MICE GIVEN *SALMONELLA*-Tox C

IL-4 is a growth and differentiation factor for B cells, and in addition this cytokine induces differentiation of T cells toward a Th2 phenotype.[34-36] Others have shown that CD4⁺ T cells isolated from naive IL-4 gene-disrupted (IL-4⁻/⁻) mice fail to produce Th2-derived cytokines and subsequent immune responses dependent on these cytokines after *in vitro* stimulation.[37] In order to understand the precise role of IL-4 in induction of antigen-specific mucosal and systemic immune responses, we immunized IL-4⁻/⁻ mice with live, attenuated *S. typhimurium* BRD 847, expressing Tox C. In order to provide a comparison of immune responses, we included a second vaccine regimen, TT coadministered with CT as adjuvant.

The live, attenuated *S. typhimurium* expressing Tox C of TT induced TT-specific mucosal IgA and serum IgG responses in IL-4⁻/⁻ mice. These responses were comparable to those in normal (IL-4⁺/⁺) mice. On the other hand, IL-4⁻/⁻ mice orally immunized with TT and mucosal adjuvant CT showed significantly lower levels of mucosal IgA anti-TT responses when compared with IL-4⁺/⁺ mice. Inasmuch as IL-4 is thought to be a key cytokine for the induction of Th2-type responses that promote not only mucosal IgA but

TABLE 1. TT-Specific Th1 and Th2 Cytokine Profiles of CD4$^+$ T Cells from IL-4$^{-/-}$ and IFN-$\gamma^{-/-}$ Mice

		Th1-type		Th2-type			Mucosal
		IFN-γ	IL-2	IL-4	IL-5	IL-10	IgA
IL-4$^{-/-}$	r*Salmonella*	+	+	−	−	+	+
	TT + CT	+	+	−	−	−	−
IFN-$\gamma^{-/-}$	r*Salmonella*	−	−	+	+	+	+
	TT + CT	−	+	+	+	+	+
Normal	r*Salmonella*	+	+	−	−	+	+
	TT + CT	−	+	+	+	+	+

also serum IgG1 and IgE responses, we investigated TT-specific IgG subclasses and IgE responses in IL-4$^{-/-}$ mice immunized with r*Salmonella* Tox C or with TT and CT as adjuvant. When TT-specific IgG subclasses were assessed in IL-4$^{-/-}$ mice, both groups showed IgG2a and IgG2b antibody responses. However, there were no detectable levels of IgG1 antibodies. Further, neither total nor TT-specific IgE responses were induced in IL-4$^{-/-}$ mice immunized with either vaccine preparation, confirming the notion that IL-4 plays a necessary role for the induction of antigen-specific IgG1 and IgE responses.[37] By contrast, sera from IL-4$^{+/+}$ mice immunized with TT and CT showed increases in both total and TT-specific IgE responses. These results revealed the capacity of oral *Salmonella* vaccines to potentiate mucosal IgA responses to expressed proteins even in the absence of IL-4.

It is well known that cytokines play an important role for the regulation of antibody isotypes induced during immune responses.[4] In order to determine which cytokines contribute to the induction of vaccine antigen-specific mucosal IgA responses, PP and SP CD4$^+$ T cells from IL-4$^{-/-}$ mice orally immunized with r*Salmonella*-Tox C or with TT plus CT were restimulated with TT-coated latex beads in the presence of feeder cells *in vitro*. After an appropriate incubation period, supernatants were assessed by cytokine-specific ELISA. TABLE 1 summarizes the cytokine profile of IL-4$^{-/-}$ mice orally immunized with *Salmonella* expressing Tox C. As expected, IL-4 was not detected in culture supernatants, and in addition no IL-5 was produced. However, significant levels of the Th2-type cytokine IL-10 was induced. On the other hand, IL-4$^{-/-}$ mice orally immunized with TT plus CT showed no increase in Th2-type cytokines (IL-5 or IL-10). Further, IL-4$^{-/-}$ mice immunized with TT plus CT did not undergo TT-specific mucosal IgA responses.[38] These results indicate that IL-4 is necessary for the development of vaccine antigen-specific mucosal IgA responses when TT is coadministered with the mucosal adjuvant CT. In this regard it has been shown that IL-4$^{-/-}$ mice also fail to respond to soluble protein antigens, keyhole-limpet hemocyanin, and ovalbumin, given orally with CT as a mucosal adjuvant.[39] However, IL-4 was not an essential cytokine for the induction of antigen-specific mucosal IgA antibody when the vaccine was delivered to mucosa-associated tissues by recombinant live vector (*e.g., Salmonella*). Taken together, our study demonstrates that oral immunization with *Salmonella* expressing a foreign antigen induces antigen-specific mucosal IgA responses without IL-4 production.

IMMUNE RESPONSES IN IFN-$\gamma^{-/-}$ MICE ORALLY IMMUNIZED WITH *SALMONELLA*-TOX C OR WITH TT AND CT

Oral immunization with *S. typhimurium* BRD 847 expressing Tox C resulted in significant cell-mediated immune responses (CMI or DTH) and dominant Th1-type responses (*e.g.*, IFN-γ and IL-2 production) in both systemic and mucosal compartments. It has been shown that IFN-γ is rapidly produced by T lymphocytes in gut-associated lymphoreticular tissues (GALT) and SP following oral *S. typhimurium* infection and that IFN-γ is essential in host resistance to *S. typhimurium.*[28] In addition, CD4$^+$ T cells from both tissues synthesize IFN-γ, IL-2, and IL-10 as Th1 and Th2 cytokines, respectively, which resulted in high titers of mucosal IgA and serum IgG2a and IgG2b responses. Thus, we next immunized IFN-$\gamma^{-/-}$ mice with live, attenuated *S. typhimurium* BRD 847, expressing Tox C or soluble TT with CT as adjuvant to examine the importance of IFN-γ in the development of vaccine antigen-specific mucosal IgA responses.

Immunized IFN-$\gamma^{-/-}$ mice showed increased serum titers of TT-specific IgM, IgG, and IgA antibodies when compared with IFN-$\gamma^{+/+}$ mice. Interestingly, the IgG-subclass profile revealed a shift from IgG2a in IFN-$\gamma^{+/+}$ mice to IgG1 in IFN-$\gamma^{-/-}$ mice. Titers of IgG2a and IgG3 antibodies were also noted in IFN-γ gene-disrupted mice. A shift from IgG2a to IgG1 in TT-specific immune responses could be explained by a dominant IL-4 response in immunized IFN-$\gamma^{-/-}$ mice. Thus, it was important to investigate whether the absence of IFN-γ resulted in an increase of IL-4 synthesis by antigen-specific CD4$^+$ T cells, which lead to TT-specific IgG1 and IgE antibodies. The results showed that despite the increase in IgG1 antibodies in sera from IFN-$\gamma^{-/-}$ mice orally immunized with *Salmonella*, TT-specific IgE responses were not detected. However, sera of IFN-$\gamma^{-/-}$ mice immunized with TT plus CT showed increased titers of TT-specific IgE responses. In the case of mucosal IgA responses, similar titers of IgA antibodies were found in both IFN-$\gamma^{-/-}$ and normal (IFN-$\gamma^{+/+}$) mice. These results indicated that vaccine antigen delivered by recombinant *Salmonella* induced mainly antigen-specific mucosal IgA and serum IgG1 responses without IgE even in a Th2 cell-dominant environment (*e.g.*, IFN-$\gamma^{-/-}$ mice). Because r*Salmonella* did not induce antigen-specific IgE antibodies in normal mice in the presence of mucosal IgA and serum IgG responses, this live antigen-delivery system can be considered as an optimal vehicle for mucosal vaccination.

When cytokine profiles from CD4$^+$ T cells from GALT and SP of IFN-$\gamma^{-/-}$ mice orally immunized with r*Salmonella* expressing Tox C were evaluated by Th1 and Th2 cytokine-specific ELISPOT and ELISA, no IFN-γ or IL-2 production were noted following *in vitro* restimulation of CD4$^+$ T cells with TT antigen in the presence of accessory cells. However, there were notable increases in Th2 cytokines, IL-4, IL-5, and IL-10. These results showed that the loss of IFN-γ resulted in a shift from induction of memory Th1-type cells to traditional Th2-type cells following oral immunization with r*Salmonella* Tox C. Further, IFN-$\gamma^{-/-}$ mice orally immunized with TT plus CT also developed a classical Th2-type response that was similar to that induced in normal mice. In both antigen delivery systems, there were increases in Th2-type IL-4, IL-5, and IL-10 in IFN-$\gamma^{-/-}$ mice (TABLE 1). These results suggested that the lack of Th1-type IFN-γ-producing cells did not affect the development of mucosal IgA responses observed with these two vaccine regimens.

SUMMARY

We have used cytokine-knockout mice to help determine the precise requirements for CD4$^+$ Th cell regulation of IgA responses. In these studies, we have used two different oral delivery systems to induce mucosal and systemic antibody responses to the vaccine

TT. In normal mice, oral administration of TT with CT as adjuvant induces Th2 cells and cytokines, which give rise to mucosal IgA and serum IgG1, IgA, and IgE responses. On the other hand, oral immunization with r*Salmonella* expressing Tox C results in Th1-type responses as well as Th2 cell-derived IL-10 and macrophage-derived IL-6, which correlate with mucosal IgA and serum IgG2a antibody responses.

Two major conclusions can be drawn from our studies with these two regimens in normal, IFN-$\gamma^{-/-}$, and IL-4$^{-/-}$ mice. First, oral administration of r*Salmonella,* which elicits classical Th1-type responses also induces significant mucosal IgA responses when given to mice with defective Th1- (IFN-$\gamma^{-/-}$) or Th2- (IL-4$^{-/-}$) cytokine pathways. Interestingly, we detect Th2-type cells producing IL-10 and macrophage-secreting IL-6 in both normal and cytokine-deficient mice, and we postulate that these two cytokines are of most importance for murine IgA responses. Second, oral administration of TT plus CT as adjuvant induces classical Th2-type responses in both normal and IFN-$\gamma^{-/-}$ mice. Further, lack of IL-4 results in failure to induce mucosal IgA responses. Thus, the IL-4 pathway is necessary for the CT adjuvant effect for mucosal IgA responses after oral immunization with a protein vaccine.

REFERENCES

1. MESTECKY, J. & J. R. McGHEE. 1987. Immunoglobulin A (IgA): molecular and cellular interactions involved in IgA biosynthesis and immune response. Adv. Immunol. **40:** 153-245.
2. McGHEE, J. R., J. MESTECKY, C. O. ELSON & H. KIYONO. 1989. Regulation of IgA synthesis and immune response by T cells and interleukins. J. Clin. Immunol. **9:** 175-199.
3. HANSON, L. A. & P. BRANDTZAEG. 1989. The mucosal defence system. *In* Immunobiological Disorders in Infant and Children. E. R. Stiehm, Ed.: 116-155. W. B. Saunders Company. Philadelphia, PA.
4. MOSMANN, T. R. & R. L. COFFMAN. 1989. Th1 and Th2 cells: different patterns of lymphokine secretion lead to different functional properties. Annu. Rev. Immunol. **7:** 145-173.
5. BEAGLEY, K. W., J. H. ELDRIDGE, F. LEE, H. KIYONO, M. P. EVERSON, W. J. KOOPMAN, T. HIRONO, T. KISHIMOTO & J. R. McGHEE. 1989. Interleukins and IgA synthesis. Human and murine interleukin 6 induce high rate IgA secretion in IgA-committed B cells. J. Exp. Med. **169:** 2133-2148.
6. BEAGLEY, K. W., J. H. ELDRIDGE, W. K. AICHER, J. MESTECKY, S. DiFABIO, H. KIYONO, H. & J. R. McGHEE. 1991. Peyer's patch B cells with memory cell characteristics undergo terminal differentiation within 24 hours in response to interleukin-6. Cytokine **3:** 107-116.
7. FUJIHASHI, K., J. R. McGHEE, C. LUE, K. W. BEAGLEY, T. TAGA, T. HIRANO, T. KISHIMOTO, J. MESTECKY & H. KIYONO. 1991. Human appendix B cells naturally express receptors for and respond to interleukin 6 with selective IgA1 and IgA2 synthesis. J. Clin. Invest. **88:** 248-252.
8. MURRAY, P. D., D. T. McKENZIE, S. L. SWAIN & M. F. KAGNOFF. 1987. Interleukin 5 and interleukin 4 produced by Peyer's patch T cells selectively enhance immunogloblin A expression. J. Immunol. **139:** 2669-2674.
9. COFFMAN, R. L., B. SHRADER, J. CARTY, T. R. MOSSMAN & M. W. BOND. 1987. A mouse T cell product that preferentially enhances IgA production. I. Biologic characterization. J. Immunol. **139:** 3685-3690.
10. BOND, M. W., B. SHRADER, T. R. MOSSMAN & R. L. COFFMAN. 1987. A mouse T cell product that preferentially enhances IgA production. II. Physicochemical characterization. J. Immunol. **139:** 3691-3696.

11. HARRIMAN, G. R., D. Y. KUNIMOTO, J. F. ELLIOTT, V. PAETKAU & W. STROBER. 1988. The role of IL-5 in IgA B cell differentiation. J. Immunol. **140:** 3033-3039.

12. LEBMAN, D. A. & R. L. COFFMAN. 1988. The effects of IL-4 and IL-5 on the IgA response by murine Peyer's patch B cell subpopulations. J. Immunol. **141:** 2050-2056.

13. RAMSAY, A. J., A. J. HUSBAND, I. A. RAMSHAW, S. BAO, K. I. MATTHAEI, G. KOHLER & M. KOPF. 1994. The role of interleukin-6 in mucosal IgA antibody responses *in vivo*. Science **264:** 561-563.

14. JACKSON, R. J., K. FUJIHASHI, J. XU-AMANO, H. KIYONO, C. O. ELSON & J. R. MCGHEE. 1993. Optimizing oral vaccines: induction of systemic and mucosal B-cell and antibody responses to tetanus toxoid by use of cholera toxin as an adjuvant. Infect. Immun. **61:** 4272-4279.

15. XU-AMANO, J., H. KIYONO, R. J. JACKSON, H. F. STAATS, K. FUJIHASHI, P. D. BURROWS, C. O. ELSON, S. PILLAI & J. R. MCGHEE. 1993. Helper T cell subsets for immunogloblin A responses: oral immunization with tetanus toxoid and cholera toxin as adjuvant selectively induces Th2 cells in mucosa associated tissues. J. Exp. Med. **178:** 1309-1320.

16. XU-AMANO, J., R. J. JACKSON, K. FUJIHASHI, H. KIYONO, H. F. STAATS & J. R. MCGHEE. 1993. Helper Th1 and Th2 cell responses following mucosal or systemic immunization with cholera toxin. Vaccine **12:** 903-911.

17. MARINARO, M., H. F. STAATS, T. HIROI, M. COSTE, R. J. JACKSON, P. N. BOYAKA, N. OKAHASHI, M. YAMAMOTO, H. KIYONO, M. BLÜTHMANN, K. FUJIHASHI & J. R. MCGHEE. 1995. The mucosal adjuvant effect of cholera toxin in mice results from induction of T helper 2 (Th2) cells and IL-4. J. Immunol. In press.

18. CURTISS III, R., S. M. KELLY & J. O. HASSAN. 1993. Live oral avirulent *Salmonella* vaccines. Vet. Microbiol. **37:** 397-405.

19. CHATFIELD, S. N., M. ROBERTS, P. LONDON, I. CROPLEY, G. DOUCE & G. DOUGAN. 1993. The development of oral vaccines based on live attenuated *Salmonella* strains. FEMS Immunol. Med. Microbiol. **7:** 1-7.

20. ROBERTS, M., S. N. CHATFIELD & G. DOUGAN. 1994. *Salmonella* as carriers of heterologous antigens. *In* Novel Delivery Systems for Oral Vaccines. D. T. O'Hagan, Ed.: 27-58. CRC Press. Ann Arbor, ME.

21. CHATFIELD, S. N., I. G. CHARLES, A. J. MAKOFF, M. D. OXER, G. DOUGAN, D. PICKARD, D. SLATER & N. F. FAIRWEATHER. 1992. Use of the nirB promoter to direct the stable expression of heterogous antigens in *Salmonella* oral vaccine strains: development of a single dose oral tetanus vaccine. Biotechnology **10:** 888-892.

22. LOCKSLEY, R. M. & P. SCOTT. 1991. Helper T-cell subsets in mouse *Leishmaniasis:* induction, expansion and effector function. Immunol. Today **12:** A58-A61.

23. SCOTT, P. 1991. IFN-γ modulates the early development of Th1 and Th2 responses in a murine model of cutaneous *Leishmaniasis*. J. Immunol. **147:** 3149-3155.

24. ZHONG, G. M. & L. M. DE LA MAZA. 1988. Activation of mouse peritoneal macrophages *in vitro* or *in vivo* by recombinant murine gamma IFN inhibits the growth of *Chlamydia trachomatis* serotype L1. Infect. Immun. **56:** 3322-3325.

25. FLESCH, I. & S. H. E. KAUFMANN. 1987. Mycobacterial growth inhibition by interferon-gamma activated bone marrow macrophages and differential susceptibility among strains of *M. tuberculosis*. J. Immunol. **138:** 4408-4413.

26. MUOTIALA, A. & H. P. MAKELA. 1990. The role of IFN-γ in murine *Salmonella typhimurium* infection. Microb. Pathog. **8:** 135-141.

27. RAMARATHINAM, L., D. W. NIESEL & G. R. KLIMPEL. 1993. *Salmonella typhimurium* induces IFN-γ production in murine splenocytes. Role of natural killer cells and macrophages. J. Immunol. **150:** 3937-3981.

28. RAMARATHINAM, L., R. A. SHABAN, D. W. NEISEL & G. R. KLIMPEL. 1991. Interferon gamma (IFN-γ) production by gut-associated lymphoid tissue and spleen following oral *Salmonella typhimurium* challenge. Microb. Pathog. **11:** 347-356.

29. MASTROENI, P., B. VILLARREAL-RAMOS & C. E. HORMAECHE. 1992. Role of T cells, TNF-α and IFN-γ in recall of immunity to oral challenge with virulent *Salmonella* in

mice vaccinated with live attenuated aro-*Salmonella* vaccines. Microb. Pathog. **13:** 477-491.

30. VANCOTT, J. L., H. F. STAATS, D. W. PASCUAL, M. ROBERTS, S. N. CHATFIELD, M. YAMAMOTO, P.B. CARTER, H. KIYONO & J. R. MCGHEE. 1995. Regulation of mucosal and systemic antibody responses by T helper cell subsets, macrophages and derived cytokines following oral immunization with live recombinant *Salmonella*. J. Immunol. In press.

31. COFFMAN, R. L., K. VARKILA, P. SCOTT & R. CHATELAIN. 1991. Role of cytokines in the differentiation of CD4⁺ T-cell subsets *in vivo*. Immunol. Rev. **123:** 189-207.

32. BEAGLEY, K. W., J. H. ELDRIDGE, H. KIYONO, M. P. EVERSON, W. J. KOOPMAN, T. HONJO & J. R. MCGHEE. 1988. Recombinant murine IL-5 induces high rate IgA synthesis in cycling IgA-positive Peyer's patch B cells. J. Immunol. **141:** 2035-2042.

33. BRIERE, F., J.-M. BRIDON, D. CHEVET, G. SOUILLET, F. BIENVENU, C. GURET, H. MARTINEZ-VALDEZ & J. BANCHEREAU. 1994. Interleukin 10 induces B lymphocytes from IgA-deficient patients to secrete IgA. J. Clin. Invest. **94:** 97-104.

34. LEGROS, G., S. Z. BEN-SASSON, R. SEDER, F. D. FINKELMAN & W. E. PAUL. 1990. Generation of interleukin-4 (IL-4)-producing cells *in vivo* and *in vitro:* IL-2 and IL-4 are required for *in vitro* generation of IL-4-producing cells. J. Exp. Med. **172:** 921-929.

35. SWAIN, S. L., A. D. WEINBERG, M. ENGLISH & G. HUSTON. 1990. IL-4 directs the development of Th2-like helper effectors. J. Immunol. **145:** 3796-3806.

36. SAD, S. & T. R. MOSMANN. 1994. Single IL-2-secreting precursor CD4 T cell can develop into either Th1 or Th2 cytokine secretion phenotype. J. Immunol. **153:** 3514-3522.

37. KOPF, M., G. L. GROS, M. BACHMANN, M. C. LAMERS, H. BLÜTHMANN & G. KOHLER. 1993. Disruption of the murine IL-4 gene blocks Th2 cytokine responses. Nature **362:** 245-248.

38. OKAHASHI, N., M. YAMAMOTO, J. L. VANCOTT, S. N. CHATFIELD, M. ROBERTS, H. BLÜTHMANN, T. HIROI, H. KIYONO & J. R. MCGHEE. 1995. Oral immunization of IL-4 knockout mice with r*Salmonella* or cholera toxin reveals that CD4⁺ Th2 cells producing IL-6 and IL-10 are associated with mucosal IgA responses. Submitted to Infect. Immun.

39. VAJDY, M., M. H. KOSCO-VILBOIS, M. KOPF, G. KOHLER & N. LYCKE. 1995. Impaired mucosal immune responses in interleukin 4-targeted mice. J. Exp. Med. **181:** 41-53.

Studying Immunological Tolerance by Physically Monitoring Antigen-specific T Cells *in Vivo*[a]

A. KHORUTS AND M. K. JENKINS

Department of Microbiology
University of Minnesota Medical School
420 Delaware Street S.E.
Minneapolis, Minnesota 55455

INTRODUCTION

Challenge of the immune system with an antigen may result in states of antigen-specific immunity or tolerance. Understanding the mechanisms that lead to these opposite effects has constituted one of the fundamental problems in immunology. However, because physical detection of lymphocytes specific for any particular antigen *in vivo* has been technically impossible, due to their exceedingly low frequency, study of the variables involved in immunity and tolerance have relied on short-term polyclonal cell cultures, or cloned lymphocyte lines or hybridomas *in vitro*. These methods have yielded a great deal of information and still remain indispensable to immunologists; yet, by their nature, they do not allow the direct study of the intact immune system.

Recently, new technologies have emerged that have overcome this problem, by allowing direct visualization of antigen-specific lymphocytes. One method relies on super-antigens, which cross-link class II MHC molecules and certain T-cell receptor (TCR) V_β segments independent of the TCR V_α chain. Therefore, it is possible to track superantigen-specific T cells, purely on the basis of TCR V_β expression by flow cytometry. The second method uses transgenic technology to produce animals that express transgenic antigen receptors of known antigen specificity that can be detected with anticlonotypic TCR antibodies.

Using these new tools, it has been finally possible to demonstrate physical elimination of autoreactive lymphocytes as they develop within the primary lymphoid organs, over 30 years after clonal deletion was originally proposed.[1] Clonal deletion has been established for self-reactive B cells in the bone marrow and T cells in the thymus. The same methods have also been used to study extrathymic T-cell lymphopoiesis within the intestinal epithelium, which seems to be at least partially responsible for the generation of intraepithelial lymphocytes and T cells found in the lamina propia.[2] Although it is unknown if dietary antigens may play a role in lymphocyte maturation in the intestine, work with superantigen and TCR transgenic systems has shown negative selection can be driven there by self-antigens.[2]

Although central tolerance established within the primary lymphoid organs is certainly a major, and the best understood, mechanism of generating immune tolerance, it cannot explain self-tolerance to antigens expressed exclusively in the periphery or to developmen-

[a] This work was supported by NIH Grants AI-27998 and AI-35296. A. Khoruts was supported by NIH Training Grant DK07654.

tally regulated antigens that appear in the organism after the T-cell repertoire has been established. Thus, there exist a number of mechanisms that lead to maintenance of peripheral tolerance, which are now amenable to direct study *in vivo*. The proposed possibilities in the past have included clonal anergy (functional inactivation), deletion, exhaustion, and ignorance, as well as generation of antigen-specific regulatory cells that suppress the immune response. By visualizing the antigen-specific lymphocytes *in vivo*, it is now possible to directly study these various mechanisms. In this paper we will discuss the recent advances made in understanding peripheral tolerance, particularly to exogenously administered antigens, a topic that has been the recent focus of research in our laboratory.

TOLERANCE IN TRANSGENIC MODELS OF EXCLUSIVE EXTRATHYMIC ANTIGEN EXPRESSION

Generation of an immune response is normally a highly orchestrated process involving different subsets of lymphocytes, antigen-presenting cells (APC), and effector cells. Therefore, initial activation of lymphocytes probably takes place within the secondary lymphoid tissues (*e.g.*, lymph node), where all these cells are present in close proximity. Indeed, naive T cells are essentially confined to the secondary lymphoid tissues, thus maximizing a productive encounter with an antigen brought there from the entry site by mobile APC (*e.g.*, macrophages and dendritic cells).[3] Thus, it may not be surprising that several attempted models of autoimmunity where potential antigen was targeted to a certain parenchymal tissue did not result in immunopathology even in mice that contained T cells expressing transgenic TCRs specific for the transgenic antigen. For example, Ohashi *et al.*[4] studied double transgenic mice expressing lymphocytic choriomeningitis virus glycoprotein (LCMV-GP) in the pancreas and TCR specific for LCMV-GP in the context of H-2D^b. No diabetes resulted in these mice, and the transgenic cells were not deleted and performed equally well *in vitro* compared to T cells from TCR single-transgenic mice. These data strongly support ignorance as the chief mechanism of tolerance operating in this system.[4] Tolerance could be easily broken by active LCMV infection,[4,5] probably through antigen delivery to the draining lymphoid tissues. Once activated, T cells exit lymphoid tissues and are able to travel freely throughout the periphery, where further effector functions may be exercised upon local encounter with the antigen.[3] Similarly, autoimmune encephalitis is seen in mice expressing transgenic TCR specific for the immunodominant peptide of myelin basic protein (MBP), but only when the animals are housed in a conventional facility, suggesting that ignorance of the self-antigen is maintained until some T cells are activated by a cross-reacting antigen.[6]

Although ignorance clearly is a major mechanism of tolerance, there are also models where the T cells do encounter parenchymally expressed antigen. Arnold and co-workers[7,8] have constructed transgenic mice expressing class I MHC K^b molecules under the control of various tissue-specific promoters. K^b is expressed primarily in the targeted tissue and cannot be detected by PCR in the thymus. Inasmuch as the mice are also transgenic for a TCR specific for K^b, the specific T cells in these mice can be monitored *in vivo*. Interestingly, depending on the amount of antigen expressed, the T cells become increasingly anergic because of decreased CD8 and TCR expression.[7-9]

The requirement for high levels of antigen expression by parenchymal tissues to achieve interaction with the T-cell population was also seen for CD4$^+$ helper T cells by Guerder *et al.*[10] in mice expressing transgenic I-E molecules exclusively on pancreatic β cells and within the kidney. Such expression of antigens results in I-E-specific unresponsiveness in the CD4$^+$ T cells. On the other hand, providing costimulation to T cells through coexpression of transgenic I-E and B7-1 molecules leads to insulitis and destruction of the pancreas, whereas pancreatic expression of transgenic B7-1 molecules alone on pancreatic β cells does not lead to autoimmunity. It thus appears likely that because most peripheral tissues express relatively low levels of class I MHC molecules (and in the absence of inflammation few express class II MHC molecules), effective interaction with T cells is normally rare. Furthermore, inasmuch as parenchymal tissues are deficient in costimulatory molecules, any engagement of the TCRs on T cells that do access these tissues will result in T-cell unresponsiveness.

ANIMAL MODELS OF PERIPHERAL TOLERANCE TO EXOGENOUSLY ADMINISTERED ANTIGENS

Immunologists have known for several decades that tolerance is induced by injecting soluble antigens into routes that result in systemic delivery.[11] This is an example of peripheral tolerance because it is equally well induced in thymectomized animals.[12] Conversely, generation of immunity toward soluble antigens typically requires that the antigen be delivered in an adjuvant (e.g., complete Freund's adjuvant (CFA) composed of heat-killed mycobacteria and mineral oil). Several groups have used superantigen or TCR transgenic systems to study the mechanisms that lead to tolerance under these conditions.[13] In our laboratory, we have used mice of the BALB/c background expressing a transgenic TCR specific for ovalbumin 323-339 bound to I-A^d class II MHC molecules.[14] The transgenic T cells can be identified by the KJ1-26 monoclonal antibody that exclusively recognizes the transgenic TCR. During establishment of the system, we noted that TCR transgenic mice responded differently than normal BALB/c mice to antigen challenge in vivo. No enhanced responsiveness of T cells from draining lymph nodes following immunization could be demonstrated in the TCR transgenic mice, and tolerance was poorly induced after systemic administration of the ovalbumin peptide without CFA. We overcame this problem by adoptively transferring limiting numbers of T cells from TCR transgenic animals into normal BALB/c recipients, such that the resultant transgenic T-cell frequency in the lymph nodes of the recipients was 0.2-0.5 percent. In this case the TCR transgenic T cells could still be detected with the KJ1-26 monoclonal antibody (mAb), but were not the dominant T-cell population, thus avoiding the artifactual situation encountered in the intact TCR transgenic mice.

Physical tracking of KJ1-26$^+$ cells with the antibody allowed the study of the in vivo behavior of antigen-specific T cells during primary and secondary responses following subcutaneous immunization with ovalbumin 323-339 peptide in CFA or intravenous tolerization with the peptide alone. Both routes of peptide challenge resulted in initial proliferation of KJ1-26$^+$ cells in vivo. However, proliferation was transient after intravenous peptide administration and was followed by rapid disappearance of transgenic cells from the lymph nodes. This was contrasted by sustained accumulation of KJ1-26$^+$ cells within the draining lymph nodes after subcutaneous immunization that reached a plateau two days after the peak observed with the intravenous peptide. After allowing the cells to rest in vivo, their functional status was tested in vitro. Transgenic cells exposed to intravenous peptide proliferated poorly and had an IL-2 production defect characteristic of the anergic cells, whereas transgenic T cells exposed to peptide subcutaneously in CFA were hypersensitive to antigenic stimulation as would be expected for memory cells.[3]

T-cell anergy has been best defined and studied in mature T-cell clones, which by definition have been propagated for multiple generations in vitro.[15-17] It can be induced upon stimulation of the TCR in the absence of costimulatory signals, which results in poor IL-2 production and lack of subsequent T-cell proliferation.[18] However, Davis and Lipsky[19] have shown that previously activated T cells are more susceptible to anergy induction than naive cells. Thus, it is likely that after intravenous injection of antigen, dendritic cells expressing abundant costimulatory and class II MHC molecules are able to initiate proliferation of naive antigen-specific T cells. However, this may be insufficient to generate immunity, and an additional signal or continued antigen presentation by another APC may be needed. The previously activated T cells (and now tolerizable) may become anergic if such subsequent antigen presentation occurs in the absence of costimulation.

ROLE OF B CELLS IN GENERATION OF T-CELL ACTIVATION AND TOLERANCE

Immunohistochemical analysis of lymph nodes from animals given a tolerogenic form of the peptide revealed that proliferation of the antigen-specific T cells occurred exclusively within the T cell-rich paracotrical area.[14] On the other hand, lymph nodes from animals immunized with the peptide/CFA demonstrated movement of antigen-specific T cells into the B cell-rich follicles after first proliferating in the paracortex.[14] This finding strongly suggests that antigen-specific T cells must interact with B cells for effective T-cell priming to occur. This idea is supported by the earlier finding that mice treated from birth with anti-IgM antibody (thus rendered B-cell deficient) showed defects in T-cell priming that could be rescued by injection of purified B cells shortly prior to immunization with antigen.[20–22]

On the other hand, much evidence suggests that antigen presentation by *resting* B cells results in T-cell tolerance.[23,24] Resting B cells lack costimulatory molecules but are very efficient at internalizing specific antigen compared to other APCs, which lack antigen-specific receptors.[25,26] Thus, B cells may also be critical for specific T-cell tolerance induction. When antigen is in monomeric form and injected intravenously, there is perhaps little opportunity for B-cell activation. Thus, one of the main functions of the adjuvant may be to activate B cells and convert them to APC that support immunity instead of tolerance. In fact, Liu and Janeway[27] have shown that several components of adjuvants lead to the induction of costimulatory molecules on B cells. In addition, T-cell immunity is generated when antigens are targeted to activated B cells *in vivo* in a situation where anti-IgD antibodies serve as the T-cell antigen and the B-cell activator.[28] It should be noted, however, that Fuchs and Matzinger[24] showed that B cells activated *in vitro* with lipopolysaccharide still induced T-cell tolerance when injected into naive hosts.

ORAL ANTIGEN ADMINISTRATION AND INDUCTION OF SYSTEMIC PERIPHERAL TOLERANCE

It has been observed as early as the beginning of this century that feeding antigens can result in antigen-specific systemic tolerance.[29] The intestine contains a highly organized immune system referred to as gut-associated lymphoid tissue (GALT), which is composed of Peyer's patches, isolated lymphoid follicles, intraepithelial lymphocytes, and other immune cells within lamina propria, as well as intestinal epithelial cells that are capable of antigen presentation. Inasmuch as the gut is exposed to the greatest variety of foreign antigens, most of which are nonpathogenic components of diet, it may be particularly well suited to induce tolerance. Indeed, many efforts to use GALT to induce systemic immunity, especially to pathogens, which gain access to the host through mucosal surfaces, have been hampered by the tolerance phenomenon.[30]

How orally administered antigen gets processed and presented to the peripheral immune system remains unclear. Studies with horseradish peroxidase have demonstrated that small amounts of intact antigen can traverse intestinal epithelial cells and reach lamina propria, mesenteric lymph, and the portal vein.[31,32] Peyer's patches are particularly adapted to sample luminal antigens by virtue of specialized membranous (M) cells, which are capable of absorbing a wide array of material ranging from macromolecules to microorganisms and latex beads.[33] The reported amounts of intact orally administered antigen that can be systemically absorbed have been estimated to be as high as 2 percent.[34] Therefore, it is possible that orally administered antigen may directly reach distant lymphoid tissue to be presented there by resident APC. It is also possible that antigen is internalized by the abundant APC present within GALT and carried by these cells to peripheral lymphoid tissues. Both Peyer's patches and the lamina propria are particularly rich in B cells, which are located closer to the lumen than T cells within the microarchitecture of these organs. It is thus conceivable that these B cells would be able to carry antigens picked up in the GALT to the peripheral lymphoid tissue and present them to distal T cells, resulting in systemic tolerance.

Mucosal immunity, rather than tolerance, can be generated by feeding antigens together with adjuvants.[30] Perhaps the best known such mucosal adjuvant is cholera toxin. Cholera toxin is an oligomeric protein (composed of five B subunits (CT-B) and a toxic A subunit (CT-A), which is responsible for adenyl cyclase activation by way of ADP ribosylation of a stimulatory G protein. The mechanisms by which cholera toxin may enhance immunogenicity have been the subject of intense investigation. As in the case of lipoidal adjuvants used for subcutaneous immunization, cholerla toxin induces inflammation, as evidenced by the induction of IL-1 production by macrophages and epithelial cells.[35,36] Cholerla toxin also affects B cells. Recombinant CT-B, which binds ganglioside GM1, up-regulates B-cell expression of MHC class II molecules.[37] Furthermore, cholerla toxin induces the costimulatory molecule, B7-1, on the M12 B cell-lymphoma line.[38] This effect is also seen in B cell-lymphoma lines stimulated with dibutyryl-cAMP and forskolin, agents that increase intracellular cAMP levels like cholera toxin.[39]

Although there is reasonable consensus that the dominant mechanism leading to tolerance in animals fed with a high antigen dose is direct inactivation of antigen-specific T cells, evidence for cellular suppression has been found when animals are fed multiple low doses of antigen.[40] This regimen of feeding is thought to lead to selective generation of antigen-specific cells that produce immunosuppressive cytokines (*e.g.,* IL-10, TGF-β). Naive T cells can differentiate into cells that preferentially secrete selected cytokines. Two main phenotypes of cytokine-secreting T cells are currently recognized: Th1 and Th2.[41] Whereas Th1 cytokines (IL-2, IFN-γ, TNF-β) are particularly important in mediating cellular immunity against intracellular parasites, Th2 cytokines (IL-4, IL-5, IL-6, IL-10, IL-13) are more important for humoral immunity and the clearance of extracellular eukaryotic parasites.[41] It is also recognized that some Th2 cytokines may down-regulate production of cytokine Th1 cells, and vice versa.[41] Th2 phenotype induction seems to be favored in the GALT,[30] and the induction of Th2 cells by feeding antigens has been proposed as a possible mechanism of disease prevention in an animal model of multiple sclerosis, experimental autoimmune encephalomyelitis (EAE).[40,42] Chen *et al.*[43] reported inhibition of active EAE by a Th2 clone and by a CD4+ T-cell clone that secreted TGF-β, both of which were specific for neuroantigens used for inducing disease by subcutaneous immunization. Clearly, the possibility of using suppressor cells is very attractive for clinical applications, as this approach may not require comprehensive knowledge of all possible antigens involved in a given disease. However, clear identity of such suppressor cells is still lacking, as is the understanding of mechanisms that may lead to their generation. Hopefully, further work with systems where antigen-specific T cells can be tracked may help to gain further knowledge in this area.

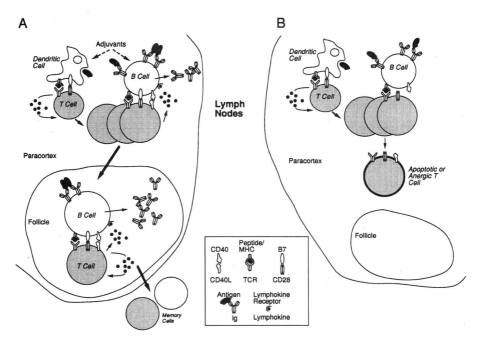

FIGURE 1. Schematic view of the microanatomy of the induction of immunity (**A**) or peripheral tolerance (**B**). **A:** Following the injection of antigen and adjuvant, lymph node–dendritic cells pick up, process, and present a peptide fragment bound to class II MHC to an antigen-specific T cell in the paracortex. This T cell then produces IL-2, proliferates, and is further stimulated by an antigen-presenting, activated, paracortical B cell. The B cell could have been activated either by a component of the adjuvant or by having its surface immunoglobulin cross-linked by aggregated antigen. Both the activated T and B cells then migrate into a follicle. Here, the B cell secretes antibody, undergoes isotype switching and somatic hypermutation. Both memory T and B cells are generated and leave the lymph node. **B:** Following injection of monomeric antigen in the absence of adjuvant, the T-cell response is initiated in the paracortex by dendritic cell antigen presentation but does not proceed further because antigen-presenting B cells do not become activated. In this case the T cells either die or become functionally inactivated in the paracortex and never enter follicles.

SUMMARY

Generation of antigen-specific immunity or tolerance are different outcomes of a highly complex interaction between antigen, antigen-specific lymphocytes, and APC. Clearly, full understanding of this process must include the study of antigen-specific lymphocytes *in vivo,* under conditions known to result in immunity or tolerance. This has now become possible with the advent of methods that allow direct detection of antigen-specific T cells.

One of the most striking observations made thus far is the seemingly critical cross-talk between T and B cells. It is well established that B-cell responses are to a high degree dependent on T-cell help, which consists of CD40/CD40 ligand interaction and delivery of various T cell-derived cytokines. Several lines of evidence now point to equal dependency of T-cell responses on interaction with B cells. T helper-cell priming in lymph nodes has only been observed when these cells migrate into B cell-rich follicles.[14] In addition, T-cell priming does not occur in anti-IgM-treated B cell-depleted mice, and adoptive transfer of B cells back into these animals before immunization results in restoration of T-cell responses.[20-22] Finally, when antigen presentation is targeted to occur exclusively through B cells, the effect on T cells seems to depend on the activation state of B cells. T-cell immunity results when B cells are activated, whereas tolerance is induced when the B cells are resting.

The following model outlines possible events that can lead to tolerance or immunity (FIG. 1), with an emphasis on the role of B-cell APC. Tolerance is induced when monomeric soluble antigens are injected without adjuvants (FIG. 1B). Antigen is taken up by dendritic cells that constitutively express costimulatory molecules (e.g., B7) and are thus able to stimulate IL-2 production and some T-cell proliferation. T-cell proliferation is short lived, and T cells are restricted to the paracortex, where they subsequently encounter resting B cells that present antigen leading to tolerance. In the case of oral tolerance, it is also possible that the GALT is the major source of B cells that carry antigen throughout the peripheral lymphoid tissues. Because antigens picked up in the GALT are predigested in the gut lumen, activation of B cells by cross-linking their surface immunoglobulin receptors may be particularly unlikely. Adjuvants, however, are able to shift the sequence toward immunity by activating B cells (FIG. 1A) to express costimulatory molecules. Adsorption of antigens to alum may do the same thing by enhancing cross-linking of B cell-surface immunoglobulins. It is also conceivable that signals generated by the antigen and adjuvant may directly act on T cells and promote migration to the follicles, where interaction with activated B cells would be more likely to take place. This would lead to further activation and proliferation of T cells (that subsequently would leave the lymph node and migrate toward the tissues) and stimulation of antibody production by the B cells.

This model places great emphasis on the role of adjuvants in the induction of immunity to soluble antigens. How then is immunity ever induced to infectious agents that obviously do not enter the body emulsified in CFA? The answer probably is that molecules with adjuvant properties (such as lipopolysaccharide, peptidoglycan, or double-stranded RNA) are intrinsic components of all microbes that the innate immune system has come to recognize. If this model is correct, then peripheral tolerance is actually the default pathway that the immune system will follow unless the antigen in question is recognized in an inflammatory context. The advantage of this strategy is that any newly expressed self-protein will induce tolerance, and only antigens that are recognized in the context of inflammation will induce immunity.

REFERENCES

1. NOSSAL, G. J. V. 1994. Cell **76:** 229-239.
2. POUSSIER, P. & M. JULIUS. 1994. Annu. Rev. Immunol. **12:** 521-553.
3. MACKAY, C. R. 1991. Immunol. Today **12:** 189-192.
4. OHASHI, P. S., S. OEHEN, K. BUERKI, H. PIRCHER, C. T. OHASHI, B. ODERMATT, B. MALISSEN, R. M. ZINKERNAGEL & H. HENGARTNER. 1991. Cell **65:** 305-317.
5. OLDSTONE, M. B. A., M. NERENBERG, P. SOUTHERN, J. PRICE & H. LEWICKI. 1991. Cell **65:** 319-331.
6. GOVERMAN, J., A. WOODS, L. LARSON, L. P. WEINER, L. HOOD & D. M. ZALLER. 1992. Cell **72:** 551-560.
7. ARNOLD, B., G. SCHONRICH & G. J. HAMMERLING. 1993. Immunol. Today **14:** 12-14.
8. HAMMERLING, G. J., G. SCHONRICH, I. FERBER & B. ARNOLD. 1991. Immunol. Rev. **122:** 47-67.

9. SCHONRICH, G., U. KALINKE, F. MOMBURG, M. MALISSEN, A.-M. SCHMITT-VERHULST, B. MALISSEN, G. J. HAMMERLING & B. ARNOLD. 1991. Cell 65: 293-304.
10. GUERDER, S., J. MEYERHOFF & R. FLAVELL. 1994. Immunity 1: 155-166.
11. DRESSER, D. W. 1961. Nature 191: 1169-1171.
12. MITCHISON, N. A. 1968. Immunology 15: 509-530.
13. KISIELOW, P., W. SWAT, B. ROCHA & H. VON BOEHMER. 1991. Immunol. Rev. 122: 70-85.
14. KEARNEY, E. R., K. A. PAPE, D. Y. LOH & M. K. JENKINS. 1994. Immunity 1: 327-339.
15. JENKINS, M. K. & R. H. SCHWARTZ. 1987. J. Exp. Med. 165: 302-319.
16. QUILL, H. & R. H. SCHWARTZ. 1987. J. Immunol. 138: 3704-3712.
17. MUELLER, D. L., M. K. JENKINS & R. H. SCHWARTZ. 1989. Annu. Rev. Immunol. 7: 445-480.
18. DESILVA, D. R., K. B. URDAHL & M. K. JENKINS. 1991. J. Immunol. 147: 3261-3267.
19. DAVIS, L. & P. E. LIPSKY. 1993. Cell. Immunol. 146: 351-361.
20. RON, Y., P. DEBASTSELIRE, E. TZEHOVAL, J. GORDON, M. FELDMAN & S. SEGAL. 1983. Eur. J. Immunol. 13: 167-171.
21. RON, Y. & J. SPRENT. 1987. J. Immunol. 138: 2848-2856.
22. KURT-JONES, E. A., D. LIANO, K. A. HAYGLASS, B. BENACERAF, M.-S. SY & A. K. ABBAS. 1988. J. Immunol. 140: 3773-3778.
23. EYNON, E. E. & D. C. PARKER. 1992. J. Exp. Med. 175: 131-138.
24. FUCHS, E. J. & P. MATZINGER. 1992. Science 258: 1156-1159.
25. JENKINS, M. K., E. BURRELL & J. D. ASHWELL. 1990. J. Immunol. 144: 1585-1590.
26. LANZAVECCHIA, A. 1985. Nature 314: 537-539.
27. LIU, Y. & C. A. JANEWAY, JR. 1991. Int. Immunol. 3: 323-332.
28. MORRIS, S. C., A. LEES & F. D. FINKELMAN. 1994. J. Immunol. 153: 3777-3785.
29. WELLS, H. G. 1911. J. Infect. Dis. 8: 147-171.
30. MCGHEE, J. R. & H. KIYONO. 1993. Infect. Agents Dis. 2: 55-73.
31. CORNELL, R., W. A. WALKER & K. J. ISSELBACHER. 1971. Lab. Invest. 25: 42-48.
32. WARSHAW, A. L., W. A. WALKER, R. CORNELL & K. J. ISSELBACHER. 1971. Lab. Invest. 25: 675-684.
33. KEREN, D. F. 1992. Semin. Immunol. 4: 217-226.
34. MOWAT, A. MC.I. 1987. Immunol. Today 8: 93-98.
35. BROMANDER, A., J. HOLMGREN & N. LYCKE. 1991. J. Immunol. 146: 2908-2914.
36. BROMANDER, A., M. KJERRULF, J. HOLMGREN & N. LYCKE. 1993. Scand. J. Immunol. 37: 452-458.
37. FRANCES, M. L., J. RYAN, M. G. JOBLING, R. K. HOLMES, J. MOSS & J. J. MOND. 1992. J. Immunol. 148: 1999-2005.
38. WATTS, T. H., N. ALAVERDI, W. F. WADE & P. S. LINSLEY. 1993. J. Immunol. 150: 2192-2202.
39. NABAVI, N., G. J. FREEMAN, A. GAULT, D. GODFREY, L. M. NADLER & L. H. GLIMCHER. 1992. Nature 360: 266-268.
40. WEINER, H. L. 1994. Proc. Natl. Acad. Sci. USA 91: 10762-10765.
41. PAUL, W. E. & R. A. SEDER. 1994. Cell 76: 241-251.
42. KHOURY, S. J., W. W. HANCOCK & H. L. WEINER. 1992. J. Exp. Med. 176: 1355-1364.
43. CHEN, Y., V. K. KUCHROO, J. INOBE, D. A. HAFLER & H. L. WEINER. 1994. Science 265: 1237-1240.

Parenteral and Oral Administration of Tolerogens: Protein-IgG Conjugates

Y. BOREL,[a,b,d] R. FRITSCHE,[a] H. BOREL,[b]
U. DAHLGREN,[c] A. DALHMAN-HÖGLUND,[c] AND
L. A. HANSON [c]

[a]Nestec Ltd.
Research Centre
Lausanne, Switzerland

[b]Fondation pour Recherches Medicales
University of Geneva
Geneva, Switzerland

[c]Department of Clinical Immunology
University of Göteborg
Göteborg, Sweden

INTRODUCTION

Interest in immunologic tolerance, discovered by Medawar almost half a century ago,[1] has increased for two main reasons: (1) Several of its mechanisms, such as clonal deletion,[2] anergy,[3] and regulatory T cells[4] have been uncovered. (2) Both systemic and oral tolerance,[5,6] the topic of this volume, can be induced to, it is hoped, prevent either autoimmune or allergic diseases. For example, several strategies have been used in trying to prevent allergy, including administration of modified allergen,[7] allergen linked to nonimmunogenic carriers,[8] single peptides,[9] or an allergen-antibody complex.[10]

It is known that antigen presentation can influence the type of immune response. Not only haptens,[11,12] but also proteins covalently linked to a carrier molecule naturally tolerated by the host, such as isologous immunoglobulin, can induce unresponsiveness to these proteins.[13,14] In this paper, the results from the parenteral administration in rats of tolerogens made of either β-lactoglobulin (βLG) or ovalbumin (OVA) linked to isologous immunoglobulin will be briefly reviewed.[15,17] In addition, new data on the administration of OVA-IgG conjugates given either intraperitoneally or orally to neonatal rats will be shown. The results suggest that tolerogenic conjugates given either parenterally or orally could provide a way to prevent certain diseases.

MATERIAL AND METHODS

Protein immunoglobulin conjugates were made, as previously described, using disuccinimidyl suberate to covalently link βLG or OVA to rat immunoglobulin.[14,15] Following

---

[d]Address correspondence to Dr. Yves Borel, Fondation pour Recherches Medicales, 64 Av. de la Roseraie, 1211 Geneva 4, Switzerland.

chromatography on Sephacryl (S300), only the fraction corresponding to monomeric IgG was used because it was shown to be the most effective to induce unresponsiveness.[15] The standard experimental protocol, unless otherwise mentioned in the text, was as previously described.[15] Briefly a single dose (2 mg/rat) of conjugate or appropriate controls (uncoupled βLG or OVA in 1/1 molar ratio mixed together with rat IgG (*i.e.*, control mixture) were given to adult male Sprague Dawley rats (3-4 weeks old) four days before immunization. The rats were bled 14 days later, and serum anti-βLG and anti-OVA antibodies of the IgE and IgG classes were assayed with ELISA.[15] Delayed hypersensitivity was measured by increase in ear thickness, as previously described.[18]

In this paper we examined whether a conjugate of OVA-rat IgG, as compared to free OVA together with IgG (*i.e.*, control mixture), could induce unresponsiveness to OVA if given either intraperitoneally or orally at two different ages in neonatal rats. Thus 14- and 20-day-old female Sprague-Dawley rats were divided into three groups and were injected intraperitoneally (ip) or orally fed with 2 mg of conjugate, 2 mg of control mixture, or phosphate buffer saline (PBS). Four days later all rats were immunized subcutaneously at two different sites on the back with 0.1 mg OVA in complete Freund's adjuvant and 0.1 mg βLG in Freund's complete adjuvant. Two weeks later both delayed-type hypersensitivity (DTH) and IgE, as well as IgG antibody responses against OVA and βLG were measured.

STATISTICS

The data were tested for statistical significance by the Mann-Whitney U. test.

RESULTS

Our previous observations can be summarized as follows. Administration of βLG, a major bovine milk protein allergen, linked to isologous gamma globulin specifically prevents sensitization to βLG in rats. This effect is antigen specific inasmuch as the immune response to the unrelated control antigen, OVA, was unaffected.[15] A single dose (2 mg) of βLG-rat IgG conjugate given intravenously (iv) suppressed not only IgE antibody, but also IgG and IgA antibody formation. It down-regulated the IgE and IgG antibody production in sensitized animals both in the primary and secondary immune responses. The suppression of the IgE antibody production by intravenous administration of βLG-rat IgG conjugate decreased mast cell mediator release (serotonin) *in vivo*. This effect was also seen using passively sensitized mast cells *in vitro*.[15] In addition, the βLG-IgG conjugate, which induced unresponsiveness *in vivo,* appears to be less antigenic *in vitro* than βLG. First, it had a reduced capacity to bind to reaginic antibody, inasmuch as there is a 10-fold reduction in the capacity of conjugated βLG versus intact βLG to trigger serotonin release by rat mast cells. Second βLG-IgG appears to be less immunogenic than βLG in eliciting T-cell proliferation. Thus, the covalent binding of βLG to IgG decreased the immunogenicity of the allergen at both arms of the immune system.[16]

More recently, we extended these observations to another food allergen, that is, OVA. We showed that not only IgE and IgG antibodies were suppressed by the administration of OVA-rat IgG conjugate given intravenously, but also DTH, as measured by an increase in ear thickness. Thus, both T and B cell-mediated immune responses appeared to be suppressed by parenteral administration of a protein conjugated to isologous IgG.[16,17]

In this paper we determined whether the conjugate (OVA-rat IgG) was also effective if given ip or orally in female rats treated at 2 or 3 weeks of age. The results for the humoral antibody response was as follows. In the group with ip-injected 14-day-old rats, the conjugate induced a significantly lower igG (p = 0.004) anti-OVA antibody response compared to the mixture (OVA together with igG) and the PBS control rats (FIG. 1). The IgE anti-OVA antibody response was slightly affected (p = 0.037). In the orally fed 14-day-old rats the conjugate induced a significantly lower level of IgG anti-OVA antibody (p = 0.016) compared to rats fed with the mixture or PBS.

All 20-day-old rats injected ip either with the conjugate or the mixture also had a significantly lower level of IgG (p = 0.007 and IgE p = 0.006) antibody to OVA compared to the control rats (FIG. 2). The 20-day-old rats given the conjugate or the mixture orally showed a significantly lower level of IgE and IgG antibody to OVA (IgG, p = 0.004 and IgE, p < 0.02) for both isotypes, compared to the rats given PBS.

The results for the T cell-mediated response to OVA (FIG. 3) were as follows. Twenty-day-old rats had a reduced immune response to OVA as compared to the PBS control, regardless of whether OVA was given as a conjugate or was free in a mixture. By contrast, in 14-day-old rats, the conjugate given either ip or orally seemed to be more effective than the mixture (OVA + IgG) in suppressing the DTH reaction. All groups showed a similar DTH response to the control antigen (results not shown).

Thus, this study demonstrated that 20-day-old rats given a single oral dose or ip injection of OVA got a suppressed immune response against OVA, regardless whether the OVA was conjugated or just mixed with rat IgG. However, in 14-day-old rats the conjugate was more effective to suppress the DTH and IgG antibody response to OVA than the mixture, when injected ip or fed orally.

DISCUSSION

Our previous studies[15–17] have clearly shown that the allergens given parenterally (iv) have to be conjugated to isologous gamma globulin to induce tolerance. To successfully induce tolerance, with a protein-Ig conjugate, as for a hapten linked to IgG, three conditions are critical: the mode of linkage of the antigen to IgG (in the present case by disuccinimidyl suberate),[14] the molar concentration of the antigenic determinant linked to IgG, and an intact monomeric IgG molecule.[11,15] When these conditions are fulfilled, a single iv dose of either βLG-IgG or OVA-IgG conjugate (2 mg/rat) can specifically suppress both T and B cell-mediated immune responses in rats.

The results presented above confirm and extend these observations. They indicate that the conjugate of OVA-IgG could suppress both delayed hypersensitivity and IgG antibody formation if given not only iv, but also ip or orally in neonatal rats at either 2 or 3 weeks of age. By contrast, IgE antibody production was not suppressed at 2 weeks of age, but it was at 3 weeks of age by oral administration of either the conjugate or OVA (mixed with igG). These data suggest that both age and route of administration might be more important for IgE than for IgG antibody suppression, because the intravenous mode of administration of the tolerogen is more efficient to suppress IgE than IgG.[16,17]

Perhaps the most interesting results are that at 2 weeks of age only the OVA-IgG conjugate administered by the oral route (or ip) did induce suppression of both DTH and IgG antibody formation. How did orally given conjugate of OVA-IgG induce tolerance at 2 weeks of age? We postulate an active transport of the conjugate through the intestinal mucosa.

This hypothesis is based on several observations: rat, mouse, or human IgG, in contrast to IgM and IgA, have been shown to cross the intestinal membrane in 5- to 14-day-old rats.[19] IgG has been observed in transport vesicles in the intestinal epithelium of neonatal rats.[20] This uptake is an active process mediated by the Fc portion of the IgG molecule, inasmuch as an Fc receptor structurally related to MHC class I antigen has been described

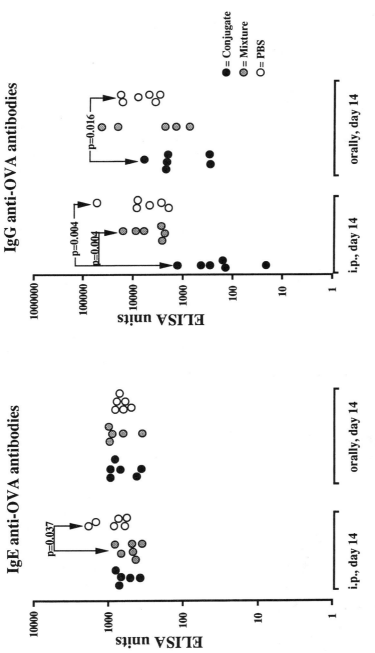
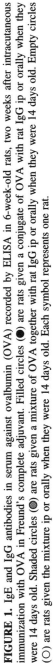

FIGURE 1. IgE and IgG antibodies in serum against ovalbumin (OVA) recorded by ELISA in 6-week-old rats, two weeks after intracutaneous immunization with OVA in Freund's complete adjuvant. Filled circles (●) are rats given a conjugate of OVA with rat IgG ip or orally when they were 14 days old. Shaded circles (◉) are rats given a mixture of OVA together with rat IgG ip or orally when they were 14 days old. Empty circles (○) are rats given the mixture ip or orally when they were 14 days old. Each symbol represents one rat.

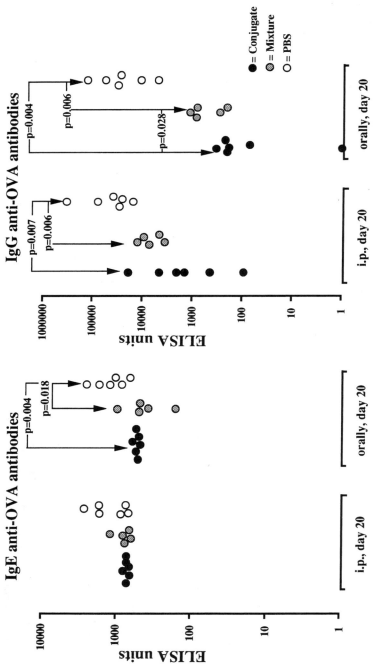

FIGURE 2. IgE and IgG antibodies in serum against ovalbumin (OVA) recorded by ELISA in 6-week-old rats, two weeks after intracutaneous immunization with OVA in Freund's complete adjuvant. Filled circles (●) are rats given the conjugate ip or orally when they were 20 days old. Shaded circles (◉) are rats given mixture ip or orally when they were 20 days old. Empty circles (○) are rats given a mixture ip or orally when they were 20 days old. Each symbol represents one rat.

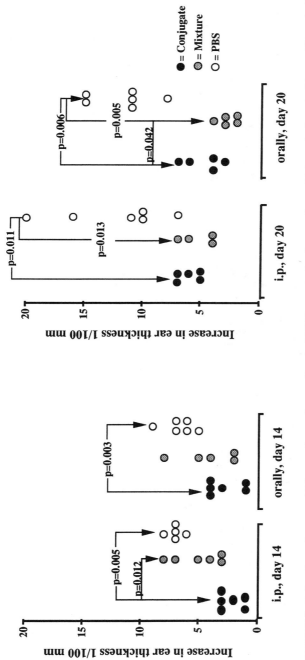

FIGURE 3. Delayed-type hypersensitivity reaction against ovalbumin (OVA) measured as increase in ear thickness in 6-week-old rats. All rats had been immunized intracutaneously with a mixture of OVA and βLG in Freund's complete adjuvant two weeks earlier. Filled circles (●) are rats given conjugate ip or orally when they were 14 or 20 days old. Shaded circles (◉) are rats given mixture ip or orally when they were 14 or 20 days old. Empty circles (○) are rats given mixture ip or orally when they were 14 or 20 days old. Each symbol represents one rat.

in the intestinal mucosa of neonatal rats.[21,22] In human placenta, an Fc receptor has been identified as an alkaline phosphatase.[23] In this regard, it is interesting to note that a single dose of 2 mg of OVA-IgG conjugate given intravenously during the last week of pregnancy in rat dams can suppress DTH to OVA in the offspring at six weeks of age (our unpublished results). Because it is known that IgG antibodies are actively transported over the placenta or intestinal mucosa in rats,[22] one can take advantage of these physiologic events in two ways for the administration of either food or airborn allergen-IgG conjugates: induce tolerance by parenteral administration of tolerogens in pregnant rats, and induce neonatal tolerance orally at birth in rats. If these findings are applicable in humans, perhaps a synergy of both therapies might be even more beneficial to prevent either cow's milk or egg allergy in atopic children. Furthermore the administration of the conjugate by gavage at birth might also reduce the dose of antigen necessary to induce oral tolerance at an age where antigen alone is ineffective.

In conclusion, these results suggest that a tolerogen made of an allergen-IgG conjugate given either by parenteral or oral route could provide a means for disease prevention in the field of allergy and autoimmunity.

REFERENCES

1. BILLINGHAM, R. E., L. BRENT & P. B. MEDAWAR. 1953. Actively acquired tolerance of foreign cells. Nature **172:** 603-606.
2. KAPPLER, J. W., N. ROEHN & P. MARRACK. 1987. T cell tolerance by clonal elimination in the thymus cell. Cell **49:** 273-280.
3. JENKINS, M. K. & R. H. SCHWARTZ. 1987. Antigen presentation by chemically modified splenocytes induces antigen specific T cell unresponsiveness *in vitro* and *in vivo*. J. Exp. Med. **165:** 302-319.
4. GERSHON, R. K. & K. KONDO. 1971. Infectious immunologic tolerance. Immunology **21:** 903-914.
5. CREMER, M. A., A. D. HERNANDEZ, A. S. TOWNES, J. M. STUART & A. H. KANG. 1983. Collagen induced arthritis in rats: antigen specific suppression of arthritis and immunity by intravenously injected native type II collagen. J. Immunol. **131:** 2995-3000.
6. WEINER, H. L., A. FRIEDMAN, A. MILLER, S. J. KHOURY, A. AL-SABBGLH, L. SANTOS, M. SAYEGH, R. B. NUSSENBLATT, D. E. TRENTHAM & D. A. HAFLER. 1994. Oral tolerance: Immunologic mechanisms and treatment of animal and organ—specific autoimmune diseases by oral administration of auto antigens. Annu. Rev. Immunol. **12:** 809-837.
7. LEE, W. A. & A. H. SEHON. 1977. Abrogation of reaginic antibodies with modified allergens. Nature **267:** 618-649.
8. KATZ, D. H., J. M. DAVIE, W. E. PAUL & B. BENACERRAF. 1971. Carrier function in antihapten antibody response. IV. Experimental conditions for the induction of hapten specific tolerance or for the stimulation of antihapten anamnestic responses by "non-immunogenic" hapten-polypeptides conjugates. J. Exp. Med. **134:** 201-203.
9. MUCKERHEIDE, A., A. J. PESCE & J. G. MICHAEL. 1977. Immunosuppressive properties of a peptic fragment of BSA. J. Immunol. **119:** 1340-1345.
10. MACHIELS, J. J., M. A. SOMVILLE, P. M. LEBRUN, S. J. LEBECQUE, M. G. JACQUEMIN & J. M. R. SAINT-REMY. 1990. Allergic bronchial asthma due to *Dermatophagoides pteronyssinus* hypersensitivity can be efficiently treated by inoculation of allergen antibody complexes. J. Clin. Invest. **85:** 1024-1035.
11. BOREL, Y. 1989. Natural immunologic tolerance and the construction of tolerogens to treat autoimmune diseases. Therapy of Autoimmune Diseases. *In* Concepts in Immunopathology. J. M. Cruse & R. E. Lewis, Eds.: 7: 145-161. Karger. Basel.
12. SEHON, A. H. 1982. Suppression of IgE antibody responses with tolerogenic conjugates of allergens and haptens. Prog. Allergy **32:** 161-202.

13. FILION, L. G., W. Y. LEE & A. H. SELON. 1980. Suppression of the IgE antibody response to ovalbumin in mice with a conjugate of ovalbumin and isologous gammaglobulins. Cell Immunol. **54:** 115-128.

14. BOREL, H. & Y. BOREL. 1990. A novel technique to link either proteins or peptides to gammaglobulin to construct tolerogens. J. Immunol. Methods **126:** 159-168.

15. FRITSCHÉ, R. & Y. BOREL. 1994. Prevention of allergic sensitization to β-lactoglobulin with conjugates made of β-lactoglobulin coupled to isologous immunoglobulin G. J. Allergy Clin. Immunol. **93:** 778-786.

16. BOREL, Y. & R. FRITSCHÉ. 1995. Induction of systemic tolerance by tolerogens. 34th Nestlé Nutrition Workshop: Intestinal Immunology and Food Allergy. **34:** 179-189. Raven Press. New York.

17. BOREL, Y., R. FRITSCHÉ, H. BOREL, U. DAHLGREN, A. DALHMAN-HÖGLUND, E. TELEMO & L. A. HANSON. 1995. Food allergens transformed into tolerogens. CIA Symposium. Nantucket. Int. Arch. Allergy Immunol. **107:** 264-267.

18. DAHLMAN, A., S. AHLSTEDT, L. A. HANSON, E. TELEMO, A. E. WOLD & U. DAHLGREN. 1992. Induction of IgE antibodies and T cell reactivity to ovalbumin in rats colonized with *Escherichia coli* genetically manipulated to produce ovalbumin. Immunology **76:** 225-228.

19. JONES, E. A. & T. A. WALDMANN. 1972. The mechanisms of intestinal uptake and transcellular transport of IgG in the neonatal rat. J. Clin. Invest. **51:** 2916-2927.

20. RODEWALD, R. & J. P. KRAEHENBUHL. 1984. Receptor mediated transport of IgG. J. Cell Biol. **99:** 159-162.

21. SIMISTER, N. E. & K. E. MOSTOV. 1989. An Fc receptor structurally related to MHC class I antigens. Nature **337:** 184-187.

22. STORY, C. M., J. E. MIKULSKA & N. E. SIMISTER. 1994. A major histocompatibility complex class I like Fc receptor cloned from human placenta: possible role in transfer of immunoglobulin G from mother to fetus. J. Exp. Med. **180:** 2377-2381.

23. MAKIYA, R. & T. STRIGBRAND. 1992. Placenta alkaline phosphatase has a binding site for the human immunoglobulin-G Fc portion. Eur. J. Biochem. **205:** 341-346.

Neonatal Oral Tolerance[a]

STEPHAN STROBEL

Division of Cell and Molecular Biology
Institute of Child Health
30 Guilford Street
London WC1N 1EH, United Kingdom

INTRODUCTION

The gastrointestinal tract of the human newborn is rapidly exposed to a wide range of bacterial, occasionally viral, and food-related antigens. The human diet consists of a multiplicity of complex animal and plant antigens, all of which are non-self antigens and, as such, potentially immunogenic. Exposure of the newborn to these antigens occurs through direct oral administration or indirectly during breast-feeding through mother's milk. The ensuing immune responses of the developing gut-associated lymphoid tissues (GALT) in the neonate have to be seen in the context of highly complex interactions between physiological functions of the mucosa and immunological interactions, which in the majority of adult rodents leads to oral tolerance (a state of specific immunological hyporesponsiveness after prior oral (mucosal) exposure). Tolerance to self and foreign antigens is acquired and maintained by thymic and peripheral events. Oral tolerance to food antigens is the paradigm for peripheral tolerance induction and is controlled by several, not mutually exclusive, immunological principles. The existence of oral tolerance is well described in laboratory rodents,[1-4] other species,[5-7] and humans.[8]

From the clinical point of view, food-sensitive diseases, such as food-induced enteropathies, and immediate[9,10] and delayed responses to foods[9,11,12] are a feature of infancy.[11,13] Despite this fact, very little is known, that is, which variables are important for the induction or failure of oral tolerance in the neonatal period. Contrary to the commonly held view that neonatal administration of antigen is particularly prone to tolerance induction (by intravenous injection of antigens or cells[14-16]), oral administration of antigen in the neonatal period is more likely to sensitize. These observations are in keeping with the results of studies in human infants where early postnatal milk exposure, especially in children from an allergic family background, has been associated with clinical reactions (*e.g.,* milk protein sensitive enteropathy, atopic eczema) to milk in later life (reviewed in refs. 17-19).

Extrapolation from results obtained in animal studies to humans and human conditions can only be made with extreme caution. Despite these caveats, evidence obtained from laboratory rodents has greatly enhanced our understanding of human immune responses, especially in those conditions where such studies would be ethically unacceptable.

[a] The work summarized in this article has been funded in major part by the following institutions whose support I gratefully acknowledge: Deutsche Forschungsgemeinschaft (DFG), Ministry of Health, R.O.C., Medical Research Council of Great Britain (MRC), and the Child Health Research Appeal Trust (CHRAT).

NEONATAL INDUCTION OF ORAL TOLERANCE IN RODENTS

Definition of the Term "Neonatal"

The term "neonatal" is not clearly defined, and rodents up to,[20] and after, the age of weaning (around 3 weeks) have been termed neonatal. Our[21-23] and other experiments in rodents[24-26] have clearly shown that the first 14 days of life are associated with rapid changes in their mucosal and systemic immune responsiveness after an antigen feed. The loose definition of "neonatal" in the literature has added to the confusion regarding the existence of neonatal tolerance versus priming after oral antigen encounter. If animals are fed during the first 3-5 days of life, systemic tolerance is generally not induced, and under certain conditions priming of subsequent immune responses is reported. To avoid confusion in the future, the exact time after birth at which the neonate is treated should be clearly stated in the protocol.

Antigens

In adult mice, virtually all investigated (mostly soluble) antigens have been shown to induce tolerance, including tolerance to skin-sensitizing agents,[27] sheep erythrocytes,[28,29] and nickel.[30] It is unclear how these observations extend to proteins with unusual mucosal binding characteristics, such as cholera toxin B and "superantigens" (see below). For the investigation of neonatal oral tolerance, hen's egg albumin (ovalbumin, OVA) and bovine serum albumin (BSA) have long been used, with the recent addition of gluten[31] and autoantigens such as myelin basic protein (MBP).[32]

Time Course

In adult rodents (*i.e.,* after weaning at ~3 weeks of age), immune suppression (deviation) affects IgG (IgG2a >> IgG1), IgE, and delayed hypersensitivity (DTH) responses very early (within 2 days) after a protein feed[33] and is well established after 7-14 days (*i.e.,* the interval between feeding and immunization as used by most investigators).

We have investigated, in a series of experiments, the immune responses of neonates after a timed and standardized feed of ovalbumin and bovine serum albumin. Neonatal animals (BALB/c) within one litter were fed a single feed of either 1 mg/g body weight antigen or saline by way of gavage and suckled by their dams. At 4 weeks of age, all animals were immunized with 100 μg of antigen emulsified in 50 μL of complete Freund's adjuvant and their IgG, and cell-mediated immune responses were measured by ELISA and a footpad swelling test.[21,22] The results of a series of experiments are summarized in FIG. 1. They demonstrate clearly that there is a transition from priming to tolerance induction at around 7-10 days of age, affecting antibody and cell-mediated responses. This is in contrast to the tolerogenic responses obtained after neonatal antigen injection (see above). Several authors have reported similar observations,[24-26] including an animal model of experimental autoimmune encephalomyelitis (EAE).[32] The authors fed MBP to neonatal rats. In parallel to the results obtained with ovalbumin, this procedure did not induce tolerance for MBP but primed for later immune responses. When these neonates were immunized after weaning with the MBP in adjuvant, they exhibited an increased disease activity.

The choice of antigen plays an important role in determining the subsequent response. Oral administration of human gamma globulin (HGG) or bovine gamma globulin to

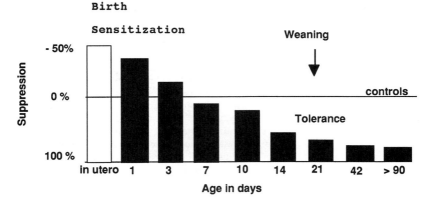

FIGURE 1. Priming and suppression after neonatal and adult antigen administration. Summary graph of a series of experiments assessing the effects of a single feed of ovalbumin (1 mg/g/ body weight) on systemic cell mediated-immune responses (delayed hypersensitivity). Ages ranged from 12 hours after birth to 3–4 months of age. Some mice had been exposed to ovalbumin *in utero* ~2 days before birth by injecting the antigen into the amniotic sac. IgG antibody responses showed a similar pattern, although the results were less consistent.

neonatal mice and rats did induce tolerance.[24,34] A possible (Fc) receptor-mediated antigen uptake could be the explanation.[35] This would also indicate that neonatal animals are principally capable of a suppressive immune response. The experimental design did not address the question of whether administration of the Fab' fragment of HGG would also be capable of immune suppression.

Weaning and Weaning Period

The amount of nutritional antigen uptake increases dramatically when breast milk is replaced by other forms of foods. At weaning there is a rapid change of intestinal morphological parameters, which are mirrored to some extent in the immunological function of the gut. Bacterial flora and antigen-driven changes include a lengthening of crypts; increases in epithelial cell kinetics, intraepithelial lymphocytes, mucosal mast cells, and eosinophils; and an increase in jejunal goblet cell numbers.[23,36–40]

We have demonstrated in mice that the weaning period leads to a short disruption of the general ease of tolerance induction in the young adult mouse (> 4 months of age). When a new antigen (OVA) was introduced (at 1 mg/g/body weight) into the weanling's diet by single gavage, systemic tolerance was reduced in those animals that were fed at the day of weaning, compared to those age-matched animals where weaning and separation from the mothers was delayed for 3 days.[21,41] These experiments did not examine the dose effect that is likely to play an important role in the inductive process.[1,42–45]

Feeding with repeated doses of 100 μg antigen every other day for 2 weeks is effective for IgG and IgE suppression. A single dose of 1 mg/mouse is suppressive for IgG and cell-mediated responses, whereas 100 μg/mouse was not, and a dose of around 10 μg/ mouse resulting in priming for cell-mediated responses.[1,45]

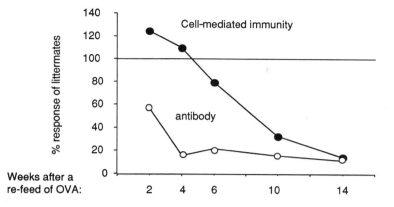

FIGURE 2. Persistence of priming. Neonatal mice at day 1 were fed ovalbumin once (1 mg/g/body weight), suckled by their dams, and re-fed with a single antigen dose after 2, 4, 6, 10, and 14 weeks. Responses are given as percent of littermates who received saline as a re-feed. The priming effects after a neonatal feed of ovalbumin were longer lasting when compared with antibody responses.

Immune Responses after Refeeding of Antigen after an Initial Sensitizing Feed in the Neonatal Period

In view of the priming observed after a single feed, it was important to identify whether repeated antigen administration within the first 14 days of life could enhance priming or would induce hyporesponsiveness. FIGURE 2 summarizes a series of experiments that demonstrate that (1) repeated antigen administrations after a sensitizing feed are capable of suppressing immune responses (DTH >> IgG), and (2) multiple feeds with the same total antigen dose as a single feed are more likely to overcome the initial priming effect.[21] A comparable dose-dependent down-regulation of immune responses in adults after immunization with antigen in adjuvant has also been demonstrated (see refs. 46 and 47).

Effects of High- and Low-dose Antigen Feeds

Whatever constitutes a high or low antigen dose in rodents has not been clearly defined. Recent reports suggest a definition on the basis of the immunoregulatory response and the underlying suppressive principles. "High" doses (> 1 mg/g/body weight) have been associated with the induction of clonal anergy and unresponsiveness of the Th1 function.[48,49]

"Low" doses (> 0.1 mg/g/body weight) are likely to generate antigen-specific regulatory (suppressor) cells after presentation through the GALT (see above). Similar observations have been made in an aerosol model of respiratory tract sensitization.[50] Aerosol-(low-dose) induced tolerance was transferable by T lymphocytes (α,β+) supporting the notion of dose-dependent induction of regulatory mechanisms.[51]

We investigated the effects of high- (1 mg/g/body weight) and low-dose (0.1 mg/g/body weight) ovalbumin administration on the development of oral tolerance as assessed by antibody- and cell-mediated immunity in earlier studies. High-dose oral tolerance, which affected antibody- and cell-mediated immunity, was not abrogated by cyclophosphamide

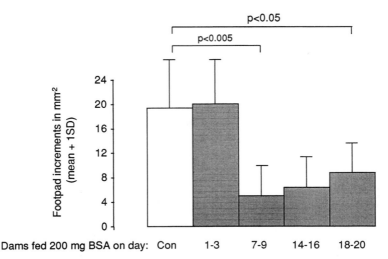

FIGURE 3. Effects of antigen transfer from breast milk. Suckling dams on an egg- and milk-free chow were fed 200 mg of BSA for a period of 3 days as indicated. Cell-mediated immunity in offspring immunized at 4 weeks of age clearly demonstrated the lack of tolerance induction when dams were fed from days 1–3. (Similar results were obtained with ovalbumin.)

injected 2 days before oral antigen administration. Cell-mediated tolerance induced with low doses of antigen (without affecting antibody suppression) could be reversed by cylophosphamide, which is believed to abrogate active suppression (elimination of cyclophosphamide/radiosensitive "suppressor" cells).[23,42,52–54] Regulatory effects differ for antibody and cell-mediated immunity and are evidence of a separate regulation of these immune responses. Similar effects have been observed in a serum transfer model of oral tolerance, adding further evidence for a regulatory "uncoupling" of antibody and cell mediated-immune responses.[55–58]

We have analyzed the effects of antigen dose during induction of neonatal tolerance in an indirect (physiological) way by maternal antigen transfer from breast milk after timed and short-term maternal feeds.

Neonatal Oral Antigen Exposure by Way of Gavage or Breast Milk

As outlined, antigen feeds by gavage lead to systemic priming of systemic immunity in neonates. Based on the clinical and epidemiological observations of a protective effect of breast milk against food-sensitive and possible autoimmune diseases in infants, it was important to investigate whether antigen administration from breast milk would have a tolerizing effect. Suckling mothers were fed for 3 days with 200 mg of ovalbumin/animal/day at several time points between giving birth and 18 days of age, that is, before weaning. Results for bovine serum albumin (BSA) are shown in FIGURE 3. Kinetics of immune responses observed after administration of antigen from breast milk were comparable to those after direct antigen administration (gavage). It has to be stressed, however, that antigen dose requirements were different. Whereas gavaged animals received 1 mg/g/body weight, suckling animals received an approximate dose of antigen that was around

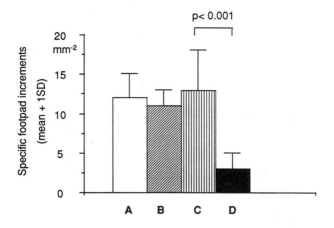

FIGURE 4. Delayed hypersensitivity response in neonates after reconstitution with adult spleen cells. Several groups of neonates received either no treatment (A) or an intraperitoneal injection of 10×10^6 spleen cells (B). In another group (C), only the dams were fed 200 mg of BSA on days 2 and 3, and a further group (D) received spleen cells 24 h prior to their dams' antigen feeds (combination of B + C). Adult spleen cell reconstitution resulted in suppression of cell-mediated immunity during a period where neonates were otherwise not susceptible to tolerance induction.

10^{-3} lower (1-10 µg/g/body weight). This is particularly interesting inasmuch as doses in this range have been associated with sensitization/priming when given directly.[45] It remains to be seen whether a similar mechanism could be the explanation for the protective effects of breast-feeding in human infants. In further attempts to delineate the underlying mechanisms, we examined whether injection of adult spleen cells at birth followed by an antigen feed from breast milk could reverse the priming effect.

Groups of neonatal animals received 10 million adult spleen cells ip on day 1, and suckling dams were fed 200 mg BSA on days 2 and 3. This was followed by an immunization 4 weeks later and measurement of immune responses *in vivo* 3 weeks after immunization (FIG. 4). Transfer of adult spleen prior to antigen transfer from breast milk cells did result in suppression of cell-mediated immunity without reducing antibody responses.[55] In several experiments, antibody responses were significantly primed. In general, all effects described here could be seen after a feed of BSA or OVA.

Mucosal Sensitization and Response to Antigen Challenge after Neonatal Antigen Administration

Priming of systemic antibody and cell mediated-immune responses after a postnatal feed of antigen (1-7 days) has been demonstrated without being able to address the question of whether priming is also seen in local mucosal cell mediated-immune responses. Using sensitive stathmokinetic techniques measuring crypt-cell turnover, we could show that a feed during the first day of life combined with a 4-week rest and a subsequent 10-day oral challenge leads to an increase in intraepithelial lymphocytes and a rise in the crypt-cell production rate, compatible with a mucosal cell mediated-immune response.[23]

A similar effect was seen after prevention of tolerance induction by administration of cyclophosphamide (100 mg/kg/body weight).[23,52]

Regulatory Mechanisms of (Neonatal) Oral Tolerance

Apart from the genetic background, the dose, frequency, and age at first antigen administration play an important part in tolerance induction. The major underlying mechanisms have been identified as clonal anergy and suppression ("immune deviation"). Whereas clonal deletion is unequivocally shown in thymic tolerance induction,[59,60] its existence in peripheral tolerance induction after oral (not intravenous injection) antigen (not superantigen) administration is less certain.[61] Recently, antigen-specific programmed cell death (apoptosis) has been suggested as a mechanism for peripheral deletion of antigen-reactive cells in (oral) tolerance.[62]

MHC Class II Expression

Clonal anergy is likely to occur when antigen is presented by "nonprofessional" antigen-presenting cells in a context of appropriate MHC antigen without a costimulatory signal by way of the CD28/CD80 pathway.[63] Mucosal epithelial cells in mature animals or adults constitutively express low levels of class II antigens on their lumenal and basolateral sides. Class II expression of enterocytes in neonatal rodents is very low/absent at around 1 week of age and increases sharply after weaning.[64] Low levels of class II expression have also been reported in human neonates.[65] The physiological role of the constitutively low MHC class II expression of enterocytes for the induction of tolerance is far from clear.

Suppressor T Cells in Oral Tolerance

Suppressor cells (Ts) have been implicated and their effects demonstrated in several models of oral tolerance either directly by cell transfer[66-69] or indirectly by eliminating cells that exert a suppressive activity.[23,42,52,54] Systemic tolerance can be transferred with Ts cells (e.g., spleen cells, CD4⁻8⁺) during the early (inductive) phase of tolerance. Spleen cells taken from animals several weeks after tolerance induction fail to suppress immune response in recipients, although, as a rule, control animals remain tolerant (ref. 70, and Strobel, unpublished observation).

Two important facts emerge from these and other reports: Suppression by Ts mainly affected cell-mediated immunity, and active cells were of the CD8⁺, TCR α^+, β^+ phenotype. The exact nature of the T-cell receptor (TCR) expressed during tolerance induction remains to be defined. Ts induced by aerosol inhalation[51] or isolated from intraepithelial lymphocytes, after administration of sheep red blood cells,[71] carry the unusual γ,δ form of the TCR. Recent reports of suppression of immune responses in CD8 knockout mice,[72] using the recombinant cholera toxin B subunit, highlight the likely existence of mutually inclusive "fail-safe mechanisms" of this fundamental immunological process.

Clonal Anergy and Suppression/Elimination of Antigen-responsive Cells

Recent studies have shown that clonal anergy and/or suppression are, to a certain extent, antigen-dose related.[43,49,73] Tolerance induction is likely to be a dynamic process, and suppressive activities at the induction stage may not be active once suppression is established. Early reports of suppressed delayed hypersensitivity responses without the presence of antigen-reactive Ts also suggest the existence of clonal anergy (silencing).[74]

Modulation of Antigen Responsiveness by Antigen Analogues

Recently antigen analogues have been used to treat or ameliorate experimental autoimmune disease.[75] These studies were designed to test the idea that a non-(encephalitogenic) peptide could compete with a disease-inducing peptide for binding to the same MHC restriction element. There is, however, also evidence that the effect may not be simply due to MHC blockade and that there is an antigen-specific component as well (review in ref. 75).

Tolerance and Cytokines

Preferential induction of certain cytokines may be of critical importance in the regulation and induction of oral tolerance. Investigation of cytokine secretion in bulk cultures may be misleading in view of the general low frequency of circulating antigen-reactive cells.[76,77] The dissociation of humoral-antibody suppression from suppression of cell-mediated immunity, a variable effect on mucosal IgA responses (suppressed or unaffected), make immunoregulatory involvement of cytokines in the mucosal microenvironment likely. Weiner's group suggests that T(s) in vitro (from rats primed in vivo with MBP) inhibit responses of primed T cells, including those to a third party antigen (bystander suppression). The active cytokine was identified as TGF-beta.[78]

While investigating the role of bystander suppression in a model of experimental autoimmune uveitis (EAU), it was recently shown that bystander suppression was observed in the periphery (hind leg), whereas the acute inflammation of the eye, the target organ, was not affected.[79] In autoimmune diseases that have a more chronic course (e.g., arthritis, diabetes), pathogenic cells are constantly generated and could still be the target for suppressor cells at the site of inflammation. Interferon-γ and in vivo depletion of IL-4 can reduce delayed hypersensitivity responses in mice. Injection of high doses of monoclonal anti-IL4 antibodies (20 mg) was able to suppress IgE responses in mice infected with Nippostrongylus brasiliensis,[80] whereas a dose of 1-2 mg failed to do so. It has been shown that mouse T-helper cells can be divided (according to their cytokine secretion pattern) into Th1 (e.g., IL-2, IFN-γ) and Th2 (e.g., IL-4, IL-5, IL10) cells. The importance of the Th2 response for tolerance induction has been suggested by several authors (review in refs. 4 and 81). Reviewing the published evidence, there is, however, no doubt that antigen feeds suppress IgG (IgG2a), delayed hypersensitivity, and IgE responses and as such are affecting both Th1 and Th2 immunoregulatory pathways. However sophisticated the in vitro methodology for analysis of tolerance might be, it cannot control or allow for the local mucosal cytokine microenvironment. Results obtained in vitro should be confirmed with in vivo functional analysis.

Intestinal Antigen Processing and Induction of Tolerance

Absorption of small amounts of immunologically intact whole proteins into the circulation is a common occurrence in humans[82] and rodents.[56] There is now substantial evidence that antigen processing by the GALT is critical for tolerance induction. In a series of experiments, we and others have demonstrated that serum removed from the circulation

TABLE 1. Experimental Conditions That Affect the Generation of a Transferable Tolerogenic Fragment(s) after Adoptive Serum Transfer

Experimental condition for mice injected ip[a]	Effects on delayed hypersensitivity responses after adoptive transfer into BALB/c
Antigen collected after 5 minutes	not suppressive
Antigen collected after 60 minutes	suppressive
Antigen collected from BALB/c mice after lethal (100 Gy) irradiation	not suppressive
Antigen collected 4 days after lethal irradiation and immediate spleen cell reconstitution	suppressive
Serum spiked with native antigen	not suppressive
Antigen collected after 5 and 60 minutes from SCID[b] mice	not suppressive
Antigen collected after 60 min from outbred mice (Swiss)	suppressive
Antigen (iv[c]) injected into mice and collected after 60 min	not suppressive
Antigen injected ip and collected after 60 min	not suppressive
Serum spiked with native antigen and vortexed for 60 min at 37°C	not suppressive

[a] ip, intraperitoneal.
[b] SCID, severe combined immunodeficient.
[c] iv, intravenous.

1 hour after a feed of a soluble protein antigen and ip injected into naive recipients is likely to suppress delayed hypersensitivity responses in the recipient (TABLE 1).[56–58,83,84] Retrieval of antigen after short-term "processing" (< 5 minutes) failed to suppress delayed hypersensitivity responses in recipient mice after adoptive transfer.[56] It is unknown whether the intestinal epithelium or the local lymphoid tissues (or both) are the site of processing. Further experiments have shown that a functional gut-associated lymphoid immune system is a necessary requirement to generate the active ovalbumin-derived moiety inasmuch as animals with irradiation-induced damage and severe-combined immunodeficient mice fail to generate such a "tolerogen".[83,85] The tolerogenic material can be detected in the circulation after 20-30 minutes; it can be eluted from the serum by anti-ovalbumin-affinity chromatography without losing its activity. The tolerogenic activity in a series of experiments has been associated with the occurrence of a 21-24 kDa peptide on SDS-PAGE analysis.[86] It seems unlikely that simple filtration or deaggregation of ovalbumin are responsible for this observation, especially in view of a lack of correlation with circulating immunoreactive amounts of antigen.[56] Furthermore, (1) iv injection of antigen and retrieval from the circulation[47,87] as well as (2) intraperitoneal filtration and "processing," retrieval, and injection into recipients fail to suppress a delayed hypersensitivity response in recipients (Furrie and Strobel, unpublished observation). Subtle conformational changes or changes in charge may be responsible for this activity. Luminal proteolytic digestion seems not to be essential for the induction of tolerance,[49] (Strobel unpublished, and FIGURE 5) although this point remains currently controversial.[88]

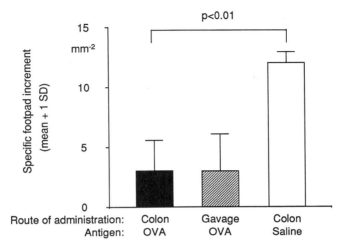

FIGURE 5. Suppression of cell-mediated immunity after administration of ovalbumin *per rectum*. Administration of ovalbumin rectally (1 mg/g/body weight) was as effective in suppressing cell-mediated immunity as an oral gavage (p < 0.01). Antibody responses were similarly suppressed (p < 0.01, not shown).

Antigen Presentation

The role of antigen presentation has been investigated by several groups.[1,22,64,89,90] Activity and the nature of antigen-presenting cells appear to be critical in modulating the immunological response after antigen feeding. Conditions and substances known to affect the reticuloendothelial system, such as graft-versus-host disease, injection of the adjuvant muramyl dipeptide at the time of feeding, estrogen administration, injection of interferon-γ, or feeding a second antigen shortly after administration of the first[91] have all been shown to interfere with tolerance induction.

CONCLUSION AND SUMMARY

Investigations into the underlying mechanism of neonatal oral tolerance in rodents have demonstrated that antigen administration directly after birth or within 5–7 days does not lead to suppression of systemic immunity but primes for subsequent humoral and at times delayed hypersensitivity responses. This contrasts the effects seen after neonatal iv injection of cells or soluble antigens. Antigen transfer from breast milk induces tolerance in the young; however, the antigen dose required for tolerance induction is 2–3 log steps lower. It remains to be seen whether the inability of the neonatal rodent to be tolerized by the oral route is related to a lack of antigen-processing capacity of the GALT or an underlying immunological immaturity. Some results would support the latter possibility because tolerance for delayed hypersensitivity can be reestablished within 24 hours after the injection of syngeneic, naive adult spleen cells (see Fig. 4). Intestinal epithelial cells may be involved in the presentation of antigen in a suppressive way in postweanling rodents and humans. It remains to be seen whether mucosal epithelial class II expression, which is low in the early neonatal period, plays a role in the inability of the neonatal rodent to be tolerized to antigens whose uptake is not receptor mediated. Indeed, IFN-γ, a cytokine also known to increase class II expression on enterocytes is associated with prevention of tolerance induction.[92]

Further elucidation of the cytokine pathways involved in the generation of tolerance by immune deviation (suppression, peptide antagonists), clonal anergy, and possible peripheral deletion (*e.g.,* antigen-specific apoptosis *in vivo?*) are certainly needed to understand a major immunological principle and to develop it for successful use in human allergic and autoimmune diseases.

REFERENCES

1. MOWAT, A. M. 1987. The regulation of immune responses to dietary antigen. Immunol. Today **8:** 93-98.
2. STROBEL, S. 1993. Food allergy-role of mucosal immune regulation and oral tolerance: facts, fiction, and hypotheses. *In* Immunophysiology of the gut. W. A. Walker, P. R. Harmatz & B. K. Wershil, Ed.: 336-357. Academic Press, San Diego. V. Moreno, Ed. Brystol Meyers/Squibb/Mead Johnson Nutrition Sumposia).
3. STROBEL, S. 1992. Dietary manipulation and induction of tolerance. J. Pediatr. **121:** S74-79.
4. WEINER, H. L., A. FRIEDMAN, A. MILLER, *et al.* 1994. Oral tolerance: immunologic mechanisms and treatment of animal and human organ-specific autoimmune diseases by oral administration of autoantigens. Annu. Rev. Immunol. **12:** 809-838.
5. PERI, B. A. & R. M. ROTHBERG. 1987. Mucosal immunity and tolerance in neonatal rabbits. Adv. Exp. Med. Biol.
6. WEAVER, L. T., T. N. KORITZ & R. R. COOMBS. 1987. Tolerance to orally induced anaphylactic sensitization to cow's milk proteins and patency of the intestinal mucosa in the neonatal guinea pig. Int. Arch. Allergy Appl. Immunol. **83:** 220-2.
7. HEPPEL, L. M. & P. J. KILSHAW. 1982. Immune responses in guinea pigs to dietary protein. I. Induction of tolerance by feeding ovalbumin. Int. Arch. Allergy Appl. Immunol. **68:** 54-61.
8. HUSBY, S., J. MESTECKY, Z. MOLDOVEANU, S. HOLLAND & C. O. ELSON. 1994. Oral tolerance in humans. T cell but not B cell tolerance after antigen feeding. J. Immunol. **152:** 4663-70.
9. HILL, D. J., R. P. FORD, M. J. SHELTON & C. S. HOSKING. 1984. A study of 100 infants and young children with cow's milk allergy. Clin. Rev. Allergy **2:** 125-42.
10. PASTORELLO, E. A., V. PRAVETTONI, A. BIGI, *et al.* 1987. IgE-mediated food allergy. Ann. Allergy. **59.**
11. WALKER-SMITH, J. A. 1988. Diseases of the small intestine in childhood (3rd ed.). Butterworths, London:
12. KUITUNEN, P., J. V. VISAKORPI, E. SAVILAHTI & P. PELKONEN. 1975. Malabsorption syndrome with cows' milk intolerance. Clinical findings and course in 54 cases. Arch. Dis. Child. **50:** 351-356.
13. STROBEL, S. 1993. Epidemiology of food sensitivity in childhood—with special reference to cow's milk allergy in infancy. Monogr. Allergy. **31.**
14. EID, A., S. MORECKI & S. SLAVIN. 1988. Induction of transplantation tolerance by intraportal injection of allogeneic bone marrow cells. Possible implications for intrauterine bone marrow transplantation across major histocompatibility barriers. Transplant. Int. **1:** 109-12.
15. IDEYAMA, S., M. HOSONO, S. IMAMURA, M. TOMANA & Y. KATSURA. 1991. Intrathymic induction of neonatal tolerance to Mls-1a determinant: clonal deletion and clonal anergy by haematolymphoid cells. Immunology **74:** 240-5.

16. VEGH, P., L. BARANY & T. JANOSSY. 1990. Induction of transplantation tolerance and development of lymphomas in mice: lack of interdependence. Cell. Immunol. **129:** 56-66.

17. American Academy of Pediatrics Committee on Nutrition: Hypoallergenic Infant Formulas. 1989. Pediatrics **83:** 1068-9.

18. AGGETT, P. J., F. HASCHKE, W. HEINE, et al. 1993. Comment on antigen-reduced infant formulae. ESPGAN Committee on Nutrition. Acta Paediatr. **82:** 314-9.

19. BUSINCO, L., S. DREBORG, R. EINARSSON, et al. 1993. Hydrolysed cow's milk formulae: Allergenicity and use for treatment and prevention. An ESPACI position paper. Pediatr. Allerg. Immunol. **3:** 101-111.

20. PEPPARD, J. V. 1992. Feeding neonatal rats with IgG antibodies leads to humoral hyporesponsiveness in the adult. Immunology **77:** 256-61.

21. STROBEL, S. & A. FERGUSON. 1984. Immune responses to fed protein antigens in mice. 3. Systemic tolerance or priming is related to age at which antigen is first encountered. Pediatr. Res. **18:** 588-94.

22. STROBEL, S., A. M. MOWAT & A. FERGUSON. 1985. Prevention of oral tolerance induction to ovalbumin and enhanced antigen presentation during a graft-versus-host reaction in mice. Immunology **56:** 57-64.

23. STROBEL, S. & A. FERGUSON. 1986. Modulation of intestinal and systemic immune responses to a fed protein antigen, in mice. Gut **27:** 829-37.

24. HANSON, D. G. 1981. Ontogeny of orally induced tolerance to soluble proteins in mice. I. Priming and tolerance in newborns. J. Immunol. **127:** 1518-1524.

25. TELEMO, E., I. JAKOBSSON, B. R. WESTROM & H. FOLKESSON. 1987. Maternal dietary antigens and the immune response in the offspring of the guinea-pig. Immunology **62:** 35-8.

26. TRONCONE, R. & A. FERGUSON. 1988. In mice, gluten in maternal diet primes systemic immune responses to gliadin in offspring. Immunology **64:** 533-7.

27. ASHERSON, G. L., M. A. PERERA, W. R. THOMAS & M. ZEMBALA. 1979. Contact-sensitizing agents and the intestinal tract: the production of immunity and unresponsiveness by feeding contact-sensitizing agents and the role of suppressor cells. In Immunology of breast milk. Raven Press. New York.

28. KAGNOFF, M. F. 1980. Effects of antigen feeding on intestinal and systemic immune responses. IV. Similarity between the suppressor factor in mice after erythrocyte-lysate injection and erythrocyte feeding. Gastroenterology **79:** 54-61.

29. DAVID, M. F. 1977. Prevention of homocytotropic antibody formation and anaphylactic sensitisation by prefeeding antigens. J. Allergy. Clin. Immunol. **60:** 180-187.

30. VAN HOOGSTRATEN, I. M., D. BODEN, M. E. VON BLOMBERG, G. KRAAL & R. J. SCHEPER. 1992. Persistent immune tolerance to nickel and chromium by oral administration prior to cutaneous sensitization. J. Invest. Dermatol. **99:** 608-16.

31. TRONCONE, R. & A. FERGUSON. 1988. Gliadin presented via the gut induces oral tolerance in mice. Clin. Exp. Immunol. **72:** 284-7.

32. MILLER, A., O. LIDER, O. ABRAMSKY & H. L. WEINER. 1994. Orally administered myelin basic protein in neonates primes for immune responses and enhances experimental autoimmune encephalomyelitis in adult animals. Eur. J. Immunol. **24:** 1026-32.

33. CHALLACOMBE, S. J. & T. B. J. TOMASI. 1980. Systemic tolerance and secretory immunity after oral immunization. J. Exp. Med. **152:** 1459-72.

34. BURTLES, S. S. & D. C. HOOPER. 1992. The effect of neonatal tolerance to bovine gamma globulin (BGG) on BGG-reactive CD4+ T lymphocytes. Immunology **72:** 311-7.

35. BRAMBELL, F. W., W. A. HEMMINGS, C. L. OAKLEY & P. P. PORTER. 1960. The relative transmission of the fractions of papain hydrolysed homologous γ-globulin from the uterine cavity to the foetal circulation in the rabbit. Proc. R. Soc. (Biol.) **151:** 478-482.

36. MOREAU, M. C. & G. CORTHIER. 1988. Effect of the gastrointestinal microflora on induction and maintenance of oral tolerance to ovalbumin in C3H/HeJ mice. Infect. Immun. **56:** 2766-8.

37. MOWAT, A. M., A. BORLAND & D. M. V. PARROTT. 1986. The delayed type hypersensitivity reaction in the small intestine. VII. Induction of the intestine phase of the murine graft versus host reaction by Lyt 2-T cells activated by I-A alloantigens. Transplantation **41:** 192-198.

38. TRONCONE, R. & A. FERGUSON. 1991. Animal model of gluten induced enteropathy in mice. Gut **32:** 871-5.

39. FERGUSON, A. 1987. Models of immunologically-driven small intestinal damage. *In* Immunopathology of the small intestine. N. Marsh, Ed.: 225-252. John Wiley and Sons. Chichester.

40. STROBEL, S. 1990. Immunologically mediated damage to the intestinal mucosa. Acta Paediatr. Scand. Suppl. 365.

41. STROBEL, S. 1984. Modulation of the immune response to fed antigens in mice. [Doctoral Dissertation] Edinburgh.

42. STROBEL, S., A. M. MOWAT, H. E. DRUMMOND, M. G. PICKERING & A. FERGUSON. 1983. Immunological responses to fed protein antigens in mice. II. Oral tolerance for CMI is due to activation of cyclophosphamide-sensitive cells by gut-processed antigen. Immunology **49:** 451-6.

43. GREGERSON, D. S., W. F. OBRITSCH & L. A. DONOSO. 1993. Oral tolerance in experimental autoimmune uveoretinitis. Distinct mechanisms of resistance are induced by low dose vs. high dose feeding protocols. J. Immunol. **151:** 5751-61.

44. MELAMED, D. & A. FRIEDMAN. 1993. Modification of the immune response by oral tolerance: antigen requirements and interaction with immunogenic stimuli. Cell Immunol. **146:** 412-20.

45. LAMONT, A. G., A. M. MOWAT & D. M. PARROTT. 1989. Priming of systemic and local delayed-type hypersensitivity responses by feeding low doses of ovalbumin to mice. Immunology **66:** 595-9.

46. LAMONT, A. G., M. G. BRUCE, K. C. WATRET & A. FERGUSON. 1988. Suppression of an established DTH response to ovalbumin in mice by feeding antigen after immunization. Immunology **64:** 135-9.

47. PENG, H. J., M. W. TURNER & S. STROBEL. 1989. The kinetics of oral hyposensitisation to a protein antigen are determined by immune status and the timing, dose and frequency of antigen administration. Immunology **67:** 425-431.

48. MELAMED, D. & A. FRIEDMAN. 1994. *In vivo* tolerization of Th1 lymphocytes following a single feeding with ovalbumin: anergy in the absence of suppression. Eur. J. Immunol. **24:** 1974-81.

49. WHITACRE, C. C., I. E. GIENAPP, C. G. OROSZ & D. M. BITAR. 1991. Oral tolerance in experimental autoimmune encephalomyelitis. III. Evidence for clonal anergy. J. Immunol. **147:** 2155-63.

50. HOLT, P. G. 1993. Regulation of antigen-presenting cell function(s) in lung and airway tissues. Eur. Respir. J. **6:** 120-9.

51. MCMENAMIN, C., B. CHILNA & P. G. HOLT. 1993. Phenotypic and functional analysis of mucosal T cells isolated from tissue explants of rat upper respiratory tract. J. Immunol. Methods **160:** 219-26.

52. MOWAT, A. M. & A. FERGUSON. 1981. Hypersensitivity in the small intestinal mucosa. V. Induction of cell-mediated immunity to a dietary antigen. Clin. Exp. Immunol. **43:** 574-82.

53. MOWAT, A. M., S. STROBEL, H. E. DRUMMOND & A. FERGUSON. 1982. Immunological responses to fed protein antigens in mice. I. Reversal of oral tolerance to ovalbumin by cyclophosphamide. Immunology **45:** 105-13.

54. HOYNE, G. F., M. G. CALLOW, J. KUHLMAN & W. R. THOMAS. 1993. T-cell lymphokine response to orally administered proteins during priming and unresponsiveness. Immunology **78:** 534-40.

55. PENG, H. J., M. W. TURNER & S. STROBEL. 1989. Failure to induce oral tolerance to protein antigens in neonatal mice can be corrected by transfer of adult spleen cells. Pediatr. Res. 26: 486-90.

56. PENG, H. J., M. W. TURNER & S. STROBEL. 1990. The generation of a 'tolerogen' after the ingestion of ovalbumin is time-dependent and unrelated to serum levels of immunoreactive antigen. Clin. Exp. Immunol. 81: 510-5.

57. LAMONT, A. G., M. GORDON & A. FERGUSON. 1987. Oral tolerance in protein-deprived mice. II. Evidence of normal 'gut processing' of ovalbumin, but suppressor cell deficiency, in deprived mice. Immunology 61: 339-43.

58. BRUCE, M. G. & A. FERGUSON. 1986. Oral tolerance to ovalbumin in mice: studies of chemically modified and 'biologically filtered' antigen. Immunology 57: 627-30.

59. MOUNTZ, J. D., H. BLUETHMANN, T. ZHOU & J. WU. 1994. Defective clonal deletion and anergy induction in TCR transgenic lpr/lpr mice. Semin. Immunol. 6: 27-37.

60. ZACHARCHUK, C. M., M. MERCEP, C. H. JUNE, A. M. WEISSMAN & J. D. ASHWELL. 1991. Variations in thymocyte susceptibility to clonal deletion during ontogeny. Implications for neonatal tolerance. J. Immunol. 147: 460-5.

61. SPRENT, J. & S. R. WEBB. 1995. Intrathymic and extrathymic clonal deletion of T cells. Curr. Opinion Immunol. 7: 196-205.

62. LIBLAU, R. S., C. I. PEARSON, K. SHOKAT, R. TISCH, X-D. YANG & H. O. McDEVITT. 1994. High-dose soluble antigen: peripheral T-cell proliferation or apoptosis. Immunol. Rev. 142: 193-208.

63. BOUSSIOTIS, V. A., J. G. GRIBBEN, G. J. FREEMAN & L. M. NADLER. 1994. Blockade of the CD28 co-stimulatory pathway: a means to induce tolerance. Curr. Opin. Immunol. 6: 797-807.

64. BLAND, P. W. & L. G. WARREN. 1986. Antigen presentation by epithelial cells of the rat small intestine. II. Selective induction of suppressor T cells. Immunology 58: 9-14.

65. BRANDTZAEG, P., T. S. HALSTENSEN, H. S. HUITFELDT, P. KRAJČI, D. KUALE, H. SCOTT & P. S. THRANE. 1992. Epithelial expression of HLA, secretory component (poly-Ig receptor), and adhesion molecules in the human alimentary tract. Ann. N.Y. Acad. Sci. 664: 157-179.

66. LIDER, O., L. M. SANTOS, C. S. LEE, P. J. HIGGINS & H. L. WEINER. 1989. Suppression of experimental autoimmune encephalomyelitis by oral administration of myelin basic protein. II. Suppression of disease and in vitro immune responses is mediated by antigen-specific CD8+ T lymphocytes. J. Immunol. 142: 748-52.

67. MOWAT, A. M. 1985. The role of antigen recognition and suppressor cells in mice with oral tolerance to ovalbumin. Immunology 56: 253-60.

68. THOMAS, H. C. & D. PARROTT. 1974. The induction of tolerance to a soluble protein antigen. Immunology 27: 631-639.

69. THOMPSON, H. S. & N. A. STAINES. 1990. Could specific oral tolerance be a therapy for autoimmune disease? Immunol. Today 11: 396-9.

70. RICHMAN, L. K., A. S. GRAEFF, R. YARCHOAN & W. STROBER. 1981. Simultaneous induction of antigen-specific IgA helper T cells and IgG suppressor T cells in the murine Peyer's patch after antigen feeding. J. Immunol. 126: 2079-2083.

71. FUJIHASHI, K., T. TAGUCHI, W. K. AICHER et al. 1992. Immunoregulatory functions for murine intraepithelial lymphocytes: gamma/delta T cell receptor-positive (TCR+) T cells abrogate oral tolerance, while alpha/beta TCR+ T cells provide B cell help. J. Exp. Med. 175: 696-707.

72. SUN, J. B., J. HOLMGREN & C. CZERKINSKY. 1994. Cholera toxin B subunit: an efficient transmucosal carrier-delivery system for induction of peripheral immunological tolerance (see comments). Proc. Natl. Acad. Sci. USA 91: 10795-9.

73. MELAMED, D. & A. FRIEDMAN. 1983. Direct evidence for anergy in T lymphocytes tolerized by oral administration of ovalbumin. Eur. J. Immunol. 23: 935-42.

74. HANSON, D. G. & S. D. MILLER. 1982. Inhibition of specific immune responses by feeding protein antigens. V. Induction of the tolerant state in the absence of specific suppressor cells. J. Immunol. **128:** 2378-2381.

75. SETTE, A., J. ALEXANDER, J. RUPPERT et al. 1994. Antigen analogs/MHC complexes as specific T cell receptor antagonists. Annu. Rev. Immunol. **12:** 63-84.

76. WENNERAS, C., A. M. SVENNERHOLM & C. CZERKINSKY. 1994. Vaccine-specific T cells in human peripheral blood after oral immunization with an inactivated enterotoxigenic *Escherichia coli* vaccine. Infect. Immun. **62:** 874-9.

77. ISOLAURI, E., H. SUOMALAINEN, M. J. T. KAILA, E. SOPPI, E. VIRTANEN & H. ARVILOMMI. 1992. Local immune response in patients with cow's milk allergy: follow up of patients retaining allergy or becoming tolerant. J. Pediatr. **120:** 9-15.

78. SANTOS, L. M., A. AL SABBAGH, A. LONDONO & H. L. WEINER. 1994. Oral tolerance to myelin basic protein induces regulatory TGF-beta-secreting T cells in Peyer's patches of SJL mice. Cell. Immunol. **157:** 439-47.

79. WILDNER, G. & S. R. THURAU. 1995. Orally induced bystander suppression in experimental autoimmune uveoretinitis occurs only in the periphery and not in the eye. Eur. J. Immunol. **25:** 1292-1297.

80. FINKELMAN, F. D., I. M. J. U. KATONA, G. M. SNAPPER, J. OHARA & W. E. PAUL. 1986. Suppression of *in vivo* polyclonal IgE responses by monoclonal antibody to the lymphokine, BSF1. Proc. Natl. Acad. Sci. USA **83:** 9675-9678.

81. MOSMAN, T. R. & R. L. COFFMAN. 1989. Th1 and Th2 cells: different patterns of cytokine excretion lead to different functional properties. Annu. Rev. Immunol. **7:** 145-173.

82. HUSBY, S., J. C. JENSENIUS & S. E. SVEHAG. 1985. Passage of undegraded dietary antigen into the blood of healthy adults. Quantification, estimation of size distribution and relation of uptake levels of specific antibodies. Scand. J. Immunol. **22:** 83-92.

83. BRUCE, M. G., S. STROBEL, D. G. HANSON & A. FERGUSON. 1987. Transferable tolerance for cell mediated immunity after feeding is prevented by radiation damage and restored by immune reconstitution. Clin. Exp. Immunol. **70:** 611-618.

84. TRONCONE, R., K. ZIEGLER, S. STROBEL & A. FERGUSAN. 1993. Gliadin, intestinal hypersensitivity, and food protein-sensitive enteropathy. *In* Nutrient modulation of the immune response. S. Cunningham-Rundles, Ed.: 319-337. Marcel Dekker, Inc. New York.

85. FURRIE, E., M. W. TURNER & S. STROBEL. 1994. Scid mice fail to generate a tolerogen after feeding of ovalbumin: the role for a functioning GALT in oral tolerance induction. Immunology **83:** 562-567.

86. FURRIE, E., M. W. TURNER & S. STROBEL. 1995. Partial characterization of a circulating tolerogenic moiety which, after a feed of ovalbumin, suppresses delayed hypersensitivity in recipient mice. Immunology **86:** In press.

87. PENG, H. J. 1989. Regulation of systemic immune responses to fed proteins in mice. Doctor of Philosophy. London.

88. HANSON, D. G., M. J. ROY, G. M. GREEN & S. D. MILLER. 1993. Inhibition of orally-induced immune tolerance in mice by prefeeding an endopeptidase inhibitor. Reg. Immunol. **5:** 76-84.

89. ZHANG, Z. & J. G. MICHAEL. 1990. Orally inducible unresponsiveness is abrogated by IFN-γ treatment. J. Immunol. **144:** 4163-4165.

90. MAYER, L., A. PANJA, Y. LI, E. SIDEN, A. PIZZIMENTI, F. GERARDI & N. CHANDSWANG. 1992. Unique features of antigen presentation in the intestine. Ann. N.Y. Acad. Sci. **664:** 39-46.

91. STOKES, C. R., T. NEWBY & F. J. BOURNE. 1983. The influence of oral immunization on local and systemic immune responses to heterologous antigens. Clin. Exp. Med. **52:** 399-406.

92. ZHANG, Z. Y. & J. G. MICHAEL. 1990. Orally inducible immune unresponsiveness is abrogated by IFN-gamma treatment. J. Immunol. **144:** 4163-5.

Induction of Anergy in Th1 Lymphocytes by Oral Tolerance

Importance of Antigen Dosage and Frequency of Feeding

AHARON FRIEDMAN

Department of Animal Sciences
Hebrew University of Jerusalem
P.O. Box 12
Rehovot 76100 Israel

ORAL TOLERANCE IS A FORM OF ANTIGEN-DRIVEN PERIPHERAL TOLERANCE

Cells of the acquired (clonotypic) immune system undergo a series of processes that prevent reactivity to self-antigens; the outcome of these processes is a state of immune tolerance (*i.e.,* immunological unresponsiveness) to self.[1,2] Immunologic tolerance is not programmed into the germline but is acquired during maturation of the immune system by mechanisms that delete or inactivate antigen-reactive lymphocyte clones; there are three basic mechanisms to explain antigen-driven tolerance: clonal deletion,[3,4] clonal anergy,[5–8] and active or cytokine-mediated suppression.[9] Tolerance of T lymphocytes is acquired in the thymus and peripheral (postthymic or extrathymic) environments, and tolerance of B lymphocytes is acquired in bone marrow as well as the periphery.[9–12] Peripheral tolerance is of major importance for protection of self, inasmuch as many antigens (self and those absorbed by the gut) are not encountered in the thymus or bone marrow.[10–13]

Oral tolerance follows the exogenous administration of antigen to the peripheral immune system by way of the gut (see refs. 14 and 15 for extensive reviews). As such, it is a form of antigen-driven peripheral immune tolerance. Achievement of peripheral tolerance by feeding has been known for over a 100 years[10,16] and is considered to be a biologically relevant pathway for inducing peripheral tolerance against dietary antigens.[14] Induction of oral tolerance to external antigens may be experimentally demonstrated by feeding a protein antigen in solution and by testing immune responsiveness directed against the same antigen after parenteral immunization.[10,14,17] Similar results may be obtained by the inhalation of aerosolized antigen or antigen "dust."[18,19] The unresponsive state obtained by feeding or inhaling antigen is antigen specific, systemic, and mediated by T lymphocytes.[14,15] Other factors such as age,[20] genetic background,[21,22] and nutritional status[23] were also shown to be important for induction of tolerance.

ANERGY IS A MECHANISM FOR ORAL TOLERANCE

The primary mechanisms associated with oral tolerance are anergy and cytokine-mediated suppression,[14,15] although there is little evidence that orally administered antigen induces clonal deletion. Because anergy and cytokine-mediated suppression were demon-

TABLE 1. Anergy- or Cytokine-mediated Suppression Are Determined by Antigen Dosage and Frequency of Feeding[27]

Feeding Regimen	Characteristics of Oral Tolerance
Single high dose (20 mg/ feeding)	1. Anergy—responsive to culture in rIL-2. 2. Low levels of TGF-β. 3. No suppression of antigen-specific proliferation.
Multiple low doses (1-5 μg/feeding—5 intermittent feedings)	1. No anergy—nonresponsive to culture in rIL-2. 2. High levels of TGF-β. 2. Suppression of antigen-specific proliferation.

strated independently,[24-26] we combined efforts to define conditions delineating between the two.[27] Our studies clearly indicated that both mechanisms were not mutually exclusive and could be coexpressed. It became apparent that the dominant mechanism was not determined by inherent properties of the immune system, but rather by external parameters, particularly antigen dosage and frequency of feeding.[27] Thus, single high doses (20 mg/ mouse) of ovalbumin (OVA) or hen egg lysozyme (HEL) induced a state of tolerance characterized mainly by anergy, whereas multiple small dosages (1-5 μg/mouse/feeding) of these antigens induced a state of tolerance characterized mainly by suppression (TABLE 1).

Evidence supporting suppression as a mechanism for oral tolerance will be reviewed elsewhere (see paper by Chen *et al.,* this volume), and the remainder of this article will present evidence for anergy as a mechanism for oral tolerance, particularly in Th1 lymphocytes. Anergy is defined as a state of T-lymphocyte unresponsiveness, characterized by absence of proliferation, IL-2 production, and diminished expression of IL-2R.[28,29] Anergic T lymphocytes were shown to have a defect in the antigen-induced transcription of the IL-2 gene,[30] which could be overcome by exposure to exogenous IL-2.[28] Thus, anergy may be experimentally differentiated from clonal deletion by demonstrating the presence of antigen-specific TcR clonotypes, or by release from the anergic state, which is accomplished by preculture of cells in IL-2.

To investigate the level of tolerance generated *in vivo* by a single feeding of antigen, we studied production of OVA-specific Th1- and Th2-dependent immune responses. A single feeding of 20 mg/mouse of OVA resulted in selective tolerization of Th1-type responses and intact Th2-type responses as detected by antibody production *in vivo* (IgG1 and IgG2) and by cytokine production *in vitro* (IL-2, IFNγ, and IL-4) (TABLE 2). Tolerance was also confirmed by frequency analysis of OVA-specific IL-2-producing cells; the frequency estimates of IL-2-producing cells for OVA-fed mice were $\frac{1}{412000}$ (95% confidence limits = $\frac{1}{187000}$-$\frac{1}{980000}$), as compared to $\frac{1}{6000}$ (95% confidence limits = $\frac{1}{1500}$-$\frac{1}{19000}$) in control-immunized mice. Hence, a single-feeding regimen induces selective Th1 tolerance with intact Th2 responses;[31] in fact, Th2 responses might even be elevated under these conditions as indicated by (1) increased IL-4 gene expression in mice tolerant for hen egg white lysozyme,[32] (2) up-regulation of IL-4 in brains of rats fed myelin-basic protein prior to induction of EAE,[33] and (3) increased secretion of IL-4 by spleen cells of lysozyme or OVA-fed mice[27] (Melamed and Friedman, unpublished observations). However, tolerance

TABLE 2. Effects of a Single Feeding on Generation of Oral Tolerance[31]

Parameter	Assay	Response[a]	
		Controls	Tolerant
Antibody production	IgG2a	++++	−
	IgG1	++++	+++
Cytokine secretion	IL-2	++++	−
	IFN-γ	++++	−
	IL-4	++++	+++

[a] ++++, maximal response; +++, slightly less than maximal; −, no response.

can be extended to include Th2-type responses by increasing the length of time mice are exposed to high antigen dosages (Melamed et al., submitted for publication).

To investigate whether tolerized Th1 lymphocytes were in a state of anergy, we reversed the anergic state by culturing lymphocytes in the presence of recombinant IL-2 (rIL-2).[24] Cells recovered from these cultures were used for frequency analysis of IL-2-producing cells, cytokine production (see below), or adoptive cell transfer.

Culture of tolerant popliteal lymph node cells with rIL-2 significantly increased their ability to secrete both IL-2 and IFNγ specifically in response to OVA (TABLE 3). Limiting-dilution analysis of IL-2-producing T lymphocytes showed the following frequency estimates of IL-2-producing cells: for OVA-fed mice, $\frac{1}{5,500}$ (95% confidence limits = $\frac{1}{2,200}$-$\frac{1}{15,900}$); for mice primed by complete Freund's adjuvant (CFA) alone, $\frac{1}{400,000}$ (95% confidence limits = $\frac{1}{170,000}$-$\frac{1}{900,000}$); and for mice primed by OVA-CFA, $\frac{1}{720}$ (95% confidence limits = $\frac{1}{330}$-$\frac{1}{1,710}$). These frequencies indicated (1) a 75-fold increase in frequency of IL-2-producing cells in cultures derived from OVA-fed mice, (2) a nonaltered frequency of IL-2-producing cells in cultures derived from mice primed by CFA alone, and (3) an 8-fold increase in frequency of IL-2-producing cells in cultures derived from OVA-CFA-primed mice. The data indicate that the increase in frequency of OVA-specific IL-2-producing cells in cultures derived from OVA-fed mice reflects a reversal of anergy rather

TABLE 3. Culture in rIL-2 Releases Anergic T Lymphocytes for OVA-driven Cytokine Secretion

Group	IL-2 (pg/mL)[a]		IFN-γ (ng/mL)[a]	
	Before[b]	After[b]	Before	After
Tolerant	11	84	3.5	45
Immunized controls	95	105	58	65
Naive controls	<10	<10	<3	<3

[a] Cytokine secretion was determined by ELISA, as described.[31]
[b] Before or after indicate capacity of cells to secrete cytokines in response to OVA prior to, or after, culture in the presence of rIL-2, respectively. Response to OVA was specific: secretion in presence of human serum albumin was less than 10 pg/mL and 3 ng/mL for IL-2 and IFN-γ, respectively.

TABLE 4. Culture in rIL-2 Releases Anergic T Lymphocytes for *in Vivo* Priming: Antibody Production and T-lymphocyte Proliferation

Cell source	Proliferation $(OD_{570-630})^a$		IgG2a $(mg/mL)^a$	
	Before[b]	After[b]	Before	After
Tolerant	0.084	0.751	0.6	3.2
Immunized controls	0.658	0.847	2.2	3.5
Naive controls	0.074	0.065	<0.5	<0.5

[a] Proliferation and IgG2a were determined, as described.[31]

[b] *Before* or *after* indicate capacity of adoptively transferred cells to induce OVA-specific immune responses prior to, or after, culture in the presence of rIL-2, respectively.

than expansion of covert primary OVA-specific T-lymphocyte clones. Taken together, these findings indicated a state of OVA-specific Th1 anergy in PLN cells of OVA-fed mice.[31]

To demonstrate that reversal of anergy was not unique to an *in vitro* system, sublethally irradiated mice were reconstituted with spleen cells taken from OVA-fed and naive donors either prior to, or after culture with rIL-2. Reconstituted mice were then primed by OVA-CFA, and T-lymphocyte responses to OVA *in vitro* and antibody production *in vivo* were measured. Results show that Th1 tolerance to OVA was effectively transferred into irradiated mice by spleen cells taken from OVA-fed donors: T lymphocytes remained unresponsive to OVA *in vitro,* and IgG2a production remained diminished (TABLE 4). However, when the tolerant spleen cells were incubated in the presence of rIL-2 prior to transfer, a complete restoration of OVA-specific Th1 responses was observed in the adoptively transferred recipients, as manifested by both proliferation *in vitro* and IgG2a production *in vivo* (TABLE 4).

ROLE OF ABSORBED ANTIGEN IN GENERATION OF ORAL TOLERANCE

The precise site in which tolerance is generated following the oral route is not known. Several previous studies have provided evidence that suppression is generated in lymphoid tissue along the intestinal tract,[34,35] and a major question is whether this is the same site for anergy induction.[14,15] As anergy of OVA-responsive cells was induced within 24 hours after feeding,[36] it is unlikely to be explained by activation, differentiation, and proliferation of effector cells, or by rapid turnover of OVA-responsive clones through the intestinal lymphoid tissue. Although dietary antigens are degraded by the time they reach the small intestine, studies in humans and rodents have indicated that degradation is partial and that some intact antigen is absorbed.[37-39] The absorption of intact antigen appears to be rapid and occurs within minutes after feeding[40] (Bar Shira and Friedman, unpublished). We favor the notion that the fed antigen, or its fragments, are absorbed into the circulation and directly induce peripheral anergy of Th1 lymphocytes in a manner similar to that observed following the iv or ip administration of antigen.[6,41] Absorbed antigen, either undegraded or partially degraded, might have an important role in the generation of oral tolerance, inasmuch as serum containing antigen absorbed from the gut one hour after feeding transfers tolerance as measured by suppression of systemic DTH responses. Serum

TABLE 5. Obstruction of Oral Tolerance to OVA by Anti-OVA Antibodies[a]

Antibody Source	Antigen Fed	Response to OVA	Response to HSA
—	OVA	0.123	—
	None	0.682	
Naive serum	OVA	0.168	—
	None	0.752	
Serum from CFA-im-	OVA	0.107	—
munized mice	None	0.715	
Serum from OVA-hy-	OVA	0.407	—
perimmunized mice	None	0.782	
Purified IgG anti-OVA	OVA	0.683	—
	None	0.813	0.765
	HSA	—	0.103

[a] The experimental design is similar to that described in ref. 31. Responses were determined by *in vitro* T-cell proliferation in response to OVA and HSA, as described.[24] (Units of measurement are as described in TABLE 4.)

from animals injected systemically with OVA did not suppress, which suggested that there might be unique tolerogenic properties of antigen that pass throughout the gut.[38–40] The use of protease inhibitors, administered together with antigen, results in a higher degree of unresponsiveness[25] (Bar-Shira and Friedman, unpublished observations), probably due to the availability of higher concentrations of absorbed intact antigen.[40] Once in the circulation, soluble external antigen should be no different than self-protein antigens for the induction and maintenance of tolerance.[42–44] The mechanism that distinguishes between anergy or immune response has not been clearly defined but involves the capacity of the antigenic signal to induce costimulatory molecules on responding lymphocytes;[45] if antigen is presented without induction of these molecules, anergy occurs.[13] Thus, soluble external antigen, when presented by resting B lymphocytes[46] or macrophages in the absence of costimulatory molecules,[41] could induce peripheral anergy of Th1 lymphocytes,[47] and should depend upon the presence of antigen for persistence.[43,44] Definition of this pathway is of major importance because it emphasizes the role of antigen in generation of either tolerance or immunity. Deciphering the role of antigen in the distinction between tolerance and immunity is crucial in approaches designed to use orally administered antigen as a means to induce tolerance against autoimmunity, allergy, or graft rejection, or, in contrast, as a means to vaccinate against pathogens.[16]

To address this issue we initiated experiments designed to evaluate the role of absorbed antigen in the generation of anergy in oral tolerance. In these studies, induction of oral tolerance to OVA was obstructed by injecting recipient mice iv with a polyvalent anti-OVA antiserum or with polyvalent-purified anti-OVA IgG (TABLE 5). Anti-OVA antibodies significantly inhibited the induction of oral tolerance to OVA; purified IgG was more effective (84% tolerance inhibition) than whole antiserum (52% inhibition). Naive or CFA hyperimmune serum had no effect on the induction of oral tolerance to OVA, thereby indicating the specificity of the anti-OVA antiserum and IgG. Anti-OVA antibodies had no effect on the establishment of oral tolerance to human serum albumin, thus minimizing effects of nonspecific serum factors on abrogation of tolerance. These results indicate that absorbed OVA, in a form recognizable by anti-OVA antibodies, was directly involved in induction of oral tolerance and dissemination of the tolerogenic stimulus. The identical purified anti-OVA IgG fraction is now being used to purify OVA fragments from serum of fed animals to directly investigate biochemical and tolerogenic properties of these fragments (Bar Shira and Friedman, unpublished work).

SUMMARY

Oral tolerance, a biologically relevant pathway for inducing peripheral tolerance in T lymphocytes, occurs by two distinct mechanisms. Multiple low doses of antigen induce regulatory T lymphocytes that secrete immunosuppressive cytokines, whereas feeding a single high dose of antigen induces anergy of antigen-specific Th1 lymphocytes (diminished IgG2a, IL-2, and IFNγ) with intact Th2 responses (IgG1 and IL-4). Anergy was demonstrated by the ability to reverse the tolerant state after culturing tolerant cells in rIL-2. Reversal of the tolerant state was established *in vitro* by increase in frequency of IL-2-secreting cells, and *in vivo* by specific IgG2a production in irradiated mice adoptively transferred with cells cultured in rIL-2. Inasmuch as the induction of anergy was inhibited by the presence of antibodies specific for the tolerizing antigen, it appears that the oral induction of anergy might depend on the systemic dissemination of antigen (or its fragments) absorbed from the gut. It is suggested that tolerance is insured by the fact that this absorbed antigen is presented to Th1 lymphocytes in draining lymph nodes in the absence of inflammatory and costimulatory molecules.

REFERENCES

1. JANEWAY, C. A. 1992. The immune response evolved to discriminate infectious nonself from noninfectious self. Immunol. Today **13:** 11-16.
2. KROEMER, G. & C. MARTINEZ-A. 1992. Mechanisms of self tolerance. Immunol. Today **13:** 401-404.
3. JONES, L. A., T. CHIN, D. L. LONGO & A. M. KRUISBEEK. 1990. Peripheral clonal elimination of functional T cells. Science **250:** 1726-1729.
4. WEBB, S., C. MORRIS & J. SPRENT. 1990. Extrathymic tolerance of mature T cells: clonal elimination as a consequence of immunity. Cell **63:** 1249-1256.
5. BURKLY, L. C., D. LO, O. KANAGAWA, R. L. BRINSTER & R. A. FLAVEL. 1989. T cell tolerance by clonal anergy in transgenic mice with nonlymphoid expression of MHC class II I-E. Nature **342:** 564-566.
6. RAMMENSEE, H. G., R. KROSCHEWSKI & B. FRANGOULIS. 1989. Clonal anergy induced in mature Vβ6[+] T lymphocytes on immunizing Mls-1[b] mice with Mls-1[a] expressing cells. Nature **339:** 541-544.
7. RAMSDELL, F., T. LANTZ & B. J. FOWLKES. 1989. A nondeletional mechanism of thymic self tolerance. Science **246:** 1038-1041.
8. RAMSDELL, F. & B. J. FOWLKES. 1990. Clonal deletion versus clonal anergy: the role of the thymus in inducing self tolerance. Science **248:** 1342-1348.
9. MILLER, J. F. A. P. & G. MORAHAM. 1992. Peripheral T cell tolerance. Annu. Rev. Immunol. **10:** 51-70.
10. MOWAT, A. M. 1987. The regulation of immune responses to dietary protein antigens. Immunol. Today **8:** 93-98.
11. GOODNOW, C. C. 1992. Transgenic mice and analysis of B-cell tolerance. Annu. Rev. Immunol. **10:** 489-518.
12. ABO, T. 1992. Extrathymic differentiation of T lymphocytes and its biological function. Biomed. Res. **13:** 1-25.
13. JOHNSON, J. G. & M. K. JENKINS. 1993. Accessory cell-derived signals required for T cell activation. Immunol. Res. **12:** 48-64.

14. FRIEDMAN, A., A. AL-SABBAGH, L. M. B. SANTOS, J. FISHMAN-LOBELL, M. POLANSKI, M. PRABHU-DAS, S. J. KHOURY & H. L. WEINER. 1994. Oral tolerance: a biologically relevant pathway to generate peripheral tolerance against external and self antigens. Chem. Immunol. **58:** 259-290.

15. WEINER, H. L., A. FRIEDMAN, A. MILLER, S. J. KHOURY, A. AL-SABBAGH, L. SANTOS, M. SAYEGH, R. B. NUSSENBLATT, D. E. TRENTHAM & D. A. HAFLER. 1994. Oral tolerance: Immunologic mechanisms and treatment of animal and human organ-specific autoimmune diseases by oral administration of autoantigens. Annu. Rev. Immunol. **12:** 809-838.

16. MESTECKY, J. & J. R. McGHEE. 1989. Oral immunization: past and present. Curr. Top. Microbiol. Immunol. **146:** 3-12.

17. CHILLER, J. M. & A. L. GLASEBROOK. 1988. Oral tolerance and the induction of T cell unresponsiveness. Monogr. Allergy **24:** 256-265.

18. HOLT, P. G., J. E. BATTY & K. J. TURNER. 1981. Inhibition of specific IgE response in mice by pre-exposure to inhaled antigen. Immunology **42:** 409-417.

19. HOLT, P. G. & S. LEIVERS. 1982. Tolerance induction via antigen inhalation: isotype specificity, stability, and involvement of suppressor T cells. Int. Archs. Allergy Appl. Immunol. **67:** 155-160.

20. HANSON, D. G. 1981. Ontogeny of orally induced tolerance to soluble proteins in mice. I. Priming and tolerance in newborns. J. Immunol. **127:** 1518-1524.

21. LAMONT, A. G., A. M. MOWAT, M. J. BROWNING & D. M. PARROTT. 1988. Genetic control of oral tolerance to ovalbumin in mice. Immunology **63:** 737-739.

22. VAZ, N. M., M. J. RIOS, L. M. LOPES, C. M. GONTIJO, E. B. CASTANHEIRA, F. JACQUEMART & L. A. ANDRADE. 1987. Genetics of susceptibility to oral tolerance to ovalbumin. Braz. J. Med. Biol. Res. **20:** 785-790.

23. LAMONT, A. G., M. GORDON & A. FERGUSON. 1987. Oral tolerance in protein deprived mice. II. Evidence of normal "gut processing" of ovalbumin, but suppressor cell deficiency, in deprived mice. Immunology **61:** 339-343.

24. MELAMED, D. & A. FRIEDMAN. 1993. Direct evidence for anergy in T lymphocytes tolerized by oral administration of ovalbumin. Eur. J. Immunol. **23:** 935-942.

25. WHITACRE, C. C., I. E. GIENAPP, C. G. OROSZ & D. BITAR. 1991. Oral tolerance in experimental autoimmune encephalomyelits. III. Evidence for clonal anergy. J. Immunol. **147:** 2155-2163.

26. MILLER, A., O. LIDER & H. L. WEINER. 1991. Antigen-driven bystander suppression following oral administration of antigens. J. Exp. Med. **174:** 791-798.

27. FRIEDMAN, A. & H. L. WEINER. 1994. Induction of anergy or active suppression following oral tolerance is determined by antigen dosage. Proc. Natl. Acad. Sci. USA **91:** 6688-6692.

28. SCHWARTZ, R. H. 1990. A cell culture model for T lymphocyte clonal anergy. Science **248:** 1349-1356.

29. DeSILVA, D. R., K. B. URDAHL & M. K. JENKINS. 1991. Clonal anergy is induced *in vitro* by T cell receptor occupancy in the absence of proliferation. J. Immunol. **147:** 3261-3267.

30. GILBERT, K. M. 1994. T cell clonal anergy. Chem. Immunol. **58:** 92-116.

31. MELAMED, D. & A. FRIEDMAN. 1994. *In vivo* tolerization of Th1 lymphocytes following a single feeding with ovalbumin: anergy in the absence of suppression. Eur. J. Immunol. **24:** 1974-1981.

32. FISHMAN-LOBELL, J., A. FRIEDMAN & H. L. WEINER. 1994. Different kinetic patterns of cytokine gene expression *in vivo* in orally tolerant mice. Eur. J. Immunol. **24:** 2720.

33. KHOURY, S. J., W. W. HANCOCK & H. L. WEINER. 1992. Oral tolerance to myelin basic protein and natural recovery from experimental autoimmune encephalomyelitis are associated with downregulation of inflammatory cytokines and differential upregulation of transforming growth factor β, interleukin 4, and prostaglandin E expression in the brain. J. Exp. Med. **176:** 1355-1364.

34. BRANDTZAEG, P. 1989. Overview of the mucosal immune system. Curr. Top. Microbiol. Immunol. **146:** 13-28.
35. Mattingly, J. A. 1984. Immunologic suppression after oral administration of antigen. III. Activation of suppressor-inducer cells in the Peyer's patches. Cell. Immunol. **86:** 46-52.
36. MELAMED, D. & A. FRIEDMAN. 1993. Modification of the immune response by oral tolerance: antigen requirements and interaction with immunogenic stimuli. Cell. Immunol. **146:** 412-420.
37. HUSBY, S., J. C. JENSENIUS & S. E. SVEHAG. 1986. Passage of undegraded dietary antigen into the blood of healthy adults. Further characterization of the kinetics of uptake and the size distribution of the antigen. Scand. J. Immunol. **24:** 447-452.
38. BRUCE, M. G. & A. FERGUSON. 1986. The influence of intestinal processing on the immunogenicity and molecular size of absorbed, circulating ovalbumin in mice. Immunology **59:** 295-300.
39. BRUCE, M. G. & A. FERGUSON. 1987. Oral tolerance produced by gut-processed antigen. Adv. Exp. Med. Biol. **216A:** 721-731.
40. PENG, H. J., M. W. TURNER & S. STROBEL. 1990. The generation of a "tolerogen" after the ingestion of ovalbumin is time-dependent and unrelated to serum levels of immunoreactive antigen. Clin. Exp. Immunol. **81:** 510-515.
41. BURSTEIN, H. J., C. M. SHEA & A. K. ABBAS. 1992. Aqueous antigens induce *in vivo* tolerance selectivity in IL-2- and IFN-γ-producing (Th$_1$) cells. J. Immunol. **148:** 3687-3691.
42. GOODNOW, C. C., J. CROSBIE, H. JORGENSEN, R. A. BRINK & A. BASTEN. 1989. Induction of self-tolerance in mature peripheral B lymphocytes. Nature **342:** 385-91.
43. RAMSDELL, F. & B. J. FOWLKES. 1992. Maintenance of *in vivo* tolerance by persistence of antigen. Science **257:** 1130.
44. ROCHA, B., C. TANCHOT & H. VANBOEHMER. 1993. Clonal anergy blocks *in vivo* growth of mature T cells and can be reversed in the absence of antigen. J. Exp. Med. **177:** 1517.
45. JUNE, C. H., J. A. BLUESTONE, L. M. NADLER & C. B. THOMPSON. 1994. The B7 and CD28 receptor families. Immunol. Today **321:** 321-331.
46. GILBERT, K. M. & W. O. WEIGLE. 1992. B cell presentation of a tolerogenic signal to Th clones. Cell. Immunol. **139:** 58-71.
47. AZUMA, M., M. CAYABYAB, J. H. PHILLIPS & L. L. LANIER. 1993. Requirements for CD28-dependent T-cell-mediated cytotoxicity. J. Immunol. **150:** 2091-2101.

Dose-dependent Activation and Deletion of Antigen-specific T Cells following Oral Tolerance

YOUHAI H. CHEN[a] AND HOWARD L. WEINER

Center for Neurological Diseases
Department of Medicine
Brigham and Women's Hospital
Harvard Medical School
Boston, Massachusetts 02115

Oral tolerance refers to a state of specific immunological hyporesponsiveness to orally administered antigens. It was first described in 1911 by Wells, who showed that systemic anaphylaxis to ovalbumin (OVA) could be prevented by previous feeding with hen's egg protein.[1] The immunological relevance of this phenomenon was established in the 1940s by Chase using the contact sensitizing agent, DNFB.[2] Subsequent research in the 1970s and 1980s led to the recognition that oral tolerance is a form of antigen-driven peripheral immunological tolerance that may be responsible for preventing adverse immune responses to dietary antigens. It is possible that failure to generate oral tolerance to food antigens is associated with intestinal hypersensitivity, as exemplified by food-sensitive enteropathies.[3–7] Recent studies by several laboratories, including our own, have shown that oral tolerance can be used as a form of immune therapy for autoimmune disease models, including experimental autoimmune encephalomyelits (EAE),[8,9] uveitis,[10,11] collagen-[12,13] and adjuvant-induced arthritis,[14] and diabetes[15,16] (reviewed in ref. 17). Oral tolerance is also being applied for the treatment of autoimmune diseases, such as multiple sclerosis[18] and rheumatoid arthritis.[19]

TWO PATHWAYS OF ORAL TOLERANCE

The mechanisms of oral tolerance include active suppression, clonal anergy, and clonal deletion. The concept of active suppression in oral tolerance was first proposed in the 1970s.[20] Investigations supporting a role for active suppression include (1) the ability to adoptively transfer specific oral tolerance to syngeneic recipients by purified T cells,[4,20] and (2) abrogation of oral tolerance by treatment of animals with cyclophosphamide, which may selectively delete suppressor cells.[4,21] However, despite extensive research on the phenomenon of *suppressor T* (Ts) cells during the past two decades, the cellular and molecular basis of immune suppression remains unclear. Part of the problem may be due to the misconception that all forms of suppression were mediated by Ts cells that suppress by releasing antigen-specific factors. We have found that suppression associated with oral tolerance is mediated by subsets of T cells that secrete antigen-nonspecific cytokines after antigen-specific triggering.[22]

---

[a] Present address: Stellar-Chance Laboratory, University of Pennsylvania, 422 Curie Boulevard, Room 401B, Philadelphia, PA 19104.

The possibility that oral antigen directly anergizes specific T cells was implicated by the work of Whitacre et al.[23] and demonstrated directly by Melamed et al. in 1993.[24] Thus when high-dose antigen is administered orally, the frequency of specific T cells (determined by limiting dilution analysis) and the specific immune response in treated animals are dramatically reduced. This state of hyporesponsiveness was partially reversible in vitro by incubating T cells from tolerized animals with recombinant IL-2.[24,25] This was taken to suggest that in orally tolerized animals, there exist T cells with anergic characteristics, as described by Jenkins et al.[26,27] Clonal deletion was not demonstrated until very recently when TcR transgenic mice were used to study oral tolerance. We found that when OVA-TcR-transgenic mice were fed with a high dose of OVA (5-500 mg per feeding), the frequency of T cells in Peyer's patch, mesenteric lymph node, spleen, and thymus were all reduced, and apoptotic T cells were detected in most of these lymphoid organs.[60] Thus, oral tolerance can be mediated by clonal deletion and clonal anergy, as well as by active suppression.

The relative role of these three mechanisms in oral tolerance is primarily determined by the dose of antigen fed.[28,29] Thus, depending on the antigen dose used, oral tolerance may follow either of the two pathways (FIG. 1). A low dose of antigen preferentially activates TGF-β and TH2 cells, which suppress TH1-cell function through releasing antiinflammatory cytokines; this leads only to *TH1 tolerance*. By contrast, a high dose of antigen directly anergizes or deletes antigen-specific T cells (including TH1 and TH2 cells), leading to both *TH1 and TH2 tolerance*. The recognition of these forms of oral tolerance has important implications for immune therapy mediated by oral tolerance; it also explains why a high-dose feeding regimen failed to induce active suppression, and vice versa.[23,28,29]

In addition to dose, other factors, such as the nature of the antigen, the genetic makeup and immunological state of the recipient,[30,31] and the presence of adjuvants,[32–36] may also be important in determining which pathway of oral tolerance will dominate. As an example, in mice and rats, feeding 0.25-1 mg of OVA or myelin basic protein (MBP) induces active suppression,[37,38] whereas for type-II collagen, 0.003 mg is optimal for inducing active suppression.[14,22,39]

CLONAL DELETION AND HIGH-DOSE ORAL TOLERANCE

Clonal deletion has been difficult to study in conventional animals because of the low frequency of antigen-reactive cells. We therefore used ovalbumin-specific T cell-receptor transgenic BALB/c mice to investigate whether peripheral deletion occurred following oral administration of antigen. TcR transgenic mice were fed up to five times with increasing doses of OVA (0.5 to 500 mg). After each feeding, the percentage of CD4[+], Vβ8.2[+] T cells in Peyer's patches was determined by flow cytometry. As shown in FIGURE 2A, depending on the dosage and the frequency of feeding, there was either an increase or a decrease in the number of CD4[+], Vβ8.2[+] T cells in the Peyer's patches. In untreated animals the percentage of CD4[+], Vβ8.2[+] cells was approximately 20% of total cells obtained from the Peyer's patches. In animals fed 500 mg, by the third feeding the percentage of CD4[+], Vβ8.2[+] T cells was less than 1.5%. A decrease in the percentage of CD4[+], Vβ8.2[+] cells was also seen in animals fed 5 milligrams. However, in animals fed 0.5 mg, there was a progressive increase in the percentage of the T cells, which reached 40% by the fifth feeding. A representative FACS contour plot of the 500-mg dose shows a marked decrease in the number of CD4[+], Vβ8.2[+] cells (0.8%) as compared to a control animal (19%) (FIGURES 2B and C). The decrease of T-cell frequency in Peyer's patches was not the result of an increase in the non-T-cell population, as feeding was also associated with a 10-25% decrease in the total number of Peyer's patch cells. In mice fed 500 mg

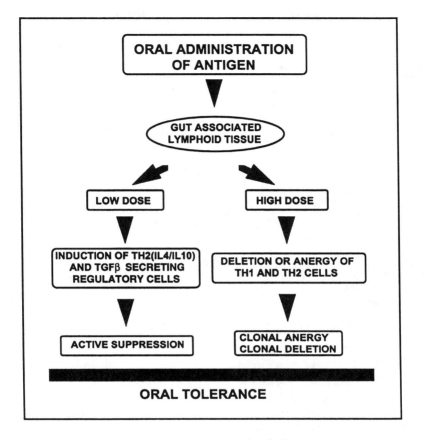

FIGURE 1. Two pathways of oral tolerance.

OVA five times, we also observed a 10-20% reduction of CD4+, Vβ8.2+ T cells in the spleen, thymus, and all other lymphoid tissues examined (axillary, cervical, inguinal, mesenteric, periaortic, and popliteal lymph nodes).

To determine whether the loss of CD4+, Vβ8.2+ cells occurred by deletion of antigen-reactive cells, we measured the percentage of apoptotic cells in the Peyer's patches by flow cytometry. In animals fed 500 mg there was a marked increase in the percentage of apoptotic cells following the second feeding, which returned to background levels by the third feeding. In the animals fed 5 mg, there was a progressive increase in the percentage of apoptotic cells, which reached 8% by the fifth feeding, whereas there was only minimal induction of cells undergoing apoptosis in animals fed with the 0.5 mg dose. To directly visualize the cells undergoing apoptosis, immunohistochemical staining of Peyer's patches was performed by labeling cells that contained degraded DNA. Using this *in situ*-labeling technique, we detected a large percentage (up to 10%) of cells undergoing programmed cell death in the dome area of Peyer's patches from mice fed 500 mg OVA. This was not seen in control animals and was only minimally present in animals fed low doses of OVA.

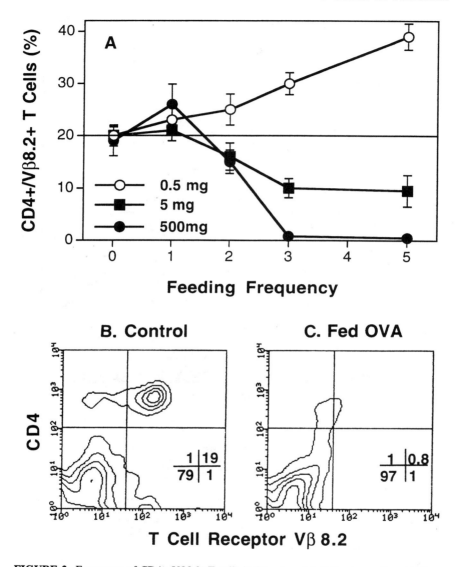

FIGURE 2. Frequency of CD4+, Vβ8.2+ T cells in Peyer's patch following antigen feeding. OVA-TcR transgenic mice were fed 0.5–500 mg of OVA every other day for a total of five feedings. Mice were sacrificed prior to the initiation of feeding or 24 h after each feeding. Peyer's patches (5–8 per mouse) were harvested from the small intestine, and a single cell suspension was prepared. Cells were first centrifuged through a Ficoll-Isopaque gradient and then stained for CD4 (with PE-conjugated YTS 191.1 mAb, Caltag, San Francisco, CA) and Vβ8.2 (with FITC-conjugated MR5-2 mAb, Pharmingen, San Diego, CA). Fluorescence was analyzed on a Beckson-Dickson FACSort using Lysis II software. Data collection was gated on live cells through propidium iodide exclusion, and data represent 10,000 events presented as probability (15%) contours. **A:** Percentage of CD4+, Vβ8.2+ T cells in the Peyer's patches. **B and C:** FACS contour plots of Peyer's patches from animal fed PBS or OVA (500 mg) 5 times.

Previous studies have demonstrated that cells secreting TGF-β or TH2 cytokines (IL-4 and IL-10) are preferentially generated following oral administration of antigens.[29,40] In order to determine whether such cytokine responses were generated following oral administration of antigen in OVA TcR transgenic animals, spleen cells were stimulated *in vitro* after feeding OVA. With high-dose antigen feeding (500 mg), there was enhancement of secretion of both TH1 (IFN-γ) and TH2 (IL-4 and IL-10) cytokines followed by complete loss of the production of these cytokines with continued feeding. IL-2 secretion decreased without prior enhancement. When 5 mg was fed, a similar pattern of IFN-γ, IL-4, and IL-10 secretion was observed. In marked contrast, with low-dose antigen feeding (0.5 mg), there was progressive enhancement of the production of Th2 cytokines (IL-4 and IL-10) with each feeding and minimal effects on the production of Th1 cytokines (IL-2 and IFN-γ).[60] Thus, the induction of peripheral tolerance following oral administration of high- but not low-dose antigen involves clonal deletion of antigen-reactive T cells, and this affects both Th1 and Th2 subsets.

In the transgenic model described here, in addition to deletion, evidence of anergy was also observed in mice fed 500 mg OVA. Specifically, the reduced splenic T-cell proliferative responses could be partially reversed (from $3,432 \pm 52$ to $24,227 \pm 1468$ cpm) by preculture of cells with recombinant IL-2. Thus, in addition to deletion of antigen-reactive T cells, anergy may be partially responsible for oral tolerance in high dose-fed animals. The relationship between anergy and deletion pathways in high-dose oral tolerance is unclear. It is likely that anergized T cells will eventually undergo apoptosis, and anergy may simply represent a preapoptotic step of the clonal-deletion pathway; alternatively, anergy and deletion may follow different pathways that are regulated by different costimulators and cytokines. Further studies are needed to resolve this issue.

ACTIVE SUPPRESSION AND LOW-DOSE ORAL TOLERANCE

In contrast to high-dose oral tolerance, oral administration of low-dose antigen induced no clonal deletion; to the contrary, the frequency of antigen-reactive T cells in the Peyer's patches of OVA-TcR transgenic mice was increased after repeated low-dose feeding (FIG. 2). Consistent with these findings, cytokines such as TGF-β, IL-4, and IL-10 are up-regulated in low-dose fed transgenic as well as conventional animals. As these cytokines are known to be suppressors of TH1 cells, a role for cytokine-mediated immune suppression in oral tolerance was suggested.

This notion is also strongly supported by the unique characteristics of oral tolerance.[4,21,41,42] Oral tolerance is primarily directed to cellular (TH1) responses, whereas humoral (TH2) immune responses are more resistant. Indeed, mucosal IgA production is almost always increased in orally tolerized animals.[4,43,44] This type of immune deviation has been referred to as "split tolerance." One exception to this rule is IgE production, which is prone to suppression by oral tolerance,[4] suggesting that mechanisms other than TH2 deviation may exist in oral tolerance.

The first evidence that cytokines were directly involved in oral tolerance was generated in the Lewis rat model of EAE orally tolerized to guinea pig MBP.[37] When splenic T cells were isolated from rats fed with a low dose of MBP, it was found that they were capable of suppressing proliferation of TH1 cells *in vitro*. The suppression was dependent on the presence of MBP but not restricted to MBP-specific cells. Thus, when OVA-specific T cells were co-cultured with splenic T cells from tolerized rats, their proliferation was also suppressed, but only when MBP was present in the culture. Addition of antibodies to TGF-β reversed the suppression.[37] Thus, oral administration of antigen induces regulatory T cells secreting TGF-β, which mediate *bystander suppression*. The *in vivo* relevance of bystander suppression was confirmed by the demonstration that (1) injection of anti-

TGF-β mAb into animals reversed oral tolerance induced by low-dose antigen[45] and (2) feeding MBP suppressed EAE induced not only by MBP but also by proteolipid protein (PLP).[46]

In the Lewis rat, splenic T cells producing TGF-β were found to be CD8[+], which recognized MBP peptides different from encephalitogenic epitopes.[37] This most probably relates to the fact that they are MHC class I restricted. How these class I-restricted T cells are generated *in vivo* is not clear at this time. CD8[+] T cells predominate in gut epithelium,[47–49] and gut epithelia cells express MHC class I molecules and are capable of presenting antigen to T cells, at least *in vitro*.[50] It is tempting to speculate that CD8 cell-epithelia interaction in the gut activates TGF-β, producing class I-restricted T cells that mediate immune suppression. The cloning of CD8[+] cells will allow the characterization of these regulatory lymphocytes.

When similar studies were extended to a mouse system, it was found that not only CD8[+] but also CD4[+] cells were responsible for active suppression, both *in vivo* and *in vitro*.[40,51] Thus, when a low dose of MBP was administered orally to SJL/J mice, TH1 but not TH2 immune responses were suppressed. In fact, TH2 cytokines (IL-4, IL-10) and TGF-β were significantly increased in mice fed with low doses of MBP. Furthermore if animals are fed MBP and then immunized intraperitoneally with the same antigen, one enhances the production of IL-4 and IL-10, as well as of TGF-β.[40] McGhee and colleagues have also found that exposure of soluble antigens to the gut preferentially generates TH2-type responses as judged by increased IL-4 and IL5 production.[52] Thus, in the gut, immune responses to soluble antigen are preferentially of a TH2 type and involve the generation of cells that secrete TGF-β. Why a TH2-type response is preferentially generated in the gut is unknown but may relate to antigen presentation or the cytokine milieu. When cells from mice fed and immunized with MBP were further studied *in vitro*, it was found that both CD4 and CD8 cells secreted TGF-β, whereas only CD4 cells secreted IL-4 and IL-10.[40] This is consistent with our studies in the Lewis rat in which CD8 cell populations secreted TGF-β. However, it was clear in the SJL model that a population of TGF-β-secreting CD4[+] cells were also generated and amplified in the gut following the feeding and subsequent immunization with MBP.

We then cloned regulatory CD4[+] T cells from the mesenteric lymph nodes of the MBP-fed mice. In all, 48 MBP-specific CD4[+] T-cell clones were generated from mice fed and immunized with MBP. Cytokine production for each individual clone after activation with MBP or anti-CD3 monoclonal antibody was determined by ELISA. TABLE 1 illustrates the cytokine profiles of representative T-cell clones. We found that the majority of T-cell clones (42 out of the 48) produced active TGF-β in addition to varying amounts of one or the other TH2-type cytokines (IL-4 and IL-10). The amount of cytokines produced by different clones varied greatly, and we thus classified TGF-β-secreting clones as TGF-β[lo]IL4/IL10[hi], TGF-β[hi]IL4/IL10[lo], or TGF-β[lo]IL4/IL10[lo]. There was little production of IFN-γ or IL-2 by most TGF-β-secreting clones. It also appeared that the TGF-β clones were different from classic TH2-type cells, as there was a general correlation between the secretion of IL-4 and IL-10 in an individual clone, whereas this was dissociated for TGF-β and IL-4/IL-10.

Mucosally derived CD4[+] clones were further characterized for their epitope specificity, MHC restriction, and TCR usage.[40] Three clones were selected for detailed analysis, all of which were found to recognize MBP peptide 84-102 and MHC class II I-A[s]. The cDNA clones were also generated from all the three T-cell clones. Sequence analyses revealed that they used either Vα1 or Vα3, and Vβ4 or Vβ17, all of which were also used by encephalitogenic TH1 cells.[53] Most interestingly, one of our mucosal TH2 clones used identical TCR Vα and Vβ chains as one of the encephalitogenic TH1 clones. The encephalitogenic T-cell clones generated, following immunization of MBP in complete Freund's adjuvant in SJL mice, have been studied in detail.[53] These autopathogenic CD4[+] T-

TABLE 1. Cytokine Profiles of MBP-specific CD4$^+$ T-Cell Clones (pg/mL)

Clones	TGF-β	IFN-γ	IL-2	IL-4	IL-10
TGFβ^{hi} IL4/IL10^{lo} (TH3 type)					
1C1	**6193**	<50	<50	101	179
1E1-N	**4868**	<50	<50	<75	<100
1F2	**3226**	<50	<50	<75	169
2F9-L1	**2030**	<50	<50	<75	157
1H8-L	**1822**	<50	<50	114	718
2E9	**1408**	<50	ND	<75	159
2H11	**1369**	<50	ND	85	165
1H4-S	**1261**	<50	<50	<75	513
1H9-L2	**1102**	<50	<50	223	729
TGFβ^{lo} IL4/IL10^{hi} (TH2 type)					
1B1-T	154	<50	<50	**3566**	**2471**
1D3	633	<50	<50	**1739**	<100
1H1-G	742	<50	<50	**1430**	**1684**
5E12-D	<100	<50	<50	**1370**	**2695**
1D9-E	234	<50	<50	**1102**	945
5D2-C	<100	<50	<50	**1034**	**2037**
TH1 type					
1D4	389	**3944**	**1895**	98	<100
2G11	<100	**2195**	ND^a	84	123
2H2	178	**2130**	**1324**	<75	<100
2E5	240	**2051**	**1403**	97	<100
2H4-B	<100	**1684**	ND	<75	<100

^{a} Not determined.

cell clones react to the immunodominant epitope of MBP 84-102, are I-A^s restricted, predominantly use TcR Vβ4 and 17, and produce Th1 cytokines. These Th1 cytokines have been implicated as the primary mediators of EAE. The regulatory T-cell clones generated in our study have striking similarities with the encephalitogenic CD4$^+$ TH1-cell clones because of their epitope specificity, TcR V gene usage, and MHC restriction. However, they can be distinguished from the latter by the fact that they produce suppressive cytokines (TGF-β and IL-4/IL-10) following antigen-specific activation. This difference in the cytokine patterns of the regulatory T-cell clones may be due to exposure of antigens to the gut-associated immune system.

To test whether the mucosally derived TH2 cells generated by oral tolerance have any immune suppressive activity *in vivo*, SJL mice were immunized with MBP to induce EAE, and at the time of immunization 2×10^6 regulatory T-cell clones were injected. This resulted in the suppression of EAE with a decreased disease incidence, day of onset, maximum disease score, and fatality.[40] *In vitro*, these cloned cells suppressed the proliferation and cytokine production of MBP-specific TH1 cells, and this suppression was abrogated by antibodies to TGF-β and IL-10 (unpublished data).

As noted earlier, bystander suppression in oral tolerance is mediated by cells secreting suppressive cytokines, such as TGF-β following antigen-specific triggering, and the suppression can be directed to adjacent cells in the microenvironment. To test this with the CD4$^+$ mucosal-derived, MBP-specific regulatory T-cell clones, we immunized animals with PLP for the induction of EAE. PLP-induced disease was also suppressed by injection of these MBP-specific T-cell clones, and this suppression was abrogated by *in vivo* injection of anti-TGF-β monoclonal antibody.[40]

Thus, regulation of immune response and cells capable of regulating immune response are not dependent on unique T-cell receptors, or MHC restriction, but are conventional T cells whose major difference relates to the cytokine profile. The profile appears stable and is uniquely generated depending on the environment in which they are induced. Bloom *et al.* reported CD8⁺ regulatory T-cell clones generated in leprosy and showed that immune suppression was mediated by IL-4.[54] Swanborg *et al.* characterized regulatory T cells in rats recovering from EAE and established that the suppression was mediated by TGF-β.[55] It thus appears that regulatory T cells are not phenotypically different in that they are generated normally during the course of immune responses. However, the primary determinant of the induction of these cells relates to the immune microenvironment in which they are generated, and these cells have an important biologic function in the ability to down-regulate autoimmune processes.

One of the unique features of mucosally derived TH2 cells is their ability to produce TGF-β. TGF-β is a member of a growing family of growth factors important for cell proliferation and differentiation.[56,57] Three isoforms, that is, TGF-β1, TGF-β2, and TGF-β3 have thus far been identified in mammals.[56] All the TGF-β isoforms were shown to be multifunctional and suppress the function of activated T lymphocytes while selectively enhancing IgA production by B lymphocytes.[56,57,58] In fact, TGF-β is the only known IgA-switching factor for B cells.[57] IL-4 and IL-10 are known to promote humoral immune responses while suppressing cellular immune responses.[59] The combination of these cytokines may lead to systemic suppression of most immune responses while sparing the IgA production by B cells, leading to the phenomenon of split tolerance.

An unanswered question is whether the mucosally derived CD4 clones represent a unique subset or type of CD4 cell (TH3) or are more closely related to classic TH2 cells. The production of TGF-β by TH2 cells has not been reported. In a separate study we have derived a number of TH2 cells following peripheral immunization and have found that only an occasional TH2 clone produces TGF-β. However, in other ongoing experiments with PLP, significant proportions of T-cell clones derived following oral administration of PLP secreted TGF-β. The final classification of mucosal-derived TGF-β secreting TH2-type cells will await further characterizations of them, as well as their activation requirements and comparison to large numbers in the study of classically derived TH2 cells.

REFERENCES

1. WELLS, H. 1911. Studies on the chemistry of anaphylaxis. III. Experiments with isolated proteins, especially those of hen's egg. J. Infect. Dis. **9:** 147–51.
2. CHASE, M. W. 1946. Inhibition of experimental drug allergy by prior feeding of the sensitizing agent. Proc. Soc. Exp. Med. **61:** 257–59.
3. EMANCIPATOR, S. N. & M. E. LAMM. 1988. Oral tolerance as a protective mechanism against hypersensitivity disease. Monogr. Allergy **24:** 244–250.
4. MOWAT, A. M. 1987. The regulation of immune responses to dietary protein antigens. Immunol. Today **8:** 93–8.
5. STROBEL, S. 1990. Mechanisms of gastrointestinal immunoregulation and food induced injury to the gut. Eur. J. Clin. Nutr. **45** (suppl. 1): 1–9.
6. STROBEL, S. 1990. Immunologically mediated damage to the intestinal mucosa. Acta Paediatr. Scand. (Suppl.) **365:** 46–57.
7. JOHNSON, R. B., J. T. LABROOY & J. H. SKERRITT. 1990. Antibody responses reveal differences in oral tolerance to wheat and maize grain protein fractions. Clin. Exp. Immunol. **79**(1): 135–40.

8. HIGGINS, P. & H. L. WEINER. 1988. Suppression of experimental autoimmune encephalomyelitis by oral administration of myelin basic protein and its fragments. J. Immunol. **140:** 440–445.

9. BITAR, D. & C. C. WHITACRE. 1988. Suppression of experimental autoimmune encephalomyelitis by the oral administration of myelin basic protein. Cell. Immunol. **112:** 364–370.

10. NUSSENBLATT, R. B., R. R. CASPI, R. MAHDI et al. 1990. Inhibition of S-antigen induced experimental autoimmune uveoretinitis by oral induction of tolerance with S-antigen. J. Immunol. **144**(5): 1689–1695.

11. SINGH, V. K., H. K. KALRA, K. YAMAKI & T. SHINOHARA. 1992. Suppression of experimental autoimmune uveitis in rats by the oral administration of the uveitopathogenic S-antigen fragment and a cross-reactive homologous peptide. Cell. Immunol. **139**(1): 81–90.

12. THOMPSON, H. & N. STAINES. 1986. Gastric administration of type II collagen delays the onset and severity of collagen-induced arthritis in rats. Clin. Exp. Immunol. **64:** 581–86.

13. NAGLER-ANDERSON, C., L. A. BOBER, M. E. ROBINSON, G. W. SISKIND & F. J. THORBEKE. 1986. Suppression of type II collagen-induced arthritis by intragastric administration of soluble type II collagen. Proc. Natl. Acad. Sci. USA **83:** 7443–7446.

14. ZHANG, Z. Y., C. S. LEE, O. LIDER & H. L. WEINER. 1990. Suppression of adjuvant arthritis in Lewis rats by oral administration of type II collagen. J. Immunol. **145**(8): 2489–93.

15. ZHANG, J., L. DAVIDSON, G. EISENBARTH & H. WEINER. 1991. Suppression of diabetes in NOD mice by oral administration of porcine insulin. Proc. Natl. Acad. Sci. USA **88:** 10252–56.

16. BERGEROT, I., N. FABIEN, V. MAGUER & C. THIVOLET. 1994. Oral administration of human insulin to NOD mice generates CD4$^+$ T cells that suppress adoptive transfer of diabetes. J. Autoimmunity **7:** 655–63.

17. WEINER, H., A. FRIEDMAN, F. MILLER et al. 1994. Oral tolerance: Immunologic mechanisms and treatment of animal and human organ-specific autoimmune diseases by oral administration of autoantigens. Annu. Rev. Immunol. **12:** 809–837.

18. WEINER, H. L., G. A. MACKIN, M. MATSUI et al. 1993. Double-blind pilot trial of oral tolerization with myelin antigens in multiple sclerosis. Science **259:** 1321–24.

19. TRENTHAM, D., R. DYNESIUS-TRENTHAM, E. ORAV et al. 1993. Effects of oral administration of collagen on rheumatoid arthritis. Science **261:** 1727.

20. TOMASI, T. JR. 1980. Oral tolerance. [Review]. Transplantation **29**(5): 353–6.

21. MOWAT, A. M., S. STROBEL, H. E. DRUMMOND & A. FERGUSON. 1982. Immunological responses to fed protein antigens in mice. I. Reversal of oral tolerance to ovalbumin by cyclophosphamide. Immunology **45**(1): 105–13.

22. WEINER, H., A. FRIEDMAN, F. MILLER et al. 1994. Oral tolerance: Immunologic mechanisms and treatment of murine and human organ specific autoimmune diseases by oral administration of autoantigens. Annu. Rev. Immunol. **12:** 809–837.

23. WHITACRE, C. C., I. E. GIENAPP, C. G. OROSZ & D. M. BITAR. 1991. Oral tolerance in experimental autoimmune encephalitomyelitis. III. Evidence for clonal anergy. J. Immunol. **147**(7): 2155–63.

24. MELAMED, D. & A. FRIEDMAN. 1993. Direct evidence for anergy in T lymphocytes tolerized by oral administration of ovalbumin. Eur. J. Immunol. **23**(4): 935–42.

25. MELAMED, D. & A. FRIEDMAN. 1993. Modification of the immune response by oral tolerance: antigen requirements and interaction with immunogenic stimuli. Cell. Immunol. **146:** 412–420.

26. JENKINS, M., C. CHEN, G. JUNG, D. MUELLER & R. SCHWARTZ. 1990. Inhibition of antigen-specific proliferation of type 1 murine T cell clones after stimulation with immobilized anti-CD3 monoclonal antibody. J. Immunol. **144**(1): 16–24.

27. SCHWARTZ, R. H. 1990. A cell culture model for T lymphocyte clonal anergy. Science **248:** 1349–1356.

28. GREGERSON, D. S., W. F. OBRITSCH & L. A. DONOSO. 1993. Oral tolerance in experimental autoimmune uveoretinitis. Distinct mechanisms of resistance are induced by low versus high dose feeding protocols. J. Immunol. **151**(10): 5751-61.

29. FRIEDMAN, A. & H. WEINER. 1994. Induction of anergy or active suppression following oral tolerance is determined by frequency of feeding and antigen dosage. Proc. Natl. Acad. Sci. USA **91**: 6688.

30. LAMONT, A. G., A. M. MOWAT, M. J. BROWNING & D. M. PARROTT. 1988. Genetic control of oral tolerance to ovalbumin in mice. Immunology **63**(4): 737-739.

31. MILLER, A., O. LIDER, A. AL-SABBAGH & H. WEINER. 1992. Suppression of experimental autoimmune encephalomyelitis by oral administration of myelin basic protein. V. Hierarchy of suppression by myelin basic protein from different species. J. Neuroimmunol. **39**: 243-250.

32. KHOURY, S. J., O. LIDER, A. AL-SABBAGH & H. L. WEINER. 1990. Suppression of experimental autoimmune encephalomyelitis by oral administration of myelin basic protein. III. Synergistic effect of lipopolysaccharide. Cell. Immunol. **131**: 302-310.

33. REVILLARD, J. P., G. COZON & C. CZERKINSKY. 1992. Oral administration of immunomodulators and the mucosal immune system. Dev. Biol. Stand. **77**: 31-7.

34. PIERRE, P., O. DENIS, H. BAZIN, E. MBONGOLO MBELLA & J. P. VAERMAN. 1992. Modulation of oral tolerance to ovalbumin by cholera toxin. Eur. J. Immunol. **22**(12): 3179-82.

35. BURNS, D., M. SCOTT, J. PHILLIPS & S. BROD. 1993. Oral administration of type I interferons prevents sensitization to MBP in acute EAE. J. Immunol. **150**(8,II): 1111A.

36. SUN, J.-B., C. HOLMGREN & C. CZERKINSKY. 1994. Cholera toxin B subunit: an efficient transmucosal carrier-delivery system for induction of peripheral immunological tolerance. Proc. Natl. Acad. Sci. USA **91**: 10795-9.

37. MILLER, A., O. LIDER & H. L. WEINER. 1991. Antigen-driven bystander suppression following oral administration of antigens. J. Exp. Med. **174**: 791-798.

38. SANTOS, L., A. AL-SABBAGH, A. LONDONO & H. WEINER. 1994. Oral tolerance to myelin basic protein induces TGF-β secreting T cells in Peyer's patches. Cell. Immunol. **157**: 439-447.

39. YOSHINO, S., E. QUATTROCCI & H. WEINER. 1995. Arthritis Rheum. In press.

40. CHEN, Y., V. K. KUCHROO, J.-I. INOBE, D. A. HAFLER & H. L. WEINER. 1994. Regulatory T cell clones induced by oral tolerance: suppression of autoimmune encephalomyelitis. Science **265**: 1237-1240.

41. STROBEL, S., A. M. MOWAT, H. E. DRUMMOND, M. G. PICKERING & A. FERGUSON. 1983. Immunological responses to fed protein antigens in mice. II. Oral tolerance for CMI is due to activation of cyclophosphamide-sensitive cells by gut-processed antigen. Immunology **49**(3): 451-6.

42. MICHALEK, S. M., J. R. McGHEE, H. KIYONO, D. E. COLWELL, J. H. ELDRIDGE, M. J. WANNEMUEHLER & W. J. KOOPMAN. 1983. The IgA response: Inductive aspects, regulatory cells, and effector functions. Ann. N.Y. Acad. Sci. **409**: 48-71.

43. MATTHEWS, J. B., B. H. FIVAZ & H. F. SEWELL. 1981. Serum and salivary antibody responses and the development of oral tolerance after oral and intragastric antigen administration. Int. Arch. Allergy Appl. Immunol. **65**(1): 107-113.

44. SILVERMAN, G. A., B. A. PERI & R. M. ROTHBERG. 1982. Systemic antibody responses of different species following ingestion of soluble protein antigens. Dev. Comp. Immunol. **6**(4): 737-746.

45. MILLER, A., O. LIDER, A. B. ROBERTS, M. B. SPORN & H. L. WEINER. 1992. Suppressor T cells generated by oral tolerization to myelin basic protein suppress both *in vitro* and *in vivo* immune responses by the release of TGFβ following antigen specific triggering. Proc. Natl. Acad. Sci. USA **89**: 421-425.

46. AL-SABBAGH, A., A. MILLER, L. M. B. SANTOS & H. L. WEINER. 1994. Antigen-driven tissue-specific suppression following oral tolerance: orally administered myelin basic protein suppresses proteolipid induced experimental autoimmune encephalomyelitis in the SJL mouse. Eur. J. Immunol. **24**: 2104-9.

47. JALKENEN, S. 1990. Lymphocyte homing to the gut. Springer Semin. Immunopathology **12:** 153-164.
48. MOWAT, A. M. 1990. Human intraepithelial lymphocytes. Springer Semin. Immunopathology **12:** 165-190.
49. GUY-GRAND, D., N. CERF-BENSUSSAN, B. MALISSEN, M. MALASSIS-SERIS, C. BRIOTTET & P. VASSALLI. 1991. Two gut intraepithelial CD8+ lymphocyte populations with different T cell receptors: a role for the gut epithelium in T cell differentiation. J. Exp. Med **173:** 471-481.
50. SANTOS, L., O. LIDER, J. AUDETTE, S. KHOURY & H. WEINER. 1990. Characterization of immunomodulatory properties and accessory cell function of small intestinal epithelial cells. Cell. Immunol. **127:** 26-34.
51. CHEN, Y., J.-I. INOBE & H. L. WEINER. 1995. Induction of oral tolerance to MBP in CD8-depleted mice: both CD4 and CD8 cells mediate the active suppression component of oral tolerance. J. Immunol. **155:** 910-916.
52. XU-AMANO, J., W. K. AICHER, T. TAGUCHI, H. KIYONO & J. R. MCGHEE. 1992. Selective induction of Th₂ cells in murine Peyer's patches by oral immunization. Int. Immunol. **4**(4): 433-445.
53. ZAMVIL, S. S. & L. STEINMAN. 1990. The T lymnphocyte in experimental allergic encephalomyelitis. Annu. Rev. Immunol. **8:** 579-621.
54. SALGAME, P., J. ABRAMS, C. CLAYBERGER, H. GOLDSTEIN, J. CONVIT & R. MODLIN. 1991. Differing lymphokine profiles of functional subsets of human CD4 and CD8 T cell clones. Science **254:** 279-82.
55. KARPUS, W. & R. SWANBORG. 1991. CD4+ suppressor cells inhibit the function of effector cells of experimental autoimmune encephalomyelitis through a mechanism involving transforming growth factor beta. J. Immunol. **146:** 1163-68.
56. ROBERTS, A. & M. SPORN. 1993. Physiological actions and clinical applications of transforming growth factor beta (TGFb). Growth Factors **8**(1): 1-9.
57. WAHL, S. 1992. Transforming growth factor beta (TGFb) in inflammation: a cause and a cure. J. Clin. Immunol. **12:** 61-74.
58. KIM, P.-H. & M. F. KAGNOFF. 1990. Transforming growth factor-β1 is a costimulatory for IgA production. J. Immunol. **144:** 3411-3416.
59. MOSMANN, T. & R. COFFMAN. 1989. Heterogeneity of cytokine secretion patterns and functions of helper T cells. Adv. Immunol. **46:** 111-47.
60. CHEN, Y., J.-I. INOBE, R. MARKS, P. GONNELLA, V. K. KUCHROO & H. L. WEINER. 1995. Peripheral deletion of antigen-reactive T cells in oral tolerance. Nature **376:** 177-180.

Inactivation of Th1 and Th2 Cells by Feeding Ovalbumin[a]

ALLAN McI MOWAT, MARGARET STEEL,
ELIZABETH A. WORTHEY, PETER J. KEWIN, AND
PAUL GARSIDE

Department of Immunology
University of Glasgow
Western Infirmary
Glasgow, Scotland G11 6NT

INTRODUCTION

Oral tolerance to protein antigens has many practical implications, including the ability to inhibit antigen-specific immunopathology.[1] In addition, oral tolerance is likely to be the physiological mechanism that prevents food hypersensitivities, such as gluten-sensitive enteropathy,[2] and it provides a useful model for studying peripheral immune tolerance in mature animals. For these reasons, it would be important to document the mechanisms responsible for the induction and maintenance of oral tolerance.

Earlier studies strongly implicated active mechanisms, such as CD8[+] suppressor T cells, in the regulation of immunity to dietary antigens.[2] Although the existence of this population thereafter came under increasing doubt, more recent work has suggested that production of inhibitory cytokines, such as γ interferon (γIFN) and transforming growth factor β (TGFβ), by CD8[+] T cells may play an important role.[1,3,4] Conversely, other findings have suggested that oral tolerance is associated with preferential production of interleukins 4 and 10, and TGFβ, by the Th2 subset of CD4[+] T cell, leading to cross-regulation of Th1 cell-mediated effector functions.[5,6] Finally, however, a number of studies have provided indirect evidence for the possibility that there is direct anergy of antigen-reactive T lymphocytes in orally tolerized mice.[7] In view of these discrepant results, often obtained using different doses of antigens in different species, we have analyzed directly the contributions of CD8[+] T cells, T cell–derived cytokines, and clonal inactivation in a single, well-established model of oral tolerance to OVA in mice.

MATERIAL AND METHODS

Mice

Female BALB/c and C57B1/6 (B6) mice were obtained from Harlan Olac, Bicester, Oxon, United Kingdom. Mice were specific pathogen free and were maintained under standard animal house conditions until use at 6-8 weeks of age.

[a]This work was supported by the BBSRC (UK) and by a postgraduate studentship from the Yamanouchi Research Institute awarded to Margaret Steel.

IL-4$^{-/-}$ mice (129Sv × C57B16) and IL4$^{+/+}$ controls obtained originally from Dr. H. Bluethmann, F. Hoffman La Roche, Basel,[8] were bred and maintained under conventional conditions by Dr. J. Alexander, Department of Immunology, University of Strathclyde.

Induction and Assessment of Oral Tolerance

As we have described in previous studies,[2,9] oral tolerance was induced with a single feed of 25 mg OVA (Fraction V, Sigma, Poole, U.K.). Ten days later, systemic antibody, delayed-type hypersensitivity (DTH) and local proliferative/cytokine responses were re-stimulated by immunization in the footpad with 100 μg OVA in complete Freund's adjuvant (CFA). To induce systemic cytotoxic T cell (CTL) activity, mice were immunized with 10 μg OVA in ISCOMS intraperitoneally.[10] Draining popliteal lymph nodes (PLN) were examined for antigen-specific proliferation and cytokine production 14 days later, whereas serum antibodies and DTH responses were assessed 21 days after parenteral immunization. Splenic CTL activity was assessed 7 days after challenge.

Depletion of CD4$^+$ and CD8$^+$ T cells In Vivo

Animals were injected iv with 0.5 mg of anti-CD4 (YTS-169) or anti-CD8 (YTS-191) antibody four days before and on the day of oral administration of OVA.

Measurement of OVA-specific Immune Responses In Vivo

OVA-specific total IgG, IgG1, and IgG2a antibodies were measured in serum using specific ELISAs,[9] whereas DTH responses were assessed by measuring the increment in footpad thickness 24 hours after challenge with 100 μg heat-aggregated OVA.

Measurement of OVA-specific CTL Activity

As described previously,[10] spleen cells from mice immunized with OVA ISCOMS were restimulated for 5 days with EG7.OVA cells *in vitro*, before being assayed against ^{51}Cr-labeled EG7.OVA cells for 4 hours in a conventional microcytotoxicity assay.

Measurement of OVA-specific Immune Reactivity In Vitro

An OVA-specific proliferative activity was assessed in single cell suspensions of PLN by culture with 1 mg/mL OVA. Control wells contained 10 μg/mL Con A (Sigma, Poole, U.K.), 50 μg/mL PPD, or medium alone. Supernatants from parallel cultures were harvested for measurement of the levels of IL-2, IL-3, IL-4, IL-5, IL-10, γIFN, and TGFβ, using sandwich ELISAs, as described in detail elsewhere.[9] Cytokine concentrations in test supernatants were determined with reference to a standard curve constructed, using serial dilutions of recombinant standard cytokines.

Morphometric and Cytological Analysis of Tolerized Lymphocytes

At intervals after culture *in vitro*, PLN cells from tolerant and control mice were harvested. Their viability was assessed by phase-contrast microscopy and stained with

Giemsa for morphometric examination. Lymphocytes stained with directly conjugated anti-CD4 or anti-CD8 monoclonal antibodies (Pharmingen, San Diego, CA) were analyzed by flow cytometry. DNA content of cultured lymphocytes was determined by flow cytometry after staining with propidium iodide.

Statistical Analysis

Results are represented as the mean $\pm$ 1 SEM where indicated and were analyzed using Student's t test. Antibody-isotype dilution curves were analyzed using probit analysis.

RESULTS

Effects of Oral Tolerance on Immune Effector Functions In Vivo

As anticipated, mice fed 25 mg OVA before immunization with OVA/CFA had significantly suppressed DTH and total serum IgG antibody responses compared with control mice (data not shown). The IgG1 and IgG2a isotypes of OVA-specific antibody were reduced to similar extents in OVA-fed mice (FIG. 1). The effects of oral tolerance was not confined to these classically CD4 T cell–dependent activities, as the CTL activity induced by immunization with OVA in ISCOMS was also completely abolished in mice fed OVA before challenge (data not shown). Previous work has shown these CTL to be CD8+ class I MHC–restricted T cells that recognize the octamer motif OVA 257-264 + H-2K^b.[10]

CD4+ but Not CD8+ T Cells Are Required for Induction of Oral Tolerance

In parallel with the ability of feeding OVA to tolerize CD8+ T cells, depletion of CD8+ T cells at the time of feeding OVA had no effect on the induction of tolerance of IgG or DTH responses. However, depletion of CD4+ T cells completely abrogated the tolerance.[11]

Tolerance of T-lymphocyte Function In Vitro

Compared with cells from control immunized mice, PLN cells from tolerized mice had markedly inhibited proliferative responses after restimulation with OVA *in vitro,* but responded well to PPD (data not shown). In addition, the antigen-specific production of IL-2, IL-3, IL-4, IL-5, IL-10, and γIFN was significantly reduced or abolished in supernatants from PLN cells of tolerant animals, compared with that from control cells (FIG. 2). The defective production of cytokines by tolerant cells was antigen-specific, as it was not found using PPD or Con A as a stimulus (data not shown).

Th2 Cells Are Not Required for Oral Tolerance

As functions of Th1 and Th2 CD4+ cells were equally sensitive to oral tolerance, these findings suggest that Th2 cells could not mediate the inhibition of effector T-cell functions *in vivo.* This was supported by experiments in IL-4^{-/-} mice, which showed that tolerance of IgG and DTH responses was induced normally in these animals, despite their lack of Th2 cells.[9]

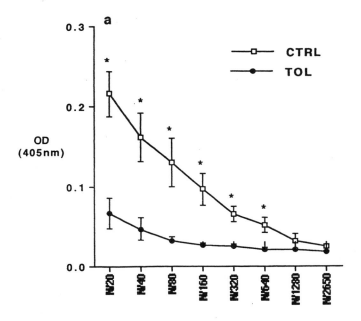

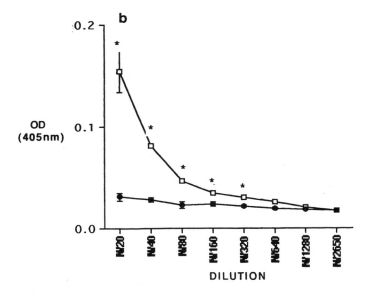

FIGURE 1. Suppression of systemic IgG isotype production by feeding ovalbumin. OVA-specific serum IgG1 (a) and IgG2a (b) antibody responses in mice immunized OVA/CFA after feeding OVA or saline as a control. The results shown are mean OD ±1 SEM for serum dilutions of sera from 5 mice per group (*p < 0.05 versus tolerant).

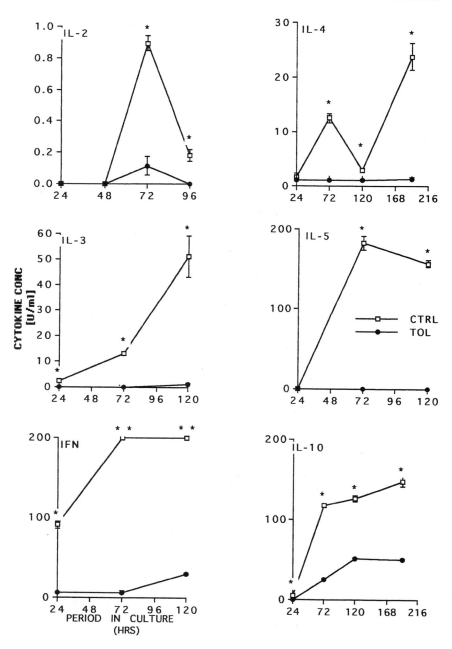

FIGURE 2. Suppression of Th1 and Th2 cytokine production by feeding ovalbumin. Antigen-specific cytokine production by draining popliteal lymph node cells taken 2 weeks after subcutaneous immunization with OVA/CFA in mice fed OVA and in controls. The results shown are mean cytokine levels ± 1 SEM of quadruplicate samples from supernatants of cells pooled from 5 mice per group (*p < 0.05 versus tolerant).

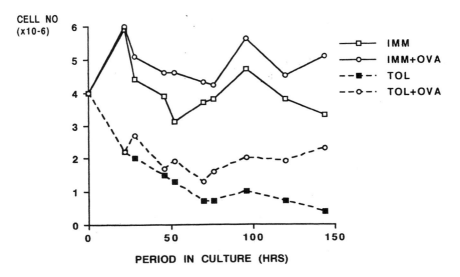

FIGURE 3. Death of tolerant lymphocytes during culture *in vitro*. PLN cells from OVA-fed mice die rapidly when cultured *in vitro* 14 days after subcutaneous challenge with OVA/CFA (TOL). This is partly prevented when tolerant cells are cultured with 1 mg/mL OVA (TOL + OVA). Immunized control PLN cells remain healthy when cultured alone (IMM) or with OVA (IMM + OVA). Results shown are mean viable cell numbers assessed by phase-contrast microscopy.

Tolerized Lymphocytes Undergo Apoptosis **In Vitro**

In parallel with the loss of all T-cell functions, PLN cells from tolerized mice died rapidly when cultured *in vitro* (FIG. 3). This cell loss affected both CD4+ and CD8+ T cells (data not shown) and was partly reduced when tolerant cells were cultured in the presence of OVA. Within 24–48 hours, lymphocytes in cultures of tolerant cells showed morphological evidence of apoptosis, with nuclear condensation and cytoplasmic shrinkage. Large numbers of activated macrophages containing apoptotic bodies could also be seen in these cultures, which ultimately took on the appearance of a stromal cell monolayer. DNA analysis confirmed the presence of large amounts of hypodiploid DNA in cultured tolerant cells compared with control cells, consistent with the development of apoptosis (FIG. 4). Again, these features could be partly inhibited by culture in the presence of OVA (data not shown).

Oral Tolerance Does Not Cause Global Inactivation of Lymphocytes and Is Preceded by Transient Immune Priming

The loss of functional lymphocytes from tolerant populations *in vitro* was not global; as in the first 24 hours of culture with OVA, these cells secreted significant amounts of TGFβ (TABLE 1). In addition, the development of tolerance was preceded by a period of T-cell priming *in vivo*, as spleen cells taken from mice in the first 4 days after feeding OVA

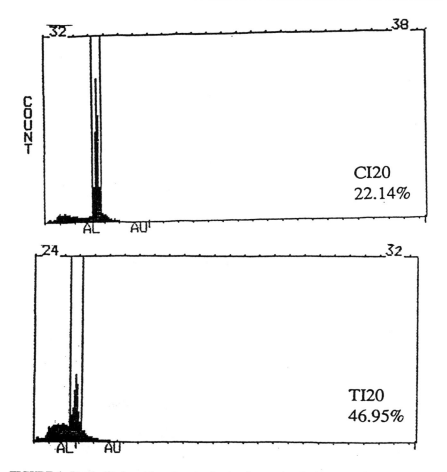

FIGURE 4. Death of tolerant lymphocytes *in vitro* is associated with apoptosis. DNA content of OVA-fed (T120) and immunized-control (C120) PLN cells taken 14 days after subcutaneous challenge with OVA/CFA and cultured for 120 hours in the absence of antigen. Flow cytometry of PI-stained cells show that tolerant cells have a large proportion of hypodiploid cells compared with control cells under the same conditions.

and without further challenge *in vivo* showed OVA-specific proliferation and production of IL-3 and γIFN when restimulated *in vitro* (FIG. 5).

DISCUSSION

These results show that feeding a relatively high dose of OVA (25 mg) suppresses the majority of T-cell functions *in vivo* and *in vitro*, including CD8+ T cells and both functional subsets of CD4+ T cells. The induction of tolerance predisposes lymphoid cells

TABLE 1. Production of TGFβ by Orally Tolerant Cells[a]

Group	OVA	TGFβ Production (pg/mL)
Control	–	49.4
Control	+	<5
Tolerant	–	<5
Tolerant	+	247.5

[a] Levels of TGFβ in supernatants of PLN cells taken 14 days after subcutaneous challenge with OVA/CFA in OVA-fed and control mice. PLN cells were cultured alone or in the presence of 1 mg/mL OVA. TGFβ levels were measured by ELISA.

to undergo apoptosis when removed from antigen, and there is selective production of TGFβ when tolerant cells are restimulated with OVA *in vitro*.

Many older studies implicated CD8+ suppressor T cells in oral tolerance, whereas more recent experiments have suggested that production of TGFβ or γIFN by CD8+ T cells regulates other immune functions in antigen-fed animals.[2-4] However, we found that class I MHC-restricted CTL activity was readily suppressed by feeding 25 mg OVA and, in other work, have been unable to detect any priming of these cells in OVA-fed mice.[11] In addition, depletion of CD8+ T cells did not influence the induction of tolerance. Together these findings indicate that, irrespective of their function, CD8+ T cells are unlikely to play a role in this model of tolerance. One possible explanation for the discrepancies between our own and other work is that CD8+ T cells may produce transient amounts of inhibitory cytokines at certain phases of oral tolerance. It would be important to follow the activation of CD8+ T cells at all times after feeding and parenteral challenge with antigen.

In our hands, CD4+ T cells were essential for the induction of tolerance by feeding OVA. Although this would be consistent with reports that preferential activation of Th2 CD4+ T cells by orally administered antigen may be responsible for down-regulating other T-cell responses,[1,4-6] our additional experiments argue against this interpretation. Thus, we found that Th2-dependent responses, such as IgG1 antibody production and secretion of IL-4, IL-5, and IL-10 were suppressed by feeding 25 mg OVA to the same extent as Th1-dependent production of IgG2a, IL-2, and γIFN. In addition, tolerance could be induced normally in IL-4-knockout mice lacking Th2 cells. In addition to all T-cell functions being abrogated by feeding OVA, lymphocytes from tolerized mice died rapidly *in vitro*, showing features of apoptosis. These results suggest that oral tolerance is associated with clonal anergy and/or deletion of antigen-reactive lymphocytes. T-cell anergy is a well-documented mechanism in other models of peripheral tolerance and has been implicated indirectly in oral tolerance.[7,12] However, clonal deletion is rarely seen in peripheral tolerance to nominal antigens, and it would now be important to determine if apoptosis of OVA-specific T lymphocytes occurs *in vivo* after feeding antigen.

A number of features of our work suggests that true deletion of OVA-specific lymphocytes may not occur *in vivo*. The death of tolerant cells in culture was partly prevented by addition of antigen, indicating that, *in vivo*, antigen-reactive lymphocytes may be maintained alive if antigen persists. Furthermore, the ability of tolerant cells to produce TGFβ when stimulated with OVA shows that the appropriate lymphocytes are still present after feeding and challenge *in vivo*. Finally, the number of apoptotic cells we observed in cultures of tolerized cells is much greater than could be explained by selective clonal

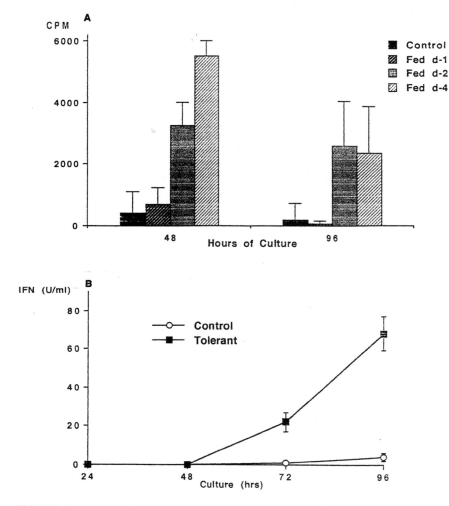

FIGURE 5. Priming of T-cell functions by feeding tolerogenic doses of ovalbumin. OVA-specific proliferation (A) and γIFN (B) production by spleen cells taken in the first 4 days after feeding 25 mg OVA and in unfed controls.

deletion of the low proportion of OVA-specific T cells that would be anticipated in these populations. For these reasons, we consider that oral tolerance in our model reflects the preferential stimulation of TGFβ production by fed OVA, leading to anergy of all antigen-specific T-cell functions. In addition, if present in sufficiently large concentrations in local microenvironments (as may occur during culture *in vitro*), this TGFβ may produce widespread cytostasis and ultimately death of neighboring lymphocytes. This "spreading anergy" may be analogous to the TGFβ-mediated bystander suppression reported in other models of oral tolerance.[1] Nevertheless, this bystander phenomenon has been identified under circumstances in which low doses of fed antigen produced active suppression and selective preservation of Th2 function. By contrast, higher doses of antigen, more similar to that used here, appeared to produce anergy and no surviving T-cell functions.[1,13,14] We would propose that these differences could be resolved if higher doses of fed antigen simply stimulate higher levels of TGFβ production, with consequently more rapid and profound loss of T-cell function after reintroduction of antigen. If confirmed, our data suggest that the clonal anergy and active suppression implicated by different studies of oral tolerance may simply be separate aspects of TGFβ production. This idea needs testing by examining the requirements for endogenous TGFβ in oral tolerance induced by feeding a range of doses of different antigens.

The reason why feeding antigen appears to inactivate T cells *in vivo* remains to be elucidated, but it may reflect association of fed antigen with relatively nonstimulatory antigen-presenting cells, leading to partial activation of T cells. This would be consistent with the transient proliferative activity and production of some cytokines we found immediately after feeding OVA, and we suggest that the selective production of TGFβ may be a consequence of antigen-specific T cells being held in this state of partial activation for long periods *in vivo*.

SUMMARY

Several different mechanisms have been implicated in oral tolerance to protein antigens, depending on the nature and dose of antigen used and the species under study. Here, we have investigated the basis of unresponsiveness in a well-established model of oral tolerance in mice fed 25 mg ovalbumin (OVA). Our results show that CD8+ T-cell activity is suppressed by feeding OVA and that these cells are not required for the induction of tolerance. CD4+ T cells are essential for tolerance to occur, but both Th1 and Th2 cell-dependent functions are tolerized equally in OVA-fed mice. Peripheral lymph node cells from tolerized mice rapidly undergo apoptosis when cultured *in vitro* but produce substantial amounts of transforming growth factor β (TGFβ) in response to OVA. The appearance of tolerance *in vivo* is preceded by a transient phase of T-cell priming, and we propose that this model of oral tolerance reflects partial activation of T cells by fed antigen, leading to selective production of TGFβ and consequent inactivation of all effector T cells. These findings indicate that the active suppression and clonal anergy identified previously in mice with oral tolerance may not be mutually exclusive phenomena.

REFERENCES

1. MOWAT, A. McI. 1987. The regulation of immune responses to dietary protein antigens. Immunol. Today **8**: 93.
2. WEINER, H. L., A. FRIEDMAN, A. MILLER, S. J. KHOURY, A. AL-SABBAGH, L. SANTOS, M. SAYEGH, R. B. NUSSENBLATT, D. E. TRENTHAM & D. A. HAFLER. 1994. Oral tolerance: Immunologic mechanisms and treatment of animal and human organ-specific autoimmune diseases by oral administration of autoantigens. Annu. Rev. Immunol. **12**: 809.
3. MCMENAMIN, C. & P. G. HOLT. 1993. The natural immune response to inhaled soluble protein antigens involves major histocompatibility complex (MHC) class I-restricted CD8+ T cell-mediated but MHC class II-restricted CD4+ T cell-dependent immune deviation resulting in selective suppression of immunoglobulin E production. J. Exp. Med. **178**: 889.
4. MILLER, A., O. LIDER, A. B. ROBERTS, M. SPORN & H. L. WEINER. 1992. Suppressor T cells generated by oral tolerization to myelin basic protein suppress both *in vitro* and

in vivo immune responses by the release of TGF-β following antigen specific triggering. Proc. Natl. Acad. Sci. USA **89:** 421.

5. KHOURY, S. J., W. W. HANCOCK & H. L. WEINER. 1992. Oral tolerance to myelin basic protein and natural recovery from experimental autoimmune encephalomyelitis are associated with downregulation of inflammatory cytokines and differential upregulation of transforming growth factor β, interleukin 4 and protaglandin E expression in the brain. J. Exp. Med. **176:** 1355.

6. CHEN, Y., V. K. KUCHROO, J. INOBE, D. A. HAFLER & H. L. WEINER. 1994. Regulatory T cells clones induced by oral tolerance: Suppression of autoimmune encephalomyelitis. Science **265:** 1237.

7. MELAMED, D. & A. FRIEDMAN. 1994. *In vivo* tolerization of Th1 lymphocytes following a single feed with ovalbumin: anergy in the absence of suppression. Eur. J. Immunol. **24:** 1974.

8. KOPF, M., G. LEGROS, M. BACHMANN, M. C. LAMERS, H. BLUETHMANN & G. KOHLER. 1993. Disruption of the murine IL-4 gene blocks Th2 cytokine responses. Nature **362:** 245.

9. GARSIDE, P., M. STEEL, E. A. WORTHEY, A. SATOSKAR, J. ALEXANDER, H. BLUETHMANN, F. Y. LIEW & A. McI. MOWAT. 1995. Th2 cells are subject to high dose oral tolerance and are not essential for its induction. J. Immunol. **154:** 3549-55.

10. MOWAT, A. McI., A. M. DONACHIE, G. REID & O. JARRETT. 1991. Immune-stimulating complexes containing Quil A and protein antigen prime class I MHC-restricted T lymphocytes *in vivo* and are immunogenic by the oral route. Immunology **72:** 317.

11. GARSIDE, P., M. STEEL, F. Y. LIEW & A. McI. MOWAT. 1995. CD4⁺ but not CD8⁺ T cells are required for the induction of oral tolerance. Int. Immunol. **7:** 501-4.

12. WHITACRE, C. C., I. E. GIENAPP, C. G. OROSZ & D. M. BITAR. 1991. Oral tolerance in experimental autoimmune encephalomyelitis III. Evidence for clonal anergy. J. Immunol. **147:** 2155.

13. GREGERSON, D. S., W. F. OBRITSCH & L. A. DONOSO. 1993. Oral tolerance in experimental autoimmune uveoretinitis: Distinct mechanisms of resistance are induced by low dose vs. high dose feeding protocols. J. Immunol. **151:** 5751.

14. FRIEDMAN, A. & H. L. WEINER. 1994. Induction of anergy or active suppression following oral tolerance is determined by antigen dose. Proc. Natl. Acad. Sci. USA **91:** 6688.

The Role of Chemokines in Oral Tolerance

Abrogation of Nonresponsiveness by Treatment with Antimonocyte Chemotactic Protein-1[a]

WILLIAM J. KARPUS[b] AND NICHOLAS W. LUKACS [c]

[b]Department of Microbiology and Immunology
Northwestern University Medical School
303 Chicago Avenue, 6-721 Tarry Building
Chicago, Illinois 60611

[c]Department of Pathology
University of Michigan Medical School
Ann Arbor, Michigan

INTRODUCTION

Peripheral, antigen-specific tolerance can be induced by oral administration of both protein and hapten antigens.[1] Oral tolerance has been used to prevent the induction of experimental autoimmune diseases[2-6] and is currently being used in clinical trials for treatment of human autoimmune diseases.[7,8] The mechanism of oral tolerance is not completely understood. There have been reports suggesting that feeding antigen induces both anergy and regulatory T cells.[9-13] More recently, the mechanism of oral tolerance has been reported to be induction of anergy/deletion by feeding a high dose of antigen[14] or regulatory T cells that secrete TGF-β by feeding multiple, small doses of antigen.[15,16] Introduction of antigen into mucosal surfaces appears to inhibit peripheral cell-mediated immune responses[9,17] but primes mucosal antibody responses[18] and also peripheral antibody responses.[19,20] Events at the intestinal mucosa that modulate antigen uptake and processing (*e.g.,* inhibition of oral tolerance induction by introduction of cholera toxin and antigen) also appear to have an influence on whether feeding antigen induces peripheral tolerance or primes a peripheral immune response.[17,21-27] Additionally, the ability to generate an IL-4 response at the time of feeding also determines whether oral tolerance can be induced.[28] Whether introduction of antigen by feeding leads to peripheral tolerance or primes a peripheral immune response, it appears that migration of lymphoid cells in and out of the mucosal immune system to and from the peripheral immune system is a necessary component of oral tolerance.[11,29,30]

Lymphocytes leave the circulation, migrate, and accumulate at sites of inflammation in response to chemoattractants. Historically, leukotrienes, platelet-activating factor (PAF), and C5a have been defined as nonspecific chemoattractants responsible for mononuclear cell recruitment. Recently, several laboratories have identified specific chemoattractant cytokines (chemokines) for neutrophils as well as mononuclear and lymphoid cells. The

[a]This work was supported in part by NIH Grant AI35934.

133

potent factors are divided into two highly conserved gene families: C-x-C and C-C, designated by the position of the first two cysteines.[31,32] The C-x-C (or α) chemokines are primarily chemotactic for neutrophils.[33] The prototypic C-x-C chemokine is IL-8. The C-C (or β) chemokines are primarily chemotactic for mononuclear cells, basophils, and eosinophils.[33-35] Representatives of this family include macrophage inflammatory protein (MIP)-1α and monocyte chemotactic protein (MCP)-1. The cellular source of the C-C chemokines has only recently been elucidated. MIP-1α has been shown to be expressed primarily by mononuclear cells, neutrophils, and inflammatory fibroblasts[36] and also has been shown to up-regulate ICAM-1,[37-40] demonstrating the importance of this factor in the migration of mononuclear cells. Another member of the C-C family, MCP-1, was first identified as an early response gene (JE) in murine fibroblasts treated with PDGF.[41] MCP-1 expression has been demonstrated in monocytes, lymphocytes, endothelial cells, epithelial cells, and smooth muscle cells[36,42] and has been identified as a chemotactic factor for CD4[+] T cells.[43,44] Recently, infection of intestinal epithelia has been shown to induce the production of MCP-1.[45]

Inasmuch as migration of lymphocytes seems to be an important consequence or oral tolerance induction, we hypothesized that C-C chemokines might be important factors in the induction of oral tolerance. In the present report, we tested the *in vivo* role of MIP-1α and MCP-1 in the induction of oral tolerance to human gamma globulin (HGG).

MATERIAL AND METHODS

Mice

Inbred female SJL/J (H-2^s) mice were purchased from Harlan Sprague Dawley (Indianapolis, IN) and housed according to Northwestern University and NIH guidelines.

Antigens

HGG was purchased from Sigma (St. Louis, MO). Bovine MBP was a kind gift of Dr. Stephen D. Miller (Northwestern University).

In Vitro *T-cell Proliferation/Cytokine Assays*

In vitro proliferative responses of lymph node T cells were measured according to established methods using [^{3}H]TdR incorporation.[46] Single cell suspensions from pooled lymph nodes were cultured at a density of 2×10^6 cells/mL in Dulbecco's modified Eagle medium (DMEM) containing 5% FCS, 1 mM glutamine, 1% Pen-Strep, 1 mM nonessential amino acids, and 5×10^{-5} M 2-ME (complete DMEM-5, all components from Sigma) in the presence or absence of 5 μg/mL HGG. Antigen-induced cytokine production was assayed from 24-, 48-, and 72-h culture supernatants. Duplicate samples were tested for the presence of IL-2, IL-4, and IL-10 by ELISA, using cyto*screen*™ ELISA kits (Biosource International, Camarillo, CA). Transforming growth factor (TGF)-β was analyzed from supernatants of cells grown in serum-free medium using a modified ELISA as previously described.[15] IFN-γ production was measured by capture ELISA using recombinant cytokine as a standard.[46] Measurement of MIP-1α and MCP-1 was performed on cell culture supernatants, as previously described.[36]

Induction of Antigen-specific DTH

Prechallenge ear thickness in metofane-anesthetized animals was measured with a Mitotoyo dial thickness gauge. Five μg of antigen (in 10 μL PBS) was injected intradermally into the dorsal surface of the ear using a 100 μL Hamilton syringe fitted with a 30 g needle. Ear swelling was measured 24 h later and expressed in units of 10^{-4} inches. HGG-induced ear-swelling responses are the result of mononuclear cell infiltration and show typical delayed-type hypersensitivity (DTH) kinetics (*i.e.*, minimal swelling at 4 h, maximal swelling at 24-48 h).

In Vivo *Administration of Antibodies*

Mice were administered 0.5 mL of either rabbit anti-MIP-1α or rabbit anti-MCP-1 intraperitoneally (ip) using a 25 gauge needle. The rabbit polyclonal antisera was specific for its respective chemokine and did not cross-react with other known chemokines or cytokines, as tested by ELISA. The sera had titers > 10^6.

RESULTS

Intragastric Administration of HGG Inhibits HGG-specific T-cell Proliferation and DTH

Two groups of three mice were either given 20 mg HGG or myelin basic protein (MBP) (as a control) intragastrically (ig) seven days prior to immunization with 25 μg HGG emulsified in CFA containing 2 mg/mL *Mycobacterium tuberculosis*. Seven days following immunization, draining lymph node cells were pooled and cultured with HGG; proliferation was measured by thymidine incorporation. FIGURE 1 shows that draining lymph node cells from control mice fed MBP and immunized with HGG make a recall T cell-proliferative response (open squares). By contrast, draining lymph node cells from mice fed HGG have a significantly decreased recall T cell-proliferative response (open circles; p < 0.01, Student's *t* test) through a 2 log dose-response range.

To determine the effect of ig administration of HGG on *in vivo*, cell-mediated immune responses, we tested DTH in groups of mice fed either HGG or MBP (control) and subsequently immunized with HGG/CFA. Seven days following immunization, mice from both groups were tested for HGG-specific DTH. Prechallenge ear thickness was measured, 5 μg of HGG was injected into each ear, and 24 h later the increased ear swelling was measured as an indication of DTH. In FIGURE 2 oral administration of 20 mg HGG seven days prior to immunization with HGG/CFA resulted in a significant decrease (p < 0.05) in *in vivo* DTH responses compared to control (MBP)-fed mice.

Effect of Intragastric Administration of HGG on Chemokine and Cytokine Responses

To test whether ig administration of HGG had an effect on the production of chemokines and cytokines, we fed mice either HGG or a control antigen (MBP) seven days prior to immunization with HGG/CFA. One week following immunization, draining lymph node cells from each group of mice were pooled and cultured in the presence or absence of HGG *in vitro*. The presence of chemokines and cytokines in the culture supernatants was

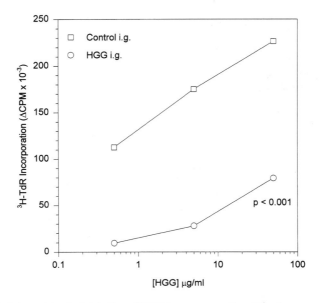

FIGURE 1. Intragastric administration of HGG decreases recall proliferative responses. Groups of three mice were fed 20 mg of either HGG or MBP (control) seven days prior to immunization with 25 μg HGG in CFA. Seven days later, draining lymph node cells were pooled and tested for proliferative responses in the presence or absence of 5 μg/mL HGG. The background proliferation for each group was less than 5000 cpm, and the standard deviation of each data point was less than 10% of the mean.

determined by specific ELISA.[36,46–48] Administration of ig HGG results in an antigen-specific decrease in IL-2 and IFN-γ, and an increase in IL-4 and IL-10 production (not shown), consistent with what has been reported in the literature.[49] In FIGURE 3 administration of 20 mg HGG ig also resulted in a decrease in MIP-1α production by lymph node cells from HGG-fed mice when compared to control-fed mice. However, to our surprise, ig administration of HGG had the opposite effect on production of MCP-1. FIGURE 4 shows that lymph node cells from mice fed 20 mg HGG 7 days prior to immunization produce a significantly greater amount of MCP-1. These results suggest that chemokines are important factors in the induction of oral tolerance.

Anti-MCP-1 Treatment in Vivo Abrogates Oral Tolerance Induction

The differential recall production of MIP-1α (FIG. 3) and MCP-1 (FIG. 4) suggested that MCP-1 production *in vivo* might be important in the induction of oral tolerance. As a test of this hypothesis, we fed mice either HGG or ovalbumin (OVA; as a control) and treated ip with either normal rabbit serum (NRS) or antiserum to MIP-1α or MCP-1 on days 0 and 2, relative to feeding. Seven days after ig administration of antigen, all mice were immunized with HGG/CFA. One week following immunization, cells from the draining lymph nodes were pooled from the three mice in each group, and antigen-specific recall proliferation was measured. FIGURE 5 shows the result of this experiment. Cells

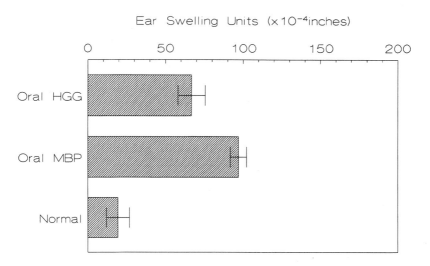

FIGURE 2. Intragastric administration of HGG results in decreased DTH responses. Mice were treated as in FIGURE 1. Seven days after immunization with HGG in CFA, the two groups of mice were challenged with 5 μg of HGG in PBS in each ear. Twenty-four hours later, ear swelling was used as a measure of DTH. The results are displayed as the mean ear swelling ± SD of three mice per group (6 ears). The DTH response in the oral HGG groups is statistically different (p < 0.05) than the DTH response for the control-fed group (oral MBP).

from mice fed OVA, treated with NRS, and immunized with HGG/CFA showed a substantial antigen-specific T cell-proliferative response (group A). By contrast, cells from mice fed HGG, treated with NRS, and immunized with HGG/CFA showed a significantly decreased proliferative response (group B; p < 0.01 when compared to group A). Cells from mice fed HGG, treated with anti-MIP-1α, and immunized with HGG/CFA (group D) also showed a decreased proliferative response when compared to its control group (group C; p < 0.01). The proliferative response of cells from group D is not significantly different than that from group B, suggesting that *in vivo* neutralization of MIP-1α does not have an effect on the induction of oral tolerance. However, cells from mice fed HGG, treated with anti-MCP-1, and immunized with HGG/CFA (group F) did not show a significantly different proliferative response than cells from the control-fed group (group E). Moreover, the proliferative response of the lymph node cells from mice fed HGG, treated with anti-MCP-1, and immunized with HGG-CFA (group F) was significantly greater (p < 0.01) than that of mice fed HGG and treated with either NRS (group B) or anti-MIP-1α (group D). These data suggest that induction of oral tolerance can be abrogated by treating recipients *in vivo* with anti-MCP-1, but not anti-MIP-1α.

DISCUSSION

Feeding protein antigens can result in the antigen-specific inhibition of peripheral immune responses[50,51] as well as the priming of antigen-specific gut responses.[18] In the present report, we demonstrated that feeding a high dose of HGG can inhibit T cell-

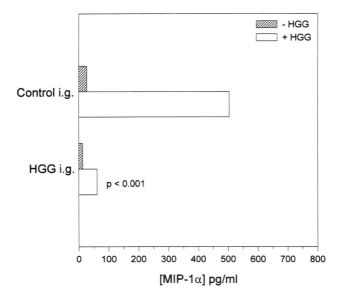

FIGURE 3. Intragastric (ig) administration of HGG results in the antigen-specific reduction in recall MIP-1α production *in vitro*. Lymph node cells from the mice in FIGURE 1 were cultured in the presence or absence of 5 μg/mL HGG. MIP-1α production was measured by ELISA, using recombinant MIP-1α as a standard, and the data are shown as pg/mL.

proliferative (FIG. 1) and DTH (FIG. 2) responses. Moreover, oral tolerance induction by feeding HGG selectively inhibited MIP-1α production (FIG. 3) and increased MCP-1 production (FIG. 4) by peripheral lymphoid cells. MCP-1 was found to be an important chemokine in the induction of oral tolerance because treatment with anti-MCP-1, but not MIP-1α, at the time of feeding HGG abrogated oral tolerance (FIG. 5). The mechanism or oral tolerance induction in the present report appears to be a combination of inhibition of Th1 and priming of Th2 cytokine responses (data not shown). Moreover, we have recently shown that feeding a high dose of the immunodominant peptide epitope of proteolipid protein results in peripheral tolerance by inducing both anergy of Th1 responses and priming of Th2 responses (manuscript submitted). Our results are consistent with what has been reported for inducing oral tolerance by feeding ovalbumin.[9,10]

One possibility that might explain why treatment with anti-MCP-1 would abrogate oral tolerance induction is that MCP-1 is an important factor in the generation of a Th2-like response after feeding HGG. We do not favor this interpretation because analysis of lymphocytes from mice treated with anti-MCP-1 revealed that there was no difference in IL-4 and TGF-β production by peripheral T cells when compared to T cells from control-treated mice (data not shown). Moreover, addition of either recombinant MCP-1 or MIP-1α to cultures of HGG-specific T cells did not alter the cytokine production pattern (data not shown). A more likely interpretation of the data in the present report is that MCP-1 is an important chemotactic factor in the gut and/or periphery and is selectively involved in the chemotaxis of Th2-like regulatory cells in and out of the gut, as well as the spleen. A recent report has suggested that MCP-1 production is induced in intestinal epithelial cells following infection.[45] It is possible that oral administration of antigens induces MCP-

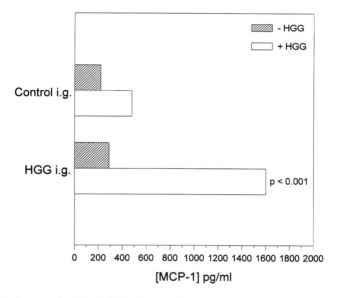

FIGURE 4. Intragastric (ig) administration of HGG results in the antigen-specific increase in recall MCP-1 production *in vitro*. Lymph node cells from the mice in FIGURE 1 were cultured in the presence or absence of 5 μg/mL HGG. MCP-1 production was measured by ELISA, using recombinant MCP-1 as a standard, and the data are shown as pg/mL.

1, which in turn induces the chemoattraction of Th2-like regulatory cells. By blocking the chemotactic effects of MCP-1 at the site of antigen intake, the influx of regulatory cells might be prevented, thereby preventing the induction of peripheral tolerance. Alternatively, MCP-1 might be involved in the efflux of regulatory cells from the gut to the periphery, and neutralization of MCP-1 in the gut would prevent the migration of these cells to the periphery. These possibilities are currently being tested.

In addition to MCP-1,[43] MIP-1α is also a chemotactic factor for T cells.[35] It is interesting that anti-MIP-1α did not abrogate the induction of oral tolerance (FIG. 5) in the present report. If the hypothesis is that oral tolerance induces a regulatory T-cell population that emigrates from the gut to the periphery to effect nonresponsiveness, one might predict that anti-MIP-1α would also abrogate induction of oral tolerance. We have previously shown that anti-MIP-1α treatment inhibits granuloma formation in both a schistosomiasis model[47] and a central nervous system demyelinating disease model, experimental autoimmune encephalomyelitis (EAE).[52] Both of these inflammatory disease models are induced by Th1-dominated responses. It is possible that MIP-1α is a preferential chemoattractant in Th1-dominated responses and that MCP-1 is a preferential chemoattractant in Th2-dominated responses. The data in the present report suggest that MCP-1 is an important chemotactic cytokine in the induction of oral tolerance, which has been reported to be mediated in part by a Th2-like response.[49]

SUMMARY

Peripheral antigen-specific tolerance can be induced by feeding protein antigens. The mechanism has been described as either clonal anergy/deletion or induction of antigen-

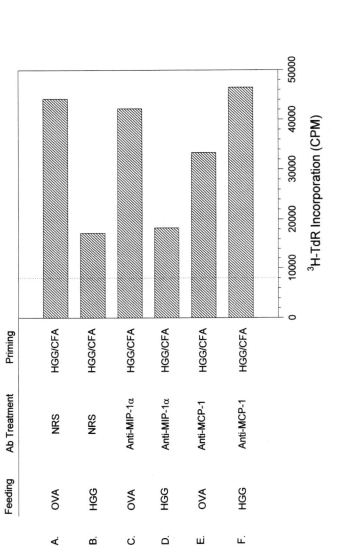

FIGURE 5. Anti-MCP-1 treatment abrogates oral tolerance induction. Six groups (A–F) of mice (3 per group) were fed either OVA (control) or HGG seven days prior to immunization and treated with either NRS, anti-MIP-1α, or anti-MCP-1 on days 0 and 2, relative to feeding. All mice were immunized with 25 μg HGG emulsified in CFA. Seven days after immunization, the draining lymph node cells were pooled from the three mice in each group, and recall proliferative responses were tested in the presence or absence of 5 μg/mL HGG. The results are displayed as mean thymidine incorporation (cpm) of triplicate wells. Statistical analysis was performed using ANOVA. The standard deviation was less than 10% of the mean in all groups and was left out of the FIGURE for clarity.

specific regulatory cells that produce transforming growth factor (TGF)-β, depending on the dose of antigen fed. Experimental autoimmune encephalomyelitis (EAE), an animal model for multiple sclerosis, can be prevented by feeding myelin basic protein (MBP) or proteolipid protein (PLP). We decided to address the role of chemokines in the induction of oral tolerance. We have used a model antigen system of feeding a high dose of human gamma globulin (HGG) to mice that have been subsequently immunized with HGG emulsified in CFA. The result was decreased recall proliferative, delayed-type hypersensitivity (DTH) and Th1 cytokine responses. By contrast, Th2 cytokine responses were enhanced. Interestingly, macrophage inflammatory protein (MIP)-1α production was decreased, whereas monocyte chemotactic protein (MCP)-1 production was enhanced. Induction of oral tolerance was prevented by the administration of anti-MCP-1 to mice fed HGG. These results show that chemokines play an important role in the induction of oral tolerance.

ACKNOWLEDGMENTS

The authors would like to thank Drs. S. D. Miller, R. M. Strieter, and S. L. Kunkel for their support.

REFERENCES

1. WEINER, H. L. 1994. Oral tolerance. Proc. Natl. Acad. Sci. USA **91:** 10762–10765.
2. LIDER, O., L. M. SANTOS, C. S. LEE, P. J. HIGGINS & H. L. WEINER. 1989. Suppression of experimental autoimmune encephalomyelitis by oral administration of myelin basic protein. II. Suppression of disease and *in vitro* immune responses is mediated by antigen-specific CD8+ T lymphocytes. J. Immunol. **142:** 748–752.
3. BITAR, D. M. & C. C. WHITACRE. 1988. Suppression of experimental autoimmune encephalomyelitis by the oral administration of myelin basic protein. Cell. Immunol. **112:** 364–370.
4. NUSSENBLATT, R. B., R. R. CASPI, R. MAHDI, C.-C. CHAN, F. ROBERGE, O. LIDER & H. L. WEINER. 1990. Inhibition of S-antigen induced experimental autoimmune uveoretinitis by oral induction of tolerance with S-antigen. J. Immunol. **144:** 1689–1695.
5. ZHANG, Z. Y., C. S. LEE, O. LIDER & H. L. WEINER. 1990. Suppression of adjuvant arthritis in Lewis rats by oral administration of type II collagen. J. Immunol. **145:** 2489–2493.
6. WANG, Z.-Y., J. HUANG, T. OLSSON, B. HE & H. LINK. 1995. B cell responses to acetylcholine receptor in rats orally tolerized against experimental autoimmune myasthenia gravis. J. Neurol. Sci. **128:** 167–174.
7. WEINER, H. L., G. A. MACKIN, M. MATSUI, E. J. ORAV, S. J. KHOURY, D. M. DAWSON & D. A. HAFLER. 1993. Double-blind pilot trial of oral tolerance with myelin antigens in multiple sclerosis. Science **259:** 1321–1323.
8. TRENTHAM, D. E., R. A. DYNESIUS-TRENTHAM, E. J. ORAV, D. COMBITCHI, C. LORENZO, K. L. SEWELL, D. A. HAFLER & H. L. WEINER. 1993. Effects of oral administration of type II collagen on rheumatoid arthritis Science **261:** 1727–1730.
9. MILLER, S. D. & D. G. HANSON. 1979. Inhibition of specific immune responses by feeding protein antigens. IV. Evidence for tolerance and specific active suppression of cell-mediated immune responses to ovalbumin. J. Immunol. **123:** 2344–2350.
10. HANSON, D. G. & S. D. MILLER. 1982. Inhibition of specific immune responses by feeding protein antigens. V. Induction of the tolerant state in the absence of specific suppressor cells. J. Immunol. **128:** 2378–2381.
11. ASHERSON, G. L., M. ZEMBALA, M. A. C. C. PERERA, B. MAYHEW & W. R. THOMAS. 1977. Production of immunity and unresponsiveness in the mouse by feeding contact

sensitizing agents and the role of suppressor cells in the Peyer's patches, mesenteric lymph nodes and other lymphoid tissues. Cell. Immunol. **33:** 145-155.

12. STROBEL, S., A. M. MOWAT, H. E. DRUMMOND, M. G. PICKERING & A. FERGUSON. 1983. Immunological responses to fed protein antigens in mice. Oral tolerance for CMI is due to activation of cyclophosphamide-sensitive cells by gut-processed antigen. Immunology **49:** 451-456.

13. RICHMAN, L. K., J. M. CHILLER, W. R. BROWN, D. G. HANSON & N. M. VAZ. 1978. Enterically induced immunologic tolerance. I. Induction of suppressor T lymphocytes by intragastric administration of soluble proteins. J. Immunol. **121:** 2429-2434.

14. WHITACRE, C. C., I. E. GIENAPP, C. G. OROSZ & D. M. BITAR. 1991. Oral tolerance in experimental autoimmune encephalomyelitis. III. Evidence for clonal anergy. J. Immunol. **147:** 2155-2163.

15. MILLER, A., O. LIDER, A. B. ROBERTS, M. B. SPORN & H. L. WEINER. 1992. Suppressor T cells generated by oral tolerization to myelin basic protein suppress both *in vitro* and *in vivo* immune responses by the release of transforming growth factor β after antigen-specific triggering. Proc. Natl. Acad. Sci. USA **89:** 421-425.

16. FRIEDMAN, A. & H. L. WEINER. 1994. Induction of anergy or active suppression following oral tolerance is determined by antigen dosage. Proc. Natl. Acad. Sci. USA **91:** 6688-6692.

17. KAY, R. A. & A. FERGUSON. 1989. The immunological consequences of feeding cholera toxin. II. Mechanisms responsible for the induction of oral tolerance for DTH. Immunology **66:** 416-421.

18. MICHALEK, S. M., J. R. MCGHEE, H. KIYONO, D. E. COLWELL, J. H. ELDRIDGE, M. J. WANNEMUEHLER & W. J. KOOPMAN. 1983. The IgA response: Inductive aspects, regulatory cells, and effector functions. Ann. N.Y. Acad. Sci. **409:** 48-71.

19. ENOMOTO, A., M. KONISHI, S. HACHIMURA & S. KAMINOGAWA. 1993. Milk whey protein fed as a constituent of the diet induced both oral tolerance and a systemic humoral response, while heat-denatured whey protein induced only oral tolerance. Clin. Immunol. Immunopathol. **66:** 136-142.

20. HUSBY, S., J. MESTECKY, Z. MOLDOVEANU, S. HOLLAND & C. O. ELSON. 1994. Oral tolerance in humans. T cell but not B cell tolerance after antigen feeding. J. Immunol. **152:** 4663-4670.

21. ELSON, C. O. & W. EALDING. 1984. Cholera toxin feeding did not induce oral tolerance in mice and abrogated oral tolerance to an unrelated protein antigen. J. Immunol. **133:** 2892-2897.

22. FARIA, A. M., G. GARCIA, M. J. RIOS, C. L. MICHALAROS & N. M. VAZ. 1993. Decrease in susceptibility to oral tolerance induction and occurrence of oral immunization to ovalbumin in 20- to 38-week-old mice. The effect of interval between oral exposures and rate of antigen intake in the oral immunization. Immunology **78:** 147-151.

23. HANSON, D. G., M. J. ROY, G. M. GREEN & S. D. MILLER. 1993. Inhibition of orally-induced immune tolerance in mice by prefeeding an endopeptidase inhibitor. Reg. Immunol. **5:** 85-93.

24. MICHALEK, S. M., H. KIYONO, M. J. WANNEMUEHLER, L. M. MOSTELLER & J. R. MCGHEE. 1982. Lipopolysaccharide (LPS) regulation of the immune response: LPS influence on oral tolerance induction. J. Immunol. **128:** 1992-1998.

25. RUSSEL, G. & C. COSTALOS. 1980. Oral tolerance of Caloreen in babies. Arch. Dis. Child. **55:** 886-887.

26. DOMEN, P. L., A. MUCKERHEIDE & J. G. MICHAEL. 1987. Cationization of protein antigens. III. Abrogation of oral tolerance. J. Immunol. **139:** 3195-3198.

27. SUN, J.-B., J. HOLMGREN & C. CZERKINSKY. 1994. Cholera toxin B subunit: An efficient transmucosal carrier-delivery system for induction of peripheral immunological tolerance. Proc. Natl. Acad. Sci. USA **91:** 10795-10799.

28. VAJDY, M., M. H. KOSCO-VILBOIS, M. KOPF, G. KÖHLER & N. LYCKE. 1995. Impaired mucosal immune responses in interleukin 4-targeted mice. J. Exp. Med. **181:** 41-53.

29. Suzuki, I., H. Kiyono, K. Kitamura, D. R. Green & J. R. McGhee. 1986. Abrogation of oral tolerance by contrasuppressor T cells suggests the presence of regulatory T-cell networks in the mucosal immune system. Nature **320:** 451–454.

30. Suh, E. D., B. P. Vistica, C. C. Chan, J. M. Raber, I. Gery & R. B. Nussenblatt. 1993. Splenectomy abrogates the induction of oral tolerance in experimental autoimmune uveoretinitis. Curr. Eye Res. **12:** 833–839.

31. Schall, T. J. 1991. Biology of the RANTES/SIS cytokine family. Cytokine **3:** 165–183.

32. Miller, M. D. & M. S. Krangel. 1992. Biology and biochemistry of the chemokines: a family of chemotactic and inflammatory cytokines. Crit. Rev. Immunol. **12:** 17–46.

33. Oppenheim, J. J., C. O. C. Zachariae, N. Mukaida & K. Matsushima. 1991. Properties of the novel proinflammatory supergene "intercrine" cytokine family. Annu. Rev. Immunol. **9:** 617–648.

34. Ernst, C. A., Y. J. Zhang, P. R. Hancock, B. J. Rutledge, C. L. Corless & B. J. Rollins. 1994. Biochemical and biologic characterization of murine monocyte chemoattractant protein-1. J. Immunol. **152:** 3541–3549.

35. Davatelis, G., P. Tekamp-Olson, S. D. Wolpe, K. Hermsen, C. Luedke, C. Gallegos, D. Coit, J. Merryweather & A. Cerami. 1988. Cloning and characterization of a cDNA for murine macrophage inflammatory protein (MIP), a novel monokine with inflammatory and chemokine properties. J. Exp. Med. **167:** 1939–1944.

36. Lukacs, N. W., S. W. Chensue, R. E. Smith, R. M. Strieter, K. Warmington, C. Wilke & S. L. Kunkel. 1994. Production of monocyte chemoattractant protein-1 and macrophage inflammatory protein-1 alpha by inflammatory granuloma fibroblasts. Am. J. Pathol. **144:** 711–718.

37. Butcher, E. C. 1991. Leukocyte-endothelial cell recognition: three (or more) steps to specificity and diversity. Cell **67:** 1033–1036.

38. Springer, T. A. 1994. Traffic signals for lymphocyte recirculation and leukocyte emigration: the multistep paradigm. Cell **76:** 301–314.

39. Vaddi, K. & R. C. Newton. 1994. Regulation of monocyte integrin expression by β-family chemokines. J. Immunol. **153:** 4721–4732.

40. Tanaka, Y., D. H. Adams, S. Hubscher, H. Hirano, U. Sienbenlist & S. Shaw. 1993. T-cell adhesion induced by proteoglycan-immobilized cytokine MIP-1β. Nature **361:** 79–82.

41. Rollins, B. J., E. D. Morriso & C. D. Stiles. 1988. Cloning and expression of JE, a gene inducible by platelet-derived growth factor and whose product has cytokine-like properties. Proc. Natl. Acad. Sci. USA **85:** 3738–3742.

42. Van Damme, J., P. Proost, W. Put, S. Arens, J.-P. Lenaerts, R. Conings, G. Opdenakker, H. Heremans & A. Billiau. 1994. Induction of monocyte chemotactic proteins MCP-1 and MCP-2 in human fibroblasts and leukocytes by cytokines and cytokine inducers. Chemical synthesis of MCP-2 and development of a specific RIA. J. Immunol. **152:** 5495–5502.

43. Carr, M. W., S. J. Roth, E. Luther, S. S. Rose & T. A. Springer. 1994. Monocyte chemoattractant protein 1 acts as a T-lymphocyte chemoattractant. Proc. Natl. Acad. Sci. USA **91:** 3652–3656.

44. Loetscher, P., M. Seitz, I. Clark-Lewis, M. Baggiolini & B. Moser. 1994. Monocyte chemotactic proteins MCP-1, MCP-2, and MCP-3 are major attractants for human CD4+ and CD8+ T lymphocytes. FASEB J. **8:** 1055–1060.

45. Jung, H. C., L. Eckmann, S.-K. Yang, A. Panja, J. Fierer, E. Morzycka-Wroblewska & M. F. Kagnoff. 1995. A distinct array of proinflammatory cytokines is expressed in human colon epithelial cells in response to bacterial invasion. J. Clin. Invest. **95:** 55–65.

46. Peterson, J. D., W. J. Karpus, R. J. Clatch & S. D. Miller. 1993. Split tolerance of Th1 and Th2 cells in tolerance to Theiler's murine encephalomyelitis virus. Eur. J. Immunol. **23:** 46–55.

47. LUKACS, N. W., S. L. KUNKEL, R. M. STRIETER, K. WARMINGTON & S. W. CHENSUE.
     1993. The role of macrophage inflammatory protein 1α in Shistosoma mansoni egg-
     induced granulomatous inflammation. J. Exp. Med. **177:** 1551-1559.
48. KARPUS, W. J., J. D. PETERSON & S. D. MILLER. 1994. Anergy *in vivo:* down-regulation
     of antigen-specific CD4+ Th1 but not Th2 cytokine responses. Int. Immunol. **6:** 721-730.
49. CHEN, Y., V. K. KUCHROO, J. INOBE, D. A. HAFLER & H. L. WEINER. 1994. Regulatory
     T cell clones induced by oral tolerance: Suppression of autoimmune encephalomyelitis.
     Science **265:** 1237-1240.
50. TOMASI, T. B., JR. 1980. Oral tolerance. Transplantation **29:** 353-356.
51. WEINER, H. L., A. FRIEDMAN, A. MILLER, S. J. KHOURY, A. AL-SABBAGH, L. SANTOS,
     M. SAYEGH, R. B. NUSSENBLATT, D. E. TRENTHAM & D. A. HAFLER. 1994. Oral
     tolerance: immunologic mechanisms and treatment of animal and human organ-specific
     autoimmune diseases by oral administration of autoantigens. Annu. Rev. Immunol. **12:**
     809-837.
52. KARPUS, W. J., N. W. LUKACS, B. L. MCRAE, R. M. STRIETER, S. L. KUNKEL & S. D.
     MILLER. 1995. An important role for the chemokine macrophage inflammatory protein-
     1α in the pathogenesis of the T-cell mediated autoimmune disease, experimental autoim-
     mune encephalomyelitis. J. Immunol. **155:** 5003-5010.

Effect of Oral Beta Interferon on Subsequent Immune Responsiveness

PATRICIA A. NELSON,[a] YEVGENYA AKSELBAND,[a]
SUSAN M. DEARBORN,[a] AHMAD AL-SABBAGH,[a]
Z. JANE TIAN,[a] PATRICIA A. GONNELLA,[b]
SCOTT S. ZAMVIL,[b] YOUHAI CHEN,[b] AND
HOWARD L. WEINER [b]

[a]*AutoImmune Inc.*
128 Spring Street
Lexington, Massachusetts 02173

[b]*Center for Neurologic Disease*
Brigham and Women's Hospital
221 Longwood Avenue
Boston, Massachusetts 02115

INTRODUCTION

Oral administration of antigen has long been shown to be an effective means of reducing immune (Th1) responses to subsequent immunization with the same antigen.[1] We are using oral autoantigens to suppress autoimmune responses in both animal models and in clinical trials with patients with autoimmune disease. Although oral autoantigens are effective in some treated individuals, not all of the patients that do show reduced disease are affected to the same extent. We would like to be able to broaden the effectiveness of oral tolerance therapy by enhancing the ability of autoantigens to induce tolerance when given by the oral route. Several factors have been shown to modulate oral tolerance, although by potentially different mechanisms. Gamma interferon (γIFN) treatment of animals interfered with oral tolerance as measured by antibody responses to orally administered bovine serum albumin (BSA), possibly by favoring Th1 over Th2 responses.[2] Orally administered lipopolysaccharide (LPS), but not systemic, enhances the protection in experimental autoimmune encephalomyelitis (EAE) by orally administered myelin basic protein (MBP).[3] In the EAE model, IL-4 secreting Th2-type cells may also play a role following oral tolerization. Immunohistochemical studies in the Lewis rat EAE model showed that orally fed MBP is associated with increased expression of TGFβ in the brain without IL-4, whereas MBP plus LPS is associated with both IL-4 and TGFβ.[4]

It had been previously reported that injected rat interferon (IFN) (likely to be type I because of fibroblast origin) suppressed disease onset and severity in a rat EAE model.[5,6] Our recent experiments, as well as others,[7,8] have indicated that beta interferon (βIFN) given orally can also serve as a synergist for oral tolerogens. We are thus exploring the possibility of feeding the autoantigens in conjunction with other agents that may enhance the induction of tolerance. The work presented here shows enhancement of oral tolerance induction in the EAE disease model *in vivo* by the oral administration of βIFN. In order to detect a synergistic effect with potential enhancing compounds, a suboptimal feeding regimen was used. Feeding proteins five or more times has been shown to be effective at inducing oral tolerance, whereas feeding low doses three times is less effective, thus

145

suboptimal. An unexpected modulation of *in vitro* cytokine profile induced by oral administration of βIFN was observed.

MATERIAL AND METHODS

Animals

Female Lewis rats, 6-8 weeks of age, were obtained from Charles River Laboratory
(Wilmington, MA). These animals were housed in Harvard Medical School Animal Care
Facilities. (PLJ/J × SJL/J)F$_1$ and SJL/J mice, 6-8 weeks of age, were obtained from the
Jackson Laboratory, Bar Harbor, ME and housed in the AutoImmune Animal Facilities.
All animals were maintained on standard laboratory chow and water ad libitum, with care
in accordance with the guidelines outlined by the Committee on Care of Laboratory
Animals of the Laboratory Research Council (Pub. #DHEW:NIH, 85-23, revised 1985).

Induction and Clinical Evaluation of EAE

Guinea pig (gp), murine, and bovine (b) MBP were purified from brain tissue by a
modified method of Deibler *et al.*[9] Protein content and purity were checked by gel
electrophoresis and amino acid analysis. Rats were immunized in the footpad with 25 μg
of gpMBP in 50 μL of PBS emulsified in an equal volume of complete Freund's adjuvant
containing 100 μg of *Mycobacterium tuberculosis* (Difco). Mice were immunized subcutaneously and in the footpad with 250 μg gpMBP in 50 μL of PBS emulsified in an equal
volume of complete Freund's adjuvant containing 100 μg of *Mycobacterium tuberculosis*
(Difco). Animals were evaluated in a coded fashion for signs of EAE beginning approximately 10 days after immunization. Clinical severity was scored on a scale of 0-5 as
follows: 0, no disease; 1, limp tail; 2, hind-limb paralysis; 3, hind-limb paraplegia, inconti-
nence; 4, tetraplegia; and 5, death.

Oral Administration of Protein

Oral proteins were administered to the animals every 2-3 days on a Monday-Wednes-
day-Friday schedule from 3 to 7 times prior to immunization, as indicated in the individual
experiments. MBP was orally administered by gastric intubation using an 18-gauge stainless steel needle (Thomas Scientific, Swedesboro, NJ). Ovalbumin (OVA) was obtained
from Sigma (OVA #A7641, St. Louis MO). Cytimmune mouse interferon beta (βIFN)
and Cytimmune rat type I interferon were obtained from Lee Biomolecular Research, Inc.
(San Diego, CA; murine βIFN = 1. 1 × 10^7 U/mg, and rat type I (α + β mix) = 3.5 × 10^6
U/mg).

In Vitro *Cell Culture*

Spleens, lymph nodes, and Peyer's patches were harvested from animals 10-12 days
following immunization. Culture medium consisted of DMEM (Gibco, Grand Island, NY),
containing penicillin (50 U/mL) and streptomycin (50 μg/mL), L-glutamine (2 mM), 2
ME (5 × 10^{-5}M), 10% heat-inactivated FCS, and HEPES (10 mM). Organs were teased
into single-cell suspensions, washed by centrifugation, counted, and cultured at a concentra-

TABLE 1. Effect of Oral MBP and Type I Interferon on Induction of Tolerance in Lewis Rat EAE[a]

Groups Treated	Incidence	Day of Onset	Mean Max Score
HEL[b] 1 mg	5/5	12.0	2.0
IFN 20,000 U	4/5	13.0	1.0
IFN 10,000 U	5/5	12.0	1.4
IFN 5,000 U	5/5	12.6	1.0
MBP 1.0 mg	5/5	12.4	1.0
MBP 1.0 mg + IFN 20,000 U	4/5	13.2	0.8

[a] Female Lewis rats, 150 to 200 grams, were fed with 1 mg of guinea pig brain myelin basic protein (MBP), varying doses of rat type I interferon, or a combination of MBP and interferon. Oral proteins were given a total of seven times every other day, 4 preimmunization and 3 postimmunization with 25 μg gpMBP for the induction of EAE. Animals were scored for signs of paralysis beginning on day 9, on a scale of 0 to 5.

[b] Hen-egg lysozyme.

tion of 5×10^5 cells/well/96-well microtiter plates. Proliferative responses were evaluated by [^{3}H]thymidine harvested at 96 hours. For cytokine analysis, 5×10^6 cells/well/24-well plate were cultured for various lengths of time, depending on the cytokines to be analyzed. Supernatants were harvested at 40 hours for gamma interferon (γIFN) and at 72 hours for TGFβ. Cytokines were quantified used ELISA kits from Genzyme (γIFN #1557-00, Cambridge MA), Endogen (IL-4 #KMIL4, Cambridge, MA), and Promega (TGFβ #G1230, Madison, WI).

RESULTS

EAE Suppression with Rat Type I-IFN Feeding

We have previously found that injected type I IFN synergizes with oral autoantigen in both the rat and mouse EAE models.[8] In an initial oral dose-response experiment, rats were treated a total of seven times with 5000, 10,000, and 20,000 units oral rat type I interferon or gpMBP alone, or a combination of 20,000 U interferon with MBP. As had been found in our previously published works,[10] MBP is suppressive if fed a total of seven times as measured by the mean maximum disease score (TABLE 1). As interferon treatments alone were suppressive, no synergy was detectable when the two were combined in the feeding regimen. This experiment demonstrated the need for a treatment regimen in which the autoantigen and the interferon were not immunosuppressive when given alone.

EAE Suppression with Murine βIFN

Animals were treated three times with 5000 units of oral βIFN (equivalent to ~450 ng) alone, 250 μg MBP, or 5,000 U βIFN and 250 μg of MBP three times. It can be seen that three oral treatments of autoantigen or interferon alone are not optimal for

TABLE 2. Synergy of Protein and βIFN in the Induction of Oral Tolerance in the SJL/J Mice EAE Study

Groups Treated	Incidence	Day of Onset	Mean Max Score
HEL 0.25 mg	5/5	15.8	2.3
βIFN 5,000 U	4/5	17.2	2.1
gpMBP 0.25 mg	4/5	18.8	1.8
gpMBP 0.25 mg + βIFN 5,000 U	2/5	17.5	0.9

[a] Female SJL mice were fed, with 0.25 mg, the guinea pig brain protein myelin basic protein (MBP) with or without 5,000 units of murine βIFN three times prior to immunization with 200 μg proteolipid protein and 200 μg MT for the induction of EAE. Animals were scored for signs of paralysis beginning on day 9, on a scale of 0 to 5.

suppression of EAE (TABLE 2). The same degree of disease severity was found in the groups given MBP and βIFN individually. Disease suppression was observed only when the oral myelin antigen was combined with oral βIFN for the three feedings.

Effect of βIFN on In Vitro OVA Proliferative Response and Cytokine Production

To study the mechanism of the synergistic effect seen *in vivo* in the suppression of disease, experiments were set up feeding antigen three times to the mice *in vivo* with and without concomitant βIFN. All mice were immunized subcutaneously with 250 μg of OVA in CFA two days after the last feeding. Because disease had been suppressed *in vivo* with a combination of antigen and βIFN orally, it was expected that the *in vitro* proliferative response would also be decreased. However, the *in vitro* anti-OVA proliferative response was not suppressed. Instead, as seen in FIGURE 1A, both the spleen and the lymph node cell response, as measured by tritiated thymidine incorporation, was the same as the unfed control or even enhanced (markedly so in the case of the lymph node cells from animals only given 5000 U of βIFN). The surprising result was the high production of γIFN by the cells from the animals fed with βIFN, as shown in FIGURE 1B. Significant amounts of IL4, IL10, and TGFβ were not detected in these conventional animals (data not shown).

Kinetics of βIFN Effect on Proliferative and Cytokine Response to bMBP

Inasmuch as it was seen that βIFN in conjunction with MBP suppressed EAE, and it has been reported that feeding βIFN alone long-term is immunosuppressive,[7] an experiment examining the effect of repeated βIFN dosing was performed. In this experiment, βIFN alone was fed to SJL/J mice for either one time, three (as in the previous experiments), five, or seven times. The latter is a regimen in which 5,000 U βIFN alone is known to be immunosuppressive (TABLE 1). All animals were immunized 2 days after their last feeding with 250 μg of bMBP in CFA, and organs were harvested 10 days later. All groups were sacrificed on the same day. The results showed that the proliferative response decreases with repeated βIFN feedings in both the spleen and the lymph nodes (FIG. 2A). A key finding was that the γIFN response was shown to spike after one βIFN dose, was enhanced after three doses (as in the previous experiments), and progressively decreased with repeated dosing (FIG. 2B). These results indicate that elevation of γIFN production is not a sustained feature of feeding βIFN. With repeated doses of βIFN alone before a normally immunogenic challenge, the immunosuppressive character of this cytokine is seen. Antigen-specific TGFβ and IL-4 production were not found in detectable levels in any of the groups, although beginning immunohistochemistry analyses show some elevated IL-4 after feeding (data not shown).

DISCUSSION

Oral tolerance therapy is potentially a breakthrough treatment regimen that can be applied to the treatment of individuals with autoimmune disease.[11] The potential exists for a nontoxic chronic treatment schedule that may decrease the damage done to tissues under attack by self-reactive T lymphocytes. Suppression of inflammatory, Th1-mediated immune responses by oral administration of autoantigen has been observed in several animal models, including EAE, several arthritis models, diabetes, uveitis, thyroiditis, myasthenia gravis, and even transplantation models. Initial clinical trials in humans have shown promising results in both multiple sclerosis (MS) and rheumatoid arthritis. Larger, more extensive trials are currently underway to further explore the therapeutic potential of this novel therapy.

The possibility of using synergists or immune enhancers in conjunction with oral tolerance is attractive for several reasons. A primary goal would be to increase effectiveness of oral tolerance induction with given protein regimens and to expand the patient population responsive to oral tolerance therapy. Second, it may be possible to modulate the cytokine profile induced by oral tolerance therapy, such that the beneficial regulatory cytokines TGFβ, IL4, and IL10 are increased. It may also be feasible to reduce the protein concentration needed for oral tolerance induction, if the immune response in the gut mucosa is enhanced.

We have chosen to concentrate our initial studies on the use of synergists with oral tolerance in systems employing treatment with βIFN. βIFN injections have been recently approved for the treatment of relapsing remitting MS.[12–14] Overviews of the pharmacological effects and the rationale for its use in multiple sclerosis have been recently published.[15,16] It has been reported that βIFN *in vitro* can enhance suppressor-cell activity when added to human lymphocytes, particularly cells from progressive MS patients.[17] *In vitro* analysis of the responses of βIFN-treated patients showed reduced mitogen-driven IL-2R expression from MS patients after βIFN injection,[18] as well as a direct inhibitory effect when βIFN was added to cultured human cells. The patients had been undergoing treatment with injected βIFN for at least two months at the time of assay. It has been observed that βIFN can inhibit γIFN production by lymphocytes from MS patients and controls.[19,20] The other type I interferon, αIFN, has been used orally both in the United States and Africa for the treatment of animals and humans with certain viral infections.[21,22] Low oral doses have even been tested in the treatment of AIDS.

In an animal model of chronic relapsing EAE, Brod recently reported that feeding mice type I interferon three times a week for six weeks reduced overall disease status and *in vitro* measurements of antigen-specific responsiveness.[7] Mitogen-induced γIFN production was also reduced after long-term treatment.

In our studies, βIFN works synergistically with oral autoantigen to reduce the symptoms of EAE in both mice and rats. When MBP was given for an inadequate number of times for oral tolerance induction, the addition of type I IFN to the experimental regimen in

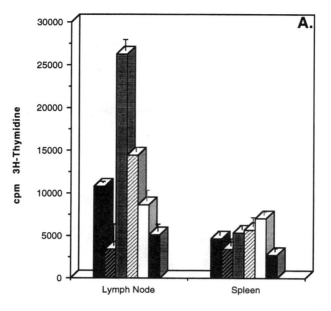

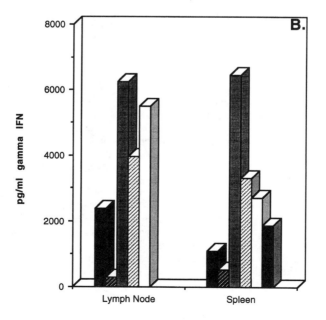

the animal models, either orally or injected (data not shown), enhanced the suppressive effects of oral protein. When dose and timing of treatment already give optimal suppression, synergy between protein and βIFN is not detectable. *In vitro* responses did not clearly correlate with *in vivo* suppression. It has been shown that the mechanism of low-dose tolerance involves the induction of cells that secrete IL-4, IL-10, and TGFβ,[23,24] and T cells preferentially producing this cytokine profile after oral induction have been recently cloned.[25]

It was thus hypothesized that the synergy of oral βIFN with autoantigen would show enhanced production of these regulatory cytokines and decreased levels of the Th1-associated cytokines IL-2 and γIFN. This was not what we observed. We found that antigen-specific γIFN production was increased compared to the positive protein immunized controls, whether or not the same antigen had been previously included in the feeding regimen. The significance of these preliminary results is not clear. Initial γIFN stimulation after oral βIFN may augment antigen presentation to the T-cell population most prevalent within the gut-associated lymphoid tissue, Th2 cells, thus leading to greater production of the down-regulatory cytokines Il-4, IL-10, and TGFβ. Preliminary experiments in transgenic animals indicate that this may be what is occurring (data not shown). The enhanced γIFN production is most pronounced shortly after one or three feedings and then steadily declines. Interestingly, the initial treatment with subcutaneous βIFN in MS patients is often associated with transient adverse effects (*e.g.*, fever, myalgias), which were side effects observed with systemic γIFN therapy.[26] A new study has found induction of γIFN producing cells in MS patients soon after commencement of βIFN injections.[27] Alternatively, the elevation in γIFN may occur secondarily in response to other cytokines induced by βIFN treatment.

These are very interesting preliminary observations that may have implications for the use of cytokines in the treatment of autoimmune disease and for their use to modulate oral tolerance. These studies indicate that βIFN treatment is compatible with oral-tolerance therapy and may have a synergistic effect if used together in humans. We are currently examining which cells are producing the elevated γIFN, whether βIFN treatment influences the frequency of these cells, and if the response is the same if different routes of administration are used. We are further investigating if the enhanced γIFN production after oral βIFN is part of the initiating events in the induction of the Th2-type regulatory cells found after antigens are given orally.

FIGURE 1. Effect of βIFN on spleen and lymph node responses to OVA *in vitro*. (PLJ × SJL)F1 mice were fed 3 times with 250 μg of OVA and/or 1,000 or 5,000 U βIFN. Two days after the last feeding, animals were immunized with 250 μg of OVA in CFA. Lymph nodes and spleens were harvested on day +10. **A:** Cultures were set up at 5×10^5/well, with 25 μg/mL OVA, incubated for 72 hours, pulsed with tritiated thymidine, and harvested 24 hours later. Results are expressed as cpm [³H]thymidine of experimental minus no-antigen control. **B:** Cultures were set up in 24-well culture plates at 5×10^6/mL with 25 μg/mL OVA and incubated for 40 hours; supernatants were collected. γIFN levels were determined using an ELISA assay. Values are expressed as net pg γIFN in wells stimulated with OVA minus media-only background values. Note that there were insufficient lymph node cells from the OVA + 1,000 U βIFN-treated group to assay for cytokine production. ■, OVA imm only; ▨, OVA po; ▨, 5K bIFN; ▨, 1K bIFN; □, OVA + 5K bIFN; ▨, OVA + 1K bIFN.

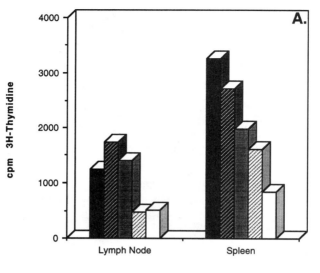

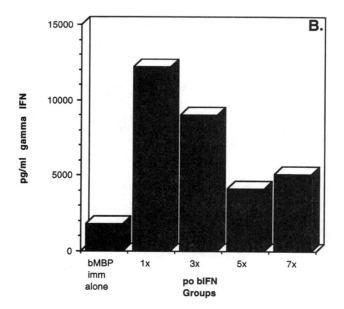

SUMMARY

Oral administration of myelin antigens reduces the incidence and severity of EAE in rat and mouse models and decreases the frequency of MBP-reactive cells and the frequency of attacks in some patients with multiple sclerosis. Low-dose oral tolerance has been shown to be mediated by Th_2-type regulatory cells that secrete TGFβ and IL-4/IL-10. Adjuvants and cytokines may modulate oral tolerance. The addition of βIFN to the experimental therapy regimen, either orally or by intraperitoneal injection, has been shown to enhance the suppressive effects of oral myelin antigens when either are fed the suboptimal dosing regimen to suppress EAE. The current studies were conducted to elucidate the mechanism of the observed *in vivo* synergy of βIFN and antigen feeding. Analysis of the *in vitro* proliferative response and cytokine production by lymphocytes from fed animals in response to specific antigen in culture shows that the synergistic effect may be related to both independent suppression of the immune response by oral βIFN and enhanced production of TGFβ and Il-4/IL-10. There was an unexpected increase in the production of γIFN by lymphocytes *in vitro* after three doses of oral βIFN *in vivo*. These observations have important implications for the use of cytokines to modulate oral tolerance.

ACKNOWLEDGMENTS

The authors wish to thank Theresa Hoffer, Christa Lajoie, Alison Coppola, Jeffrey Rego, Marise St. Charles, and Pamela Hyde for excellent technical assistance.

FIGURE 2. Kinetics of βIFN effect on spleen and lymph node response to bMBP *in vitro*. SJL mice were fed 1, 3, 5, or 7 times with 5,000 U bIFN. Two days after the last feeding, animals were immunized with 250 μg bMBP in CFA. Lymph nodes and spleens were harvested on day +10. **A:** Cultures were set up at 5×10^5/well, with 50 μg/mL bMBP, incubated for 72 hours, pulsed with tritiated thymidine, and harvested 24 hours later. Results are expressed as cpm [^{3}H]thymidine of experimental minus no-antigen control. ■, bMBP imm only; ▨, 1 × po bIFN; ■, 3 × po bIFN; ▨, 5 × po bIFN; □, 7 × po bIFN. **B:** Cultures were set up in 24-well culture plates at 5×10^6mL with 50 μg/mL bMBP and incubated for 40 hours; supernatants were collected. γIFN levels were determined using an ELISA assay. Values are expressed as net pg γIFN in wells stimulated with bMBP minus media-only background values.

REFERENCES

1. WEINER, H. L., A. FRIEDMAN, A. MILLER, S. J. KHOURY, A. AL-SABBAGH, L. SANTOS, M. SAYEGH, R. B. NUSSENBLATT, D. E. TRENTHAM & D. A. HAFLER. 1994. Oral tolerance: Immunologic mechanisms and treatment of animals and human organ specific autoimmune diseases by oral administration of autoantigens. Annu. Rev. Immunol. **12**: 809-837.
2. ZHANG, Z. & J. MICHAEL. 1990. Orally inducible immune unresponsiveness is abrogated by IFN-γ treatment. J. Immunol. **144**: 4163-4165.
3. KHOURY, S. J., O. LIDER, A. AL-SABBAGH & H. L. WEINER. 1990. Suppression of experimental autoimmune encephalomyelitis by oral administration of myelin basic protein. III. Synergistic effect of lipopolysaccharide. Cell. Immunol. **131**: 302-310.
4. KHOURY, S. J., W. W. HANCOCK & H. L. WEINER. 1992. Oral tolerance to myelin basic protein and natural recovery from experimental autoimmune encephalomyelitis are associated with down-regulation of inflammatory cytokines and differential upregulation of TGF-β, IL-4 and PGE expression in the brain. J. Exp. Med. **46**: 1355-1364.
5. ABREU, S. L. 1982. Suppression of experimental allergic encephalomyelitis by interferon. Immunol. Commun. **11**: 1-7.
6. HERTZ, F. & R. DEGHENGHI. 1985. Effect of rat and β-human interferons on hyperacute experimental allergic encephalomyelitis in rats. Agents Actions: **16**: 397-403.
7. BROD, S. A. & D. K. BURNS. 1994. Suppression of relapsing experimental autoimmune encephalomyelitis in the SJL/J mouse by oral administration of type I interferons. Neurology **44**: 1144-1148.
8. AL-SABBAGH, A., P. A. NELSON & H. L. WEINER. 1994. Beta interferon enhances oral tolerance to MBP and PLP in experimental autoimmune encephalomyelitis. Neurology (abstract) **44** (Suppl 2): A242.
9. DEIBLER, G. E., L. F. BOYD & M. W. KIES. 1984. Proteolytic activity associated with purified myelin basic protein. Experimental allergic encephalomyelitis: A useful model for multiple sclerosis. 249-256. Alan R. Liss, Inc. New York.
10. HIGGINS, P. & H. L. WEINER. 1988. Suppression of experimental autoimmune encephalomyelitis by oral administration of myelin basic protein and its fragments. J. Immunol. **140**: 440-445.
11. WEINER, H. L. 1994. Oral tolerance. Proc. Natl. Acad. Sci. USA **91**: 10762-10765.
12. GROUP, T. I. M. S. S. 1993. Interferon beta-1b is effective in relapsing-remitting multiple sclerosis: Clinical results of a multicenter, randomized, double-blind, placebo-controlled trial. Neurology **43**: 655-661.
13. ARNASON, B. G. W. 1993. Interferon beta in multiple sclerosis. Neurology **43**: 641-643.
14. PATY, D. W. 1994. The interferon-β1b clinical trial and its implications for other trials. Ann. Neurol. **36**: S113-S114.
15. FAULDS, D. & P. BENFIELD. 1994. Interferon beta-1b in multiple sclerosis: An initial review of its rationale for use and therapeutic potential. Clin. Immunother. **1**: 79-87.
16. WEINSTOCK-GUTTMAN, B., R. M. RANSOHOFF, R. P. KINKEL & R. A. RUDICK. 1995. The interferons: Biological effects, mechanisms of action, and use in multiple sclerosis. Ann. Neurol. **37**: 7-15.
17. NORONHA, A., A. TOSCAS & M. A. JENSEN. 1990. Interferon beta augments suppressor cell function in multiple sclerosis. Ann. Neurol. **27**: 207-210.
18. RUDICK, R. A., C. S. CARPENTER, D. L. COOKFAIR, V. K. TUOHY & R. M. RANSOHOFF. 1993. *In vitro* and *in vivo* inhibition of mitogen-driven T-cell activation by recombinant interferon beta. Neurology **43**: 2080-2087.
19. PANITCH, H. S., J. S. FOLUS & K. P. JOHNSON. 1987. Recombinant beta-interferon inhibits gamma interferon production in multiple sclerosis. Ann. Neurol. **22**: (abstract) 139.
20. NORONHA, A., A. TOSCAS & M. A. JENSEN. 1991. IFN-beta down-regulates IFN-gamma production by activated T cells in MS. Neurology **41**(suppl. 1): (abstract) 219.
21. CUMMINS, J. M., M. B. TOMPKINS, R. G. OLSEN, W. A. TOMPKINS & M. G. LEWIS. 1988. Oral use of human alpha interferon in cats. J. Biol. Response Modif. **7**: 513-523.

22. YOUNG, A. S. & J. M. CUMMINS. 1990. The history of interferon and its use in animal therapy. East Afr. Med. J. **67:** SS.31-SS.63.
23. MILLER, A., O. LIDER, A. B. ROBERTS, M. B. SPORN & H. L. WEINER. 1992. Suppressor T cells generated by oral tolerization to myelin basic protein suppress both *in vitro* and *in vivo* immune responses by the release of TGFβ after antigen-specific triggering. Proc. Natl. Acad. Sci. USA **89:** 421-425.
24. FRIEDMAN, A. & H. L. WEINER. 1994. Induction of anergy or active suppression following oral tolerance is determined by frequency of feeding and antigen dosage. Proc. Natl. Acad. Sci. USA **91:** 6688-6692.
25. CHEN, Y., V. K. KUCHROO, J.-I. INOBE, D. A. HAFLER & H. WEINER. 1994. Regulatory T cell clones induced by oral tolerance: Suppression of autoimmune encephalitis. Nature **265:** 1237-1240.
26. PANITCH, H. S., R. L. HIRSCH, J. SCHINDLER & K. P. JOHNSON. 1987. Treatment of multiple sclerosis with gamma interferon: Exacerbations associated with activation of the immune system. Neurology **37:** 1097-1102.
27. ARNASON, B. G. W., M. JENSEN, A. LLEDO & A. DAYAL. 1995. Interferon β (INFβ) induction in multiple sclerosis increases interferon γ (INFγ)-secreting cells. Neurology (abstract) **45** (Suppl. 4): A437.

Oral-Antigen Delivery by way of a Multiple Emulsion System Enhances Oral Tolerance[a]

CHARLES O. ELSON,[b,e] MAURIZIO TOMASI,[b]
MARK T. DERTZBAUGH,[c] GREGORY THAGGARD,[b]
ROBERT HUNTER,[d] AND CASEY WEAVER [b]

[b]*Departments of Medicine and Pathology*
University of Alabama at Birmingham
Birmingham, Alabama 35294

[c]*USAMRIID*
Ft. Detrick, Maryland

[d]*Department of Pathology*
Emory University
Atlanta, Georgia

INTRODUCTION

Over the past two decades, a number of important variables for the induction of oral tolerance have been identified[1-4] (TABLE 1). The types of antigens that have induced oral tolerance include various protein antigens, contact allergens, heterologous red blood cells, and certain killed viruses. Although eukaryotic proteins commonly induce oral tolerance, there are few reports of oral tolerance induction using purified bacterial proteins.[5] A common feature of tolerogenic antigens is that most induce T cell-dependent immune responses when given parenterally; there are few, if any, reports of oral tolerance being induced by feeding T cell-independent antigens. Other important variables in oral tolerance include antigen dose (which usually involves milligram quantities); a mucosal route of delivery; and the age, genetic background, and species of the host. Remarkably, there are very few studies on whether oral tolerance can be enhanced by varying the delivery vehicle or incorporating immunomodulators with the fed antigens. Indeed, there are only two such reports. In one report, the addition of bacterial lipopolysaccharide to a protein antigen enhanced oral tolerance to the protein.[6] In another, covalent coupling of various protein antigens to cholera toxin B subunit enhanced tolerance induction for delayed-type hypersensitivity responses.[7]

Although the phenomenon of oral tolerance is very reproducible and well established, the site of tolerance induction after feeding and the exact mechanisms underlying oral tolerance remain unclear. There are data that support the lymphoid follicles in the gut or Peyer's patches as being one site of tolerance induction.[8] However, they may not be the

[a]This work was supported by the following Grants from the National Institutes of Health: DK44240, AI35991, and UO1 AI33445.

[e]Address for correspondence: Charles O. Elson, M.D., Division of Gastroenterology and Hepatology, University of Alabama at Birmingham, UAB Station, Birmingham, AL 35294.

TABLE 1. Important Variables in the Induction of Oral Tolerance

Type of antigen
Antigen dose
Route of delivery
Age and genetic background of host
Species
? Delivery system or adjuvant

only site. Antigen presentation by gut epithelial cells *in vitro* seems to preferentially induce suppressor cells,[9,10] possibly because epithelial cells lack costimulatory molecules, such as B7.[11] Whether the epithelium is a site of induction for oral tolerance has been postulated but has not yet been proven. Multiple cellular mechanisms of oral tolerance have been demonstrated, including clonal deletion, clonal anergy, and suppression. Interestingly, a recent report indicates that large antigen doses (20 mg) preferentially induced anergy, whereas repeated small 1 mg doses preferentially induced suppression.[12]

In the present report we describe some initial studies examining the use of a multiple emulsion system to deliver antigen to intestinal lymphoid tissue. Antigen incorporation into emulsions, either water-in-oil or water-in-oil-in-water (multiple emulsions), has long been used for induction of immunity by parenteral injection.[13] However, the use of multiple emulsions for antigen delivery into the gut has not previously been examined. In the studies reported here, antigen was sequestered within microdispersed oil particles and then delivered into the gut. The oil phase was a mixture of squalene and emulsifiers that are biodegradable and nontoxic. One of the emulsifiers used was nonionic block copolymer, a poloxamer that has adjuvant activity when administered parenterally.[14] In these initial studies antigen delivered in this manner enhanced the induction of oral tolerance to various protein antigens.

MATERIAL AND METHODS

Animals

CB6F1 mice were purchased from the Jackson Laboratory, Bar Harbor, ME. Female mice were used at 6 weeks of age.

Antigens

GtfB.1 : : PhoA, a chimeric protein generated by the fusion of an oligonucleotide encoding the antigenic peptic 345-359 of the glucosyltransferase B enzyme of *Streptococcus mutans* GS-5 with the amino terminal end of the gene encoding *E. coli* alkaline phosphatase (PhoA), was prepared as described.[15] Purified cholera toxin was obtained from List Biological Labs, Inc., Campbell, CA. Bovine serum albumin and ovalbumin were obtained from Sigma Chemical Company, St. Louis, MO.

Preparation of Multiple Emulsions

To prepare 3 mL of MES, 0.5 mL of 0.9% NaCl containing 10% of nonionic block copolymer L180 was incubated for 20 min at 4 °C with the antigen dissolved in 0.3 mL

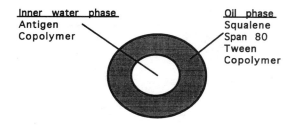

FIGURE 1. Schematic representation and constituents of the multiple emusion particles used in these experiments.

0.1 M NaHCO$_3$; 0.2-mL aliquots were then added and mixed with 0.7 mL of 90% squalene oil, 10% Span 80 in an apparatus consisting of two Luer-lock single-use syringes without a rubber gasket (Henke-Sass Wolf GmbH, Tuttelingen, Germany), which were connected by a three-way stopcock. When the emulsion was ready, as denoted by a sharp increase in the viscosity, 1.5 mL of 0.9% NaCl solution, containing 0.25% Tween 80 and 0.5% block copolymer P1003, was added and mixed to homogeneity. This preparation is referred to here as the multiple emulsion system (MES). The form and composition of an MES particle is shown schematically in FIGURE 1.

Feeding and Immunizations

For antigen feeding, 0.5 mL of a mixture containing the antigen at the indicated dose was placed in the mouse stomach using a 22-gauge ball-ended feeding needle. For intraperitoneal immunization, 50–100 μg of protein was administered in a suitable adjuvant or carrier.

Measurement of Antibody

Serum antibody was determined by enzyme-linked immunosorbent assay, as previously described.[15]

RESULTS AND DISCUSSION

Induction of Oral Tolerance to a Bacterial Protein Antigen

In the first set of experiments, groups of five mice were fed vehicle alone, the GtfB.1 : : PhoA chimera as a soluble antigen in bicarbonate at 1 mg per dose, GtfB.1 : : PhoA chimera at 0.5 mg per dose incorporated into the MES, or GtfB.1 : : PhoA chimera plus cholera toxin (CT), 10 μg per dose in the multiple emulsions. These groups of mice were fed three times at two-week intervals and subsequently immunized ip with 50 μg of antigen in alum on days 60 and 85. Sera were taken from the mice at day 92, one week after the booster dose, and serum IgG antibody to the antigen was measured

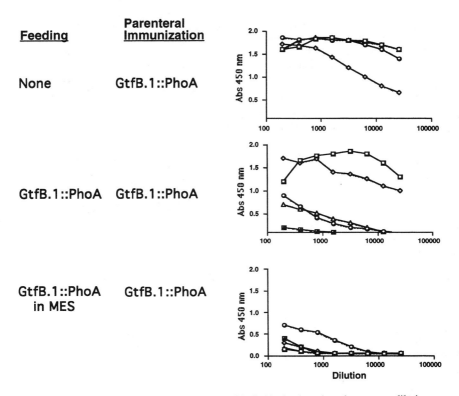

FIGURE 2. Serum IgG anti-GtfB.1 : : PhoA of individual mice plotted as serum dilution vs. ELISA optical density (Abs 450 nm). Groups of mice were fed 3 times at 2-wk intervals. The dose of GtfB.1 : : PhoA fed in soluble form was 1 mg/dose, and of GtfB.1 : : PhoA fed in MES was 0.5 mg/dose. After the feedings, all mice were primed with GtfB.1 : : PhoA, 50 μg in alum ip, and boosted 25 days later. Data shown are from sera collected 1 wk after the booster dose.

by ELISA. The results of individual mice of each group are shown in FIGURE 2 as dilution curves versus OD. Mice that were not fed the GtfB.1 : : PhoA chimera but only parenterally immunized with it had uniformly good serum IgG responses. Mice that were fed the soluble GtfB.1 : : PhoA in bicarbonate had a good deal of variability. Two of the mice were not tolerized at all; the other three were. The mice that were fed GtfB.1 : : PhoA in multiple emulsions were uniformly tolerized and had very low serum antibody responses compared to the other two groups.

This particular antigen was chosen for these experiments because in earlier work the feeding of this chimeric antigen to mice did not result in oral tolerance.[15] In that previous experiment, 3.5 mg of the purified chimera was fed three times at 10-day intervals prior to immunization of the mice. None of the animals became tolerized by this feeding. When one adds that data to the data in the equivalent group shown here, about 70% of mice fed this protein did not develop tolerance to it. Although this antigen is present in *E. coli* that are themselves present in the gut, no serum antibody to it is present in normal mice. Yet purified PhoA is a good parenteral immunogen, as witnessed by the high levels of antibody to it as shown in the top panel of FIGURE 2. The lack of oral tolerance in most mice being fed this purified antigen raises an interesting question as to whether the endogenous priming by bacteria in the gut might alter subsequent mucosal immune responses to bacterial antigens in favor of immunity and against tolerance. There is now very little data available on this point. The delicate balance between the induction of tolerance versus the induction of immunity at mucosal surfaces is illustrated by the results of the fourth group that received the GtfB.1 : : PhoA chimera along with 10 μg of CT in MES. The results are dramatically different from those obtained with mice fed only the GtfB.1 : : PhoA in MES. The addition of CT "broke" tolerance and induced instead a strong immune response in the serum and secretions (data not shown). When the mice of this group fed antigen plus CT in MES were parenterally immunized with GtfB.1 : : PhoA, serum antibody responses rose even further. The mechanisms involved in the induction of tolerance by antigen in MES remain unclear. Similar experiments have been done using a more classic oral tolerogen, bovine serum albumin (BSA), and similar results have been obtained. Three 200 μg doses of BSA in MES were able to induce oral tolerance, doses much lower than the milligram amounts that were usually required (data not shown).

Induction of Tolerance in T-cell Receptor Transgenic Mice

One of the difficulties in determining the exact cellular and molecular mechanisms underlying oral tolerance is the low frequency of T cells specific for any given antigen in a normal animal. This problem is overcome by the use of T cell-receptor transgenic mice in which the bulk of T cells in the mouse is reactive with a defined antigen. T cells from DO11.10 TcR transgenic mice[16] recognize the chicken ovalbumin peptide 323-339 in the context of I-A^d. We have recently initiated studies in these transgenic animals to determine whether we can induce oral tolerance by antigen feeding. Groups of mice were fed either vehicle, 20 mg of soluble ovalbumin, or 2 mg of ovalbumin in MES. As controls, normal BALB/c mice were fed vehicle or 20 mg of soluble ovalbumin. After two feedings one week apart, the animals were immunized intraperitoneally with 50 μg of ovalbumin (OVA) in MES. Serum was collected one week after the last dose and analyzed for IgG anti-OVA. T-cell receptor (TCR) transgenic mice receiving OVA parenterally without a feeding had a good serum IgG response, which was modestly higher than but comparable to that seen in normal BALB/c mice. Both TCR transgenic and the normal BALB/c mouse fed 20 mg of soluble OVA on two occasions developed oral tolerance, as manifested by a 10-fold lower serum IgG response to the parenteral immunization. Interestingly, transgenic mice fed 2 mg of OVA in MES, that is, a 10-fold lower dose, on two occasions also developed an equivalent level of oral tolerance. The mechanism of such tolerance is currently under investigation.

The sensitivity of such TCR transgenic mice to the induction of oral tolerance is remarkable, considering that the bulk of T cells in this mouse are reactive to this peptide, including those in peripheral lymph node and spleen, which are at a distance from the mucosal surface. One could postulate that the large dose of soluble OVA generates sufficient peptide molecules in the gut that are absorbed and thus induce anergy even in T cells at remote sites. However, this certainly would not be the case for the OVA that is delivered within the lipid particles of the multiple emulsions. It is highly likely that only a small fraction of the OVA in MES actually gets into the gut lymphoid tissue. Yet that small amount is able to tolerize the entire mouse against this peptide. These mice do represent a new tool with which the mechanisms involved in oral tolerance can be dissected and analyzed at a level that has not been previously possible.

SUMMARY

The delivery of diverse antigens by way of this multiple emulsion system enhances the induction of oral tolerance. This has been found with three different antigens, namely with GtfB.1 : : PhoA, a bacterial protein that is a weak inducer of oral tolerance when given by itself, with BSA, and with OVA. With regard to the last antigen, delivery of OVA in MES in fairly low dose is able to induce tolerance even in a T-cell receptor transgenic mouse. Based on preliminary observations, the MES appears to deliver antigen into the lymphoid follicles or Peyer's patches of the mouse intestine, and not into the epithelial layer. The mechanism of tolerance induction by MES is not yet known. However, addition of small amounts of CT to antigen in MES is able to break tolerance and switch the response to one of strong immunity.

Because the components of the MES used in these experiments are biodegradable and nontoxic, this system could potentially be used in humans. Oral tolerance has been formally demonstrated in humans after the feeding of a soluble protein antigen.[17] This result supports the notion that oral tolerance might be exploited for the treatment of autoimmune disorders.[18,19] To date, the studies of autoantigen feeding for the treatment of multiple sclerosis[20] and rheumatoid arthritis[21] have demonstrated safety, but the efficacy has been unclear. The use of MES in humans has not been tested, but this approach or others like it may increase the effectiveness of this potential therapy.

REFERENCES

1. ELSON, C. O. 1985. Induction and control of the gastrointestinal immune system. Scand. J. Gastroenterol. **114S**: 1-15.
2. BRUCE, M. G. & C. O. ELSON. 1989. Oral immunization and oral tolerance. *In* Immunology and Immunopathology of the Liver and Gastrointestinal Tract. S. R. Targan & F. Shanahan, Eds.: 171-182. Igaku-Shoin Medical Publishers, Inc. New York.
3. MOWAT, A. M. 1994. Oral Tolerance. *In* Handbook of Mucosal Immunology. P. L. Ogra, J. Mestecky, M. E. Lamm, W. Strober, J. R. McGhee & J. Bienenstock, Eds.: 391-402. Academic Press. San Diego.
4. WEINER, H. L., A. FRIEDMAN, A. MILLER, S. J. KHOURY, A. AL-SABBAGH, L. SANTOS, M. SAYEGH, R. B. NUSSENBLATT, D. E. TRENTHAM & D. A. HAFLER. 1994. Oral tolerance: immunologic mechanisms and treatment of animal and human organ-specific autoimmune diseases by oral administration of autoantigens. Annu. Rev. Immunol. **12:** 809-837.
5. STOKES, C. R., T. J. NEWBY, J. H. HUNTLEY, D. PATEL & F. J. BOURNE. 1979. The immune response of mice to bacterial antigens given by mouth. Immunology **38:** 497-502.
6. KHOURY, S. J., O. LIDER, A. AL-SABBAGH & H. L. WEINER. 1990. Suppression of experimental autoimmune encephalomyelitis by oral administration of myelin basic protein. III. Synergistic effect of lipopolysaccharide. Cell. Immunol. **131:** 302-10.
7. SUN, J.-B., J. HOMGREN & C. CZERKINSKY. 1994. Cholera toxin B subunit: an efficient transmucosal carrier-delivery system for induction of peripheral immunological tolerance. Proc. Natl. Acad. Sci. USA **91:** 10795-10799.
8. SANTOS, L. M., A. AL-SABBAGH, A. LONDONO & H. L. WEINER. 1994. Oral tolerance to myelin basic protein induces regulatory TGF-beta-secreting T cells in Peyer's patches of SJL mice. Cell. Immunol. **157:** 439-47.
9. BLAND, P. W. & D. M. KAMBARAGE. 1991. Antigen handling by the epithelium and lamina propria macrophages. Gastroenterol. Clin. North Am. **20:** 577-96.
10. MAYER, L., D. EISENHARDT & R. SHLIEN. 1988. Selective induction of antigen nonspecific suppressor cells with normal gut epithelium as accessory cells. Monogr. Allergy **24:** 78-80.

11. SANDERSON, I. R., A. J. OUELLETTE, E. A. CARTER, W. A. WALKER & P. R. HARMATZ. 1993. Differential regulation of B7 mRNA in enterocytes and lymphoid cells. Immunology **79:** 434-438.
12. FRIEDMAN, A. & H. L. WEINER. 1994. Induction of anergy or active suppression following oral tolerance is determined by antigen dosage. Proc. Natl. Acad. Sci. USA **91:** 6688-92.
13. HERBERT, W. J. 1965. Multiple emulsions. A new form of mineral-oil antigen adjuvant. Lancet **2:** 771.
14. HUNTER, R. L. 1991. Nonionic block copolymers: new preparations and review of the mechanism of action. *In* Topics in Vaccine Adjuvant Research. D. R. Spriggs & W. C. Koff, Eds.: 89-97. CRC Press. Boca Rotan, FL.
15. DERTZBUAGH, M. T. & C. O. ELSON. 1993. Comparative effectiveness of the cholera toxin B subunit and alkaline phosphatase as carriers for oral vaccines. Infect. Immun. **61:** 48-55.
16. MURPHY, K. M., A. B. HEIMBERGER & D. Y. LOH. 1990. Induction by antigen of intrathymic apoptosis of CD4+CD8+TCR[lo] thymocytes *in vivo*. Science **250:** 1720-1723.
17. HUSBY, S., J. MESTECKY, Z. MOLDOVEANU, S. HOLLAND & C. O. ELSON. 1994. Oral tolerance in humans. T cell but not B cell tolerance after antigen feeding. J. Immunol. **152:** 4663-70.
18. THOMPSON, H. S. G. & N. A. STAINES. 1990. Could oral tolerance be a therapy for autoimmune disease? Immunol. Today **11:** 396-9.
19. WEINER, H. L. 1993. Treatment of autoimmune diseases by oral tolerance to autoantigens. Autoimmunity **15:** 6-7.
20. WEINER, H. L., G. A. MACKIN, M. MATSUI, E. J. ORAV, S. J. KHOURY, D. M. DAWSON & D. A. HAFLER. 1993. Double-blind pilot trial of oral tolerization with myelin antigens in multiple sclerosis [see comments]. Science **259:** 1321-4.
21. TRENTHAM, D. E., R. A. DYNESIUS-TRENTHAM, E. J. ORAV, D. COMBITCHI, C. LORENZO, K. L. SEWELL, D. A. HAFLER & H. L. WEINER. 1993. Effects of oral administration of type II collagen on rheumatoid arthritis. Science **261:** 1727-1730.

Effects of Oral Antigen in T-cell Receptor Transgenic Mice

STEPHEN D. HURST, HAE-OCK LEE,
MICHAEL P. SMITH, JASON G. ROSENBERG, AND
TERRENCE A. BARRETT

Veterans Administration Lakeside Medical Research Center
and
Northwestern University Medical School
Department of Medicine
Section of Gastroenterology
Chicago, Illinois 60611

INTRODUCTION

It has been suggested that oral tolerance is mediated through effects on T cells. In support of this hypothesis, several different systems have demonstrated the induction of T-cell anergy or suppression following antigen feeding.[1,2] It has been proposed that anergy occurs when fed antigen is inappropriately presented in the periphery and involves the inactivation and ultimate demise of the T cell by deletion.[3] The induction of anergy has been measured by a decrease in proliferative responses or cytokine production. Suppression, on the other hand, involves T-cell differentiation in response to oral antigen.[4] This differentiation is thought to yield a T-cell phenotype capable of producing cytokines that downregulate immune responses of effector T cells in a bystander fashion. Although these two models are not mutually exclusive, confusion has arisen about their respective roles in oral tolerance. For example, evidence of T cells with suppressor function has been found following low-dose antigen administration, whereas T-cell anergy has been detected following high doses.[5] Another confounding factor in assessing oral tolerance has been the criteria used to define the tolerant state *in vivo*. For example, oral tolerance has been defined as a decrease in antibody responses.[6] However, upon closer examination, it has been shown that only those antibody isotypes that are associated with T-helper type-1 (TH-1) cytokines, such as IFN-γ and IL-2, are suppressed by oral antigen.[7] Alternatively, oral tolerance has been defined as the ability to decrease delayed-type hypersensitivity responses (DTH) to subsequent antigenic challenge. These results implicate the absence, or functional inactivation, of a TH-1 subset of antigen-specific T cells. Lastly, more precise measurements of T-cell function have used specific cytokine ELISAs to define the cytokine production induced by oral antigen. These studies have demonstrated that oral antigen induces TGF-β production in the absence of IFN-γ or IL-4.[8] Taken together, it appears that multiple pathways may be involved in the induction and maintenance of oral tolerance, depending on the specific antigen, the dosage, the prior immune status of the host, and the functional assay used to measure tolerance.

THE T-CELL RECEPTOR TRANSGENIC SYSTEM

To address the response of systemic T cells to oral antigen, we have used a T-cell receptor transgenic (TCR) mouse model. The alpha and beta TCR transgenes expressed

163

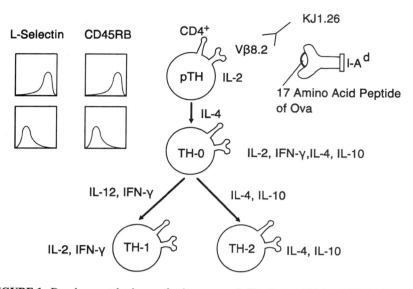

FIGURE 1. Developmental scheme of naive transgenic T cells into TH-1 and TH-2 effectors. CD4[+], precursor T-helper cells (pTH) from transgenic mice express a Vβ8.2 TCR, specific to the 17 amino acid peptide of chicken ovalbumin (OVA) in the context of class II I-A[d]. The TCR clonotype is detectable by the mAb KJ1.26. Naive pTH cells secrete large amounts of IL-2 with activation. Activation of pTH cells in the presence of IL-4 induces an intermediate subset that has a down-regulated L-selectin and CD45RB surface phenotype. Repeated stimulation of TH cells in the presence of exogenous cytokines, such as IL-12 or IL-4, can lead to the differentiation of TH cells into TH-1 or TH-2 effector phenotypes, respectively.

by the DO11.10 mice were derived from a CD4[+] T-cell clone specific for a 17 amino acid peptide of chicken ovalbumin (OVA), presented in the context of the major histocompatibility complex class II molecule I-A[d].[9] T cells expressing the transgenic TCR can be identified with the clonotypic monoclonal antibody (mAb) KJ1-26.1. These mice provide a source of naive, antigen-specific T cells that have a single TCR with homogeneous affinity for the OVA peptide. In previous studies, the transgenic T cells isolated from the spleen of these mice have been shown to express a naive IL-2-producing cytokine profile.[10] We have also found that naive splenic T cells express high levels of L-selectin and CD45RB, and low levels of CD44 and CD69, consistent with the overall naive phenotype. Once activated, the antigen-specific, naive T cells can be differentiated into both TH-1 and TH-2 subsets, with repeated stimulation in the presence of IFN-γ or IL-4, respectively. As illustrated in FIGURE 1, this functional differentiation into TH-1 and TH-2 subsets passes through an obligate intermediate TH-0 stage.[11] This TH-0 cell type produces IL-2, IFN-γ, and IL-4, although TH-0 clones have been described with variations on this scheme. In the DO11.10 transgenic mouse model, we have found that transgenic T cells isolated from the intestinal lamina propria compartment express low levels of L-selectin and CD45RB and high levels of CD44 and CD69, consistent with an activated phenotype. Lamina propria T cells isolated from unimmunized transgenic mice predominately produce IFN-γ along with IL-4 and IL-2, suggesting that they have functionally differentiated from the naive phenotype observed for splenic T cells of the same animals. Thus, it

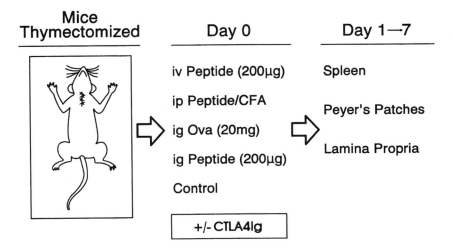

FIGURE 2. Transgenic T-cell trafficking: experimental design. Transgenic mice were thymectomized to prevent new T cells from obscuring the trafficking phenomena. Mice were injected or fed OVA peptide or whole OVA with or without CTLA4Ig as shown. Mice were sacrificed between day 1 and day 7 for time-course studies, at which point spleen, Peyer's patch, and lamina propria compartments were recovered and analyzed for percent transgenic T cells versus control mice. Data are described in the text.

appears that in unimmunized transgenic mice, T cells have functionally differentiated and localized to nonlymphoid peripheral tissues.

First, we used these mice as an *in vivo* model of T-cell responses to oral and systemic antigen (FIG. 2). Transgenic mice were thymectomized to avoid dilution by thymic émigrés during the course of the experiments. Mice were then given 20 mg of whole OVA intragastric (ig), a 200 μg intravenous (iv) injection of OVA peptide, or a 200 μg intraperitoneal (ip) injection of OVA peptide in complete Freund's adjuvant (CFA). The different dosages between whole and peptide OVA represent equal molar amounts of the critical antigenic peptide. In order to study the affect of B7-mediated costimulation on each of these regimens, the initial antigen administration was performed with and without a 0.2 mg ip injection of CTLA4Ig.[12] Following antigen administration, transgenic T cells were examined in the spleen, Peyer's patch, and lamina propria. In addition, we have also used the adoptive transfer model as proposed by M. K. Jenkins.[13] In this system, splenic T cells are isolated from the OVA-specific DO11.10 transgenic mice. After assessment of T-cell purity, 2.5 million transgenic T cells were then injected into nontransgenic, syngeneic BALB/c recipients. Transgenic T-cell numbers were then followed with the clonotypic mAb. We used the same antigen administration schedule and compared transgenic T-cell phenotypes in these mice to that of the unmanipulated, adoptively transferred control mice. The adoptive transfer model was used to examine functional differentiation in the spleen under more physiologically relevant conditions, with a lower precursor frequency, compared to intact transgenic mice.

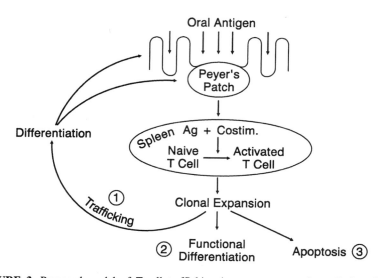

FIGURE 3. Proposed model of T-cell trafficking in response to antigen. Oral antigen is transported across the intestinal epithelia and is delivered to the Peyer's patch and circulation. Antigen is presented to T cells in peripheral lymphoid tissue, such as the spleen. Three outcomes of this activation event occur: (1) trafficking to the gut, accompanied by differentiation into effector T-cell subsets, (2) local functional differentiation in the periphery where antigen was first encountered, and (3) apoptosis. These three outcomes are not mutually exclusive and appear to be partially dependent upon antigen dosage.

MODEL OF T-CELL RESPONSES TO ANTIGEN

As we will discuss in this article, FIGURE 3 illustrates the proposed scheme for oral antigen-induced T-cell responses. Initially, antigen is ingested as whole protein and undergoes digestion in the upper intestinal tract. After further digestion with luminal peptidases, protein is broken down into peptides that pass through the mucosal surface. Enteric protein antigen may be taken up by specialized epithelial cells, called M cells, which overlay the dome area of the Peyer's patches.[14] However, it is likely that peptide antigen may also be absorbed through epithelial barriers in the intervening mucosa. Once absorbed, antigen gains access to the systemic circulation. It has been demonstrated by D. G. Hanson *et al.*, and others that radiolabeled fractions derived from fed proteins may be detected as early as one hour following feeding.[15] We have, therefore, hypothesized that oral antigen may be presented to naive T cells in the spleen in a manner similar to that of intravenous peptide. Once antigen is presented with costimulation to naive T cells in the spleen, these T cells become activated and undergo blastogenesis. At this time, a subset of T cells activated by systemic antigen traffic to mucosal lymphoid and mucosal nonlymphoid tissue. We propose that these T cells undergo functional differentiation as they localize. Activated T cells observed in the splenic tissue take up BrdU, demonstrating local proliferation, and splenic T-cell numbers expand from 1 to 3 days. By day 5, these activated T cells can be found to have modulated surface markers consistent with activation. Concurrent with these surface phenotype changes, cells also undergo functional differentiation from naive T-helper cell precursors to activated TH-0 cells. These activated TH-0 cells produce IL-2 and increased levels of IL-4 and IFN-γ, compared to naive CD4+ T cells. Late in the response, a subset of activated T cells also can be found undergoing programmed cell death, as measured by apoptosis, although at any given time this percentage does not appear to exceed 8 to 10% of the splenic T-cell population. The contribution of trafficking and apoptosis ultimately results in a decrease of antigen-specific T cells of 30 to 40% by day 7.

Thus, we have found that oral antigen is rapidly absorbed through the intestine and can be shown to activate systemic T cells. This activation event induces trafficking of T cells to mucosal surfaces that express a memory phenotype. T cells remaining in the splenic lymphoid tissue undergo further functional differentiation to an activated TH-0 phenotype.

SYSTEMIC ANTIGEN INDUCES T-CELL TRAFFICKING TO MUCOSAL TISSUES

We have found that ip, iv, or ig administration of antigen leads to a rapid increase in transgenic T-cell numbers in the Peyer's patches as identified by flow cytometry. Peyer's patch transgenic T-cell numbers increased to greater than 150% of control unmanipulated mice as early as 12 hours after antigen administration. Splenic T-cell numbers, however, remained constant or increased slightly over the first four days. After four days, transgenic T-cell numbers began to decrease in the splenic tissues. As evaluated by immunohistochemistry of intestinal sections, we have also found that antigen administered by ip, iv, or ig routes can be shown to increase transgenic T-cell numbers in the lamina propria within 12 hours. Furthermore, the transgenic T cells isolated from the Peyer's patch and lamina propria tissues express activated phenotypes with decreased expression of L-selectin and CD45RB along with increased expression of CD44 and CD69, compared to naive splenic T cells. The dramatic increase in transgenic T-cell numbers in these tissues within 12 hours suggests that migration of T cells to these tissues contributed to the expansion.

As our data suggests that antigen administration induces T-cell trafficking to T-cell tissues, we also examined functional phenotypes. As discussed earlier, T cells from immunized mice in the spleen express naive surface marker phenotypes and produce mainly IL-2 but little significant IL-4 or IFN-γ. Transgenic T cells isolated from lamina propria or Peyer's patch, however, express a TH-0 cytokine profile of high IFN-γ and significant IL-2 and IL-4. In mice administered ig OVA, transgenic T cells from intestinal Peyer's patch or lamina propria compartments produced the same TH-0 pattern of cytokines as the resident cells, suggesting that newly recruited T cells may have undergone functional differentiation associated with activation and migration.

ACTIVATION OF NAIVE T CELLS IS DEPENDENT ON B7-MEDIATED COSTIMULATION

As our initial findings suggested that activation of transgenic T cells by systemic antigen led to trafficking to intestinal tissues, we next examined the requirement for costimulation for this activation. Using the identical model described in the previous section, we delivered antigen with and without coadministration of CTLA4Ig. In all examples, CTLA4Ig was found to significantly decrease antigen-induced, T-cell expansion. The most dramatic effects were found following ig administration of antigen where CTLA4Ig decreased the number of transgenic T cells induced from 200% to 50% over control animals. Likewise, transgenic T-cell numbers did not increase following iv or ig administration of antigen when CTLA4Ig was administered simultaneously. These results suggested that costimulation played a major role in the activation of systemic T cells that lead to trafficking to intestinal tissues.

Along with antigen-induced increases and mucosal T-cell numbers, we also observed cytokine production by mucosal transgenic T cells in response to oral antigen administration. At the same 12-hour point, we examined intestinal tissues for IL-2 production *in situ*. Frozen sections were stained with the anti-IL-2 mAb, S4B6, from tissue of OVA-fed and CTLA4Ig-treated, OVA-fed mice. Although dramatic increases in IL-2 staining were observed in mice fed antigen, this IL-2 production was greatly inhibited by the coadministration of CTLA4Ig. This abrogation of expansion as well as functional responses by CTLA4Ig demonstrated the critical role of costimulation during the T-cell response to oral antigen.

SPLENIC T-CELL RESPONSES TO SYSTEMIC ANTIGEN

As we had found that systemic antigen administration induced dramatic changes in mucosal tissues, we next examined the effects of antigen on splenic T-cell populations. First, we examined splenic tissues in mice given the antigen by ip, iv, or ig routes for clonal expansion. Clonal expansion was followed by detection of BrdU incorporated into transgenic T cells *in vivo*.[16] Dramatic increases in BrdU-positive T cells were observed in animals administered OVA ip or intravenously. However, at 72 hours, oral antigen-treated mice displayed a modest increase in BrdU incorporation. This modest increase of 8%, however, was associated with a more significant increase of 25% BrdU-positive transgenic T cells observed in the Peyer's patch. It is unclear whether the BrdU-positive T cells within the Peyer's patch had expanded locally or represent early trafficking T cells from other tissue. Nonetheless, coadministration of CTLA4Ig abrogated the clonal expansion induced by systemic antigen, suggesting that B7-mediated costimulation was a necessary step for optimal T-cell activation induced by systemic antigen.

INDUCTION OF SPLENIC T-CELL RESPONSES BY SYSTEMIC ANTIGEN

As our observation of T-cell trafficking and clonal expansion suggested that T cells in the spleen and other systemic and lymphoid tissue had been activated by ip, iv, or ig antigen, we next examined the functional responses induced. Isolation of spleens from these mice was followed by T-cell purification. We found that within one hour after iv or ig administration of antigen, IL-2 as well as IL-4 mRNA increased greater than 200-fold. This dramatic induction of cytokine mRNA provided further evidence of the rapid absorption and presentation of orally delivered antigen. In fact, we found little evidence for a significant lag in the response to ig compared to iv antigen, suggesting that the response rates were similar.

FUNCTIONAL DIFFERENTIATION OF SYSTEMIC T CELLS INDUCED BY ANTIGEN

Naive T cells can undergo a transition to the pluripotent TH-0 phenotype after activation in the presence of IL-4.[17] Although T-cell activation can promote this transition, it is not clear whether TCR-mediated activation is required. In the current paradigm of CD4[+]

T-cell functional differentiation, however, the TH-0 phenotype is considered an intermediate step for naive T cells to develop into TH-1 or TH-2 phenotypes. Given this scheme of T-cell functional differentiation, we hypothesized that activation of T cells by systemic antigen would induce a functional transition from naive to TH-0 phenotype. This hypothesis is distinct from some models of oral tolerance that suggest that oral antigen induces T-cell anergy. We therefore set out to test these distinct predictions using the adoptive transfer system described earlier. This model allows us to examine the effects of systemic antigen on T-cell differentiation under more physiologic conditions of low precursor frequency. After adoptive transfer, mice were given antigen by iv, ip, or ig routes as before. After five days, CD4$^+$ splenic T cells were purified, and the percentage of transgenic T cells were assessed. The results indicated that although iv peptide slightly increased transgenic T-cell numbers from 1 to 2%, the ip administration of peptide in CFA led to substantial expansion of T-cell numbers. Transgenic T cells represented 10% of the *lymphoid* gate in mice given ip antigen compared to 1% in unmanipulated mice. Transgenic T cells remained constant or slightly decreased in mice given ig antigen, compared to controls.

First, we assessed the surface phenotype of transgenic T cells isolated from mice given ip, iv, or ig OVA. The levels of L-selectin and CD45RB on gated transgenic T cells were significantly modulated by antigen. In control, unmanipulated mice, L-selectin and CD45RB were expressed at high levels, whereas in mice given OVA ip in CFA, L-selectin levels were uniformly decreased. L-selectin levels were also decreased on a major subset of transgenic T-cell mice given iv or ig OVA. Similarly CD45RB levels decreased on transgenic T cells in mice given systemic antigen. The most dramatic effect was observed in response to iv peptide,where CD45RB levels decreased uniformly compared to that observed in control mice. In addition, modulation of each of these surface markers was abrogated by coadministration of CTLA4Ig intraperitoneally. These data suggested that T cells expressing the transgenic T-cell receptor had undergone activation in response to systemic antigen administration, and that this activation was costimulation dependent. In order to assess the functional consequences of this activation, we measured cytokine production by cells in response to *in vitro* stimulation with OVA peptide. Transgenic T-cell numbers were first normalized for *in vitro* cultures. Wells were then supplemented with irradiated T cell–lysed spleen and activated with OVA peptide. In unmanipulated mice, transgenic T cells produced high levels of IL-2 (2900 pg/mL) but low levels of IL-4 (90 pg/mL) and IFN-γ (5300 pg/mL). However, cells isolated from mice given antigen ip in CFA produced nearly twice the level of IL-2 on a per cell basis. The most dramatic effect, however, was observed with regard to IL-4 and IFN-γ. Transgenic T cells produced 20-fold increased levels of IL-4 compared to unmanipulated mice and approximately 15-fold increased levels of IFN-γ. This suggested that *in vivo* activation of T cells by ip antigen in CFA had induced functional differentiation from a naive to TH-0 phenotype. Administration of peptide iv induced increases in IL-4 and IFN-γ over that seen in control mice. Both IFN-γ and IL-4 production was increased fourfold by iv antigen. A similar increase in cytokine production was measured from T cells following ig antigen administration as well. Taken together, these data suggest that systemic administration of antigen had induced functional differentiation. Interestingly, the responses of T cells isolated from mice given OVA ip in CFA were greater than that observed for iv or ig administered mice. It is important to note, however, that these results demonstrate that when antigen-specific T-cell numbers are appropriately normalized between samples, functional responses do not suggest clonal anergy. In fact, transgenic T cells produce greater levels of IL-2 after ig antigen compared to control unmanipulated mice on a per T-cell basis. Similarly, when proliferation was assessed, we found that ig, iv, or ip antigen failed to decrease T-cell responses to peptide. Conversely, ig antigen led to an increased proliferative response to OVA peptide *in vitro*. Overall, these results suggested that early in the evolution of oral tolerance, T-cell functional responses were actually up-regulated. This up-regulation of IFN-γ and IL-4 production was consistent with the hypothesis that activation of naive T cells leads to functional differentiation.

INDUCTION OF APOPTOSIS BY SYSTEMIC ANTIGEN

As we had observed that systemic antigen administration induced an initial rise in transgenic T-cell numbers followed by a decrease overall of approximately 40% of splenic transgenic T-cell numbers, we addressed whether apoptosis was occurring for this population. By using terminal deoxynucleotidyl transferase (TdT) to incorporate biotiyinylated dUTP, we detected cells with significant strand breaks by flow cytometry.[18] Transgenic T cells were surface stained prior to permeabilization to allow for gating on transgenic T cells. Although the level of the percent of apoptosis did not increase over 8%, we found ongoing apoptosis from days 3 to 7. Furthermore, ongoing apoptosis from days 3 to 7 in all mice with the highest levels of apoptosis was observed following ip antigen in CFA. Similar to that observed for clonal expansion, trafficking, and cytokine production induced by antigen, we also found a significant decrease in the percent of apoptosis induced by coadministration of CTLA4Ig, regardless of the route of antigen. Again, this difference suggested that the observed events had followed a B7-mediated activation of systemic T cells.

DISCUSSION

We have used a T-cell receptor transgenic mouse model to study the effects of distinct routes of antigen administration on systemic and intestinal T-cell populations. Our findings suggest that oral, iv, or ip injections of antigen in adjuvant lead to similar consequences when T cells are examined early after the activation event. These responses include the following (Fig 3): (1) antigen-induced blastogenesis and proliferation of systemic T cells, (2) B7-mediated activation of systemic T cells leading to induction of IL-2 and IL-4 mRNA, (3) trafficking of activated T cells to the Peyer's patch and lamina propria compartment, (4) apoptosis of an activated T-cell subset detectable in the spleen, and (5) functional differentiation of T cells activated by systemic antigen. Specifically, the differentiation of transgenic T cells activated by antigen was apparent for T cells that had trafficked to intestinal tissues as well as those cells detected in the spleen five days following antigen administration.

The results of antigen-induced up-regulation of IL-2 and IL-4 mRNA were particularly striking. The induction of IL-2 and IL-4 message by oral antigen detectable within one hour of feeding suggests that oral antigen is rapidly taken up into the systemic circulation where it activates peripheral T cells. Interestingly, the results of these RT-PCR analyses suggest that although the T-cell population in the spleen of these transgenic mice has been reported to produce IL-2 with less IL-4, our results suggest that, in fact, IL-4 production is evident immediately after activation for splenic T cells. Also, it is interesting that the amount of IL-2 mRNA made in the spleen after feeding is not reflected in the amount of splenic T-cell proliferation observed by BrdU incorporation. This finding may be the result of an antigen or cytokine threshold, or a reflection of more immediate and complete trafficking of the activated subset preferentially to ig-delivered antigen.

Another significant aspect of these studies was the critical role played by costimulation. In each assay of T-cell activation we measured, CTLA4Ig was able to abrogate or significantly diminish responses. This was true of T-cell trafficking, the clonal expansion and differentiation induced by antigen, as well as modulation of surface markers. Therefore, we have interpreted these results as suggesting that costimulation is a necessary requirement for the early time point in T-cell activation by systemic antigen. Furthermore, our observations that oral antigen induced a functional differentiation of T cells rather than clonal anergy suggest that B7-mediated costimulation is involved in the induction of a tolerizing immune response. One of the interesting aspects of these results was the dramatic trafficking observed induced by systemic antigen. This migratory event seemed to have several characteristics that were very reproducible. First, antigen-induced T-cell activation led to mucosal trafficking only when a costimulation was provided. Second, the trafficking of the T cells to the mucosal tissues was likely associated with a transition from naive to activated T-cell phenotypes. These activated T cells may have then migrated to the mucosal sites where they produce cytokine. This may have important relevance to the mucosal immune response, as it suggests that one mechanism for up-regulation of mucosal immunity may be the activation of systemic T cells and induction of a cytokine response by these cells after they have migrated out of the circulation.

We have used the DO11.10 transgenic model to examine the functional consequences of oral antigen administration. Our findings suggest that oral antigen activates systemic T cells and that activation induces functional differentiation. In previous reports from H. L. Wiener *et al.*, it has been suggested that oral antigen induces a TGF-β-producing population of T cells that mediate oral tolerance.[19] If we were to include this observation into our own paradigm, we might speculate that T cells initially undergo a transition to a TH-0 phenotype, but that oral antigen administration directs further development into a suppressive, TGF-β-producing phenotype. It is quite possible that although the initial event may be one involving activation, clonal expansion, and functional differentiation, repeated activation by oral antigen presented in distinct tissues may induce this suppressive TGF-β phenotype. In support of this possibility, recent observations by M. H. Sayegh *et al.* showed that thymic dendritic cell populations induce TGF-β production by naive T cells compared to dendritic cells isolated from spleen (ref. 20 and personal communication). This finding suggests that T cells with the ability to produce TGF-β may have trafficked through the thymus, encountered antigen on thymic-dendritic cells, and emigrated to peripheral tissues where they mediate tolerance.

We have proposed a pathway of T-cell responses to oral antigen that resembles that observed following intravenous administration of peptide antigen. In previous reports of superantigen-induced systemic tolerance, it was similarly shown that iv antigen induced an initial burst of expansion followed by a subsequent clonal elimination detectable in systemic lymphoid tissues. Although we agree with the general understanding of this response, we would add that the early events following activation of systemic T cells involve T-cell trafficking. We have used the advantages of the transgenic system to compare functional responses of antigen-specific populations. These data have yielded surprising results, suggesting that oral antigen had up-regulated cytokine production over that of controls. This is in contrast to previous reports where oral antigen was thought to have induced anergy. In our evaluation of lamina propria T cells, we have found that proliferative responses have decreased to one-tenth of that observed for naive, splenic T cells. An extrapolation of this observation would be that activated T cells inherently proliferate at lower rates compared to naive T-cell populations. We suspect, however, that although proliferation has decreased following ig antigen, cytokine production by these cells, at least at an early point has appeared to be intact, and in some instances, up-regulated.

REFERENCES

1. WHITACRE, C. C., I. E. GIENAPP, C. G. OROSZ & D. M. BITAR. 1991. Oral tolerance in EAE. III. Evidence to clonal anergy. J. Immunol. **147:** 2155-2163.
2. MILLER, A., O. LIDER & H. L. WEINER. 1991. Antigen-driven bystander suppression after oral administration of antigens. J. Exp. Med. **174:** 791-798.
3. KAWABE, Y. & A. OCHI. 1991. Programmed cell death and extrathrathymic reduction of VB8⁺ CD4⁺ T cells in mice tolerant to *Staphylococcus aureus* enterotoxin B. Nature **349:** 245-248.
4. KHOURY, S. J., W. W. HANCOCK & H. L. WEINER. 1992. Oral tolerance to MBP and natural recovery from EAE are associated with downregulation of inflammatory cytokines and differential upregulation of TGF-b, IL-4 and PgE2 expression in the brain. J. Exp. Med. **176:** 1355-1364.
5. MELAMED, D. & A. FRIEDMAN. 1993. Modification of the immune response by oral tolerance: Antigen requirements and interaction with immunogenic stimuli. Cell. Immunol. **146:** 412-420.
6. KAGNOFF, M. F. 1978. Effects of antigen-feeding on intestinal and systemic immune responses. III. Antigen-specific serum-mediated suppression of humoral antibody responses after antigen feeding. Cell. Immunol. **40:** 186-203.
7. BURSTEIN, H. L., C. M. SHEA & A. K. ABBAS. 1992. Aqueous antigens induce *in vivo* tolerance selectively in IL-2 and IFN-γ-producing (Th-1) cells. J. Immunology **148:** 3684-3686.
8. CHEN, Y., V. K. KUCHROO, J. INOBE, D. A. HAFLER & H. L. WEINER. 1994. Regulatory T cell clones induced by oral tolerance: suppression of autoimmune encephalomyelitis. Science **265:** 1237-1240.
9. MURPHY, K. M., A. B. HEIMBERGER & D. Y. LOH. 1990. Induction by antigen of intrathymic apoptosis of CD4⁺ CD8⁺ TCRˡᵒ thymocytes *in vivo*. Science **250:** 1720-1723.
10. HSIEH, C.-S., A. B. HEIMBERGER, J. S. GOLD, A. O'GARRA & K. M. MURPHY. 1992. Differential regulation of T helper phenotype development by interleukins 4 and 10 in an ab T cell receptor transgenic system. Proc. Natl. Acad. Sci USA **89:** 6065-6069.
11. MOSMANN, T. R., H. CHERWINSKI, M. W. BOND, M. A. GIELDIN & R. L. COFFMAN. 1986. Two types of murine helper T cell clones. I. Definition according to profiles of activities and secretory proteins. J. Immunol. **136:** 2348-2356.
12. LINSLEY, P. S., W. BRADY, M. URNES, L. S. GROSMAIRE, N. K. DAMLE & J. A. LEDBETTER. 1991. CTLA-4 is a second receptor for the B cell activation antigen B7. J. Exp. Med. **174:** 561-569.
13. KEARNEY, E. R., K. A. PAPE, D. Y. LOH & M. K. JENKINS. 1994. Visualization of peptide-specific T cell immunity and peripheral tolerance induction *in vivo*. Immunity **4:** 327-339.
14. OWEN, R. L., N. F. PIERCE & W. C. CRAY JR. 1983. Autoradiographic analysis of M cell uptake and transport of cholera vibrios into follicles of rabbit Peyer's patches. Gastroenterology **84:** 1267-1279.
15. HANSON, D. G. & S. D. MILLER. 1982. Inhibition of specific immune responses by feeding protein antigens. V. Induction of the tolerant state in the absence of specific suppressor T cells. J. Immunol. **128:** 2378-2381.
16. ROCHA, B., C. PENIT, C. BARON, F. VASSEUR, N. DAUTIGNY & A. A. FREITAS. 1990. Accumulation of BrdU-labeled cells in central and peripheral lymphoid organs: Minimal estimates of production and turnover rates of mature lymphocytes. Eur. J. Immunol. **20:** 1697-1708.
17. SEDER, R. A., W. E. PAUL, M. M. DAVIS & B. FRAZEKAS DE ST. GROTH. 1992. The presence of IL-4 during *in vitro* priming determines the lymphocyte-producing potential of CD4⁺ T cells from T cell receptor transgenic mice. J. Exp. Med. **176:** 1091-1098.
18. GORCZYCA, W., S. BRUNO, R. J. DARZYNKIEWICZ, J. GONG & Z. DARZYNKIWEICZ. 1992. DNA strand breaks occurring in apoptosis: Their early *in situ* detection by the terminal

deoxynucleotidyl transferase and nick translation assays and prevention by serine protease inhibitors. Int. J. Oncol. **1:** 639-648.

19. MILLER, A., O. LIDER, A. B. ROBERTS, M. B. SPORN & H. L. WEINER. 1992. Suppressor T cells generated by oral tolerization to myelin basic protein suppress both *in vitro* and *in vivo* immune responses by the release of TGF-b after antigen-specific triggering. Proc. Natl. Acad. Sci. USA **89:** 421-425.

20. KHOURY, S. J., L. GALLON, W. CHEN, K. BETRES, M. E. RUSSELL, W. W. HANCOCK, C. B. CARPENTER, M. H. SAYEGH & H. L. WEINER. 1995. Mechanisms of acquired thymic tolerance in experimental autoimmune encephalomyelitis: Thymic dendritic-enriched cells induce specific peripheral T-cell unresponsiveness *in vivo*. J. Exp. Med. **182:** 357-366.

Molecular Mechanisms Securing "Unresponsiveness" in Lamina Propria T Lymphocytes

STEFAN C. MEUER,[a] FRANK AUTSCHBACH,[b]
GUIDO SCHÜRMANN,[c] MARKUS GOLLING,[c]
JUTTA BRAUNSTEIN,[a] AND LIANG QIAO [d]

[a]Deutsches Krebsforschungszentrum
Im Neuenheimer Feld 280
69120 Heidelberg, Germany

[b]Pathologisches Institut
Im Neuenheimer Feld 220
69120 Heidelberg, Germany

[c]Chirurgische Universitätsklinik
Im Neuenheimer Feld 110
69120 Heidelberg, Germany

[d]Department of Obstetrics and Gynecology
Loyola University Medical Center
Maywood, Illinois 60153

INTRODUCTION

A major proportion of the cellular immune system homes to the intestinal environment. It is believed to represent a functional barrier that separates the host from pathogens and toxins. Nevertheless, despite the abundance of lymphocytes in mucosal and adjacent areas and a multitude of exogenous antigens in the intestine to which these cells are permanently exposed, systemic immune responses are, under normal circumstances, not generated. For example, it is virtually impossible to achieve host protection by means of oral vaccination employing antigens, which, if systemically introduced through another route, can elicit strong and long-lasting cellular immune responses *in vivo*.

The mechanisms of how the mucosal immune system can exert its protective function, yet, at the same time, remain hypo- or nonresponsive to, for example, dietary antigens, are unclear at present. Lymphocytes are known to recirculate and, therefore, local selection for or against particular recognition repertoires are rather unlikely to explain this functional peculiarity. One might rather speculate that environmental influences aimed at adjusting lymphocyte reactivity to local requirements must exist, leading to a specialized functional state of effector cells.

Besides the mode of antigen presentation by MHC, the T-cell receptor and its signal transduction apparatus[1] provide access for immunomodulatory effects. Moreover, at a second level, costimulation through constitutively expressed accessory receptors, such as CD2, CD4, CD8, and CD28, appears to be crucial for clonal expansion following antigen encounter.[2-4] The latter receptors are engaged by cell-surface "adhesion" molecules (CD58; MHC class II and class I, respectively; CD80; CD86; and CD54) whose expression and cell-surface density can vary considerably.[5] As a general rule, high expression of

174

Environment

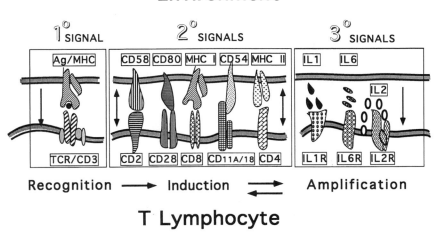

FIGURE 1. T-lymphocyte activation is regulated in at least three individual levels where specific receptors are engaged by their respective ligands. The initial signal for lymphocyte activation is mediated through the T-cell receptor/CD3 complex upon encounter of antigen/MHC. This first signal makes T cells competent to receive additional second or costimulatory signals. The latter decide whether T cell–clonal expansion and generation of effector cells occur. In the absence of costimulatory signals, T cells having encountered antigen/MHC will become unresponsive. A third level is induced by the signals received at levels 1 and 2. Some responses can be initiated through T cell-receptor triggering alone, such as interleukin-2 (IL-2) receptor expression or secretion of IFN-γ. The production of IL-2, however, and the expression of receptors for interleukin-1 and -6, is dependent on secondary signals that can be mediated through, *e.g.*, CD2, CD4, CD8, or CD28. Cytokines exert additional potent regulatory influences on the T-cell response.

these ligands for accessory receptors correlates with symptomatic immune reactions (*e.g.*, inflammatory responses), whereas low or absent expression exists in areas where no immune reactions occur.

A third regulatory level could be termed the amplification or modulation level. Here, cytokines that are secreted upon costimulation bind to their specific receptors, whose induction is controlled through activating signals (FIG. 1). This complex network of interdependent receptor levels is highly susceptible to modulation. Importantly, novel reagents allow us to specifically address the functional state of these receptors in experimental *in vitro* systems and, thus, help to elucidate the molecular basis of the specialized features of the human intestinal mucosal immune system.

SIGNALING THROUGH THE T-CELL RECEPTOR/CD3 COMPLEX IS DOWN-REGULATED IN LAMINA PROPRIA T LYMPHOCYTES

To investigate T-lymphocyte reactivity in response to antigen encounter through the T-cell receptor/CD3 complex, monoclonal antibodies directed at the CD3 ε subunit, which

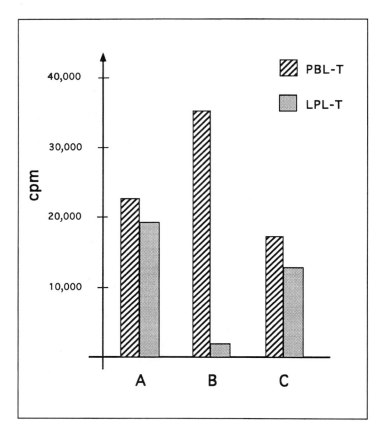

FIGURE 2. *In vitro* responses of peripheral blood T lymphocytes (PBL-T) or lamina propria T lymphocytes (LPL-T), respectively, to various stimuli. [³H]Thymidine incorporation by 2.5 × 10⁴ cells incubated with (A) a mitogenic combination of CD2 monoclonal antibodies, (B) CD3 monoclonal antibody coupled to Sepharose beads, and (C) CD28 mAb plus IL-2 (10 U/mL).

are known to be mitogenic for resting human peripheral blood T lymphocytes,[6] were employed for the stimulation of freshly isolated lamina propria mononuclear cells. As shown in FIGURE 2, CD3 antibodies, albeit highly mitogenic for PBL-T, do not trigger proliferation of LPL-T, as determined by means of [³H]thymidine incorporation. In marked contrast, activation of lamina propria T lymphocytes (LPL-T) employing mitogenic CD2[7,8] monoclonal antibodies or, alternatively, a combination of CD28-directed antibody (IgM) plus interleukin-2 (IL-2),[9,10] was possible or even enhanced as compared with PBL-T. This indicates that the impaired responses of LPL-T to CD3/T cell-receptor stimulation are not due to a general down-modulation of lymphocyte responsiveness in the LPL preparation but rather due to a particular functional state.[11-17] Moreover, it should be noted that the method of LPL preparation does not affect cellular *in vitro* reactivities because such a treatment of autologous PBL did not alter their pattern of responses to the various stimuli employed.[13]

Given that lymphocyte proliferation is highly dependent on an intact interleukin-2/interleukin-2 receptor system,[6,18] we subsequently investigated both IL-2 production of LPL as well as their capacity to respond to exogenously added IL-2 upon stimulation with CD3 monoclonal antibodies. As opposed to PBL, LPL do not produce detectable amounts of IL-2 under these experimental conditions (FIG. 3A). Importantly, even the addition of exogenous IL-2 to CD3-stimulated LPL did not result in proliferation, suggesting that one of the earliest responses following T cell-receptor triggering (FIG. 3B), namely, IL-2 receptor expression, does not occur.[11,13] This indicates that an impairment of T cell-receptor signal transduction appears to exist in LPL. Such a notion is further supported by the findings demonstrating that triggering of the T cell-antigen receptor in LPL does not lead to the characteristic increase in cytoplasmic-free calcium, known to occur in PBL, or to the generation of inositol[1,4,5]-trisphosphate (IP$_3$).[13]

THE MUCOSAL ENVIRONMENT EXERTS REGULATORY INFLUENCES ON T CELL-RECEPTOR SIGNALING

To investigate the basis of the impaired responsiveness to T cell-receptor activation in LPL, we addressed the question of whether the mucosal environment might be responsible for this functional state. To this end, PBL were incubated with isolated autologous mucosal cells and then subjected to stimulation employing the above-mentioned panel of monoclonal antibodies (CD3, CD2, CD3, plus CD28).[12,19] As shown in FIGURE 4, coculture with mucosal cells induces an analogous functional state in PBL, as previously observed to exist for freshly isolated LPL. Thus, T-cell receptor triggering is selectively down-modulated. Our subsequent experiments employing a transwell system, in which mucosal cells and the PBL population are physically separated, indicate that the influences on the functional behavior of PBL are likely due to soluble activities that are produced by mucosal cells.

To further elucidate the molecular nature of the observed activity inmucosal cell supernatants, the latter were dialyzed against culture medium employing a semipermeable membrane that allows the passage of molecules of >12 to 14 kDa. Because this treatment led to a complete loss of the functional effects, we had to conclude that the inhibitory molecules must be of lower molecular weight. Subsequently, when supernatants from mucosa were digested with proteinase K overnight at 37 °C, subsequently boiled at 100 °C, and tested on PBL-T, as described above, the down-modulating functional activities were still present (FIG. 4), suggesting that the relevant substances under investigation were not of protein or peptide nature.[19]

It is well known that reducing agents such as 2ME and DTT can enhance lymphocyte proliferation *in vitro,* whereas oxidants inhibit growth of T lymphocytes stimulated by either mitogens, such as concanavalin A, or phorbol-ester plus calcium ionophore. Therefore, it was necessary to investigate the mucosal supernatant for the presence of oxidants. To this end, PBL-T were cocultured with the mucosal supernatant in the absence or presence of catalase and superoxide-dismutase (SOD), which are scavengers for hydrogen peroxide and superoxide anion, respectively. Then PBL-T were washed and subsequently stimulated. In fact, catalase and SOD significantly reversed the inhibition of PKC activation by phorbol ester and ionomycin, as well as activation through CD3/TCR.[19]

To confirm the effects of oxydative substances on T-cell activation, T cells were preincubated with H$_2$O$_2$, then washed and stimulated with CD3 or phorbol-ester plus ionomycin. Such a treatment induced down-regulation of T-cell responses to both CD3 and PKC stimulation. Pretreatment of PBL-T with H$_2$O$_2$ in the presence of 2ME reversed the effects of H$_2$O$_2$ on T cells. To find out whether reducing agents could increase the constitutively low responsiveness of LPL-T to CD3 triggering, LPL-T were stimulated

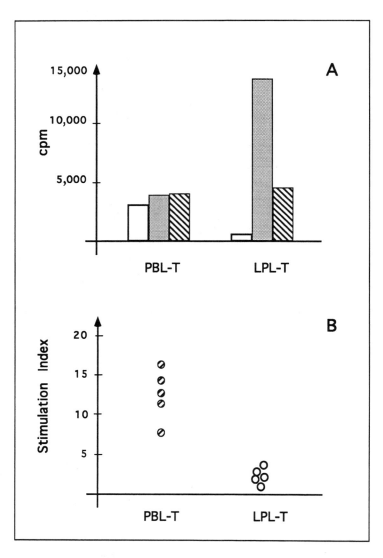

FIGURE 3. Interleukin-2 production (**A**) and responsiveness to exogenous IL-2 (**B**) following exposure of PBL-T or LPL-T to different stimuli. **A:** PBL-T or LPL-T were exposed to Sepharose-coupled CD3 mAb (open columns), a mitogenic combination of CD2 mAbs (shaded columns), or a combination of CD3⁺ CD28 mAbs (dashed columns) for 36 hours. Subsequently, supernatants were harvested and added to the murine IL-2-responsive T-cell line, CTLL-2. Results are expressed as [³H]thymidine incorporation of CTLL-2 cells. **B:** PBL-T or LPL-T from 5 different donors were exposed to Sepharose-coupled CD3 mAb in the presence of 10 U/mL of IL-2 and thymidine incorporation determined after 72 hours of *in vitro* culture. Results are expressed as stimulation index ([³H]thymidine incorporation to CD3 mAb plus IL-2 divided by [³H]thymidine incorporation in response to CD3 mAb alone).

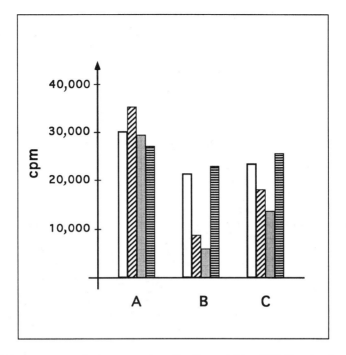

FIGURE 4. Human intestinal mucosa alters T-cell reactivities. PBL-T preincubated for 60 hours with medium (open columns), mucosal supernatant (dashed bars), or mucosal supernatant digested by proteinase K at 1 mg/mL overnight at 37° C and boiled 5 min at 100° C (shaded bars), or with medium digested by proteinase K and boiled as above (striped bars) were incubated with (A) a mitogenic combination of CD2 mAbs, (B) Sepharose-coupled CD3 mAb plus IL-2, or (C) PBU-2 plus ionomycin, respectively. Cultures were pulsed with [³H]thymidine at day 4 for 16 hours. Data are expressed as mean cpm of triplicate cultures and are representative of three independent experiments.

with CD3 monoclonal antibody plus Il-2 in the presence of 2ME. 2ME indeed enhanced the reactivity of LPL-T to CD3 stimulation up to a level of [³H]thymidine incorporation comparable to that reached with untreated PBL-T.[19]

LIGANDS FOR ACCESSORY RECEPTORS ARE DOWN-REGULATED ON MONONUCLEAR CELLS OF THE HUMAN INTESTINE

In the next set of experiments, we addressed the costimulatory level of lymphocyte activation in the human intestinal environment. To this end, mononuclear cell preparations obtained from human peripheral blood or lamina propria were subsequently incubated on plastic dishes either coated with fibronectin or panned with CD14 antibody to enrich for cells of the monocyte lineage. The resulting preparations were first investigated for their morphological characteristics. Monocytes isolated from peripheral blood are uniform and composed of CD11c⁺, CD20⁻, CD3⁻ cells (not shown) and, as a minimal contamination, few CD3⁺, CD20⁻ lymphocytes. By contrast, cells isolated from the lamina propria population are more heterogenous. Monocytes/macrophages with an immunoprofile of peripheral blood monocytes were scarce and CD3⁺ T lymphocytes somewhat more numerous. CD20⁺ B cells were very rare. As revealed employing the epithelium-specific antigen EGP34, most cytospin preparations investigated were devoid of EGP34⁺ enterocytes, indicating a very efficient depletion.

The prevailing cell population isolated from lamina propria consists of CD11c⁻ monocytoid cells that are slightly smaller in size than the CD11c⁺ blood macrophages (not shown). These cells often cluster and occasionally form spheroid clumps. These clumps of homotypically adhering cells occasionally contain a minor subset of CD3⁺ lymphocytes. The monocytoid cells express the panleukocyte antigen CD53 at various levels. They are consistently CD1c⁻, CD3⁻, CD20⁻, CD21⁻, CD38⁻, and CD57⁻. This excludes a derivation from B cells (CD20⁺), plasma cells (CD38⁺), or follicular dendritic cells (CD21⁺). In addition, this makes a T or NK derivation unlikely. Interestingly, this peculiar monocyte type differentially expresses MHC class II determinants. Most, but not all, are HLA DR⁺. The majority is also HLA-DP⁺, but HLA-DP⁻ cells are clearly more numerous than HLA⁻DR⁻ ones. HLA-DQ expression is restricted to a minor subset. Thus, the frequency of MHC class II sublocus products detected in this cell type is DR > DP > DQ. By contrast, the CD11c⁺ macrophage/monocyte population from peripheral blood evenly coexpresses these molecules at high levels. In summary, cells isolated from peripheral blood and from lamina propria differ in their composition of monocytogenic cells. The lamina propria contains predominantly CD11c⁻ monocytoid cells that are characterized by a strong propensity to form aggregates and by their differential expression of MHC class II products.

Employing monoclonal antibodies and flow cytometry, we investigated the quantitative expression of ligands that bind to receptors on the lymphocyte surface and are known to mediate costimulatory activity. As shown in FIGURE 5, neither peripheral blood monocytes (PB-MO) nor lamina propria monocytes (LP-MO) express CD80 molecules, the ligands of CD28. By contrast, CD14 expression is clearly detectable on LP-MO, albeit at approximately half the density level as peripheral blood monocytes. CD54 is also detectable but much lower in expression, and there is barely any CD58 on LP-MO as compared to peripheral blood monocytes.

Taken together, although the CD14⁺ cells isolated from lamina propria differ markedly in their immunoprofile from PB-MO, their close relationship to the monocyte lineage seems unequivocal. The above findings regarding expression of MHC class II and various adhesion molecules on lamina propria-derived cells are consistent with the results of *in situ* analysis of various families of adhesion structures in the human intestinal mucosa, which were found to be extremely low under normal conditions.[20,21]

It is well established that the density of cell-surface molecules, such as CD54, CD58, and CD80 is controlled by cytokines, such as TNF-α and/or interferon-γ,[22] whose expression, as judged by *in situ* hybridization, is also not detectable in the intestinal mucosa.[20] Given the impairment of T cell-receptor signal transduction in lamina propria T cells, which controls IFN-γ expression and secretion, these interactive cycles of cytokines and adhesion molecules up-regulating each other are apparently not operative in the normal mucosa. This situation may change considerably when, due to enhanced T-cell receptor reactivity in inflammatory processes,[23] pathways are initiated by antigen/MHC, which through cytokine production up-regulate the constitutively low levels of adhesion molecules.

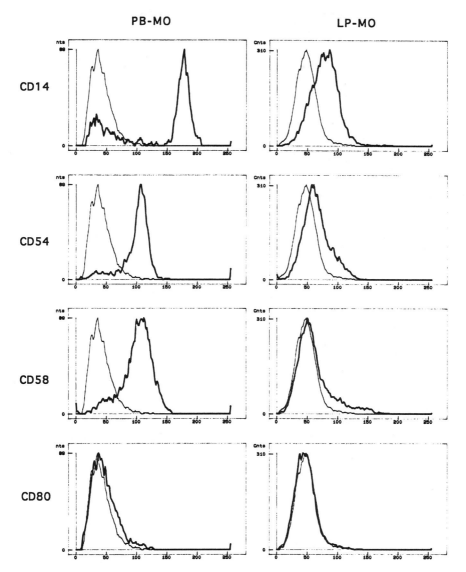

FIGURE 5. Expression of ligands for T cell–accessory receptors by PB-monocytes (PB-MO) and LP-monocytes (LP-MO), respectively. Monocytes from peripheral blood and lamina propria cell preparations were obtained as described in the text and subsequently stained with monoclonal antibodies directed at the differentiation antigens CD14, CD54, CD58, and CD80, respectively. Subsequently, goat anti-mouse FITC serum was added, and the cell preparations were washed and analyzed on a flow cytometer. Negative controls (goat anti-mouse FITC antibody in the presence of an irrelevant, nonbinding monoclonal antibody) are given by the thin lines in the various histograms, whereas antibody-staining is given by the thick curves.

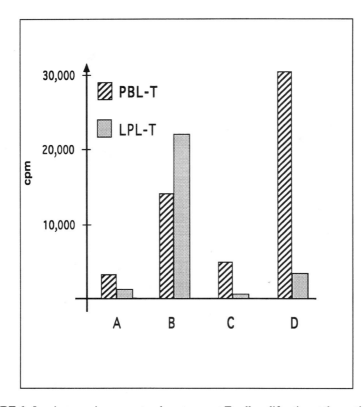

FIGURE 6. Lamina propria monocytes do not support T-cell proliferation at the costimulation level. Mononuclear cell preparations were obtained from peripheral blood and lamina propria from the same patient. Subsequently, T cells and monocytes were separated by adherence, recombined *in vitro,* and stimulated as indicated below. [³H]Thymidine incorporation was determined after 96 hours of *in vitro* culture for the subsequent 16 hours. Stimulation was as follows: (A) Sepharose-coupled CD3 mAb alone; (B) Sepharose-CD3⁺ PB-MO; (C) Sepharose-CD3⁺ LP-MO; and (D) Sepharose-CD3⁺ IL-2 (10 U/mL).

MONONUCLEAR CELLS OF THE LAMINA PROPRIA DO NOT SUPPORT T-CELL PROLIFERATION AT THE COSTIMULATION LEVEL

A functional analysis regarding costimulatory activity for human T cell-clonal expansion by lamina propria monocytes is shown in two independent experiments, which were performed in autologous *in vitro* systems. Here, purified T and "monocyte" populations derived from, respectively, lamina propria and peripheral blood were combined and exposed to suboptimal concentrations of CD3 monoclonal antibody. As shown in FIGURE 6, lamina propria monocytes have much lower costimulatory activity than the peripheral monocyte population for both PBL-T and LPL-T. This is likely due to the reduced expression of adhesion molecules by the former, which are known to be crucial for the induction of clonal T-cell expansion. Another interesting point needs to be mentioned: IL-2 receptor expression represents one of the earliest events detectable following T cell-receptor triggering. As described earlier, freshly isolated LPL-T, as opposed to PBL-T, barely respond to CD3 triggering in the presence of IL-2 (FIG. 3B).[12,13] This finding can easily be explained by the fact that T cell-receptor signal transduction is impaired. We had suggested that this functional state is mediated by oxidative influences exerted by the local environment[19] inasmuch as addition of reducing agents was capable of reverting this down-regulated reactivity in PLP-T (see above). Here, addition of peripheral blood monocytes to isolated lamina propria T cells, however, fully reconstituted their proliferative potential to IL-2 (B columns in FIG. 6) which, in fact, is even slightly higher than that of PBL-T. Explanations for these findings could be the following: (1) restoration of the CD3/T-cell receptor-mediated signal is mediated by reducing agents produced and released by peripheral blood monocytes but not by lamina propria monocytes, and (2) the enhanced proliferative responses of LPL-T in the presence of peripheral blood monocytes, as observed consistently under the experimental conditions employed here, could be due to the well-established enhanced reactivity to costimulatory signals mediated through CD2.[13,16,24]

In conclusion, the present data provide further evidence for the notion that the local intestinal environment exerts a potent regulatory influence on the functional activities of LPL-T. It seems clear that environmental conditions in the human intestine have to secure a certain degree of T-cell unresponsiveness to luminal antigens with the aim of avoiding clonal expansion and memory cell generation. Alterations of these conditions may up-regulate the adhesion molecule/cytokine cascade and promote inflammatory reactions.

Given the down-regulation of both, recognition/competence and costimulatory progression signals in T cells homing to the intestinal mucosa, it seems unlikely to expect that it is possible to induce specific tolerance in this environment inasmuch as such a mechanism would require an intact T-cell receptor-mediated signal. The observed functional state of lamina propria T cells would rather suggest local "unresponsiveness" towards antigens. Upon recirculation to other areas of the organism, T cells can immediately respond with antigen-specific proliferation when they fully encounter competent antigen-presenting cells, such as peripheral blood monocytes.

REFERENCES

1. WEISS, A. 1993. T cell antigen receptor signal transduction: A tale of tails and cytoplasmic protein-tyrosine kinases. Cell **73:** 209-212.
2. MEUER, S. C., B. SCHRAVEN & Y. SAMSTAG. 1994. An "alternative" pathway of T cell activation. Int. Arch. Allergy Appl. Immunol. **104:** 216-221.
3. LINSLEY, P. S. & J. A. LEDBETTER. 1993. The role of the CD28 receptor during T cell responses to antigen. Annu. Rev. Immunol. **11:** 191.
4. CAUX, C., B. VANBERVLIET, C. MASSACRIER, M. AZUMA, K. OKUMURA, L. L. LANIER & J. BANCHEREAU. 1994. B70/B7-2 is identical to CD86 and is the major functional ligand for CD28 expressed on human dendritic cells. J. Exp. Med. **180:** 1841-1847.
5. MEUER, S. C. 1994. Accessory receptors: Regulators of the Local Immune Response. 9-28. Academic Press Ltd.
6. MEUER, S. C. & K.-H. MEYER ZUM BÜSCHENFELDE. 1986. T cell receptor triggering induces responsiveness to interleukin-1 and interleukin-2 but does not lead to T cell proliferation. J. Immunol. **136:** 4106-12.
7. MEUER, S. C., R. E. HUSSEY, M. FABBI, D. FOX, O. ACUTO, K. A. FITZGERALD, J. C. HODGDON, J. P. PROTENTIS, S. F. SCHLOSSMAN & E. L. REINHERZ. 1984. An alternative pathway of T cell activation: A functional role for the 50 kD T11 sheep erythrocyte receptor protein. Cell **36:** 897-906.

8. T. HÜNIG, G. TIEFENTHALER, K.-H. MEYER ZUM BÜSCHENFELDE & S. C. MEUER. 1987. Binding of CD2 to its complementary cell surface molecule provides a triggering signal through the "alternative pathway" of T cell activation. Nature **326:** 298-301.

9. HARA, T., S. M. FU & J. A. HANSEN. 1985. Human T cell activation. II. A new activation pathway used by major T cell population via a disulfide-bonded dimer of a 44 kD polypeptide (9.3 antigen). J. Exp. Med. **161:** 1513-1524.

10. MORETTA, A., G. PANTALEO, M. LOPEZ-BOTET & L. MORETTA. 1985. Involvement of T44 molecules in an antigen independent pathway of T cell activation. J. Exp. Med. **162:** 823-838.

11. PIRZER, U. C., G. SCHÜRMANN, S. POST, M. BETZLER & S. C. MEUER. 1990. Differential responsiveness to CD3-Ti vs CD2-dependent activation of human intestinal T lymphocytes. Eur. J. Immunol. **20:** 2339-42.

12. QIAO, L., G. SCHUAMANN, M. BETZLER & S. C. MEUER. 1991. Down-regulation of protein kinase C activation in human lamina propria T lymphocytes: Influence of intestinal mucosa on T cell reactivity. Eur. J. Immunol. **21:** 2385-9.

13. QIAO, L., G. SCHÜRMANN, M. BETZLER & S. C. MEUER. 1991. Activation and signaling status of human lamina propria T lymphocytes. Gastroenterology **101:** 1529-36.

14. ZEITZ, M., T. C. QUINN, A. S. GRAEFF & S. P. JAMES. 1988. Mucosal T cells provide helper function but do not proliferate when stimulated by specific antigen in lymphogranuloma venereum proctitis in nonhuman primates. Gastroenterology **94:** 353-66.

15. GREENWOOD, J. H., L. L. AUSTIN & W. O. DOBBINS. 1983. *In vitro* characterization of human intestinal intraepithelial lymphocytes Gastroenterology **85:** 1023-35.

16. EBERT, E. C., A. I. ROBERTS, R. E. BROLIN & K. RASKA. 1986. Examination of the low proliferative capacity of human jejunal intraepithelial lymphocytes. Clin. Exp. Immunol. **65:** 148-57.

17. EBERT, E.C. 1989. Proliferative responses of human intraepithelial lymphocytes to various T-cell stimuli. Gastroenterology **97:** 1372-81.

18. MEUER, S. C., R. E. HUSSEY, D. A. CANTRELL, J. C. HODGDON, S. F. SCHLOSSMAN, K. A. SMITH & E. L. REINHERZ. 1984. Triggering of the T3-Ti antigen receptor complex results in clonal T cell proliferation via an interleukin-2 dependent autocrine pathway. Proc. Natl. Acad. Sci. USA **81:** 1509-1513.

19. QIAO, L., G. SCHÜRMANN, F. AUTSCHBACH, R. WALLICH & S. C. MEUER. 1993. Human intestinal mucosa regulates T cell reactivities. Gastroenterology **105:** 814-9.

20. AUTSCHBACH, F., L. QIAO, R. WALLICH, G. SCHÜRMANN & S. C. MEUER. 1995. Cytokine mRNA expression and proliferation status of intestinal mononuclear cells in non-inflamed gut and Crohn's disease. Virchows Archiv B. **426:** 51-60.

21. AUTSCHBACH, F., L. QIAO, R. WALLICH, P. MOUBAYED, K. HOLL-ULRICH, A. FELLER & S. C. MEUER. Immunohistochemical evaluation of cytokine receptor workshop antibodies. *In* Leucocyte Typing V. S. F. Schlosmann, Ed. Oxford University Press. In press.

22. SCHEIBENBOGEN, C., U. KEILHOLZ, S. C. MEUER, T. DENGLER, W. TILGEN & W. HUNSTEIN. 1993. Differential expression and release of LFA-3 and ICAM-1 in human melanoma cell lines. Int. J. Cancer **54:** 494-498.

23. QIAO, L., F. AUTSCHBACH, G. SCHÜRMANN & S. C. MEUER. 1994. T cell receptor repertoire and mitotic responses of lamina propria T lymphocytes in inflammatory bowel disease. Clin. Exp. Immunol. **97:** 303-308.

24. TARGAN, S. R., R. L. DEEM, M. LIU, S. WANG & A. NEL. 1994. Definition of a lamina propria T cell responsive state. Enhanced cytokine responsiveness of T cells stimulated through the CD2 pathway. J. Immunol. **154:** 664-675.

Cholera Toxin B Subunit as Transmucosal Carrier-Delivery and Immunomodulating System for Induction of Antiinfectious and Antipathological Immunity[a]

CECIL CZERKINSKY,[b,c] JIA-BIN SUN,[b]
MICHAEL LEBENS,[b] BIN-LING LI,[b] CAROLA RASK,[b]
MARIANNE LINDBLAD,[b] AND JAN HOLMGREN [b]

[b]Department of Medical Microbiology and Immunology
University of Göteborg
Guldhedsgatan 10A
S-413 46 Göteborg, Sweden

[c]I.N.S.E.R.M. Unité 80
Lyon, France

INTRODUCTION

Mucosal surfaces represent the largest organ system in vertebrates. Being the most frequent portals of entry of common microbes and environmental antigens, these surfaces provide a critical barrier against entry of exogenous matters. Endowed with powerful mechanical and physicochemical cleansing mechanisms, these surfaces are further protected by a specialized immune system that guards them against potential insults from the environment.

The mucosa-associated lymphoid tissue (MALT), the largest mammalian lymphoid organ system, represents a well-known example of compartmentalized immunological system as evidenced by (1) the existence of defined lymphoid microcompartments within mucosal tissues and glands; (2) phenotypically and functionally distinct B-cell, T-cell, and accessory-cell subpopulations; and (3) restrictions imposed upon lymphoid cell recirculation potential to (and from) a given mucosal site or even within various regions of the same mucosal organ.[1] Through the compartmentalization of its afferent and efferent limbs, the MALT functions essentially independently from the systemic immune apparatus, at least as regards induction of humoral immune responses. This notion explains why systemic injection of immunogens is relatively ineffective at inducing an antibody response in mucosal tissues.

The MALT has three main functions: to protect against colonization and invasion by the large number of potentially dangerous microbes; to prevent uptake of undegraded antigens, including foreign proteins derived from ingested food and commensal microorganisms; and to prevent the development of potentially harmful immune responses to

[a]The studies summarized here were supported in part by the Swedish Medical Research Council and the Institut National de la Santé et de la Recherche Médicale (France).

185

these antigens. At variance with the systemic immune apparatus, which is a sterile compartment that can respond vigorously to most invaders, the mucosal immune system guards organs that are replete with foreign matters, including microorganisms. It follows that upon encounter with a given antigen, the MALT must select appropriate effector mechanisms and regulate the intensity of its response so as to avoid bystander tissue damage and immunological exhaustion.

MUCOSAL VACCINES

Immune responses expressed in mucosal tissues are typified by secretory immunoglobulin A (SIgA), the predominant Ig class in human external secretions (and by far the most abundant class of antibodies in this species) and the best-known entity providing specific immune protection for mucosal tissues.[1] SIgA antibodies provide "immune exclusion" of bacterial and viral pathogens, bacterial toxins, and other potentially harmful molecules, and have also been reported to neutralize directly a number of viruses, to mediate antibody-dependent cell-mediated cytotoxicity (in cooperation with macrophages, lymphocytes, and eosinophils), and to interfere with the utilization of growth factors for bacterial pathogens in the mucosal environment.[1] Interestingly, SIgA not only functions well in external secretions but also can express its antimicrobial properties within the epithelial cell, that is, in the very same cell that transports newly formed IgA molecules from the subepithelial lymphoid compartment to the external side of a mucosal tissue.[1] Furthermore, being devoid of complement-activating properties and relatively inefficient as opsonin, SIgA represents a unique type of noninflammatory specific immune effector molecule.

Based on the concept of a common mucosal immune system through which a fraction of IgA-committed B cells recruited in the gut, for example, by ingestion of antigen, can disseminate immunity not only in the intestine but also to other mucosal and glandular tissues, there is currently much interest in the possibility of developing oral vaccines against, for example, infections in the buccal, ocular, respiratory, and genital mucosae.

In addition to SIgA antibody formation, cytotoxicity mediated by T lymphocytes (CTL), antibody-dependent cytotoxicity, and natural-killer activity can develop in mucosal tissues, especially in the epithelium of the gastrointestinal tract.[2-4] Oral administration of allogeneic cells and viruses has been shown to induce virus-specific CTLs in Peyer's patches and other mucosal tissues.[5] Because CTL are critical for eliminating virus-infected cells, their presence in the epithelium of mucosal tissues and their potential role as a first line of defense against invasion by viruses should be advantageous to the host, a possibility that deserves being investigated more thoroughly.

It is now almost axiomatic that in order to be efficacious, vaccines against mucosal infections must stimulate the mucosal immune system, and that this goal is usually better achieved by administering immunogens by the oral route rather than parenterally. However, stimulation of mucosal immune responses by, for example, the oral consumption, inhalation, or topical deposition of most nonviable antigens is often inefficient, requiring multiple administrations of large (milligram to gram) quantities of immunogens and yielding, if any, modest and short-lasting antibody responses. It has thus been widely assumed that only live vaccines would efficiently stimulate a mucosal immune response. The use of live attenuated recombinant bacteria and viruses that can be genetically engineered to express unrelated antigens is being advocated because natural infection with live microorganisms is known to induce persistent and strong immune responses in both mucosal and systemic compartments. However, with most live microbial vectors, a critical balance between attenuation, adequate expression, and immunogenicity is often difficult to achieve, and potential side effects associated with tissue-damaging DTH-like reactions can develop, as has been reported with vaccinia viruses and bacillus Calmette-Guérin (BCG).

Alternative strategies of antigen delivery, including liposomes, and biodegradable microspheres, such as copolymers of poly-DL-lactide-co-glycolide, polyphosphacenes, polyalginates, cellulose starch with incorporated or surface-adsorbed antigens, have been used, but their preparation generally requires relatively large amounts of antigens and/ or harsh conditions, resulting in potential denaturation of antigens. Mucosal lectin-like molecules endowed with immunostimulatory properties, such as cholera toxin (CT), the most potent mucosal immunogen and adjuvant known so far, and its analogue *Escherishia coli* heat-labile enterotoxin (LT), when coadministered with either unconjugated or conjugated antigens have been shown to promote mucosal and systemic antibody responses. This is mostly due to the ability of CT to bind avidly to G_{M1} ganglioside on cell surfaces, including epithelial M cells, a property ascribed to its B subunit, and further to the adjuvant properties of the toxin that appear to require the ADP-ribosylating action of the enterotoxic A subunit.[6] Several formulations, based on chemical coupling or genetic fusion of the cholera toxin B subunit (CTB) with selected antigens or nucleotides, are not being evaluated as potential vaccines against sexually transmitted chlamydia and HIV infections.[6]

ORAL TOLERANCE

Mucosal uptake of antigen (Ag) has far more ensuing consequences than systemic intake of Ag on the development of immune responsiveness. Not only can it induce secretory IgA antibody responses in various mucosal tissues but also, and often, systemic tolerance, or even both. Induction of either or both types of responses could be advantageous to protect the host from colonization by mucosal pathogens and from pathogenic systemic responses that may develop against absorbed Ag produced by these pathogens.

Mucosal administration of antigens is, in fact, a long-recognized method of inducing peripheral tolerance.[7] The phenomenon, often referred to as "oral tolerance" (because this state was initially documented by the effect of oral administration of Ag) is characterized by the fact that animals fed or having inhaled an antigen become refractory or have diminished capability to develop an immune response when re-exposed to that very same Ag introduced by the systemic route, for example, by injection. This phenomenon is an important natural physiological mechanism whereby we avoid developing DTH reactions to many ingested food proteins and other antigens.[8] Depending upon the dose of antigen administered, anergy of antigen-specific T cells[9,10] and/or expansion of cells producing immunosuppressive cytokines (IL-4, IL-10, and TGF-β)[11] may result in decreased T-cell immune responsiveness. It is interesting to note that the latter scenario involves cytokines that are also known to up-regulate IgA production[1,12] and is thus compatible with the observation that secretory humoral immune responses and systemic T-cell tolerance may develop concomitantly.[13] Because tolerance can be transferred by both serum and cells from tolerized animals, it is possible that humoral antibodies (IgA?), circulating undegraded antigens, or tolerogenic fragments and cytokines may act synergistically to confer T-cell unresponsiveness. Because it is exquisitely specific of the antigen initially ingested or inhaled, and thus does not influence the development of systemic immune responses against other antigens, its manipulation has become an increasingly attractive strategy for preventing and possibly treating illnesses associated or resulting from the development of untoward immunological reactions against specific antigens encountered or expressed (autoantigens) in nonmucosal tissues.

Mucosally induced immunological tolerance has earlier been proposed as a strategy to prevent or to reduce the intensity of allergic reactions to chemical drugs,[14] soluble protein antigens, and particulate antigens,[15,16] and to reduce or suppress immune responses against self-antigens.[17-20] It has thus been possible to delay the onset and/or to decrease the intensity of experimentally induced autoimmune diseases in a variety of animal systems by mucosal deposition of autoantigens onto the intestinal (by feeding) or the respiratory mucosa (by aerosolization or intranasal instillation of antigens). Pilot clinical trials of oral tolerance have recently been conducted in patients with autoimmune diseases, and promising clinical results have been reported[21] (see also H. L. Weiner, this volume). Much in the same way, oral administration of antigens had earlier been proposed to prevent and/or treat allergic reactions to common allergens, such as house dust components or substances present in grass pollen.[22,23]

Although the above examples indicate that oral tolerance offers good promise for inducing specific immunologic tolerance, its therapeutic potential remains limited by practical problems. Indeed, to be clinically broadly applicable, mucosally induced immunological tolerance must also be effective in patients in whom the disease process has already established itself and/or in whom potentially tissue-damaging immune cells already exist. This is especially important when considering strategies of tolerance induction in patients suffering from an autoimmune disease, an allergic condition, or a chronic inflammatory reaction to a persistent microorganism. Current protocols of mucosally induced tolerance have had limited success in suppressing the expression of an already established state of systemic immunological sensitization.[24,25] Most importantly, and by analogy with mucosal vaccines aimed at inducing immune responses to infectious pathogens, induction of systemic immunological tolerance by mucosal application of most antigens often requires considerable amounts (milligrams to grams) of tolerogen/antigen and, unless the tolerogen/antigen is administered repeatedly over long periods of time, is of relatively short duration. A likely explanation is that most antigens are extensively degraded before entering a mucosal tissue and/or are absorbed in insufficient quantities. It has thus been widely assumed that only molecules with known mucosa-binding properties can induce local and systemic immune responses when administered by a mucosal route, such as the oral route, without inducing systemic immunological tolerance.[26] A notable example is cholera toxin, one of the most potent mucosal immunogens known so far[27] and which when administered simultaneously with an unrelated antigen by the oral route can also prevent induction of systemic immunological tolerance to said antigen.[28] Based on these observations and as discussed above, mucosal administration of antigens coupled to mucosa-binding molecules, such as cholera toxin or its mucosa-binding fragment cholera toxin B subunit, has been proposed as a strategy to induce local and systemic immune responses rather than systemic tolerance.[29-31] Some years ago, CT and CTB attracted interest not only as potent mucosal immunogens and efficient carrier molecules for oral delivery of foreign protein antigens, but also as agents capable of abrogating oral tolerance when coadministered with various antigens/tolerogens.[28]

CHOLERA TOXIN B SUBUNIT AS TRANSMUCOSAL CARRIER-DELIVERY SYSTEM FOR INDUCTION OF SYSTEMIC TOLERANCE

We suspected that the tolerance-breaking properties attributed to both CT and CTB[28] might be selective for CT and thus, as concerns CTB, explained by low yet significant levels of contamination by CT of commercial CTB preparations used in previous studies. Consistent with this hypothesis, we have observed that physical coupling of an antigen to recombinantly produced and thus inherently uncontaminated CTB led to effects contrary to those reported previously: when given by various mucosal (oral, intranasal, vaginal, rectal) routes in the absence of CT adjuvant, CTB induced a strong mucosal IgA immune response to itself as well as to conjugated antigens in, for example, the gut, and, instead of abrogating systemic tolerance to itself and to the conjugated antigens, enhanced it profoundly.[32] Based on this unexpected finding and on the results of recent experiments

TABLE 1. Prevention of Early and Late DTH Reactions by Oral Administration of SRBC Coupled to CTB[a]

| | Specific Thickness Increment 10^{-3} cm | |
Oral Tolerogen	2 hours	24 hours
CTB-SRBC × 1	0 ± 2.8**	2 + 0.6**
CTB-HRBC × 1	9 ± 3.5	36 ± 6.1
SRBC 1	13 ± 8.0	32 ± 5.0
SRBC × 5	11 ± 4.2	38 ± 6.0
SRBC × 10	11 ± 4.8	24 ± 8.5
SRBC × 15	10 ± 2.0	12 ± 2.2*
SRBC × 20	10 ± 1.6	1.8 ± 0.4**
Saline	8 ± 3.0	38 ± 4.5

[a] BALB/c mice were fed single or daily consecutive doses of SRBC-CTB or SRBC. One week after the last oral administration, animals were primed and challenged by systemic injections of SRBC in the left footpad, followed 5 days later by injection in the right footpad. It was found that the daily oral administration of SRBC for 3 to 4 weeks was required to suppress the 24-h DTH reactions to a level comparable to that achieved by a single administration of SRBC conjugated to CTB. As many as 20 consecutive feedings with SRBC over a 4-week period had no effect on the development of the early phase (2-4 hours) of the DTH response, in contrast to the situation seen with animals fed a single dose of SRBC conjugated to CTB who failed to develop an early DTH response (*p < 0.01; **p < 0.001; Mann-Whitney U test).

with several soluble protein antigens (gamma globulins, myelin basic protein, collagen II, insulin), haptens, and particulate antigens (red blood cells, allogeneic thymocytes), we have good reasons to believe that such a mucosal delivery system, based on coupling antigens to a mucosa-binding nontoxic carrier molecule, may be extremely advantageous for inducing peripheral tolerance.

The validity of this concept has been exemplified by the use, as mentioned, of recombinant CTB as a mucosa-binding molecule and of sheep red blood cells (SRBC) as antigen/tolerogen in a murine system. This antigen was chosen as a model because it is one of the best characterized oral tolerogens with regard to both antibody formation and cell-mediated immune reactions, the latter reactions being typified by the classical delayed-type hypersensitivity (DTH) reaction. Both types of immune reactions have been implicated in the development of autoimmune diseases, allergic reactions, acute graft rejection, and in a number of chronic inflammatory conditions.

The effects of oral administration of CTB-SRBC on the development of systemic serum antibody responses and DTH reactions to systemically administered antigens can be summarized as follows. Oral administration of a single dose of CTB-SRBC suppressed *in vitro* antigen-induced proliferative responses of T cells, *in vivo* DTH reactivity to SRBC, and, although to a lower extent, serum antibody responses (not shown).[32] In the case of DTH reactivity, both early (2-4 h) and late 24-48 h) responses were either abrogated or considerably reduced (TABLE 1). By contrast, daily consecutive administration of unconjugated SRBC for 20 to 30 days was required to suppress antibody responses and DTH reactivity to levels comparable to those obtained after feeding a single dose of CTB-conjugated antigen. With respect to DTH reactivity, only late (24-48 h) reactions were suppressed with no apparent effect on the early component (TABLE 1). The latter observation is especially important, inasmuch as it suggests that the suppressive effects

TABLE 2. Inhibition of Early and Late DTH Reactions by Oral Administration of SRBC Coupled to CTB in Immune Mice[a]

Oral Tolerogen	Specific Thickness Increment $\times 10^{-3}$ cm	
	2 hours	24 hours
CTB-SRBC	0 ± 3.3**	0 ± 7.1**
CTB-SRBC + CT	20 ± 3.9	57 ± 7.8
SRBC	19 ± 2.6	22 ± 4.4
Saline	24 ± 2.3	33 ± 3.6

[a] SRBC were first injected in the left rear footpad of BALB/c mice to induce a state of primary systemic immunity. Four days later, animals were fed a single oral dose of SRBC conjugated to CTB with or without free CT (100 ng), SRBC alone, or saline. Two days after the latter feeding, animals were given a second injection of SRBC in the right footpad to elicit DTH reactions. The latter DTH responses were monitored at various times after this secondary systemic immunization. Whereas mice fed SRBC alone developed DTH responses undistinguishable from those seen in control animals fed only saline, mice fed SRBC conjugated to CTB had considerably reduced early and late DTH responses to SRBC (**$p < 0.001$; Wilcoxon rank test).

of oral administration of antigens coupled to CTB involve mechanisms that appear to be distinct from those implicated in conventional regimens of oral tolerance induction.

Most importantly, this new strategy could be employed to suppress cellular responses even in animals previously sensitized at systemic sites. Thus, when mice were first systemically sensitized (by footpad injection) with SRBC and then fed a single dose of SRBC-CTB conjugate, they failed to develop early as well as late DTH reactivity to a subsequent systemic challenge with SRBC (TABLE 2). By contrast, animals fed the same dose of unconjugated SRBC displayed normal skin DTH reactivity to SRBC (TABLE 2). Further, adding as little as 100 nanogram to 1 microgram of intact CT to the oral SRBC-CTB conjugate abrogated the tolerogenic effects of the conjugate (TABLE 2).

In more recent studies (to be published), we have been able to independently transfer suppression of the early and the late components of DTH reactions to SRBC with cells from animals orally tolerized with SRBC-CTB. The implications of the latter finding may be considerable, inasmuch as they demonstrate that this novel strategy of tolerance induction acts on the very early stages of a T cell-mediated inflammatory reaction. Identifying the cell types and regulatory molecules involved in the suppression of these early and late T cell-mediated inflammatory reactions may be rewarding when considering future therapeutic strategies for the control of autoimmune diseases, allograft rejection, allergic reactions, or chronic inflammatory reactions to exogenous microbial and environmental agents.

We have now extended the above initial finding to other antigens, including allogeneic thymocytes and a number of soluble protein antigens, including selected autoantigens, and also to trinitrophenyl (TNP) as a model of a contact irritant haptenic compound. In all instances, single or double mucosal (oral or intranasal) administration of CTB-conjugated antigens was effective at doses 100- to 1000-fold lower than those of corresponding unconjugated antigens required or known to induce similar levels of inhibition of late DTH responses. Furthermore, overexpression systems have been developed to allow large-scale production of CTB preparations amenable to simple chemical coupling procedures, thereby facilitating the preparation of tolerogenic conjugates.

TABLE 3. Oral Administration of CTB-conjugated MBP Prevents and Reverses Induction of EAE in Lewis Rats[a]

Oral Tolerogen	Feeding Day	EAE Incidence of Paralysis
CTB-MBP, 25 μg × 1	−4	0/5
MBP, 100 μg × 5	−2, −4, −6, −8, −10	5/5
MBP, 1000 μg × 5	−2, −4, −6, −8, −10	0/5
Saline × 5	−2, −4, −6, −8, −10	8/8
CTB-MBP, 50 μg × 1	+6	0/4
MBP, 50 μg × 1	+6	4/4
MBP, 1000 μg × 5	+2, +4, +6, +8, +10	0/4

[a] Female Lewis rats were injected in the rear footpads with MBP emulsified in Freund's complete adjuvant so as to induce EAE. MBP alone or conjugated to CTB was administered at the indicated doses and times before or after disease induction.

TREATMENT OF EXPERIMENTAL AUTOIMMUNE DISEASES AND ALLOGRAFT REJECTION BY MUCOSAL DELIVERY OF CTB-CONJUGATED ANTIGENS

Of special interest because of the similarity of this animal model with human multiple sclerosis, we have found that a single dose of oral cholera B subunit conjugated to myelin basic protein (MBP) prevents experimental autoimmune encephalomyelitis (EAE) in Lewis rats. Animals were injected in the hind footpad with MBP plus Freund's complete adjuvant after being pretreated with different antigens by the oral route (TABLE 3). Animals who were fed saline, an irrelevant antigen coupled to cholera B subunit, or repeated moderate doses of MBP, all developed EAE disease with severe paralysis. By contrast, rats fed repeatedly with a high dose of MBP antigen (5 × 1 mg) or with a single low (25 μg) dose of cholera B subunit-coupled MBP remained healthy. The clinical picture was in complete accordance with the presence or absence of inflammation in the central nervous system, as judged by histopathology (J-B. Sun, T. Olsson, J. Holmgren, and C. Czerkinsky, to be published). It thus appears that by using cholera B subunit-coupled MBP, one can both reduce the number of doses and dramatically decrease the amount of antigen needed for preventing this autoimmune disease, which has many similarities with multiple sclerosis in humans. Analyses of cytokine production after *in vitro* MBP challenge of lymph node cells from CTB-MBP-treated animals have disclosed that oral administration of CTB-conjugated MBP leads to profound down-regulation of IL-2 production and concurrent up-regulation of interferon-γ secretion. The latter finding is in sharp contrast with the effect of feeding repeated large doses (5 × 1 mg) of unconjugated MBP, which resulted in suppression of both IL-2 and IFN-γ production (not shown), suggesting again that CTB exerts unique immunomodulating properties on peripheral T-cell responses to co-fed antigens. Most importantly, feeding animals with CTB-MBP after (7 days) disease induction could also abrogate clinical EAE (TABLE 3).

The recombinant CTB overexpression system has by its design been provided also with unique restriction sites at the 5′ and 3′ ends of the mature CTB gene. This allows genetic fusion of foreign peptide antigens to either or both amino and carboxy ends of the CTB chain, and for a variety of systems. Our laboratory has shown that such fusion proteins are well expressed and retain most or all of the desired properties of such hybrid antigens, that is, receptor binding capacity and antigenicity. Additional sites within the CTB gene into which one can insert foreign genes in positions that are exposed on the surface of the molecule have also been identified. These developments are now being used to fuse to the CTB gene with synthetic oligonucleotides encoding selected foreign epitopes. Preliminary experiments involving oral and intranasal administrations of small doses of a CTB-fused encephalitogenic peptide derived from MBP have yielded very promising results in the Lewis rat system of EAE, and several CTB-based chimeric constructs are now being prepared along this line.

We have also been able to demonstrate the efficiency of this strategy of tolerance induction in a murine model of antigen-induced arthritis. DBA mice, having inhaled as little as 25 micrograms of collagen type II chemically coupled to CTB given one week after disease induction (by intracutaneous injection of collagen type II in Freund's adjuvant), showed considerably delayed (by approximately 30 days) onset of arthritis and had decreased disease severity (joint swelling and erosiveness) as compared to animals given comparable doses of unconjugated collagen type II or CTB alone (A. Tarkowski et al., to be published).

More recently, using the NOD mouse model of spontaneous autoimmune diabetes, we also found that a single oral dose of insulin conjugated to CTB could protect animals against diabetes. In adoptive-transfer experiments, T cell-enriched spleen cells from animals fed CTB-insulin were shown to suppress autoimmune diabetes when cotransferred with syngeneic diabetogenic T cells (C. Thivolet et al., to be published).

Furthermore, by coupling thymocytes to CTB and feeding this conjugate to mice, we have also been able to significantly prolong the survival of transplanted hearts in allogeneic mouse recipients. Again, the effect was superior to that obtained by feeding the cells alone (J-B. Sun, B-L. Li, C. Czerkinsky, and J. Holmgren, to be published).

Based upon these new findings, we are optimistic that it may be possible to use cholera B subunit as a mucosal carrier delivery system for inducing specific systemic T-cell tolerization. Although still at the early stages of animal experimentation, this new tolerization principle may lead to the development of medically useful immunotherapeutic agents in selected autoimmune and DTH-type diseases.

CONCLUSIONS

Such features should bear on the design of vaccines aimed at promoting SIgA immune responses against the numerous infectious pathogens that enter the host through mucosal membranes, and at protecting the host from developing potentially harmful cell-mediated immune responses against the same matters. The relative inefficiency of injectable vaccines to evoke secretory IgA immune responses in mucosal tissues and the fact that they can induce DTH reactivity and thereby bystander tissue damage upon subsequent encounter with the corresponding pathogen constitute two major reasons to encourage the development of alternative strategies to stimulate appropriate immune responses in MALT. Mucosal administration of antigens may theoretically result in the concomitant expression of SIgA antibody responses in various mucosal tissues and secretions, and under appropriate conditions, in the simultaneous down-regulation of cell-mediated immune reactivity at local and systemic sites. Thus, developing formulations based on efficient delivery of selected antigens/tolerogens, cytokines, and adjuvants may impact on the design of future vaccines and of specific immunotherapeutic agents to prevent and/or treat diseases or conditions associated with untoward tissue-damaging immune responses, such as certain autoimmune diseases and allograft rejection.

ACKNOWLEDGMENTS

We gratefully acknowledge the active contributions of Drs. Thomas Olsson, Charles Thivolet, and Andrej Tarkowski.

REFERENCES

1. BRANDTZAEG, P. 1995. The Immunologist 3(3): 89-96.
2. GUY-GRAND, D., D. C. GRISCELLI & P. VASSALI. 1978. J. Exp. Med. 148: 1661-1671.
3. TAGLIABUE, A., W. LUINI, D. DOLDATESCHI & D. BOTASCHI. 1981. Eur. J. Immunol. 11: 919-922.
4. MACDERMOTT, R. P., G. O. FRANKLIN, R. M. JENKINS, I. J. KODNER, G. S. NASH & I. J. WEINRIEB. 1980. Gastroenterology 78: 47-56.
5. MCGHEE, J. R. & J. MESTECKY. 1993. Mucosal vaccines: areas arising. *In* Mucosal Immunology Update. H. Kiyono & P. Ernst, Eds. Vol 4: 1-19. Raven Press. New York.
6. HOLMGREN, J., N. LYCKE & C. CZERKINSKY. 1993. Vaccine 11: 1179-1184.
7. WELLS, H. 1911. J. Infect. Dis. 9: 147-158.
8. MOWAT, A. M. 1987. Immunol. Today 8: 93-98.
9. WHITACRE, C., C. GIENAPP, I. E. OROSZ & D. BITAR. 1991. J. Immunol. 147: 2155-2163.
10. MELAMED, D. & A. FRIEDMAN. 1993. Eur. J. Immunol. 23: 935-942.
11. MILLER, A., O. LIDER, A. B. ROBERTS, M. SPORN & H. L. WEINER. 1992. Proc. Natl. Acad. Sci. USA 89: 421-425.
12. CZERKINSKY, C. & J. HOLMGREN. 1995. The Immunologist 3(3): 97-103.
13. CHALLACOMBE, S. J. & T. B. TOMASI. 1980. J. Exp. Med. 152: 1459-1472.
14. CHASE, M. W. 1946. Proc. Soc. Exp. Biol. Med. 61: 257-259.
15. THOMAS, H. C. & D. M. V. PARROT. 1974. Immunology 27: 631-639.
16. MATTINGLY, J. & B. WAKSMAN. 1978. J. Immunol. 121: 1878-1886.
17. THOMPSON, H. S. G. & N. A. STAINES. 1986. Clin. Exp. Immunol. 64: 581-587.
18. NAGLER-ANDERSON, C., L. A. BOBER, M. E. ROBINSON, G. W. SISKIND & G. J. THORBECKE. 1986. Proc. Natl. Acad. Sci. USA 83: 7443-7448.
19. BITAR, D. M. & C. C. WHITACRE. 1988. Cell. Immunol. 112: 364-373.
20. HIGGINS, P. J. & H. L. WEINER. 1988. J. Immunol. 140: 440-445.
21. WEINER, H. L., A. FRIEDMAN, A. MILLER, S. J. KHOURY, A. AL-SABBAGH, L. SANTOS, M. SAYEGH, R. B. NUSSENBLATT, D. E. TRENTHAM & D. A. HAFLER. 1993. Annu. Rev. Immunol. 12: 809-837.
22. REBIEN, W., E. PUTTONEN, H. J. MAASCH, E. STIX & U. WAHN. 1982. Eur. J. Pediatr. 138: 341-344.
23. WORTMANN, F. 1977. Allergol Immunopathol. 5: 15-26.
24. HANSSON, D. G., N. M. VAZ, L. A. RAWLINGS & J. M. LYNCH. 1979. J. Immunol. 122: 2261-2266.
25. CHILLER, J. M. & A. L. GLASEBROOK. 1988. Monogr. Allergy 24: 256-65.
26. DE AIZPURUA, H. J. & G. J. RUSSELL-JONES. 1988. J. Exp. Med. 167: 440-451.
27. ELSON, C. O. & W. EALDING. 1984. J. Immunol. 132: 2736.
28. ELSON, C. O. & W. EALDING. 1984. J. Immunol. 133: 2892.
29. MCKENZIE, S. J. & J. F. HALSEY. 1984. J. Immunol. 133: 1818-1824.
30. NEDRUD, J. G., X. LIANG, N. HAGUE & M. E. LAMM. 1987. J. Immunol. 139: 3484-3492.
31. CZERKINSKY, C., M. W. RUSSELL, N. LYCKE, M. LINDBLAD & J. HOLMGREN. 1989. Infect. Immun. 57: 1072-1077.
32. SUN, J. B., J. HOLMGREN & C. CZERKINSKY. 1994. Proc. Natl. Acad. Sci. USA 91: 10795-10799.

Induction of Tolerance in Humans

Effectiveness of Oral and Nasal Immunization Routes[a]

JIRI MESTECKY,[b] STEFFEN HUSBY,[b,c]
ZINA MOLDOVEANU,[b] F. BRYSON WALDO,[d]
A. W. L. VAN DEN WALL BAKE,[b,e] AND
CHARLES O. ELSON [b]

[b]Departments of Microbiology and Medicine
University of Alabama at Birmingham
Birmingham, Alabama 35294

[c]Department of Pediatrics
Aarhus University Hospital
Aarhus, Denmark

[d]Department of Pediatrics
University of Alabama at Birmingham
Birmingham, Alabama 35294

[e]Department of Nephrology
University Hospital
Leiden, the Netherlands

INTRODUCTION

The diversity (humoral and cellular response in the mucosal and systemic immune compartments) and dichotomy (specific response versus tolerance) of the immune responses induced by the mucosal route of antigen exposure are essential for survival of an individual in an environment rich in foreign antigens and infectious agents. Decreased or abolished antigen-specific systemic unresponsiveness achieved by preceding ingestion of the same antigen has far-reaching consequences for human health. Successful suppression of humoral as well as cellular systemic responses to environmental allergens (e.g., tree and grass pollens), autoantigens (e.g., myelin basic protein and collagen type II), and alloantigens (e.g., transplantation antigens) by ingestion of the corresponding antigens could alleviate health problems of large populations of patients with atopic and autoimmune diseases or, possibly, organ transplantation recipients.[1-6] By contrast, induction of tolerance by ingestion of oral vaccines could impair protective immune responses in mucosal tissues—the most frequent portal of entry of infectious agents.[7,8] The factors that influence the balance between the desired (protective immunity) and undesired (suppression) response to oral immunization with microbial antigens are not yet known. Why does one soluble protein antigen given orally induce systemic tolerance (e.g., ovalbumin), whereas another induces neutralizing antibodies in external secretions (e.g., glucosyltransferases of *Streptococcus mutans*)?[1,2,8] A partial answer to this paradox was obtained from studies

[a]These studies were supported by US PHS Grants AI-35991 and DE-08182.

194

of mucosal and systemic immune responses in mice orally immunized with soluble and particulate antigens.[9] These studies suggested that systemic immune unresponsiveness may coexist with active mucosal responses, manifested by the presence of antigen-specific secretory IgA antibodies, and stressed the relative independence of the systemic and mucosal compartments of the immune system.[7,10,11] Further compartmentalization has been observed even within the mucosal immune system: an allergen encountered by the respiratory route may induce an immediate-type hypersensitivity, and yet the same allergen given orally desensitizes an individual to a subsequent respiratory tract challenge.[1,5,6] Although some factors, including the nature and dose of an antigen, species, age, and genetic background of the individual, have a profound effect on the end result of an antigen encounter at a mucosal surface, many other factors remain unexplained.[1,2] Furthermore, abundant literature concerning oral tolerance deals, with a few exceptions, with animal models.[1,2]

ORAL TOLERANCE IN HUMANS

Erroneous interpretation of Dakin's[13] results from 1829 have led to a perpetuation of a story of decreased skin reactivity to poison oak and ivy by chewing leaves of these plants. Nevertheless, several investigators (for review see ref. 14) have achieved a substantial reduction in skin reactivity after a long-term ingestion of initially minute but progressively increasing doses of extracts of fresh or dry leaves. Analogous suppression of contact hypersensitivity has been observed by the feeding of low doses of haptens to volunteers;[15] specific serum and mucosal antibodies were not evaluated. However, in a typical protocol for induction of oral tolerance in animals, large doses of protein antigens are necessary to induce systemic unresponsiveness.[1,2] Thus, human newborns and adults were fed with bovine serum albumin (BSA), and sera were examined for anti-BSA antibodies.[16,17] The response varied with the age of the individuals; surprisingly, newborns were immunized rather than tolerized. However, in adults, despite continued oral stimulation with BSA, the levels of serum antibodies decreased progressively with age. Although there were marked variances in levels of serum and secretory antibodies to dietary antigens,[18] most adults usually had low levels, and the titers did not increase upon parenteral immunization despite prolonged ingestion. These results suggest that an extended exposure to common dietary antigens may indeed lead to a diminished systemic responsiveness reminiscent of an oral tolerance.

To address the question of basic importance—the induction of systemic unresponsiveness in humans by mucosal exposure—groups of volunteers were first exposed to a protein antigen by the intestinal or nasal route and subsequently immunized by the systemic route; both humoral (serum and secretory antibody levels) and cellular (T-cell proliferation and delayed-type hypersensitivity) responses were measured.[19,20] Studies carried out in humans are usually hampered by difficulties with the selection of an antigen that has not been encountered previously as a component of the diet. To avoid this problem, we used keyhole limpet hemocyanin (KLH), a potent systemic immunogen in humans and animals, and an excellent oral tolerogen in animals.

Oral Immunization[19]

A group of eight volunteers was administered 500 mg KLH orally divided in 10 doses given on days 1-5 and 15-19; subcutaneous immunization (100 μg KLH) was performed on days 26 and 36. Levels of serum, salivary, and intestinal IgG, IgM, and IgA anti-KLH antibodies (measured by ELISA) were determined on days 0, 10, 26, 36, and 44; antibody-secreting cells (ASC) were enumerated (by ELISPOT) on days 0, 26, and 44; T-cell proliferation was determined on the same days. A control group of eight volunteers received only two subcutaneous doses of KLH (100 μg).

Ingestion of 500 mg KLH did not induce significant levels of IgA, IgG, and IgM antibodies in sera or external secretions, or anti-KLH ASC in peripheral blood. However, feeding followed by systemic immunization resulted in significantly higher levels of serum and secretory antibodies and ASC in KLH-fed and systemically immunized volunteers, compared to those receiving only systemic immunization. Thus, mucosal immunization had a priming effect, manifested by higher humoral immune responses (FIG. 1). This priming effect of oral immunization was not seen when T cell-mediated responses were evaluated. Instead, T-cell proliferation and delayed-type hypersensitivity testing (10 μg KLH, intracutaneously) revealed that KLH-fed and systemically immunized volunteers displayed lower stimulation indexes (FIG. 2) and skin reactivities than volunteers who received only systemic KLH injections (TABLE 1).

These studies demonstrated that KLH given orally at this dose and by this schedule altered the outcome of a subsequent systemic immunization: a priming effect was seen in humoral serum and secretory antibody responses, but a tolerogenic effect was seen in T-cell responses (*in vitro* T-cell proliferation and *in vivo* skin reactivity). Thus, the induction of tolerance was restricted to the T-cell compartment.

Intranasal Immunization[20]

Although frequently used for stimulation of mucosal responses to viral vaccines,[7,8,21] rarely has the intranasal immunization route been considered for induction of tolerance in animal models.[12]

In humans, intranasal immunization with tetanus toxoid induced an increase of serum IgA antibodies to a subsequent intramuscular immunization.[22] Because almost all volunteers had been exposed to tetanus toxoid by previous systemic immunization, the priming effect of intranasal exposure was difficult to evaluate. Therefore, we used KLH in aerosol spray given as three to four doses (100 mg each) on days 0, 14, 28, and 42. Three months after the final intranasal immunization, the four volunteers involved in this study received 100 μg KLH subcutaneously. A control group comprised eight volunteers immunized only subcutaneously (100 μg KLH). In contrast to oral immunization, intranasal exposure to KLH resulted in the appearance of ASC of IgA, IgM, and IgG isotypes in peripheral blood 7–11 days (peak on day 9) after the first immunization. Interestingly, this response was not boosted by subsequent intranasal immunizations. Anti-KLH antibodies of IgA, IgG, and IgM isotypes were detected in sera and secretory IgA in nasal secretions after two to three intranasal immunizations (FIG. 3).

Subcutaneous immunization (100 μg KLH) carried out after a three-month hiatus resulted in an appearance of IgA and IgG ASC in peripheral blood in both experimental and control groups of volunteers. However, a boosting effect of mucosal priming seen in orally immunized individuals was not present in intranasally immunized individuals. Although not statistically significant, intranasally and subcutaneously immunized volunteers displayed a lower IgG and IgA ASC response than only subcutaneously immunized individuals. This was also reflected in lower serum IgG and IgA antibodies to KLH in the experimental group.

In agreement with orally immunized volunteers, intranasal immunization resulted in an equally profound and statistically significant decrease in delayed-type hypersensitivity, as evaluated by skin testing (TABLE 1).

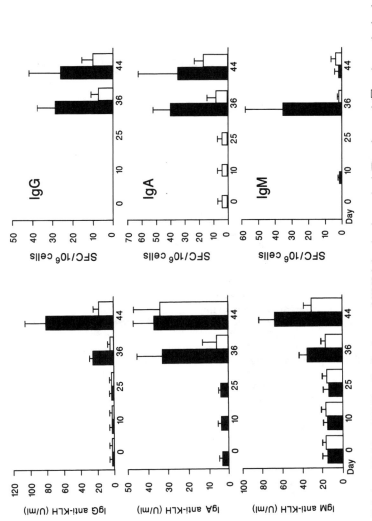

FIGURE 1. Left: IgG, IgA, and IgM anti-KLH antibodies in sera of KLH-fed and sc immunized (■) and control (□, sc immunized only) groups of volunteers. Right: Antibody (spot)-forming cells (SFC) in the peripheral blood of KLH-fed and control group volunteers. Oral immunization was administrated on days 1–5 and 15–19; subcutaneous immunization was on days 26 and 36.

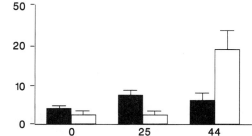

FIGURE 2. KLH-induced proliferation (SI) of peripheral blood T cells from KLH-fed ■ and control □ group volunteers.

DISCUSSION

Despite the differences in the immunization protocols, our studies have demonstrated that systemic cellular immune responses to KLH were markedly altered by previous oral or intranasal immunization with the same antigen.[19,20] Delayed-typed hypersensitivity reactions were consistently diminished in both experimental groups when compared to only systemically immunized volunteers. The most notable difference was seen in the appearance of serum antibodies. Although oral immunization with a total dose of 500 mg KLH primed volunteers for a subsequent systemic response, serum antibodies as well as ASC in peripheral blood were not induced by oral immunization. By contrast, a single intranasal dose of 100 mg KLH resulted in the appearance of both serum antibodies and peripheral blood ASC. This variance may have been due to a relatively low absorption of undigested KLH from the intestinal tract, and a marked, but not fully appreciated, difference in the compositions of immunocompetent cells in the intestinal and respiratory tracts.[23,24] Furthermore, repeated intranasal immunizations did not result in increased numbers of ASC in peripheral blood, and did not prime, in contrast to orally immunized individuals, for subsequent systemic boosting. Therefore, it appears that the primary intranasal immunization with a protein antigen in humans is perhaps even more effective in the induction of systemic tolerance than the oral administration of such antigens. It must be strongly emphasized, however, that these are only initial studies performed with a rather limited number of volunteers, a single antigen (KLH) without extensive determination of optimal doses and the most effective immunization frequencies, and evaluation of antigen-delivery systems that would induce the most profound systemic unresponsiveness.[25] Nevertheless, with these limitations, it is apparent that oral, or perhaps more correctly mucosal, tolerance defined by systemic unresponsiveness to mucosally

TABLE 1. Delayed Hypersensitivity Test Responses to Intradermally Injected KLH (10 μg) of Orally or Nasally Immunized Volunteers

Group	Mean (Range)	Number of Positive/Total
KLH oral	0 (0–0)	0/8
KLH nasal	0.05[a] (0–0.2)	1[a]/4
Controls	11.9 (0–23)	7/8

[a] Redness but not induration.

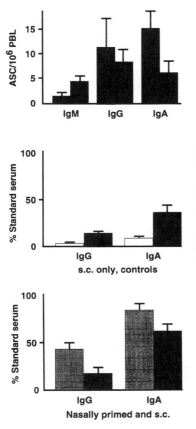

FIGURE 3. Antibody-secreting cells (ASC) and serum antibodies to KLH, nasally and sc immunized (■), and control (□, only sc immunized) groups of volunteers. Top graph: ASC were determined one week after systemic immunization (week 17 after the beginning of intranasal immunization on weeks 0, 2, 4, and 6). PBL, peripheral blood lymphocytes. Middle graph: Serum anti-KLH responses: □, preimmune; □, one week after systemic (sc) immunization. Bottom graph: Serum anti-KLH responses (□) after intranasal immunization; ■, intranasal and sc immunizations.

administered antigens can be induced not only in species such as mice and rats but also in humans.

UNRESOLVED PROBLEMS AND FUTURE STUDIES

The molecular and cellular mechanisms involved in the induction of oral tolerance in humans remain unclear;[1,2] current concepts that are beyond the scope of this communication are discussed elsewhere in this volume. Because of the enormous potential medical importance of mucosal tolerance in the prevention and treatment of immediate as well as delayed-type hypersensitivity reactions[1,5,6,14,15] and some autoimmune diseases (*e.g.,* multiple sclerosis,[3] rheumatoid arthritis,[4] and possibly others), further studies are warranted. Specifically, (1) the relative effectiveness of the oral[19] versus nasal,[20] or rectal immunization routes should be compared; (2) the types and forms of relevant antigens for optimal tolerization should be further examined; (3) optimal antigen-delivery systems, such as covalent linkage to cholera toxin B subunit,[25] should be evaluated in humans to maximize the tolerance and at the same time minimize the doses necessary to make mucosal tolerance applications economically feasible; and (4) immunization protocols should be explored that would selectively enhance or suppress the type of desired immune response. The last point deserves a particular emphasis in studies of orally or mucosally delivered microbial vaccines whose development is currently promoted by national and world health agencies.[7,8] Although, as expected, mucosally delivered viral and bacterial vaccines induce mucosal and often serum antibodies, T cell-mediated protective responses and induction of cytotoxic T cells in humans have not been adequately studied.

REFERENCES

1. Mowat, A. McL. 1994. Oral tolerance and regulation of immunity to dietary antigens. *In* Handbook of Mucosal Immunology. P. L. Ogra, J. Mestecky, M. E. Lamm, W. Strober, J. R. McGhee & J. Bienenstock, Eds.: 185-201. Academic Press. San Diego, CA.
2. Kagnoff, M. F. 1982. Oral tolerance. Ann. N.Y. Acad. Sci. **392:** 248-265.
3. Weiner, H. L., G. A. Mackin, M. Matsui, E. M. Orav, S. J. Khoury, D. M. Dawson & D. A. Hafler. 1993. Double-blind pilot trial of oral tolerization with myelin antigens in multiple sclerosis. Science **259:** 1321-1324.
4. Trentham, D. E., R. A. Dynesius-Trentham, E. J. Orav, D. Combitchi, C. Lorenzo, K. L. Sewell, D. A. Hafler & H. L. Weiner. 1993. Effects of oral administration of Type II collagen or rheumatoid arthritis. Science **261:** 1727-1730.
5. Taudorf, E., L. C. Laursen, A. Lanner, B. Björksten, S. Dreborg, M. Soborg & B. Weeke. 1987. Oral immunotherapy in birch pollen hay fever. J. Allergy Clin. Immunol. **80:** 153-156.
6. Mestecky, J., M. W. Russell & M. Kilian. 1995. The potential role of IgA-mediated mucosal immunity in the prevention of hypersensitivity reactions in the respiratory tract. *In* Progress in Allergy and Clinical Immunology. S. G. O. Johansson, Ed.: **3:**45-49. Hogrefe & Huber Publisher. Seattle.
7. McGhee, J. R. & J. Mestecky. 1990. In defense of mucosal surfaces. Development of novel vaccines for IgA response protective at the portals of entry of microbial pathogens. Infect. Dis. Clin. North Am. **4**(2): 315-341.
8. Mestecky, J. & J. R. McGhee, Eds. 1989. New strategies for oral immunization. Curr. Top. Microbiol. Immunol. **146:** 3-237.
9. Challacombe, S. J. & T. B. Tomasi, Jr. 1980. Systemic tolerance and secretory immunity after oral immunization. J. Exp. Med. **153:** 1459-1472.
10. Mestecky, J., M. W. Russell, S. Jackson & T. A. Brown. 1986. The human IgA system: A reassessment. Clin. Immunol. Immunopathol. **40:** 105-114.
11. Conley, M. E. & D. L. Delacroix. 1987. Intravascular and mucosal immunoglobulin A: Two separate but related systems of immune defense? Ann. Intern. Med. **106:** 892-899.
12. Holt, P. G., J. E. Batty & K. J. Turner. 1981. Inhibition of specific IgE response in mice by pre-exposure to inhaled antigen. Immunology **42:** 409-417.
13. Dakin, R. 1829. Remarks on a cutaneous affection, produced by certain poisonous vegetables. Am. J. Med. Sci. **4:** 98-100.
14. Stevens, F. A. 1945. Status of the poison ivy extracts. J. Am. Med. Assoc. **127:** 912-921.
15. Lowney, E. D. 1968. Immunological unresponsiveness to a contact sensitizer in man. J. Invest. Dermatol. **51:** 411-417.
16. Korenblat, P. E., R. M. Rothberg, P. Minden & R. S. Farr. 1968. Immune response of human adults after oral and parenteral exposure to bovine serum albumin. J. Allergy **41:** 226-235.
17. Rothberg, R. M. & R. S. Farr. 1965. Anti-bovine serum albumin and anti-alpha lactalbumin in the serum of children and adults. Pediatrics **35:** 571-578.

18. RUSSELL, M. W., J. MESTECKY, B. A. JULIAN & J. H. GALLA. 1986. IgA-associated renal diseases: Antibodies to environmental antigens in sera and deposition of immunoglobulins and antigens in glomeruli. J. Clin. Immunol. **6:** 74-86.

19. HUSBY, S., J. MESTECKY, Z. MOLDOVEANU, S. HOLLAND & C. O. ELSON. 1994. Oral tolerance in humans. T cell but not B cell tolerance after antigen feeding. J. Immunol. **152:** 4663-4670.

20. WALDO, F. B., A. W. L. VAN DEN WALL BAKE, J. MESTECKY & S. HUSBY. 1994. Suppression of the immune response by nasal immunization. Clin. Immunol. Immunopathol. **72:** 30-34.

21. CLEMENTS, M. L. & B. R. MURPHY. 1986. Development and persistence of local and systemic antibody responses in adults given live attenuated or inactivated influenza A virus vaccine. J. Clin. Microbiol. **23:** 66-72.

22. WALDO, F. B. 1991. Nasal immunization with tetanus toxoid increases the subsequent systemic dimeric IgA1 antibody response to intramuscular immunization. J. Clin. Lab. Immunol. **34:** 125-129.

23. BRANDTZAEG, P. 1995. Immunocompetent cells of the upper airway: Functions in normal and diseased mucosa. Eur. Arch. Oto-rhino-laryngol. **252:** S8-S21.

24. BRANDTZAEG, P. 1989. Overview of the mucosal immune system. Curr. Top. Microbiol. Immunol. **146:** 13-25.

25. SUN, J.-B., J. HOLMGREN & C. CZERKINSKY. 1994. Cholera Toxin B subunit: An efficient transmucosal carrier-delivery system for induction of peripheral immunological tolerance. Proc. Natl. Acad. Sci. USA **91:** 10795-10799.

Active Immunity or Tolerance to Foods in Patients with Celiac Disease or Inflammatory Bowel Disease

ANNE FERGUSON, HELEN GILLETT, AND
SEAMUS O'MAHONY

Gastro-Intestinal Unit
Department of Medicine
University of Edinburgh
Western General Hospital
Edinburgh EH4 2XU, United Kingdom

DEFINITIONS AND PATHOGENESIS OF IMMUNE-MEDIATED FOOD SENSITIVITY

Food Intolerance

Adverse reactions to ingested food cause a wide variety of conditions, syndromes, symptoms, and diseases for which general descriptive terms, such as food intolerance or food sensitivity, are useful. Thus *food intolerance* can be defined as a reproducible, unpleasant (*i.e.,* adverse) reaction to a specific food or food ingredient that is not psychologically based. This occurs even when the affected person cannot identify the type of food that has been given. The reaction may have a clearly defined metabolic, pharmacologic, or immunopathologic basis, but often the mechanism is unknown or disputed. The provoking agent may be a single food or ingredient, but sometimes, particularly in food allergy, many different foods are involved.

In *food allergy* or *food hypersensitivity,* there is both reproducible food intolerance and evidence of an abnormal immunological reaction to the food. The classical examples are IgE/mast cell-mediated food allergic reactions, for example, food-induced anaphylaxis or the oral allergy syndrome; and celiac disease, in which the pathogenesis of the intestinal damage is probably through delayed-type hypersensitivity (DTH) reactions to wheat gliadin and related antigens. It is also entirely possible that immune reactions to foods play a role in the pathogenesis of motility disorders and so-called idiopathic inflammatory gut diseases. Knowledge of whether and how oral tolerance (OT) fails in these and similar settings could open up entirely new avenues of therapy for an important and disabling group of diseases.

Induction and Expression of Immunity to Food Antigens

As extensively discussed by other contributers, mucosal immune functions can be separated into induction and effector phases, and this is particularly relevant physiologically in relation to food antigens. The induction of a specific immune response is critically dependent on the situation of the individual when the antigen is first encountered. In

202

humans, the first exposure to a food antigen may be as part of the infant or weaning diet, but may even be in utero to food molecules that have crossed the placenta, or possibly to antiidiotype antibodies mimicking the antigenic structure of food antigens. Certainly, in animals, the maternal diet profoundly affects later immunity.[1] Whatever the age at exposure, factors such as dose, route of encounter, and physicochemical form of antigen critically influence the type of immune response that will predominate for the rest of the life of the individual. The state of activation of antigen-processing cells and T cells in the tissues where antigen is first encountered are also important factors.

In clinical studies and research on food sensitivity, most observations concern the pathological and immune effects of reexposure to antigen, in other words the expression of an antibody-mediated or cell-mediated specific immune response, either at the site of exposure or, if the substance is absorbed or otherwise transferred around the body, at other sites or systemically. It seems very likely that in healthy people, for most or all foods, the immunological response induced by natural exposure will have been tolerance, but this remains to be proven. For example, the immune system may remain naive to some antigens that have been rapidly degraded in the gut.

Certainly, IgE antibody to foods are rarely detected, even in people with atopic diseases; methods for detection of cell-mediated immunity to foods are unsatisfactory, but there is little evidence of this occurring apart from a few specific intestinal diseases. However, serum IgG, IgA, and IgM antibodies, and gut IgA and IgM antibodies to many different food antigens can be detected in low titer in healthy individuals, and may be present in high titer in several gastrointestinal (GI) diseases and other diseases, including atopic eczema, celiac disease, and Crohn's disease.

EXPERIMENTAL WORK ON ORAL TOLERANCE

Some data from our experimental program of work on gut immunity and tolerance is relevant to these issues.

Many Chemically Disparate Antigens Induce Oral Tolerance

Like most groups, we selected cheap, fully characterized, soluble proteins, such as ovalbumin and BSA for the main lines of our work, including the phenomenon of gut-antigen processing. However, it proved necessary, in the course of the studies of several doctoral students, to examine other materials. We were surprised to find that OT, and gut-antigen processing to produce tolerogen in the blood, occurred with insoluble proteins, such as wheat gliadin[2] and (for DTH) even with cholera toxin[3] (see below).

Perhaps the most remarkable example derives from work we did as part of the safety monitoring of a food constituent, gum arabic, which had been requested by the European Community Food Safety Regulatory Body. We used a standard oral tolerance protocol[4] that showed that mice were tolerized by feeding gum arabic, a product of the acacia trees in North Africa.[5] This proteinaceous polysaccharide has a molecular weight range of 250,000–2,000,000. A typical molecule is spherical and contains 50,000 sugars in long chains, 10,000 water molecules, and 300 amino acids, which are in the form of peptides approximately 15 amino acids long, scattered within the body of the molecule. There is no degradation within stomach or small bowel; digestion of gum arabic is by bacterial enzymes, within the colon.

Separate Regulation of Serum Antibody and DTH Tolerance—the Example of Protein Malnutrition

We examined the effects of protein deprivation on the induction of oral tolerance for systemic antibody and DTH responses to ovalbumin (OVA) in mice.[6] Mice were fed 4% or 24% protein diets from weaning and given a single feed of OVA or saline at age 5 weeks. Then the presence of tolerance was assessed by comparing systemic responses of OVA and saline-prefed animals to immunization with OVA in adjuvant. There were disparate effects on the humoral and cell-mediated limbs of oral tolerance. Tolerance for serum antibody responses was more profound in protein-deprived animals than in controls. Conversely, tolerance for DTH responses was impaired in protein-deprived mice.

Impaired induction of oral tolerance for DTH responses to OVA could also be explained by changes in the gut epithelium, with failure of the processing of fed antigen. This was studied by using serum, collected one hour after feeding, which should have contained tolerogenic, "gut-processed" antigen. Suppression of DTH was transferred with one-hour serum from normal, protein-sufficient mice, and also with serum from deprived mice,[7] indicating that their capacity for intestinal antigen processing was normal. Furthermore, the quantity of absorbed antigen in the serum one hour after feeding was similar in both protein-deprived and normal groups. Our results supported the hypothesis that protein deprivation selectively depletes the population of suppressor-type T cells responsible for the fine control of DTH tolerance.

Separate Regulation of Serum Antibody and DTH Tolerance—the Example of Cholera Toxin

We found, as have several other investigators, that a single oral dose of cholera toxin (CT) in mice induced not only intestinal antibodies but also a serum antibody response. Previous experiments had shown that DTH to CT can be induced by immunization with CT in complete Freund's adjuvant (CFA), and that cholera toxoid (CTd) is a suitable agent to test for DTH by skin test.[8] However, the cellular limb of immunity (assessed by a footpad swelling test of DTH, after later, systemic immunization) was down-regulated; in other words, oral tolerance for DTH was induced at the same time as active humoral immunization.[3] Results of a typical experiment are shown in FIGURE 1. The legend gives details of the experimental protocol and an interpretation of the results. Tolerance was antigen-specific, dose-dependent, and transferable by spleen suppressor lymphocytes. Oral tolerance for DTH could also be transferred by serum obtained from mice fed CT one hour previously; thus CT is gut-processed to a tolerogenic form during absorption.[9]

Stock Mice are Immunologically Tolerant to a Protein in Their Diet (Gluten)

We studied induction of oral tolerance to gliadin, using a colony of mice reared for several generations on a gluten-free diet;[10] the insoluble antigen was incorporated in a pellet of agar for conventional protocols, and OT could be induced by a single feed of 25 or 125 μg gliadin or by feeding a gluten-containing diet for a week. However, we also showed that mice, conventionally reared on a gluten-containing diet, showed OT, with significantly lower serum antibody and DTH responses to gliadin in CFA than were found in mice from the gluten-free diet colony[2] (FIG. 2).

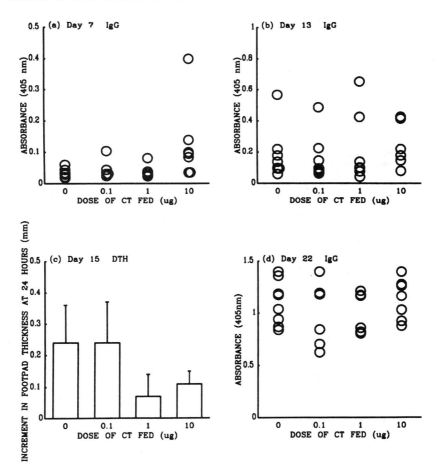

FIGURE 1. The effect of prefeeding different doses of CT. Animals were fed either ABS (inert buffer) or 0.1, 1, or 10 µg CT (day −7) one week before immunization with 1 µg CT in complete Freund's adjuvant (day 0). Two weeks later (day 14), they were challenged with 5 µg toxoid into a footpad, and their DTH responses were measured as footpad swelling after 24 h. Animals were bled on days 7, 13, and 22 of the experiment for assessment of their serum antitoxin antibody responses. The IgG antitoxin responses of animals fed either 0.1 or 1 µg CT were no different from ABS-fed controls at any time. However, animals fed 10 µg CT had significantly higher IgG antitoxin responses (p < 0.02) on day 7. By contrast, animals fed either 1 or 10 µg CT had suppressed DTH responses (p < 0.001 and p < 0.01, respectively), but a dose of 0.1 µg CT did not significantly inhibit the induction of DTH. The graphs show the IgG antitoxin antibody response in serum on days 7(a), 13(b), and 22(d) and the DTH response on day 15(c).

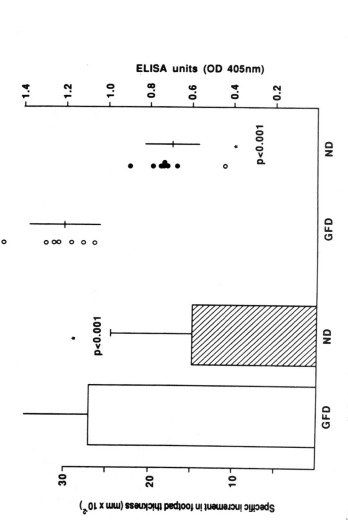

FIGURE 2. Systemic immune response to gliadin in mice reared on a gluten-containing diet. DTH (left) and antibody (right) responses three weeks after parenteral immunization with gliadin in mice from the gluten-free diet (GFD) and the normal diet (ND) colonies. DTH results are shown as mean specific increments in footpad thickness + 1 SD. Antibody results are shown as individual OD 405 readings in ELISA. Bars indicate mean + 1 SD.

HYPOTHESIS: STEPS IN THE PATHOGENESIS OF CELIAC DISEASE

In celiac disease, the presence of certain cereal proteins (gluten) in the diet causes chronic inflammation, in the small intestinal mucosa, and malabsorption. Integration of knowledge of oral tolerance with recent changes in our perspectives of gluten sensitivity in patients led us to propose the following hypothetical sequence as the pathogenesis of gluten-sensitive enteropathy (celiac disease):[11] The sequence begins with (1) failure of the development of OT for T cell-mediated immunity, either globally (many antigens) or confined to gluten. (2) The genetically predisposed individual is thus vulnerable to being actively immunized to the food antigen (gluten) if a particular combination of diet, gut permeability, and mucosal and systemic immunomodulatory signals coincide.The frequency with which this occurs in nontolerant individuals, and at what age, will depend on many intrinsic and environmental factors. (3) When active T-cell sensitization has occurred, and there is gluten in the diet, relatively subtle effects on the gut mucosa (low-grade pathology, *e.g.*, high intraepithelial lymphocyte (IEL) count with normal villi) occur, but only in a proportion of those at risk. (4a) It is then only a matter of time until a critical combination of antigen dose and activated mucosal T-effector cells occurs, and this then precipitates the evolution of severe enteropathy and malabsorption. (4b) Simultaneously with 4a, a wide range of immune effector cells are recruited and other dietary antigens, and possibly autoantigens, become involved, thus perpetuating and worsening the enteropathy, explaining why tissue damage persists for weeks or months after strict dietary exclusion of gluten, and why many immunological epiphenomena occur in celiac patients.

Differences in the proportion of those "at risk" who progress to the next step 1 → 2, 2 → 3, and 3 → 4 will explain striking differences in disease frequency in groups that share the same genetic make-up, for example, Swedes and Danes, British infants in the late 1960s, and, now, healthy and affected relatives of patients with celiac disease. Knowledge of the factors that progress the genetically predisposed individual along this sequence of stages will mean that new approaches for stopping or even reversing the process, and thus curing celiac disease, can be devised.

METHODS USED FOR CLINICAL STUDIES OF GUT ANTIBODIES

We have been developing a series of clinical protocols to facilitate the study, in humans, of immune phenomena well established in experimental animals.[12] Peroral gastrointestinal lavage with nonabsorbable fluid is now extensively used to cleanse the gastrointestinal tract prior to colonoscopy, barium enema examination, or colonic surgery. This lavage fluid contains abundant quantities of IgA, and, in disease, also IgM and IgG. After filtration and processing with protease inhibitors, ELISA and biochemical assay techniques can readily be applied.[12–14] A recently completed study of fluid intake/output data and concentrations of various substances in sequentially passed specimens has confirmed that whole gut lavage fluid (WGLF) is a gut perfusate,[12] and we have reported that in patients with intestinal inflammatory diseases, WGLF contains immunoglobulins, antibodies, plasma-derived proteins, inflammatory cells, and cytokines.[15–22]

The clinical procedure is quite simple. The lavage solution (available commercially in the U.K. as Klean-prep (Norgine, Oxford, U.K.)) has an osmolality of 260 mosm/liter. After an overnight fast, supervised and monitored by an experienced research nurse, patients or healthy volunteers drink the lavage solution, aiming for a rate of 200 mL every

12 minutes. Several formed or semiliquid stools are passed, followed by fecal-stained fluid. These are discarded until clear fluid, resembling urine, is being passed per rectum. There is a very high success rate in obtaining clear specimens when this procedure is conducted as described, more than 95% in a series of hospital inpatients ranging in age from 14 to 89 years.

Specimens are processed as follows. Twenty mL of clear fluid are filtered through GF/A (Whatman) glass fiber filters. To 10 mL of the filtered fluid the following reagents are added, with mixing after each addition (final concentrations in brackets): soya-bean trypsin inhibitor in phosphate-buffered saline (PBS) (80 μg/mL), sodium ethylene diamine tetracetic acid in PBS (15 mM), phenyl methyl sulphonyl fluoride in 95% ethanol (2 mM), sodium azide (1 mM), and newborn calf serum (5% v/v). Aliquots of processed WGLF are stored at −70 °C for later analyses.

Assay Techniques

Concentrations of immunoglobulins and of isotype-specific antibodies to the dietary proteins gliadin (GLI), β-lactoglobulin (BLG), and OVA were determined by ELISAs, previously described by us.[23] Isotype-specific antibodies to cholera toxin were assayed by a minor adaptation of a published "G_{M1}" method;[24] precoating the ELISA plates with this protein ensures optimal binding of the cholera toxin B subunit. Results were expressed as arbitrary units in relation to a reference standard that differed for each isotype; the lower limit of detection for these tests was 20 units/mL unless otherwise stated. It should be emphasized that although WGLF is dilute (in theory 28 liters produced per day), very low concentrations of materials (ng/mL) can readily be detected by immunoassay, and we are confident that differences in detection rate between serum and gut fluid cannot merely be explained on technical grounds.

As part of an extensive program of clinical research, WGLF had been obtained from healthy volunteers and from well-characterized patients with inflammatory bowel disease (IBD), or with celiac disease.[25] Stored specimens were retrieved and assayed for the antibodies listed above. We have already established that there is great variation in the rate of IgA production,[18] and preliminary analysis showed that titers of antibody were unrelated to total IgA concentration in gut fluid. Because the protocol standardizes WGLF perfusion rate at 20 mL/min, we have expressed results per unit volume.

GUT/BLOOD ANTIBODIES TO FOOD ANTIGENS: PARALLEL, RECIPROCAL, OR INDEPENDENT?

IBD Patients and Healthy Volunteers

We examined antibody data to test two theories: that active systemic immunity was the result of gut IgA antibody deficiency (in which case blood and gut antibodies would have reciprocal relationships), or that up- or down-regulation of humoral immunity to foods affected both systemic and mucosal immune systems in parallel.

Frequencies of detection of IgG antibodies in blood (serum) and of IgA antibodies to the same antigen in the gut (WGLF) in 12 healthy volunteers and in 54 patients with IBD

TABLE 1. Frequencies of Detection of IgG Antibodies in Blood (Serum) and of IgA Antibodies to the Same Antigen in the Gut (WGLF) in 12 Healthy Volunteers and in 55 Patients with IBD

Diagnosis	Antigen	Antibody in Blood	Antibody in Gut	
			Yes	No
Normal	Gliadin	yes	4	5
Volunteer		no	0	3
	β-Lactoglobulin	yes	2	9
		no	0	1
	Ovalbumin	yes	4	6
		no	1	1
Inflammatory	Gliadin	yes	12	17
bowel		no	2	23
disease	β-Lactoglobulin	yes	6	24
		no	1	23
	Ovalbumin	yes	13	16
		no	5	20

are shown in TABLE 1. It is clear that the first theory is not sustained. Neither in healthy individuals nor IBD patients were there many instances of positive gut antibodies and absent serum antibodies.

More positive results were obtained for serum than for WGLF, but a clear relationship between the two compartments emerged, both in the healthy volunteers with low frequen-

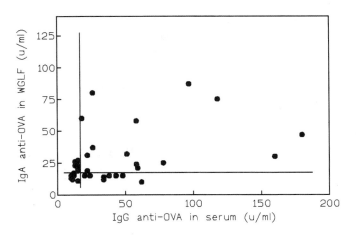

FIGURE 3. Antibodies to ovalbumin of the IgG class in serum, and of the IgA class in gut secretions, in patients with inflammatory bowel disease.

TABLE 2. Percentage Frequencies of Patterns of Antibody Detection in Blood and in Gut Secretions in Patients with Crohn's Disease, Ulcerative Colitis (GLI, BLG, and OVA Antibodies combined), and in Patients with Celiac Disease (BLG and OVA Antibodies only).

	Blood+ Gut+	Blood+ Gut−	Blood− Gut+	Blood− Gut−
Crohn's disease (105 tests)	25	35	6	36
Ulcerative colitis (57 tests)	9	37	3	50
Celiac (72 tests)	15	4	42	39

cies, and in the IBD patients with many cases of detectable antibody. In general, those cases with gut IgA antibodies also had serum IgG antibodies, and there were many cases with serum antibodies only. FIGURE 3 illustrates this for OVA antibodies in IBD patients. If these data are confirmed in more extensive studies, and if active immunity reflects a failure of OT, this would suggest that OT for antibody responses occurs to an extent in the gut as well as systemically, and that systemic tolerance is more easily abrogated systemically than in the gut. The implications for oral vaccination are self-evident.

Intestinal Antibodies in Celiac Disease

The data for IBD patients is presented in TABLE 2 as percentage frequencies, separately for Crohn's disease and ulcerative colitis patients (GLI, BLG, and OVA antibodies combined), together with results for BLG and OVA, a group of patients with celiac disease (BLG and OVA only). Distributions were similar for Crohn's disease and ulcerative colitis, but in the celiac patients, 42% of the tests showed intestinal IgA antibodies in the absence of serum IgG antibodies to the same antigen (the figures being 6% for Crohn's disease and 3% for ulcerative colitis). In the context of our hypothesis of the pathogenesis of celiac disease, it seems likely that this abnormality of regulation of humoral immunity is one of the events in 4b (above), an immunological epiphenomenon, but which may contribute to perpetuation and worsening of the enteropathy. In any even, this "experiment of nature" provides an opportunity to explore candidate gut immunoregulatory mechanisms in humans.

CIRCUMSTANTIAL EVIDENCE OF PRIOR EXPOSURE TO A GUT IMMUNOSTIMULANT IN PATIENTS WITH CELIAC DISEASE

Antibodies to Cholera Toxin in Gut Secretions

Given the profound disturbances in systemic and mucosal immunity in patients with celiac disease, it might be expected that their immune response to vaccines would differ from those of healthy volunteers. We made an attempt to study this by using the oral

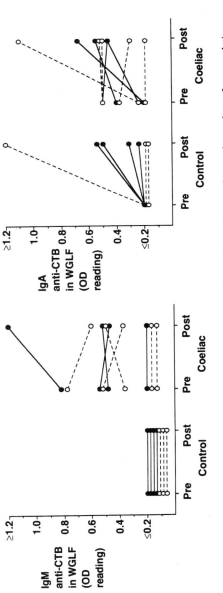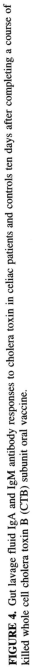

FIGURE 4. Gut lavage fluid IgA and IgM antibody responses to cholera toxin in celiac patients and controls ten days after completing a course of killed whole cell cholera toxin B (CTB) subunit oral vaccine.

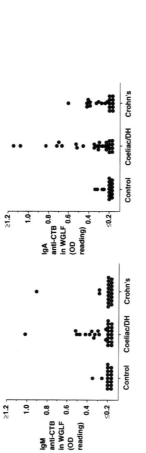
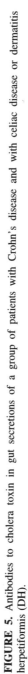

FIGURE 5. Antibodies to cholera toxin in gut secretions of a group of patients with Crohn's disease and with celiac disease or dermatitis herpetiformis (DH).

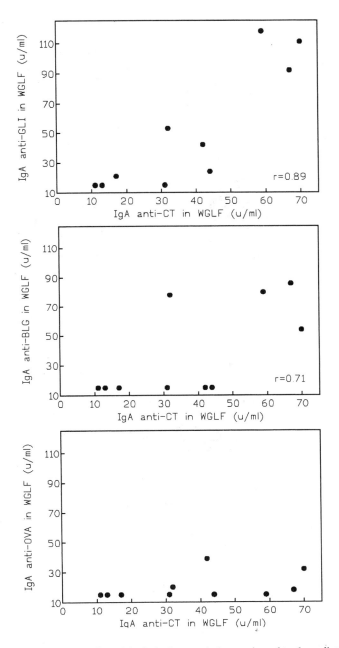

FIGURE 6. Intestinal antibodies of the IgA class to cholera toxin and to three dietary protein antigens in a group of untreated celiac patients.

cholera vaccine (combined killed while-cell/B subunit), which is known to evoke high levels of specific intestinal antibodies along with antitoxic protection. As explained below, the original aims were not achieved, but this work has opened up a new line of research on gut immunoregulation in humans.

Seven healthy volunteers and nine untreated celiac patients were studied (age range 24–46 years). All celiac patients had had a recent jejunal biopsy showing subtotal or severe partial villus atrophy, and all were taking a normal (i.e., gluten-containing) diet. The oral cholera vaccine used was a gift of Professor Jan Holmgren (Göteborg, Sweden). Each dose of vaccine contained 1 mg of B subunit and 10^{11} skilled vibrios. The vaccine was given mixed with 150 mL of a sodium bicarbonate solution. Following baseline collections of serum and gut lavage fluid, the subjects were given two or three doses of vaccine; collection of serum and gut lavage fluid was repeated 10 days after the last dose.

When antibodies were assayed, we found that before immunization, both IgM and IgA antibody levels in WGLF were significantly higher in the celiac patients (both $p < 0.03$) compared to controls. Immunization resulted in an increase in WGLF IgA antibody activity in 5 of 7 controls, and in 5 of 9 celiacs (FIG. 4). However, because the prevaccination levels of antibody differed, no conclusion could be drawn as to any possible intrinsic difference in gut immune capacity between patients with celiac disease and others.

Studies of WGLF from a larger group of celiac patients, together with IBD patients and immunologically normal controls, confirmed the high frequency of intestinal anti-CT antibodies in celiac disease and also in some IBD patients (FIG. 5).

Correlations between Intestinal Antibody Titers to Food Antigens and to CT in Celiac Disease

Some supportive evidence that CT may be a key immunostimulant in celiac disease is obtained by comparing titers of anti-CT and antibodies to food proteins in the same sample (note again, titers of antibodies per milliliter did not correlate with IgA concentration). In a group of untreated celiac patients, strong positive correlations were obtained for anti-CT versus anti-GLI and anti-BLG (FIG. 6); such relationships were not present in volunteers, IBD patients, or in celiac patients treated with a gluten-free diet.

Why should celiac patients who have never had clinical cholera or been exposed to cholera vaccine have high levels of specific intestinal antibodies? The most likely explanation is that these are antibodies to the heat-labile enterotoxin of *E. Coli,* which is antigenically very similar to cholera toxin. Whether the bacteria persist, or whether the antibodies are "footprints" left by an earlier encounter, is unknown. Nevertheless, it seems not unreasonable to postulate that the adjuvant effect of this product of the gut flora could explain the upregulation of intestinal humoral immunity to dietary antigens in untreated celiac disease. Whether infection or colonization with a toxin-producing *E. coli* is a trigger for exacerbation of enteropathy and the clinical expression of celiac disease remains to be established.

CONCLUSION

Much exciting information on the physiology of gut immunity, as well as data relevant to the mechanisms and pathogenesis of the disease, is emerging from experimental animal work and from *in vitro* and molecular studies. With ingenuity on the part of investigators, and the active cooperation of patients with GI disease, informative and ethical clinical studies of human gut immunity and tolerance are now entirely feasible.

REFERENCES

1. TRONCONE, R. & A. FERGUSON. 1988. In mice, gluten in maternal diet primes systemic immune responses to gliadin in offspring. Immunology **64:** 533-537.
2. TRONCONE, R. & A. FERGUSON. 1988. Gliadin presented via the gut induces oral tolerance in mice. Clin. Exp. Immunol. **72:** 284-287.
3. KAY, R. & A. FERGUSON. 1989. The immunological consequences of feeding cholera toxin. I. Feeding cholera toxin suppresses the induction of systemic delayed-type hypersensitivity but not humoral immunity. Immunology **66:** 410-415.
4. STROBEL, S. & A. FERGUSON. 1987. Persistence of oral tolerance in mice fed ovalbumin is different for humoral and cell-mediated immune responses. Immunology **60:** 317-318.
5. STROBEL, S. & A. FERGUSON. 1986. Induction of oral tolerance, in mice, to gum arabic. Food Addit. Contam. **3:** 43-46.
6. LAMONT, A. G., M. GORDON & A. FERGUSON. 1987. Oral tolerance in protein-deprived mice. I. Profound antibody tolerance but impaired DTH tolerance after antigen feeding. Immunology **61:** 333-37.
7. LAMONT, A. G., M. GORDON & A. FERGUSON. 1987. Oral tolerance in protein deprived mice. II. Evidence of normal "gut processing" of ovalbumin, but suppressor cell deficiency, in deprived mice. Immunology **61:** 339-343.
8. KAY, R. A. & A. FERGUSON. 1989. Systemic delayed-type hypersensitivity to cholera toxin and a detoxified derivative. Clin. Exp. Immunol. **76:** 111-116.
9. KAY, R. A. & A. FERGUSON. 1989. The immunological consequences of feeding cholera toxin. II. Mechanisms responsible for the induction of oral tolerance for DTH. Immunology **66:** 416-421.
10. TRONCONE, R. & A. FERGUSON. 1991. Animal model of gluten induced enteropathy in mice. Gut **32:** 871-875.
11. FERGUSON, A. 1995. Coeliac disease research and clinical practice—Maintaining momentum into the Twenty-first Century. *In* Howdle: Coeliac Disease. Bailliere's Clin. Gastroenterol. Rev. **9:** 395-412.
12. FERGUSON, A., J. SALLAM, S. O'MAHONY & I. POXTON. Clinical investigation of gut immune responses. Review on non-parenteral vaccines. Adv. Drug Delivery. In press.
13. GASPARI, M. M., P. T. BRENNAN, S. M. SOLOMAN & C. O. ELSON. 1988. A method of obtaining, processing, and analyzing human intestinal secretions for antibody content. J. Immunol. Methods **110:** 85-91.
14. O'MAHONY, S., J. R. BARTON, S. CRICHTON & A. FERGUSON. 1990. Appraisal of gut lavage in the study of intestinal humoral immunity. Gut **31:** 1341-1344.
15. O'MAHONY, S., E. ARRANZ, J. R. BARTON & A. FERGUSON. 1991. Dissociation between systemic and mucosal humoral immune responses in coeliac disease. Gut **32:** 29-35.
16. HODGES, M., K. KINGSTONE, W. G. BRYDON, J. SALLAM & A. FERGUSON. 1994. Use of gut lavage fluid to measure intestinal immunity in healthy Sierra Leonean children. J. Pediatr. Gastroenterol. Nutr. **19:** 65-70.
17. O'MAHONY, S., N. ANDERSON, G. NUKI & A. FERGUSON. 1992. Systemic and mucosal antibodies to klebsiella in ankylosing spondylitis and Crohn's disease. Ann. Rheum. Dis. **51:** 1296-1300.
18. FERGUSON, A., J. SALLAM, L. McLINTOCK, N. CROFT & I. POXTON. 1994. The gut as an immune organ: Intestinal anti-endotoxin antibodies. *In* Organ metabolism and nutrition: Ideas for future critical care. J. M. Kinney & H. N. Tucker, Eds.: 231-244. Raven Press Ltd. New York.
19. CHOUDARI, C. P., S. O'MAHONY, G. BRYDON, O. MWANTEMBE & A. FERGUSON. 1993. Concentrations of immunoglobulin G, albumin and alpha-1-antitrypsin in whole gut lavage fluid: objective measures of disease activity in inflammatory bowel disease. Gastroenterology **104:** 1064-1071.
20. BRYDON, W. G. & A. FERGUSON. 1992. Haemoglobin in gut lavage fluid as a measure of gastro-intestinal blood loss. Lancet **340:** 1381-1382.

21. FERGUSON, A., S. GHOSH, L. M. HANDY, C. CHOUDARI, O. MWANTEMBE & M. A. MCINTYRE. 1994. Analysis of disease distribution, activity and complications in the patient with inflammatory bowel disease. Scand. J. Gastroenterol. 29(203): 15-19.
22. HANDY, L. M., S. GHOSH & A. FERGUSON. 1995. Investigation of neutrophil migration into the gut by cytology of whole gut lavage fluid. Eur. J. Gastroenterol Hepatol. 7: 53-58.
23. ARRANZ, E. & A. FERGUSON. 1993. Intestinal antibody pattern of coeliac disease: occurrence in patients with normal jejunal biopsy histology. Gastroenterology 104: 1263-1272.
24. SVENNERHOLM, A-M., D. A. SACK, J. HOLMGREN & P. K. BARDHAN. 1982. Intestinal antibody responses after immunization with cholera B subunit. Lancet i: 305-308.
25. FERGUSON, A. & O. MWANTEMBE. Intestinal lavage test of gut inflammation and immunity. In Mucosal Immunity in the Gut Epithelium. S. Auricchio, R. Troncone & A. Ferguson, Eds.: S. Karger AG Basel. In press.

Oral Tolerance in Experimental Autoimmune Encephalomyelitis

CAROLINE C. WHITACRE, INGRID E. GIENAPP,
ABBIE MEYER, KAREN L. COX, AND
NAJMA JAVED

Department of Medical Microbiology and Immunology
2078 Graves Hall
333 West Tenth Avenue
The Ohio State University College of Medicine
Columbus, Ohio 43210

INTRODUCTION

Early work on oral tolerance focused on feeding such antigens as ovalbumin, bovine serum albumin, and sheep red blood cells, among others. These studies, performed from 1911 until the early 1980s focused on suppression of systemic anaphylaxis, contact hypersensitivity, antibody production, and T-cell proliferation. It was not until the latter half of the 1980s that attention turned to the oral administration of autoantigens as a strategy for suppression of autoimmune disease. Thompson and Staines[1] showed in 1986 that oral administration of type II collagen delayed the onset and decreased the severity of collagen-induced arthritis in rats. Nagler-Anderson *et al.*[2] reported suppression of type II collagen-induced arthritis by oral administration of type I collagen in the mouse.

We and others independently reported in 1988 that experimental autoimmune encephalomyelitis (EAE) could be suppressed by the oral administration of myelin basic protein (MBP).[3,4] This disease, induced by a single injection of myelin, MBP, or MBP peptides combined with complete Freund's adjuvant, is widely accepted to be a T cell-mediated autoimmune disease. The clinical course of EAE differs dramatically in the two species most often examined. In the Lewis rat, EAE manifests as an acute, rapidly progressive paralysis, which spontaneously remits, leaving the animal refractory to subsequent EAE reinduction. By contrast, EAE in susceptible mouse strains (SJL, B10.PL, and PL/J) is characterized by a remitting-relapsing course that is often quite unique for each experimental animal, often with periods of disease chronicity late in the disease course. We have examined the capacity of oral tolerization to affect both forms of EAE, acute and chronic-relapsing, and show that orally administered MBP provides a striking degree of protection in both forms.

ORAL TOLERANCE IN EAE

We and others examined the oral administration of guinea pig MBP to Lewis rats and showed that such treatment renders these animals refractory to subsequent induction of EAE with guinea pig MBP and complete Freund's adjuvant (CFA).[3,4] The majority of rats receiving MBP orally exhibited no clinical signs of EAE, with the remainder showing either markedly reduced signs or a substantial delay in disease onset. The central nervous system histopathologic changes observed were also significantly reduced relative to vehi-

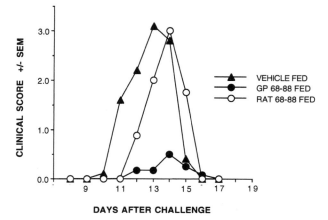

DAYS AFTER CHALLENGE

FIGURE 1. EAE is suppressed by the oral administration of the guinea pig 68-88 fragment of MBP, but not rat 68-88. Lewis rats were fed 5 mg of each peptide (1.25 mg, 4 times) suspended in bicarbonate buffer with STI, followed by challenge with rat 68-88 and CFA. Clinical signs were scored daily on a 0-4 scale.

cle-fed controls. Because of the marked lability of MBP in the presence of proteolytic enzymes known to occur naturally in the rat gastrointestinal tract, we found it necessary to feed MBP in the presence of sodium bicarbonate and a trypsin inhibitor.[3] Without such additives, the MBP-specific tolerance in male rats was not demonstrable. We examined the possibility of a gender difference in the induction of oral tolerance as well as the requirement for inclusion of soybean trypsin inhibitor (STI) for successful oral-tolerance induction. Both male and female rats exhibited a profound decrease in EAE clinical signs following oral administration of MBP in STI relative to rats fed ovalbumin or nothing. However, in the absence of STI, a gender difference was observed, such that females but not males could be rendered tolerant by oral administration of MBP alone (*i.e.*, without the addition of bicarbonate and STI). The gender differences may relate to differing amounts of glucocorticoid hormones between male and female Lewis rats, such that female rats exhibit much higher basal circadian corticosterone levels than do male rats.[5] In the course of this work in the rat, it was determined that (1) multiple feedings of MBP consistently produced a greater degree of tolerance than did single oral dosings, (2) a minimum of 10 mg MBP administered orally was necessary for tolerance induction, with 15-20 mg MBP producing more consistent tolerance, and (3) oral administration of vehicle alone (soybean trypsin inhibitor in bicarbonate buffer) had no inhibitory effect on the induction of EAE.

MBP-induced oral tolerance has been shown to be quite antigen specific. For example, oral administration of ovalbumin did not change the kinetics or clinical course of EAE following challenge with guinea pig MBP-CFA.[4] Moreover, MBP-induced oral tolerance was found to be exquisitely specific for the fed antigen, because rats fed guinea pig MBP were protected following challenge with guinea pig MBP, but not after challenge with human or rat MBP.[4] Similarly, rats fed human MBP were protected following challenge with human MBP, but not after challenge with rat or guinea pig MBP. Interestingly, rats fed rat MBP were not tolerant to rat, guinea pig, or human MBP challenge. This inability to demonstrate tolerance following oral administration of the self-MBP molecule has been extended to the peptide level[6] (Fig. 1). Lewis rats fed the major encephalitogenic epitope of guinea pig MBP (GP 68-88) were protected from EAE. However, rats fed rat 68-88, differing by a single amino acid from the guinea pig epitope, were not protected following challenge with either the rat- or guinea pig-derived peptide, although the appearance of clinical signs was somewhat delayed in this group. It should be noted that the presence of soybean trypsin inhibitor in the feeding mixture was required for the demonstration of peptide-induced tolerance.[6] These results show that (1) oral administration of a peptide autoantigen can successfully induce oral tolerance, (2) the tolerance achieved using this antigen system is dependent upon the oral administration of a non-self MBP sequence, (3) the tolerance induced following oral administration of a non-self (GP) yet closely related peptide sequence extends to the self (rat)-sequence, and (4) the gut immune system can apparently discriminate small peptide sequence differences, which will be of critical importance in the design of human trials.

Accompanying the suppression of clinical and histopathological manifestations of EAE after oral administration of MBP, we observed that MBP-specific lymphocyte proliferative responses were also profoundly suppressed.[4] Feeding as little as 5 mg MBP was seen to reduce the proliferation of lymph node lymphocytes in fed animals, with larger oral doses producing a more dramatic decrease. This suppression of the *in vitro* proliferative response was specific for MBP, inasmuch as proliferative responses to adjuvant components (PPD) or mitogens were unchanged relative to control vehicle-fed rats. Frequencies of MBP-specific TH1 cells were determined in orally tolerant and control rats using the technique of limiting dilution analysis (LDA) with secretion of IL-2 as the indicator of TH1 function. This approach revealed a 5- to 10-fold reduction in the number of MBP-reactive cells in tolerant rats relative to vehicle-fed controls.[7]

The effect of orally administered MBP on MBP-specific antibody production was also examined. Statistically significant decreases in MBP-specific serum IgG and IgA, but not IgM, are observed in MBP-fed rats, suggesting a lack of maturation of the primary antibody response.[8] It is likely that decreased amounts of specifically derived T-cell factors, that is, IL-4 and IL-5, may be, in part, responsible for the interruption in class switching observed. In contrast to the decreased levels of MBP-specific serum IgA, we observed increased levels of salivary IgA specific for the fed antigen.[8] This observation argues for a compartmentalization of the B-lymphocyte response, such that MBP-specific B cells may be selectively localized in mucosal sites.

MECHANISMS OF ORAL TOLERANCE IN EAE

Two primary mechanisms have been proposed to explain oral tolerance in EAE-active suppression following feeding of lower doses of antigen and clonal anergy or deletion following oral administration of higher antigen doses. Weiner's group was the first to propose the active or bystander suppression model, which invokes suppressor T cells as mediating MBP-induced oral tolerance.[9] In the rat, concanavalin A (Con A)-activated CD8[+] cells from either the spleen or mesenteric lymph nodes of orally tolerized rats were shown to transfer the tolerance to naive recipients.[10] These cells have been proposed as the mediators of active suppression, inasmuch as the T suppressor cells were shown to be activated in an antigen-specific means to release an antigen nonspecific factor, TGFβ1.[11] These investigators postulate that the secretion and action of TGFβ1 is at the level of the local microenvironment, that is, in the lymphoid tissue or within the target organ at the site of autoantigen localization.[12] However, in the mouse, active suppression is mediated by CD4 lymphocytes, which have also been shown to elaborate TGFβ1.[13,14]

Our laboratory has focused on the mechanism of "high-dose tolerance" in the rat and mouse. Multiple lines of evidence argue for an anergy or deletional mechanism following oral administration of 20 mg MBP (administered in multiple 5 mg feeds).[7]

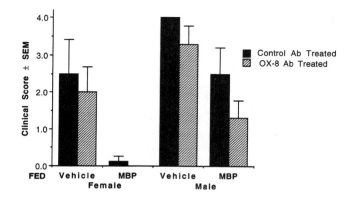

FIGURE 2. Depletion of CD8+ lymphocytes does not affect the induction of oral tolerance in the Lewis rat. Female and male Lewis rats received 2–4 mg OX-8 monoclonal antibody or MOPC isotype-matched control antibody intraperitoneally prior to and during the MBP feeding regimen. Rats were fed vehicle or 20 mg MBP suspended in bicarbonate buffer with STI (5 mg MBP, 4 times), followed by encephalitogenic challenge with MBP-CFA. Clinical signs were monitored daily using a 0–4 scale.

Using such a feeding regimen in the rat, the tolerance induced by feeding MBP is not transferable. Passive transfer of lymph node cells (LNC), splenocytes, thymocytes, mesenteric LNC, Peyer's patch lymphocytes, or serum from MBP-fed donors did not protect recipient rats from subsequently induced EAE. Second, the passive transfer of EAE was inhibited or significantly reduced when donors received MBP orally prior to MBP-CFA sensitization, indicating a reduction in MBP-reactive lymphocytes in fed rats. *In vitro* expansion of spleen cells (using Con A or MBP) or LNC (using MBP) from MBP-fed and challenged rats showed no increase in transfer activity. Third, treatment of MBP-fed rats with cyclophosphamide, using dosages known to eliminate suppressive cell populations, had no effect on MBP-induced tolerance. Fourth, in cell-mixing experiments, LNC from MBP-fed rats were cocultured with LNC from control vehicle-fed rats in the presence of specific antigen. When equal numbers of LNC were mixed together, the proliferative response was indistinguishable from that of the control LNC alone, arguing against a suppressive influence exerted by cells from tolerant animals. Fifth, we observed that EAE could be readily transferred into orally tolerant rats using MBP-specific encephalitogenic T-cell lines.[7] Finally, we have shown that interleukin 2 (IL-2) and gamma interferon levels, both indicators of TH1 cell function, are reduced in supernates derived from the culture of spleen or LNC from MBP-fed relative to control rats.[7] Taken together, these lines of evidence argue in favor of clonal anergy or deletion as responsible for the orally tolerant state following feeding of higher antigen doses.

Additional supportive evidence for anergy/deletion comes from studies in which CD8+ cells were depleted *in vivo* in Lewis rats. This cell type has been implicated as playing a causative role in oral-tolerance induction,[10] and a CD8 cell has been shown to play a role in MBP peptide-induced anergy.[15] Male and female Lewis rats received OX-8 monoclonal antibodies or isotype-matched control antibodies prior to the first MBP feeding and again during the high-dose feeding regimen. All groups were subsequently challenged with MBP-CFA. The results showed that MBP-induced oral tolerance was demonstrable in Lewis rats in the presence or absence of CD8+ cells (FIG. 2). In fact, a greater degree of protection was achieved in the absence of CD8[+] cells. CD8 levels were monitored in the spleen and lymph node compartments by flow cytometry and were dramatically reduced or absent even up until 21 days after depletion. Similar results have recently been reported in the mouse using a "low-dose" feeding regimen, that is, that oral tolerance is demonstrable following depletion of CD8[+] cells, therefore also implicating CD4[+] cells in mediating active suppression.[14]

We undertook a direct comparison of the frequency of MBP-specific lymphocytes following a low-dose versus a high-dose feeding regimen in the Lewis rat to attempt to distinguish between the different mechanisms reported. Rats were fed a typical 5 mg low-dose regimen (1 mg MBP in PBS given every other day, 5 times) or a typical 20 mg high-dose regimen (5 mg MBP in bicarbonate with STI, given every other day, 4 times), followed by encephalitogenic challenge. Frequencies of MBP-reactive cells were monitored by limiting-dilution analysis, measuring secretion of IL-2. The results, shown in FIGURE 3, indicate that MBP-reactive TH1 cells are reduced as a result of low-dose feeding (from 1/20,227 in the vehicle-fed rat to 1/50,271 in the low-dose-fed rat), but that a much more profound reduction is seen as a result of feeding high-dose MBP (1/519,596). The frequencies were corroborated by the clinical picture, where a consistently greater degree of tolerance was achieved following higher oral antigen doses.

To further investigate the mechanism(s) underlying low-dose versus high-dose oral tolerance and to distinguish between anergy and deletion in high-dose feeding regimens, we undertook *in vivo* administration of IL-2. Rats were fed either a low-dose (1 mg × 5) or a high-dose (5 mg × 4) regimen of MBP followed by intraperitoneal injection of varying doses of recombinant human IL-2 (Hoffmann-La Roche Inc.), prior to EAE challenge. The results indicated that low-dose oral tolerance could be reversed, whereas high-dose oral tolerance could not (FIG. 4). In the high-dose fed group, deletion of the MBP-reactive cells had likely occurred, inasmuch as clinical signs, proliferative responses to MBP, and cytokine secretion in response to MBP stimulation were all still profoundly suppressed at all doses of IL-2 administered. In the low-dose fed rats, return of clinical signs in the groups receiving IL-2 indicated either an anergy component or perhaps suppression of TGFβ1 production in the presence of IL-2.

ORAL TOLERANCE IN CHRONIC RELAPSING EAE

The clinical course of EAE in certain mouse strains is characterized by a relapsing-remitting or chronic paralytic pattern of EAE that is unique for each animal and that more closely approximates the course of MS in humans. Over the course of 140 days following injection of MBP/CFA and pertussis toxin, we observed that B10.PL (H-2[u]) mice exhibited as many as seven relapses or maintained chronic symptoms of paralysis. We examined whether the long-term clinical course of EAE could be changed as a result of orally administering MBP in a single 20 mg feeding, 7 days prior to neuroantigen challenge. In FIGURES 5A and 5B, the representative clinical course of mice fed vehicle or MBP is shown. A clear difference is observed between groups with total inhibition of acute disease and relapses in some MBP-fed animals. Thus far, we have observed 16/17 vehicle-fed mice exhibiting signs of acute EAE (mean highest clinical score (MHCS) = 3.6 ± 0.4), whereas 9/17 MBP-fed mice exhibited signs of acute disease (MHCS = 1.73). Moreover, the number of animals exhibiting EAE relapses, the mean number of relapses, the cumulative clinical signs during relapses, and the cumulative relapse days were significantly reduced in the MBP-fed group relative to the vehicle-fed group. Therefore, feeding MBP prior to challenge resulted in significant suppression of acute EAE as well as relapses.

It was critical to determine whether the oral administration of MBP at the time of disease onset would also prove to be suppressive. We therefore challenged groups of

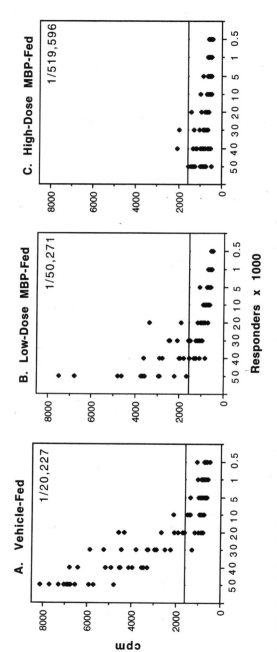

FIGURE 3. Quantitation of MBP-reactive TH1 lymphocytes shows a reduction of such cells in low-dose MBP-fed rats, but a more profound reduction in high-dose MBP-fed rats. Lewis rats were fed either vehicle, a low-dose MBP regimen (1 mg × 5), or a high-dose MBP regimen (5 mg × 4) and challenged with MBP-CFA. Lymph node cells draining the site of antigen challenge were evaluated by limiting dilution analysis for IL-2 secretion following stimulation with MBP. Responses shown are [³H]thymidine incorporation of CTLL-20 IL-2-dependent indicator cells. Frequencies of MBP-reactive cells, derived by chi-square minimization, are indicated.

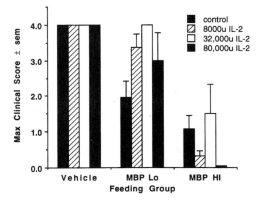

FIGURE 4. Injection of IL-2 *in vivo* reverses oral tolerance induced by low-dose but not high-dose feeding of MBP. Lewis rats were fed either a low-dose MBP regimen (1 mg × 5) or a high-dose MBP regimen (5 mg × 4). Prior to challenge, rats received either 8000, 32,000, or 80,000 units of recombinant human IL-2 intraperitoneally. Thereafter, rats were challenged with MBP-CFA and monitored for clinical signs.

B10.PL mice and fed them 20 mg MBP on the first day of clinical signs (days 10–12 after challenge). We observed that the vehicle-fed animals exhibited multiple relapses of disease throughout the 100-day examination period (FIG. 5C). However, the mice fed MBP on the first day of clinical disease often showed a blunted acute phase of EAE, with some animals exhibiting a total inhibition of relapses (FIG. 5D). In our experience with this design, 7/8 vehicle-fed mice had a mean number of relapses of 2.8 ± 0.6, whereas 3/6 MBP-fed mice showed 1.0 ± 0.6 relapses. Therefore, orally administered MBP was indeed effective in not only blunting the acute phase of EAE but was capable of reducing the incidence and severity of relapses. In these mice, MBP-reactive lymphocyte populations (specific for the immunodominant epitope) would have already been activated and expanded at the time of introduction of oral antigen. Therefore, these results signify that oral tolerance may be able to be used therapeutically to arrest the progression of already established disease. Mice fed after recovery from the initial acute attack had less severe relapses of disease, but the protective effect appeared to be less pronounced than that achieved by feeding earlier.

ORAL TOLERANCE IN MBP T CELL–RECEPTOR TRANSGENIC MICE

Goverman *et al.*[16] recently reported the generation of mice expressing the Vα2 and Vβ8.2 TCR specific for the dominant NAc1-11 epitope of the B10.PL mouse. In the transgenic animals, 100% of spleen cells express the transgenic β chain, whereas splenic T-cell expression of the transgenic α chain ranged from 50-95 percent. These animals exhibit EAE following injection with MBP peptide/CFA/pertussis, or pertussis toxin alone.[16] It is noteworthy that T-cell tolerance was not induced in the periphery of these mice, and Goverman *et al.*[16] showed the existence of functional, MBP-reactive T cells in the lymphoid tissue of the transgenic mice. Using these mice, Critchfield *et al.*[17] showed that the transgene-positive cells were deleted following administration of MBP intravenously.

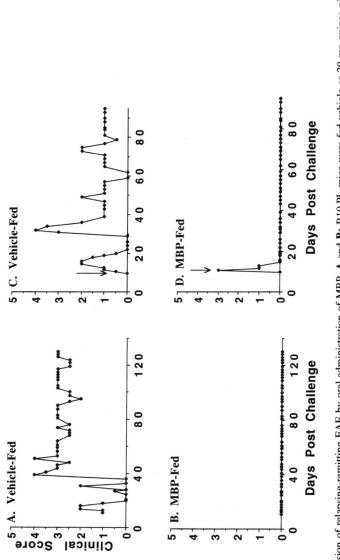

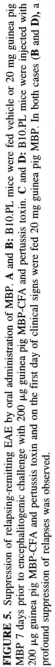

FIGURE 5. Suppression of relapsing-remitting EAE by oral administration of MBP. A and **B:** B10.PL mice were fed vehicle or 20 mg guinea pig MBP 7 days prior to encephalitogenic challenge with 200 μg guinea pig MBP-CFA and pertussis toxin. C and **D:** B10.PL mice were injected with 200 μg guinea pig MBP-CFA and pertussis toxin and on the first day of clinical signs were fed 20 mg guinea pig MBP. In both cases (**B** and **D**), a profound suppression of relapses was observed.

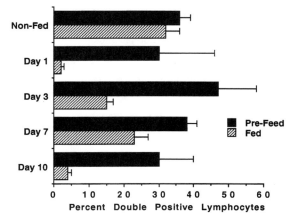

FIGURE 6. Feeding MBP to MBP-TCR transgenic mice results in a dramatic decrease in the transgenic phenotype in the peripheral blood. Data shown is from the same animals prior to and at various times after feeding 100 mg MBP. Samples from the nonfed group were obtained from unmanipulated transgenic mice and run at the same time as the fed mice.

We have examined the effects of oral administration of MBP on the fate and function of the MBP-reactive transgenic T cells. Early studies revealed that a single 20 mg feeding of MBP did not alter the T-cell repertoire of these mice. This was not surprising due to the large proportion of that repertoire that is specific for MBP. Therefore, groups of transgenic mice were fed 100 mg MBP or saline and sacrificed at varying times after feeding (1, 3, 7-8, and 10 days later) in order to determine the phenotype and MBP reactivity of the lymphoid cells. FIGURE 6 shows flow cytometric analysis of transgene positive cells in the peripheral blood of mice before and at the indicated times after oral MBP. It can be seen that there is a marked diminution in the number of transgenic cells at all times in the fed animals, with the greatest reductions observed on days 1 and 10. Similar flow analyses of lymphoid cells from multiple organs revealed that the proportion of transgenic lymphocytes was profoundly reduced in the periphery within 24 hours after antigen feeding. Specifically, $V\alpha2^+V\beta8.2^+$ lymphocytes were markedly decreased in the peripheral blood, lymph node, spleen, mesenteric lymph node, and Peyer's patch compartments. Interestingly, there was an increase in the transgenic cells shortly thereafter, that is, days 3 and 7-8 after feeding in these same compartments, followed by a final decrease on day 10. A functional assessment of the transgenic lymphocytes revealed a similar pattern to the phenotypic assessments. MBP-specific proliferative responses were profoundly reduced on days 1 and 10, with increases (relative to nonfed animals) observed on days 3 and 7.

Th1 and Th2 cytokine profiles were also examined in MBP-fed mice by determination of the frequency of IL-2- and IL-4-secreting cells using LDA. For determination of IL-2 secreting-cell frequencies, CTLL-20 cells were added to limiting-dilution microculture wells, whereas CT4.S cells were added to separate wells for determination of IL-4 secreting-cell frequencies. A large increase in the frequency of IL-2 secreting cells was observed in the LNC, spleen, and mesenteric LNC at days 1 and 3 after feeding, which decreased profoundly by days 7-10. A similar increase was observed in the frequency of IL-4 secreting cells, which remained high at days 7 and 10. Thus, there appeared to be a shift from Th1 to Th2 cytokine production in multiple lymphoid organs over time after MBP feeding.

In contrast to the' functional and phenotypic picture in the lymphoid organs, we observed that there was a large increase in transgenic cells in the lamina propria of the small intestine at all times examined. Thus, this finding suggested that cells were either trafficking into the gut secondary to specific antigen deposition at that site, or that transgenic cells already in residence in the gut were vigorously proliferating in response to antigen stimulation. Experiments are now in progress to distinguish these possibilities. Ultimately, autoreactive cells appear to be deleted from the periphery by day 10 after feeding by functional and phenotypic measures. Therefore, diverse mechanisms involving lymphocyte trafficking, shifts in cytokine secretion patterns, and deletion are involved in high-dose oral tolerance.

SUMMARY

In work performed by a number of laboratories, it has become quite clear that the oral administration of autoantigens exerts a profoundly suppressive effect on the development and long-term clinical course of autoimmune disease. Specific peptide sequences derived from the autoantigens are similarly suppressive. An interesting sidelight to emerge from specificity studies is that oral administration of a self-protein or peptide sequence (*i.e.*, rat MBP peptide administered to a rat) is markedly less tolerogenic than oral administration of a non-self or even closely related sequence (guinea pig MBP peptide administered to a rat). The dose of oral antigen is now known to play a critical role in determination of the mechanism of oral tolerance, with low doses of antigen causing active suppression with concomitant release of TGFβ1. Studies outlined here suggest that oral administration of higher antigen doses (*e.g.*, 20 mg MBP to rats or mice) results in deletion of specific antigen-reactive T lymphocytes. This conclusion stems from the fact that injections of IL-2 could not reverse high-dose oral tolerance while reversing low-dose oral tolerance. Moreover, feeding MBP to MBP-TCR transgenic mice caused trafficking of transgenic cells to the intestine followed by a profound depletion of transgene-positive cells and reduction in proliferative function in all peripheral lymphoid organs. Oral tolerance has proven to be of therapeutic benefit in other animal models of autoimmune disease as well, including uveitis, collagen-induced arthritis, adjuvant arthritis, thyroiditis, myasthenia gravis, and diabetes. Initial human trials in multiple sclerosis, rheumatoid arthritis, and uveitis show promising results.

REFERENCES

1. THOMPSON, H. S. G. & N. A. STAINES. 1986. Gastric administration of type II collagen delays the onset and severity of collagen-induced arthritis in rats. Clin. Exp. Immunol. **64:** 581.

2. NAGLER-ANDERSON, C., L. A. BOBER, M. A. ROBINSON, G. W. SISKIND & G. J. THORBECKE. 1986. Suppression of type II collagen-induced arthritis by intragastric administration of soluble type II collagen. Proc. Natl. Acad. Sci. USA **83:** 7443.

3. BITAR, D. M. & C. C. WHITACRE. 1988. Suppression of experimental autoimmune encephalomyelitis by the oral administration of myelin basic protein. Cell. Immunol. **112:** 364.

4. HIGGINS, P. J. & H. L. WEINER. 1988. Suppression of experimental autoimmune encephalomyelitis by oral administration of myelin basic protein and its fragments. J. Immunol. **140:** 440.

5. GRIFFIN, A. C. & C. C. WHITACRE. 1991. Sex and strain differences in the circadian rhythm fluctuation of endocrine and immune function in the rat: Implications for rodent models of autoimmune disease. J. Neuroimmunol. **35:** 53.

6. JAVED, N. H., I. E. GIENAPP, K. L. COX & C. C. WHITACRE. 1995. Exquisite peptide specificity of oral tolerance in experimental autoimmune encephalomyelitis. J. Immunol. **155:** 1599.

7. WHITACRE, C. C., D. M. BITAR, I. E. GIENAPP & C. G. OROSZ. 1991. Oral tolerance in experimental autoimmune encephalomyelitis. III. Evidence for clonal anergy. J. Immunol. **147:** 2155.

8. FULLER, K. A., D. PEARL & C. C. WHITACRE. 1990. Oral tolerance in experimental autoimmune encephalomyelitis: Serum and salivary antibody responses. J. Neuroimmunol. **28:** 15.

9. MILLER, A., O. LIDER & H. L. WEINER. 1991. Antigen-driven bystander suppression after oral administration of antigens. J. Exp. Med. **174:** 791.

10. LIDER, O., L. M. B. SANTOS, C. S. Y. LEE, P. J. HIGGINS & H. L. WEINER. 1989. Suppression of EAE by oral administration of MBP. II. Suppression of disease and *in vitro* immune response is mediated by antigen-specific CD8$^+$ T lymphocytes. J. Immunol. **142:** 748.

11. MILLER, A., O. LIDER, A. B. ROBERTS, M. B. SPORN & H. L. WEINER. 1992. Suppressor T cells generated by oral tolerization to myelin basic protein suppress both *in vitro* and *in vivo* immune responses by the release of transforming growth factor β after antigen-specific triggering. Proc. Natl. Acad. Sci. USA **89:** 421.

12. KHOURY, S. J., W. W. HANCOCK & H. L. WEINER. 1992. Oral tolerance to myelin basic protein and natural recovery from experimental autoimmune encephalomyelitis are associated with downregulation of inflammatory cytokines and differential upregulation of transforming growth factor β, interleukin 4, and prostaglandin E expression in the brain. J. Exp. Med. **176:** 1355.

13. CHEN, Y., V. K. KUCHROO, J. I. INOBE, D. A. HAFLER & H. L. WEINER. 1994. Regulatory T cell clones induced by oral tolerance: suppression of autoimmune encephalomyelitis. Science **265:** 1237.

14. CHEN, Y., J. I. INOBE & H. L. WEINER. 1995. Induction of oral tolerance to myelin basic protein in CD8-depleted mice: Both CD4$^+$ and CD8$^+$ cells mediate active suppression. J. Immunol. **155:** 910.

15. GAUR, A., R. HASPEL, J. P. MAYER & C. G. FATHMAN. 1993. Requirement for CD8$^+$ cells in T cell receptor peptide-induced clonal unresponsiveness. Science **259:** 91.

16. GOVERMAN, J., A. WOODS, L. LARSON, L. P. WEINER, L. HOOD & D. M. ZALLER. 1993. Transgenic mice that express a myelin basic protein-specific T cell receptor develop spontaneous autoimmunity. Cell **72:** 551.

17. CRITCHFIELD, J. M., M. K. RACKE, J. C. ZUNIGA-PFLUCKER, B. CANNELLA, C. S. RAINE, J. GOVERMAN & M. J. LENARDO. 1994. T cell deletion in high antigen dose therapy of autoimmune encephalomyelitis. Science **263:** 1139.

Mucosal Tolerance in a Murine Model of Experimental Autoimmune Encephalomyelitis[a]

BARBARA METZLER AND DAVID C. WRAITH[b]

Division of Immunology
Department of Pathology
Cambridge University
Tennis Court Road
Cambridge CB2 1QP, United Kingdom

INTRODUCTION

Oral tolerance has been studied in various models of autoimmune disease and is currently being tested as a therapeutic approach for a number of organ-specific diseases.[1,2] The phenomenon of oral tolerance is critically dependent on the dose of the administered antigen. In rat models of collagen-induced or adjuvant-induced arthritis, greater suppression of disease was achieved with lower doses of fed collagen (2.5 μg or 3 μg) than with ten times higher doses.[3,4] In a mouse model of arthritis, feeding 3 mg of collagen had no protective effect, whereas feeding 0.5 mg reduced the clinical severity of arthritis.[5] By contrast, a study on pristane-induced arthritis in mice revealed improved protection with increasing doses of intragastrically administered type II collagen.[6] A positive correlation between the amounts of fed antigen and the degree of protection from disease was also shown for Lewis rat models of experimental autoimmune uveitis (EAU) and experimental autoimmune encephalomyelitis (EAE).[7,8] Furthermore, different doses and epitopes appeared to selectively trigger distinct mechanisms. In the Lewis rat model of EAE, oral tolerance was achieved with a nonencephalitogenic fragment and, to a lesser extent, also with an encephalitogenic fragment of myelin basic protein (MBP).[8] Subsequently, the suppressive effect of antigen feeding was attributed to transforming growth factor β (TGF-β) released by CD8+ T cells following antigen-specific stimulation.[9] Only nonencephalitogenic epitopes of MBP triggered the release of TGF-β by CD8+ T cells. Nevertheless, the encephalitogenic epitopes were also capable of inducing oral tolerance by a yet-undefined mechanism.[10] Other investigators failed to demonstrate evidence for suppression in the same mode. In one report, reduced *in vitro* proliferation and IL-2 production of MBP-specific T cells and failure to transfer tolerance were interpreted as evidence for clonal anergy.[11] The discrepancies between these two studies were suspected to arise from different experimental protocols, in particular that the higher amount of fed MBP (4 × 5 mg versus 5 × 1 mg) in the latter study favored anergy induction over suppression. Recent

[a]The authors are indebted to Hoffmann-La Roche (Basel), the Wellcome Trust, and the Multiple Sclerosis Society of Great Britain and Northern Ireland for financial support.

[b]D. C. Wraith was a Senior Research Fellow of the Wellcome Trust and the Stanley Elmore Medical Research Fellow at Sidney Sussex College. Present address and address for correspondence: Department of Pathology and Microbiology, University of Bristol School of Medical Sciences, University Walk, Bristol BS8 1TD, UK.

studies on oral tolerance in EAU demonstrated that the mechanism of oral tolerance was strictly dependent on the dose of fed retinal S antigen (SAg)-derived peptides. High intragastric doses of the pathogenic peptide (5 mg/feeding) induced oral tolerance that lacked characteristics of active suppression, inasmuch as it was strictly epitope-specific (no bystander effect) and not transferrable. By contrast, low-dose feeding (250 µg/feeding) of the same peptide fulfilled the criteria for suppression.[12]

The H-2^u mouse model of EAE is well suited to address the mechanism of oral tolerance. The N-terminal nonapeptide of MBP serves as the dominant epitope for induction of EAE. Feeding the major encephalitogenic peptide Ac1-9 (or Ac1-11) should reveal whether oral tolerance requires additional suppressive epitopes. Furthermore, the higher affinity analogues of this peptide, with alanine or tyrosine at position four, provide useful tools to study the significance of higher avidity MHC-peptide-TCR interactions in oral tolerance. The N-terminal peptide of MBP, with lysine at position 4 of the peptide, displays low affinity for I-A^u, whereas analogues with alanine and tyrosine at position 4 display increasingly higher affinity for the MHC-restriction element.[13] The putative role of distinct regulatory epitopes can be tested by oral administration of whole MBP purified from pig spinal cord. This protein is highly encephalitogenic in H-2^u mice, porcine MBP and mouse MBP sharing 90% sequence homology and the N-termini being identical.[14] Additionally, whole mouse spinal cord homogenate may be fed as a rich source of homologous MBP. Finally, EAE, induced by whole myelin in this model, tends to follow a chronic or chronic-relapsing course. This model therefore offers the opportunity to assess the therapeutic effects of oral antigen administration.

In addition to oral tolerance, antigen inhalation has also been revealed as a promising tolerogenic route. Inhalation of antigen has been demonstrated to specifically down-regulate immune responses to soluble proteins such as OVA[15] and to retinal antigens in experimental autoimmune uveoretinitis,[16] and one report also mentioned that administration of MBP, as an aerosol, suppressed EAE.[17] Here we compare directly the suppressive effect of either oral administration or inhalation of peptide analogues prior to induction of EAE. To test the inhibitory potential of inhaled peptide further, we extend these studies to disease induced with whole mouse spinal cord homogenate (SCH), which induces more vigorous disease than peptide alone and also allows for the processing and presentation of additional epitopes. Finally we discuss experiments that aim to test the therapeutic influence of peptide inhalation after disease induction.

METHODS

MBP was prepared from pig spinal chords according to the procedures of Eylar, Kniskern, and Jackson.[18] Peptide antigens were synthesized using FMOC chemistry, as described previously.[19,20] Sequences of peptides were as follows: Ac1-9, acetyl-ASQKRPSQR; Ac1-11, acetyl-ASQKRPSQRHG; Ac1-11(4A), acetyl-ASQARPSQRHG; Ac1-11(4Y), Acetyl-ASQYRPSQRHG. A homogenate (SCH) was prepared from freshly isolated spinal chords by mixing with a minimal amount of water in a dounce homogenizer. The homogenate was frozen at −80 °C and lyophilized.

Mice of the H-2^u haplotype (PL/J, B10.PL or (PL/J × B10.PL)F1) were bred and housed under specific pathogen-free conditions. EAE was induced in 2- to 3-month-old mice by subcutaneous (sc) injection of 50 µg peptide or 1 mg SCH in 0.1 mL of Freund's complete adjuvant containing 400 µg *Mycobacterium tuberculosis* (H37RA). On the day of immunization and 2 days later, mice were also injected intraperitoneally with 200 ng pertussis toxin in 500 µL phosphate-buffered saline (PBS). Mice were monitored daily for disease and were scored as follows: grade 1 = flaccid tail, 2 = partial hind-limb paralysis and impaired righting reflex, 3 = total hind-limb paralysis, 4 = fore- and hind-limb paralysis, 5 = moribund.

Antigen Feeding

Mice were fed using a 1.5 × 22 G dosing cannula with a rounded tip. Peptides and proteins were given in 200 μL of 75 mM NaHCO$_3$ buffer with or without 20 mg/mL trypsin inhibitor at the doses and intervals indicated for each experiment.

Peptide Inhalation

Mice received 25 μL of peptide in PBS (4 mg/mL) intranasally while under light ether anesthesia either one week before or at a specified time after induction of EAE.

Mice were primed with antigen in CFA (sc) at the base of the tail, as described above. Ten days later, the draining lymph nodes (inguinal, popliteal, and paraaortic) were aseptically removed. Single cell suspensions were prepared and diluted to a density of 8 × 10^6 live cells/mL, and 100 μL of cell suspension was dispensed into flat-bottomed cell cuture plates containing 100 μL of antigen solution. Plates were incubated at 37 °C for a total of 90 hours and pulsed with 0.5 μcurie of tritiated thymidine in 25 μL Iscove's modification of Dulbecco's medium (IMDM) per well for the last 20 hours of incubation. The contents of the culture well were harvested onto filter mats, and the dried filters were soaked with scintillation fluid. Tritium decay was counted on a LKB Wallac 1205 betaplate liquid scintillation counter. For each experiment, samples were plated in triplicate, and the arithmentic means of antigen-specific proliferative responses were illustrated in plots of [^{3}H]thymidine uptake against a titration of antigen. The standard deviations of triplicates were between 10-15% of the means. The means and standard deviations of control values for medium only and PPD are included in the legend to FIGURE 1 or stated beside the plot symbols.

The Fisher exact probability test was used to compare the incidence of disease between groups. Differences in median day of onset were analyzed using the Mann-Whitney U test. Comparison of means was performed by using Student's t test where appropriate.

RESULTS

Oral Tolerance

Previous reports have described the use of MBP to induce oral tolerance in the Lewis rat model of EAE. In the rat model the mechanism of oral tolerance has been studied extensively.[2] Both the encephalitogenic as well as nonencephalitogenic fragments of MBP were able to induce tolerance. In our studies, however, the N-terminal epitope of MBP failed to induce tolerance when administered over a wide concentration range, when given in repeated doses, and when administered in alkaline buffer containing protease inhibitors

TABLE 1. The Encephalitogenic Epitope of MBP Fails to Induce Oral Tolerance in H-2^u Mice[a]

Group	Fed Antigen	Incidence of Disease	Median Day of Onset	Mean Maximal Grade of EAE
Experiment 1				
3 × buffer	−	6/8	14	2.6 ± 2.1
3 × 2.5 μg	Ac1-11 (4K)	5/7	14	2.0 ± 1.8
3 × 25 μg	Ac1-11 (4K)	5/9	15	2.2 ± 2.2
3 × 250 μg	Ac1-11 (4K)	6/8	13	2.5 ± 1.8
Experiment 2				
2 × buffer	−	8/8	12	1.7 ± 0.7
2 × 400 μg	Ac1-11 (4K)	6/6	11.5	2.0 ± 0.9
2 × 400 μg	Ac1-11 (4A)	6/6	10	2.0 ± 1.1

[a] Experiment 1: PL/J mice were fed the indicated amounts of Ac1-11 in 75 mM NaHCO$_3$ buffer plus 20 mg/mL trypsin inhibitor, or 200 μL buffer plus trypsin inhibitor alone, on days −7, −5, and −2. On day 0, EAE was induced with 50 μg Ac1-11/CFA. Experiment 2: On days −7 and −5, PL/J mice were fed 400 μg of either Ac1-11 or Ac1-11 (4A) in 75 mM NaHCO$_3$ buffer, including 20 mg/mL trypsin inhibitor. EAE was induced with 50 μg Ac1-11/CFA on day 0.[21]

(TABLE 1). However, high amounts (3 × 1 mg) of the highest affinity analogue (Ac1-9(4Y)) produced complete abrogation of the *in vitro* T-cell proliferative response to the encephalitogenic peptide Ac1-9(4K) and conferred full protection from peptide-induced EAE (FIG. 1).

Because the N-terminal peptide of MBP does not display demonstrable binding to class I molecules of the H-2^u haplotype,[13] we reasoned that the difficulty in inducing oral tolerance with this peptide might result from a failure to activate immunosuppressive CD8$^+$ cells in the gut. This belief would be supported by the observation that the encephalitogenic fragments of MBP, in the Lewis rat, are distinct from those that induce suppressive mechanisms in the gut.[10] With this in mind, we set up a model of EAE in the mouse using porcine MBP (pMBP) as encephalitogen. Mice were fed 3 times 1 mg pMBP, and EAE was subsequently induced with either Ac1-11(4K) or pMBP. Prior feeding of pMBP had no protective effect when disease was induced with peptide (FIG. 2a). By contrast, there was an encouraging tendency for pMBP to protect mice from EAE induced with the homologous protein (FIG. 2b). This observation was not, however, reproducible. Instead, intragastric administration of pMBP appeared to exacerbate rather than suppress disease induction (*e.g.,* FIG. 3). Finally, in the belief that feeding homologous MBP might be more tolerogenic than feeding porcine MBP, mice were fed homologous SCH. This protein mixture provided no protection from SCH-induced disease (FIG. 4).

Inhalation Tolerance

In contrast to peptide given by the oral route, inhalation of the N-terminal peptide of MBP consistently reduced the mean maximal grade of EAE observed when the homologous peptide was used as an encephalitogen (TABLE 2). Most strikingly, both the incidence of

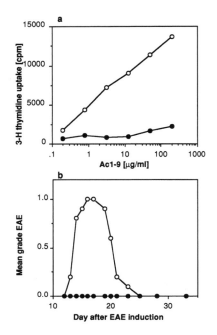

Group	Incidence of Disease[a]	Median Day of Onset	Mean Maximal-grade EAE
PBS	6/10	15.5	1.2 ± 1.1
Ac1-9(4Y)	0/10	—	0

[a] p = 0.005.

FIGURE 1. Effect of high oral doses of Ac1-9(4Y) on lymphocyte proliferation and EAE. PL/J mice were fed 1 mkg Ac1-9(4Y) on days −7, −5, and −3. Peptide was administered in 500 μL 150 mM NaHCO₃ buffer, including 2.5 mg/mL trypsin-chymotrypsin inhibitor (closed circles). Controls received 50 μL buffer plus inhibitors alone (open circles). On day 0, the mice were divided to test the effect of peptide feeding on lymphocyte proliferation (**a**) and on EAE (**b**). **a:** On day 0, mice were primed with 50 μg Ac1-9/CFA (sc) at the base of the tail. Ten days later, lymphocytes from draining lymph nodes were restimulated *in vitro* with Ac1-9, and proliferation was measured by [³H]thymidine uptake. Symbols represent the arithmetic mean of triplicates; standard deviations were less than 20% of the mean. Controls for medium/PPD in counts per minute (cpm) were 490 ± 40/39,480 ± 660 for lymphocytes from control-fed mice, and 370 ± 70/34,020 ± 1700 with lymphocytes from the peptide-fed group. **b:** on day 0, EAE was induced with 50 μg Ac1-9/CFA, as described in METHODS.

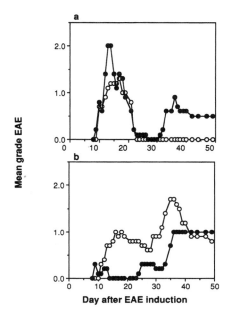

FIGURE 2. Feeding MBP before peptide-induced or MBP-induced EAE. PL/J mice received 3 × 1 mg of pMBP in PBS (closed circles) or PBS alone (open circles) on days −7, −5, and −2. On day 0, EAE was induced with either 50 μg Ac1-11/CFA (**a**) or 1 mg pMBP/CFA (**b**).

Group	Incidence of Disease	Median Day of Onset	Mean Maximal-Grade EAE
1. PBS-fed/ Ac1-11-primed	7/10	14	2.1 ± 1.3
2. MBP-fed/ Ac1-11-primed	10/11	12	2.7 ± 1.3
3. PBS-fed/ MBP-primed	8/10	18.5	2.1 ± 1.6
4. MBP-fed/ MBP-primed	4/10	>time of experiment	1.3 ± 2.0

disease and the mean maximal grade of disease were reduced when higher affinity peptide analogues were administered by inhalation. When compared with the data displayed in TABLE 1, it is clear that the intranasal route of peptide administration is more effective than the oral route. Furthermore, similar protection was observed when peptide inhalation was used to prevent EAE induced with SCH, a complex mixture of potential encephalitogenic proteins (TABLE 3). In these experiments it appears that inhalation of the wild-type peptide (Ac1-9(4K)) resulted in more mild disease as opposed to a reduction in incidence per se. More significant was the effect of peptide inhalation on late phases of disease. As shown in FIGURE 5, inhalation of the peptide analogues had a variable effect on the initial phase of disease induced with SCH. Each of the peptide analogues, however, provided protection from disease relapse.

FIGURE 3. Feeding MBP before MBP-induced EAE. PL/J mice received 3 × 1 mg of MBP in PBS (closed circles) or PBS only (open circles) on days −7, −5, and −2. EAE was induced with 1 mg pMBP/CFA on day 0.

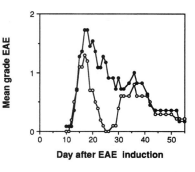

Group	Incidence of Disease	Median Day of Onset	Mean Maximal-Grade EAE
PBS	7/9	15	2.1 ± 1.3
MBP	11/11	15	2.7 ± 1.0

FIGURE 4. Oral administration of mouse spinal chord homogenate (SCH) before SCH-induced EAE. PL/J mice were fed 2 mg SCH in PBS (closed circles) or PBS alone (open circles) 7, 5, and 2 days prior to EAE induction with 1 mg SCH/CFA.

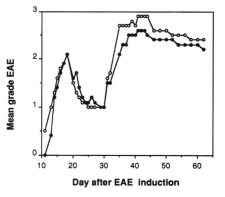

Group	Incidence of Disease	Median Day of Onset	Mean Maximal-Grade EAE
PBS	9/10	14	3.2 ± 1.8
SCH	8/8	14.5	3.6 ± 1.6

TABLE 2. The Encephalitogenic Epitope of MBP Induces Inhalation Tolerance in H-2^u Mice[a]

Antigen Inhaled	Antigen Used to Induce EAE	Incidence of Disease	Median Day of Onset	Mean Maximal Grade EAE
Experiment 1				
PBS	Ac1-11	9/9	14	4.1 ± 1.4
Ac1-11	Ac1-11	6/8	16	1.7[b] ± 1.7
Experiment 2				
PBS	Ac1-11	6/9	16	2.1 ± 1.9
Ac1-11	Ac1-11	5/9	22	1.3 ± 1.9
Ac1-11 (4A)	Ac1-11	2/10[c]	>time of experiment	0.2 ± 0.4
Experiment 3				
PBS	Ac1-11	9/10	13	1.2 ± 0.8
Ac1-11	Ac1-11	4/10[d]	>time of experiment	0.5 ± 0.7
Ac1-11 (4A)	Ac1-11	2/10[e]	>time of experiment	0.2 ± 0.4
Ac1-11 (4Y)	Ac1-11	0/10[f]	—	—

[a] Experiments 1, 2, and 3: PL/J mice inhaled 100 μg of the indicated peptide in the single 25 μL droplet, or PBS as control, under light ether anesthesia. EAE was induced with 50 μg Ac1-11/CFA seven days later.

[b] $p < 0.01$ versus PBS control.

[c] $p = 0.05$ versus PBS control.

[d] $p = 0.029$.

[e] $p = 0.0027$.

[f] $p = 0.00006$ versus PBS control.[21]

Peptide Inhalation after Disease Onset

It is likely that inhalation tolerance would be more difficult to achieve after T-cell priming when (a) the frequency of antigen-specific cells is higher, (b) most antigen-specific T cells are activated, (c) the immune response may have spread to include other T-cell epitopes, and (d) the effector arms of the immune response, such as inflammatory macrophages, have come into play. Can peptide inhalation reverse ongoing disease? Here we are fortunate, in that the H-2^u model of EAE tends to display at least a biphasic course when induced with SCH. Inhalation of peptide Ac1-11(4A) on the day of disease onset led to a reduction in clinical signs and a delay in disease onset (FIG. 6). Other experiments have emphasized the importance of the timing of peptide administration. For instance, when using Ac1-11(4Y) for inhalation, administration of peptide prior to the first signs of disease may cause a more rapid first phase of disease (FIG. 7a and b), whereas giving peptide after disease onset reduced the severity of disease over the whole course of the experiment (FIG. 7c and d). Although effects of inhalation of a single dose of peptide on early disease have proved variable, there is one optimistic conclusion. The results of these and other experiments show that peptide inhalation at the time of disease onset can lead to clear protection from later stages of disease.

TABLE 3. Protection from SCH-induced EAE by Inhalation of Analogues of the N-terminal Epitope[a]

Antigen Inhales	Antigen used to Induce EAE	Incidence of Disease	Median Day of Onset	Mean Maximal Grade EAE
Experiment 1				
PBS	SCH	9/10	9.5	2.6 ± 1.3
Ac1-9	SCH	9/11	13	1.4[c] ± 1.0
Ac1-11 (4A)	SCH	5/11[b]	>time of experiment	0.7 ± 1.0
Experiment 2				
PBS	SCH	9/9	17	2.5 ± 1.3
Ac1-11 (4A)	SCH	2/10[d]	>time of experiment	0.7 ± 1.6

[a] Experiment 1 and 2: (PL/J × B10.PL)F1 mice were given on intranasal dose of 100 μg peptide or PBS, and EAE was induced with 1 mg SCH/CFA after one week.

[b] $p = 0.042$.

[c] $p < 0.05$.

[d] $p = 0.0006$ versus PBS control.[21]

DISCUSSION

We have failed to provide evidence for oral tolerance by the major encephalitogenic peptide Ac1-11 or the higher-affinity analogue 4A in the PL/J mouse model of EAE. Only high doses of the 4Y analogue, capable of forming stable complexes with I-A^u, abrogated EAE and *in vitro* T-cell proliferative responses. To account for the possible need for antigen processing in GALT and the role of distinct regulatory epitopes involved in oral tolerance, subsequent studies included oral administration of purified porcine MBP and mouse spinal cord homogenate. These feeding regimes did not, however, show any reproducible, protective effect.

A single dose of the N-terminal peptide or its higher-affinity analogues (4A and 4Y) profoundly inhibited EAE when administered by inhalation one week prior to disease induction.[21] The positive correlation between the degree of protection from EAE and the affinity of peptides for the H-2^u molecule suggests that direct (CD8$^+$ T-independent) interactions between antigen-presenting cells (APC) and encephalitogenic T cells play a significant role in tolerance induction by the intranasal route.

The finding that inhalation of a single peptide, such as Ac1-9 or its higher affinity analogues, protected against EAE induced with SCH[21] may be explained by the large degree of dominance of Ac1-9 over other epitopes. Therefore, without the need for suppressor mechanisms, direct specific down-regulation of the dominant response may be sufficient to inhibit autoimmune responses to the whole antigen. However, amelioration of EAE induced with whole myelin, after inhalation of the dominant epitope alone, raises the possibility that lymphocyte responses to subdominant epitopes are also affected in a bystander fashion. This has been clearly shown in a mouse model of allergy to the house dust mite antigen Der P1.[22] Even though there are at least three different epitopes within Der P1, inhalation of a single dominant CD4$^+$ T-cell epitope inhibited the response to other epitopes within the same protein. This study revealed diminished IL-2 production, as well as antibody secretion, by spleen cells *in vitro*, implying a CD4$^+$ T cell-dependent

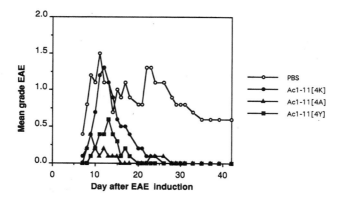

Group	Incidence of Disease[a]	Median Day of Onset	Mean Maximal-grade EAE
1. PBS	10/10	9	2.4 ± 1.3
2. Ac1-11 (4K)	8/10	10	1.6 ± 1.2
3. Ac1-11 (4A)	4/9	>time of experiment	0.5 ± 1.0
4. Ac1-11 (4Y)	6/10	13	0.8 ± 0.8

[a] Groups 1 and 3, p = 0.01. Groups 1 and 4, p = 0.04.

FIGURE 5. Inhalation of Ac1-11 and its higher affinity analogues prior to SCH-induced EAE in (PL/J × B10.PL)F1 mice. Mice were given one intranasal dose of 100 μg Ac1-11 (closed circles), Ac1-11(4A) (triangles), Ac1-11(4Y) (squares), or PBS alone (open circles). One week later, EAE was induced with 1 mg SCH/CFA.

mechanism of suppression following peptide inhalation. Taken together, these observations suggest that peptide inhalation may induce a form of "bystander regulation."

Modulation of encephalitogenic T cells by peptide inhalation 6-10 days after EAE induction with SCH was possible, but the influence on the early phase of disease appeared largely unpredictable. Treatment with 4Y induced a characteristic pattern of an exacerbated first phase of disease, after which animals were refractory to further relapses. This phenomenon is best interpreted as clonal anergy/deletion following hyperactivation of primed cells, the exacerbation of disease being accounted for by transient cytokine release from hyperactivated cells. In one experiment, however, the effect of 4Y was different and reduced disease severity during the whole course of the experiment. These findings imply differential effects of intranasally administered peptide at different stages of T-cell activation. It will now be necessary to analyze the effect of peptide inhalation on T-cell physiology at different stages of activation. Additionally, different experimental conditions, such as repeated rather than single doses of inhaled peptide, might be required to override T-cell activation in favor of tolerance.

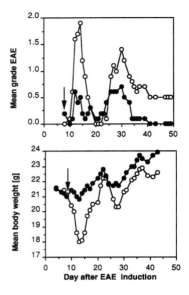

FIGURE 6. Inhalation of Ac1-11(4A) eight days after the induction of EAE. (PL/J × B10.PL)F1 mice were primed with 1 mg SCH/CFA for the induction of EAE. Eight days later, all were treated with 100 μg Ac1-11(4A) in PBS (closed circles) or PBS alone (open circles).

Group	Incidence of Disease	Median Day of Onset[a]	Mean Maximal-grade EAE[b]
PBS	10/10	11.5	2.9 ± 1.1
Ac1-11 (4A)	7/10	19.5	1.2 ± 1.0

[a] $p < 0.05$.
[b] $p < 0.01$.

There are two possible explanations for the type of suppression observed following peptide inhalation. The strong immune response to the dominant epitope is probably associated with high concentrations of IFN-γ and IL-2 at some stages of T-cell activation. Therefore, whenever T-cell responses to other subdominant epitopes are initiated within the same microenvironment, they might benefit from the high local concentrations of stimulatory lymphokines triggered by the dominant immune response. In this case, the response to a dominant T-cell epitope, such as Ac1-9, could provide bystander help for T cells specific for an adjacent subdominant epitope. Consequently, inhalation of Ac1-9 might only directly inhibit T cells specific for this same epitope and yet also indirectly impair the response to other epitopes through deprivation of bystander help. Alternatively, inhalation of the N-terminal peptide of MBP, or its higher-affinity analogues, might create a tolerogenic microenvironment that would mainly affect T cells specific for Ac1-9 but would also have an impact on adjacent T cells specific for other epitopes. For instance, it is conceivable that the intranasal route of antigen administration favors Th2- over Th1-type responses, as implied for the oral route.[23] T cells that encounter peptide administered by inhalation might be induced to produce lymphokines, such as Il-4 and IL-6, that inhibit

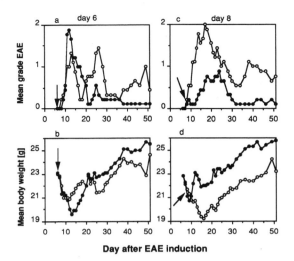

Day after EAE induction

Group	Incidence of Disease	Median Day of Onset	Mean Maximal-grade EAE[a]
1. PBS, d6	8/9	11	2.2 ± 1.1
2. Ac1-11 (4Y), d6	9/9	11	2.2 ± 1.0
3. PBS, d8	8/9	13	2.7 ± 1.3
4. Ac1-11 (4Y), d8	6/9	17	1.3 ± 1.2

[a] $p < 0.02$ for 3 versus 4.

FIGURE 7. Inhalation of Ac1-9(4Y) on day six or day eight after the induction of EAE. (PL/J × B10.PL)F1 mice were primed with 1 mg SCH/CFA for the induction of EAE. Mice received an intranasal dose of 100 μg Ac1-9(4Y) (closed circles) or PBS (open circles) on day six (**a, b**) or day eight (**c, d**) after the induction of EAE.

inflammatory Th1-mediated responses central to the manifestation of EAE *in vivo* or IFN-γ production *in vitro*. These Th2-type lymphokines might also bias the function of nearby T cells of other specificities that were attracted to the same site of antigen presentation. Other candidates for inhibitory lymphokines, such as TGF-β, could also be involved. Although the immunosuppressive role of TGF-β has mainly been discussed in the context of CD8+-suppressor T cells, TGF-β secretion by CD4+ T cells has also been shown.[23]

An argument against T cell–phenotype switching as the mechanism for inhalation tolerance comes from the observation that both Th1 and Th2 responses appear to be affected by the same treatment (our unpublished observations). This argues for some form of anergy or deletion as the mechanism involved. On the other hand, in the Der P1 model of inhalation tolerance, there is strong evidence for bystander regulation, as discussed above. Here, in cell-mixing experiments, lymph node T cells from mice treated with peptide by inhalation inhibited *in vitro* antibody production by spleen cells, containing both Der P1-primed T and B cells.[22] This implies that inhalation not only inhibits the function of T-cells but arms them with the capacity to modulate responses among adjacent T cells *in vitro*. However, as mentioned before, there is also evidence to argue in favor of T-cell anergy in the absence of immune deviation. How then would apparently anergic T cells mediate bystander regulation? In order to explain such a phenomenon, one would have to assume that anergic cells can act as competitors for antigen presentation *in vivo*. This possibility was proposed some time ago as a mechanism to explain the inhibitory properties of certain antibodies on immune responses in mice[24] and has been supported by a recent study of anergic cells *in vitro*. Anergic human T cells were shown to inhibit antigen-specific and allospecific T-cell proliferation.[25] Evidence for competition, as opposed to nonspecific cytokine release, came from the observation that anergic T cells had to be specific for the same antigen-presenting cells as the T cells that were suppressed. As yet, the only explanation for this effect is competition for the APC and/or locally produced lymphokines. However, it is also possible that the anergic cell produces an, as yet, unidentified inhibitory cytokine or has an inhibitory influence on the APC, resulting from ligation of the MHC-antigen complex on the APC. Whatever the mechanism of inhalation tolerance, it is clear from the work described above that the inhalational route of peptide administration is effective for the induction of unresponsiveness among autoreactive T cells, both before and after T-cell priming, in a complex organ-specific disease, even after inhalation of a single peptide epitope, and that the effect is related to the affinity of the peptide : MHC interaction.

SUMMARY

Attempts to induce oral tolerance in a murine model of EAE with either the dominant T-cell epitope or whole protein have failed. These results may, in part, be due to the extraordinarily low affinity for class II MHC displayed by the dominant T-cell epitope. This belief is supported by experiments using a high-affinity analogue of the peptide that was capable of inducing tolerance at a high dose. By contrast, peptide inhalation has proven an effective route for induction of mucosal tolerance in this model. Most importantly, the inhalation of a single peptide could inhibit disease induced by the complex mixture of antigens found in whole myelin. Peptide inhalation was effective both before and after disease induction, and there was a positive correlation between affinity of class II binding and tolerogenicity of a panel of analogues of the N-terminal peptide of myelin basic protein.

REFERENCES

1. THOMPSON, H. S. G. & N. A. STAINES. 1990. Could specific oral tolerance be a therapy for autoimmune disease? Immunol. Today **11:** 369-399.
2. WEINER, H. L., A. FRIEDMAN, A. MILLER, S. J. KHOURY, A. AL-SABBAGH, L. SANTOS, M. SAYEGH, R. B. NUSSENBLATT, D. E. TRENTHAM & D. A. HAFLER. 1994. Oral tolerance: Immunologic mechanisms and treatment of animal and human organ-specific autoimmune diseases by oral administration of autoantigens. Annu. Rev. Immunol. **12:** 809-837.
3. THOMPSON, H. S. G. & N. A. STAINES. 1985. Gastric administration of type II collagen delays the onset and severity of collagen-induced arthritis in rats. Clin. Exp. Immunol. **64:** 581-586.

4. ZHANG, Z. J., C. S. Y. LEE, O. LIDER & H. L. WEINER. 1990. Suppression of adjuvant arthritis in Lewis rats by oral administration of type II collagen. J. Immunol. **145:** 2489-2493.

5. NAGLER-ANDERSON, C., L. A. BOBER, M. E. ROBINSON, G. W. SISKIND & G. J. THORBECKE. 1986. Suppression of type II collagen-induced arthritis by intragastric administration of soluble type II collagen. Proc. Natl. Acad. Sci. USA **83:** 7443-7446.

6. THOMPSON, S. J., H. S. G. THOMPSON, N. HARPER, M. J. DAY, A. J. COAD, C. J. ELSON & N. A. STAINES. 1993. Prevention of pristane-induced arthritis by the oral administration of type II collagen. Immunology **79:** 152-157.

7. NUSSENBLATT, R. B., R. R. CASPI, R. MAHDI, C.-C. CHAN, F. ROBERGE, O. LIDER & H. L. WEINER. 1990. Inhibition of S-antigen induced experimental autoimmune uveoretinitis by oral induction of tolerance with S-antigen. J. Immunol. **144:** 1689-1695.

8. HIGGINS, P. J. & H. L. WEINER. 1988. Suppression of experimental autoimmune encephalomyelitis by oral administration of myelin basic protein and its fragments. J. Immunol. **140:** 440-445.

9. MILLER, A., O. LIDER, A. B. ROBERTS, M. B. SPORN & H. L. WEINER. 1992a. Suppressor T cells generated by oral tolerization to myelin basic protein suppress both *in vitro* and *in vivo* immune responses by the release of transforming growth factor β after antigen-specific triggering. Proc. Natl. Acad. Sci. USA **89:** 421-425.

10. MILLER, A., A. AL-SABBAGH, L. M. B. SANTOS, M. PRABHU DAS & H. L. WEINER. 1993. Epitopes of myelin basic protein that trigger TGF-β release after oral tolerization are distinct from encephalitogenic epitopes and mediate epitope-driven bystander suppression. J. Immunol. **151:** 7307-7315.

11. WHITACRE, C. C., I. E. GIENAPP, C. G. OROSZ & D. M. BITAR. 1991. Oral tolerance in experimental autoimmune encephalomyelitis. III. Evidence for clonal anergy. J. Immunol. **147:** 2155-2163.

12. GREGERSON, D. S., W. F. OBRITSCH & L. A. DONOSO. 1993. Oral tolerance in experimental autoimmune uveoretinitis. Distinct mechanisms are induced by low dose vs. high dose feeding protocols. J. Immunol. **151:** 5751-5761.

13. FAIRCHILD, P. J., R. WILDGOOSE, E. ATHERTON, S. WEBB & D. C. WRAITH. 1993. An autoantigenic T cell epitope forms unstable complexes with class II MHC: a novel route for escape from tolerance induction. Int. Immunol. **5:** 1151-1158.

14. FRITZ, R. B. & D. E. MCFARLIN. 1989. *In* Antigenic Determinants and Immune Regulation. E. Sercarz, Ed.: **46:** 101-125. Karger. Basel.

15. HOLT, P. G. & C. MCMENAMIN. 1989. Defence against allergic sensitization in the healthy lung: the role of inhalation tolerance. Clin. Exp. Allergy **19:** 255-262.

16. DICK, A. D., Y. F. CHENG, A. MCKINNON, J. LIVERSIDGE & J. V. FORRESTER. 1993. Nasal administration of retinal antigens suppresses the inflammatory response in experimental allergic uveoretinitis. A preliminary report of intranasal induction of tolerance with retinal antigens. Br. J. Ophtalmol. **77:** 171-175.

17. WEINER, H. L., Z. J. ZHANG, S. J. KHOURY, A. MILLER, A. AL-SABBAGH, S. A. BROD, O. LIDER, P. HIGGINS, R. SOBEL, R. B. NUSSENBLATT & D. A. HAFLER. 1991. Antigen-driven peripheral immune tolerance: Suppression of organ-specific autoimmune diseases by oral administration of autoantigens. Ann. N.Y. Acad. Sci. **636:** 227-232.

18. EYLAR, E. H., P. J. KNISKERN & J. J. JACKSON. 1974. Myelin basic protein. Methods Enzymol. **32:** 323-341.

19. WRAITH, D. C., D. E. SMILEK, D. J. MITCHELL, L. STEINMAN & H. O. MCDEVITT. 1989. Antigen recognition in autoimmune encephalomyelitis and the potential for peptide-mediated immunotherapy. Cell **59:** 247.

20. WRAITH, D. C., B. BRUUN & P. J. FAIRCHILD. 1992. Cross-reactive antigen recognition by an encephalitogenic T cell receptor. J. Immunol. **149:** 3765.

21. METZLER, B. & D. C. WRAITH. 1993. Inhibition of experimental autoimmune encephalomyelitis by inhalation but not oral administration of the encephalitogenic peptide: influence of MHC binding affinity. Int. Immunol. **5:** 1159-1165.

22. HOYNE, G. F., R. E. O'HEHIR, D. C. WRAITH THOMAS, W. R. & J. R. LAMB. 1993. Inhibition of T cell and antibody responses to house dust mite allergen by inhalation of the dominant T cell epitope in naive and sensitized mice. J. Exp. Med. **178:** 1783-1788.
23. CHEN, Y., V. K. KUCHROO, J.-I. INOBE, D. A. HAFLER & H. L. WEINER. 1994. Regulatory T cell clones induced by oral tolerance: suppression of autoimmune encephalomyelitis. Science **265:** 1237-1240.
24. WALDMANN, H. 1989. Manipulation of T-cell responses with monoclonal antibodies. Annu. Rev. Immunol. **7:** 407-444.
25. LOMBARDI, G., S. SIDHU, R. BATCHELOR & R. LECHLER. 1994. Anergic T cells as suppressor cells *in vitro*. Science **264:** 1587-1589.

Three-year Open Protocol Continuation Study of Oral Tolerization with Myelin Antigens in Multiple Sclerosis and Design of a Phase III Pivotal Trial

MARIKA J. HOHOL, SAMIA J. KHOURY,
SANDRA L. COOK, E. JOHN ORAV,
DAVID A. HAFLER, AND HOWARD L. WEINER

Center for Neurologic Diseases
Brigham and Women's Hospital
and
Harvard Medical School
221 Longwood Avenue
LMRC, Room 102A
Boston, Massachusetts 02115

Multiple sclerosis (MS) is an inflammatory disease of the central nervous system (CNS) of presumed autoimmune etiology. Until recently, most therapeutic approaches have involved nonspecific immunosuppressive drugs with inherent toxicities, which often limit their use, especially early in the disease course, a time when therapy is most likely to prove beneficial.[1] Newer strategies include more specific immunomodulatory drugs, such as interferon-beta and copolymer-1, which have been shown, in large multicenter clinical trials, to have a positive effect on the disease course.[2,3] However, these drugs require parenteral administration and are not without adverse effects.

Oral tolerization is a method of inducing specific immunologic hyporesponsiveness through oral administration of antigen. The concept has been well recognized for many years. In 1911, Wells showed that feeding hen egg protein to guinea pigs inhibited systemic anaphylaxis to the same material.[4] Oral tolerance presumably evolved to prevent systemic immune reactions to ingested proteins necessary for nutrition and thus survival. Orally administered antigen encounters gut-associated lymphoid tissue (GALT), a well-developed immune network, consisting of villi that contain epithelial cells capable of antigen presentation, intraepithelial lymphocytes, and lamina propria lymphocytes.[5] In addition, there are lymphoid nodules, known as Peyer's patches, interspersed below the villi, which are one of the primary areas in the GALT, where specific immune responses are generated. Low doses of oral antigen achieve oral tolerance by way of generation of active cellular suppression, which is mediated by the induction of regulatory T cells in the GALT. These T cells secrete suppressive cytokines (such as transforming growth factor β (TGF-β), IL-4, and IL-10) when they encounter the oral tolerogen in the microenvironment of the target organ. Oral administration of myelin basic protein (MBP) suppresses acute experimental autoimmune encephalomyelitis (EAE),[6,7] and chronic, relapsing EAE can be suppressed after the onset of disease by oral administration of MBP or myelin.[8] Theoretically, one may not need to known the autoantigen against which the autoimmune response is directed for oral tolerance to be effective as long as it is an antigen capable of inducing regulatory

243

TABLE 1. Double-blind Study of Oral Myelin in Relapsing-Remitting MS: Clinical Outcomes in Patient Subgroups

Group	Attacks[a]	Improved[b]	Stable[b]	Worse[b]
		Myelin treated		
Total	6/15	6/15	6/15	3/15
Males	0/8	5/8	3/8	0/8
Females	6/7	1/7	3/7	3/7
DR2⁻	0/6	4/6	2/6	0/6
DR2⁺	6/9	2/9	4/9	3/9
		Placebo treated		
Total	12/15	2/15	9/15	4/15
Males	3/3	0/3	1/3	2/3
Females	9/12	2/12	8/12	2/12
DR2⁻	3/4	0/4	2/4	2/4
DR2⁺	9/11	2/11	7/11	2/11

[a] Number of patients with major (nonsensory) exacerbations.
[b] Number of patients improved/worse by at least one EDSS point of baseline, or stable (within 0.5 EDSS point of baseline).

T cells that secrete suppressive cytokines when they encounter the same antigen in the target organ. In support of this theory, oral administration of MBP suppresses EAE induced by proteolipid protein (PLP).[9] Thus, even if another CNS protein is the target of the autoimmune attack, orally administered MBP could still be effective. Oral tolerance is effective in suppressing other experimental autoimmune diseases, including models of arthritis,[10-12] uveitis,[13] and diabetes,[14] without apparent toxicities.

We initially studied 30 relapsing-remitting MS patients as part of a one-year, double-blind, randomized, placebo-controlled trial, comparing 300 mg of bovine myelin to a control protein.[15] We found that 6 of 15 individuals in the myelin-treated group had one or more major exacerbations compared to 12 of 15 in the control group (TABLE 1). No toxicities or side effects were noted. The results of this trial, though not statistically significant, showed a positive trend (p = 0.06) and suggested improvement due to myelin both in terms of EDSS and attacks, particularly among males and DR2⁻ patients.[15] Upon completion of the study, patients were offered ongoing treatment with bovine myelin in an open protocol format. We report here the three-year clinical results in these patients and the design of a multicenter phase III trial based on the initial trial.

METHODS

Of the original 30 patients, 17 elected to participate in the open protocol continuation study, and some have been followed for up to six years. Nine originally received myelin; eight received the placebo. One patient was excluded from the analysis because of a long hiatus before recommencing treatment with myelin. She withdrew from the original double-blind study at the six-month point due to pregnancy and did not resume myelin until approximately two years later. Although the other five female patients delayed initiation of treatment with myelin for one year, as described below, all of these patients had

TABLE 2. Baseline Characteristics of Oral Myelin–treated Patients

Patients	Age (yrs)	Sex (No. of Females)	Disease Duration (yrs)	EDSS	No. of Attacks in Previous Two Years	HLA-DR2⁻ (No.)
Total (N = 16)	34.0	5	7.8	2.8	3.1	9
Male (N = 11)	32.3		6.3	3.0	3.8	8
Female (N = 5)	38.0		11.2	2.4	1.6	1
DR2⁻ (N = 9)	33.2	1	6.5	2.7	3.1	
DR2⁺ (N = 7)	35.1	4	9.5	2.9	3.1	

received placebo in the double-blind study and thus began treatment with myelin *de novo*. For some of the patients, myelin therapy began during the double-blind study; for others (who received placebo in the double-blind trial), it began during the open-protocol continuation study. Consequently, all 16 patients have been followed for at least three years, and we report here their three-year data. Demographics for these sixteen patients are shown in TABLE 2, where baseline characteristics represent values prior to initiating treatment with myelin. Of the patients who participated in the double-blind study and received myelin, reasons for not continuing open protocol therapy were as follows: disease course was active, and they were on other disease-modifying therapies at the time when open-label treatment was offered (4/7); pregnancy (1/7); and moved to another city (1/7). Reasons patients declined who originally received placebo: they had been stable on placebo (3/7); disease course was active and they were on another disease-modifying therapy at the time when open-label treatment was offered (2/7); planning to become pregnant (1/7); and lost to follow-up (1/7).

Male patients commenced open protocol treatment within a few months of participation in the double-blind study; however, female patients had a one-year delay in starting therapy due to a desire to manufacture a lower dose for women (30 mg compared to 300 mg for men). The rationale for the dosage difference was that, as a group, female patients did not do as well as male patients in the original double-blind study (where all patients received 300 mg of bovine myelin). In animals, oral tolerance is dose specific, and loss of clinical effect may occur with increased dosages.[8,12,14] However, after one year, females were treated with the 300-mg dose when no apparent benefit was seen at lower doses. Because of initial difficulties with supply, there were times in the open-protocol study when patients received either decreased dosages of myelin (*e.g.,* 1-3 times weekly rather than daily) or had to temporarily discontinue dosing.

Patients were examined every three months. Assessments included number of major exacerbations and disability, as measured by the Expanded Disability Status Scale (EDSS). Only significant exacerbations involving vision, strength, coordination, and/or gait were recorded. Attacks that were purely sensory or involved bowel and/or bladder function alone were not included. Patients were questioned about side effects, and toxicity was assessed through white blood counts and chemistry panels performed annually.

STATISTICAL METHODS

For the 16 patients who received myelin and had quarterly follow-up data for three years, we present mean yearly exacerbation rates, and the percentage of patients improved,

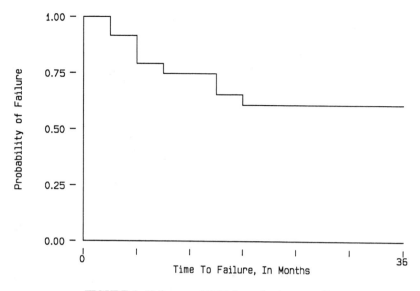

FIGURE 1. Failures on EDSS for patients on myelin.

stable, and worse at three years. To determine whether the quarterly incidence of exacerbations or change in EDSS scores were affected by the dose of myelin, sex, or DR2 status, we performed a repeated-measures logistic regression for exacerbations, and a repeated-measures linear regression for EDSS. The repeated-measures analyses implemented the generalized estimating equation technique introduced by Liang and Zeger[16] and adjusts for correlation between the quarterly data from each patient. In addition to including dose, sex, and DR2 status in each regression model, we also included baseline exacerbation count or EDSS, as appropriate.

In addition to the 16 patients with three years of follow-up, 8 patients from the original study took myelin for a briefer period of time. For these 24 patients, we also present a Kaplan-Meier curve, showing the time to failure on EDSS, where we define failure as a one point decline on EDSS that is sustained for at least six months. For patients who failed, the time of failure was recorded as the first quarter during which the EDSS declined. Of the 8 patients who had less than three years of follow-up, 2 discontinued myelin when they became pregnant and were censored from the Kaplan-Meier curve; the other 6 were counted as failures whether or not they satisfied the requirement for six-month verification of the decline in EDSS.

RESULTS

Time to Failure on EDSS

For the 24 patients that were ever on myelin, FIGURE 1 shows the Kaplan-Meier curve for time to failure on EDSS. At 12 months, a patient on myelin has a 75% (SE 9%) chance of avoiding a sustained one point increase in EDSS, whereas at 24 and 36 months, a patient has a 61% (SE 10%) chance of avoiding a sustained worsening.

TABLE 3. Oral Myelin–treated Patients: Mean Exacerbation Rate by Year of Treatment

Year of Treatment	−2	−1	1	2	3
Total (N = 16)	1.5	1.6	0.4	0.4	0.6
Male (N = 11)	1.6	2.2	0.4	0.5	0.7
Female (N = 5)	1.2	0.4	0.4	0.2	0.2
DR2⁻ (N = 9)	1.3	1.8	0.1	0.3	0.4
DR2⁺ (N = 7)	1.7	1.4	0.7	0.6	0.7

Mean Exacerbation Rate

The mean exacerbation rate by year of treatment is shown in TABLE 3. For all 16 patients, the annual exacerbation rate during the two years prior to treatment was 1.5 and 1.6, with an average value of 1.6 over the two years, compared to an average value of 0.5 during the three years on oral myelin therapy. Disability, as measured by EDSS remained unchanged after three years of treatment with myelin (mean 3.0 for all 16 patients) compared to an initial mean EDSS of 2.8. TABLE 4 shows the number of patients improved, stable, or worse at the end of three years of treatment. Thirteen of sixteen were either stable or improved, and only three were worse, as evidenced by a decline of at least one EDSS point. In the original double-blind study, subgroup analyses showed that two characteristics, gender and MHC phenotype, may have been related to treatment outcome, in that patients who were either male or lacked the HLA-DR2 phenotype did best. This finding continued in the ongoing study. HLA-DR2⁺ status predicted an increased incidence of attacks (odds of attack = 3.1 for DR2⁺ versus DR2⁻, p = .01) after adjusting for attacks prior to study, sex, and dosage. Also, as shown in TABLE 4, male and HLA-DR2⁻ patients were more likely to be stable or improved at three years compared to female or HLA-DR2⁺ patients. Linear regression showed male patients to have EDSS scores 0.1 point lower than females (p = .004), even after adjusting for baseline DR2 status and dosage of myelin. However, the contribution of sex and DR2 status remains ambiguous, because individuals were not originally randomized for gender and HLA phenotype. In the double-blind study, 6 of 8 male myelin-treated patients were HLA-DR2⁻, whereas all

TABLE 4. Disability Status[a] following Three Years of Treatment with Oral Myelin

Group	Improved	Stable	Worse
Total (N = 16)	3	10	3
Male (N = 11)	3	7	1
Female (N = 5)	0	3	2
DR2⁻ (N = 9)	3	5	1
DR2⁺ (N = 7)	0	5	2

[a] No. of patients improved/worse by at least one EDSS point of baseline, or stable (within 0.5 EDSS point of baseline).

the females were HLA-DR2$^+$. Similarly, in the open-protocol continuation study, 8 of 11 male patients but only 1 of 5 female patients were HLA-DR2$^-$.

Correlation between Clinical Outcome and Treatment

As mentioned above, there were time periods when patients were temporarily on a decreased dose of myelin or received no myelin at all due to a limited supply of the drug. Furthermore, female patients initially received 30 mg of myelin for one year at the start of the open-label study. For each three-month evaluation period, myelin doses were recorded as either full (300 mg daily), decreased, or none. Overall, patients received full-dose myelin 76% of the time, decreased dose 15% of the time, and no myelin 9% of the time. Correlations were found between clinical outcome and dosing. Specifically, when not receiving myelin, patients' EDSS worsened by an average of 0.3 point over the three-month evaluation period (p = 0.006, adjusted for baseline EDSS, sex, and DR2 status). Similarly, the risk of an attack doubled when on low dose or no myelin, although this finding was not statistically significant (odds ratio = 2.3 for no dose, p = .25; odds ratio = 2.3 for decreased dose, p = .15; adjusted for pretreatment attacks, sex, and DR2 status).

Concomitant Treatment

Patients were treated with intravenous or oral steroids during exacerbations at the discretion of their physician. Eleven of 16 patients received at least one course of steroids over the three-year period. Eight of eleven male patients received a total of 13 steroid treatments compared to 3 of 5 female patients who received a total of three courses. Five of 9 DR2$^-$ patients were treated with a total of six steroid treatments compared to 6 of 7 DR2$^+$ patients who received a total of 10 courses. Towards the end of the third year of treatment with oral myelin, a DR2$^+$ male patient entered a relapsing-progressive course of MS and was treated with cyclophosphamide and methylprednisolone with intravenous monthly boosters, in addition to continuing oral myelin. No other patients received additional disease-modifying treatments in the first three years. No side effects or toxicities were associated with myelin treatment.

DISCUSSION

This open protocol continuation study (which is ongoing) was designed to assess the long-term safety of ongoing daily bovine myelin treatment in relapsing-remitting MS. To date, the drug has been found to be safe with no toxicities. Although the original double-blind study involving 30 patients and the subsequent follow-up open-protocol trial with 16 patients demonstrated positive effects, no conclusions regarding efficacy can be made based on these small numbers of patients. Similarly, the apparent difference in clinical response to myelin observed in relation to sex and expression of DR2 phenotype cannot be adequately assessed because of small patient numbers and lack of randomization for gender and HLA phenotype prior to initiating the pilot study. To address these issues, a multicenter, double-blind, placebo-controlled trial has been initiated using the same dose of bovine myelin (Myloral) as the continuation study. In this phase III study, early relapsing-remitting MS patients will be treated for two years. The primary outcome measure will be the annual attack rate. Disability and MRI lesion load will be secondary outcome measures. MRI examination is performed prior to treatment and at yearly intervals;

TABLE 5. Design of Phase III Pivotal Trial

	Male Treated vs. Placebo	Female Treated vs. Placebo
DR2⁻	84/84	84/28
DR2⁺	84/28	84/28

MRI was not part of the pilot trial. Patients are stratified and prospectively randomized by gender and HLA phenotype, using the design shown in TABLE 5. In this design the attack rate data will be analyzed sequentially, starting with the male DR2⁻ group, then adding and reanalyzing data from the male DR2⁺, female DR2⁻, and female DR2⁺ groups, respectively. This Bauer loop method will address the question of efficacy within the whole population and in each of the four groups. Based on immunologic analysis, we found that patients in the continuation study have myelin-specific TGF-β-secreting regulatory T cells in their peripheral blood.[17] Thus the dose chosen is immunologically active. In summary, positive clinical and immunologic findings have been observed in this open-label continuation study, and the phase III study will determine the degree to which oral myelin (Myloral) is clinically effective in relapsing-remitting MS. All patients (504) have been enrolled, and the unblinding of results is scheduled for mid-1997.

REFERENCES

1. WEINER, H. L. & D. A. HAFLER. 1988. Immunotherapy of multiple sclerosis. Ann. Neurol. **23:** 211-222.
2. THE IFNB MULTIPLE SCLEROSIS STUDY GROUP AND THE UNIVERSITY OF BRITISH COLUMBIA MS/MRI ANALYSIS GROUP. 1995. Interferon beta-1b in the treatment of multiple sclerosis: Final outcome of the randomized controlled trial. Neurology **45:** 1277-1285.
3. JOHNSON, K. P., B. R. BROOKS, J. A. COHEN, C. C. FORD, J. GOLDSTEIN, R. P. LISAK, L. W. MYERS, H. S. PANITCH, J. W. ROSE, R. B. SCHIFFER, T. VOLLMER, L. P. WEINER, J. S. WOLINSKY & THE COPOLYMER 1 MULTIPLE SCLEROSIS STUDY GROUP. 1995. Copolymer 1 reduces relapse rate and improves disability in relapsing-remitting multiple sclerosis: Results of a phase III multicenter, double-blind, placebo-controlled trial. Neurology **45:** 1268-1276.
4. WELLS, H. G. 1911. Studies on the chemistry of anaphylaxis (III). Experiments with isolated proteins, especially those of the hen's egg. J. Infect. Dis. **8:** 147-171.
5. BRANDTZAEG, P. 1989. Overview of the mucosal immune system. Curr. Top. Microbiol. Immunol. **146:** 13-28.
6. HIGGINS, P. & H. L. WEINER. 1988. Suppression of experimental autoimmune encephalomyelitis by oral administration of myelin basic protein and its fragments. J. Immunol. **140:** 440-445.
7. BITAR, D. & C. C. WHITACRE. 1988. Suppression of experimental autoimmune encephalomyelitis by the oral administration of myelin basic protein. Cell. Immunol. **112:** 364-370.
8. BROD, S. A., A. AL-SABBGH, R. A. SOBEL, D. A. HAFLER & H. L. WEINER. 1991. Suppression of experimental autoimmune encephalomyelitis by oral administration of myelin antigens. IV. Suppression of chronic relapsing disease in the Lewis rat and strain 13 guinea pig. Ann. Neurol. **29:** 615-622.
9. AL-SABBAGH, A., A. MILLER, L. M. B. SANTOS & H. L. WEINER. 1994. Antigen-driven tissue-specific suppression following oral tolerance: Orally administered myelin basic

protein suppresses proteolipid induced experimental autoimmune encephalomyelitis in the SJL mouse. Eur. J. Immunol. **24:** 2104-2109.

10. NAGLER-ANDERSON, C., L. A. BOBER, M. E. ROBINSON, G. W. SISKIND & F. J. THORBEKE. 1986. Suppression of type II collagen-induced arthritis by intragastric administration of soluble type II collagen. Proc. Natl. Acad. Sci. USA **83:** 7443-7446.

11. THOMPSON, H. S. G. & N. A. STAINES. 1986. Gastric administration of type II collagen delays the onset and severity of collagen-induced arthritis in rats. Clin. Exp. Immunol. **64:** 581-586.

12. ZHANG, J. Z., C. S. Y. LEE, O. LIDER & H. L. WEINER. 1990. Suppression of adjuvant arthritis in Lewis rats by oral administration of type II collagen. J. Immunol. **145:** 2489-2493.

13. NUSSENBLATT, R. B., R. R. CASPI, R. MAHDI, C. C. CHAN, F. ROBERGE, O. LIDER & H. L. WEINER. 1990. Inhibition of S-antigen induced experimental autoimmune uveoretinitis by oral induction of tolerance with S-antigen. J. Immunol. **144**(5): 1689-1695.

14. ZHANG, J. A., L. DAVIDSON, G. EISENBARTH & H. L. WEINER. 1991. Suppression of diabetes in NOD mice by oral administration of porcine insulin. Proc. Natl. Acad. Sci. USA **88:** 10252-10256.

15. WEINER, H. L., G. A. MACKIN, M. MATSUI, E. J. ORAV, S. J. KHOURY, D. M. DAWSON & D. A. HAFLER. 1993. Double-blind pilot trial of oral tolerization with myelin antigens in multiple sclerosis. Science **259:** 1321-1324.

16. LIANG, K-Y. & S. L. ZEGER. 1986. Longitudinal data analyses using generalized linear models. Biometrika **73:** 13-22.

17. FUKAURA, H., S. C. KENT, M. J. PIETRUSEWICZ, S. J. KHOURY, H. L. WEINER & D. A. HAFLER. 1996. Antigen-specific TGFβ1 secretion with bovine myelin oral tolerization in multiple sclerosis. 1996. This volume.

Antigen-specific TGF-β1 Secretion with Bovine Myelin Oral Tolerization in Multiple Sclerosis

HIKOAKI FUKAURA, SALLY C. KENT,
MATTHEW J. PIETRUSEWICZ, SAMIA J. KHOURY,
HOWARD L. WEINER, AND DAVID A. HAFLER

Center for Neurologic Diseases
Brigham and Women's Hospital
and
Harvard Medical School
221 Longwood Avenue
Boston, Massachusetts 02115

INTRODUCTION

Multiple sclerosis (MS) is a chronic inflammatory disease characterized by lymphocyte infiltration and demyelination in the central nervous system (CNS) thought to be initiated by T lymphocytes recognizing myelin components of the CNS.[2,3] Experimental autoimmune encephalomyelitis (EAE), a model for autoimmune CNS disease, shows pathologic similarities to MS. EAE is induced by activated T cells recognizing myelin basic protein (MBP), proteolipid protein (PLP), or myelin-oligodendrocyte glycoprotein (MOG).[4] Once activated, CD4+ myelin-reactive T cells, secreting the cytokines IL-2, IFN-γ, TNF-α, and lymphotoxin, migrate into the CNS and initiate a cascade of events that can lead to clinical paralysis in the animals. In the EAE model, spontaneous recovery is associated with secretion of IL-4, IL-10, and TGF-β1 from Th2-like cells.[5]

The oral administration of antigen is a classic method of inducing tolerance to prevent systemic immune reactions by way of the gut.[6] More recently, oral tolerance has been used to suppress experimental autoimmune diseases, including collagen and adjuvant-induced arthritis, EAE, uveitis, and the nonobese diabetes model.[7-12]

Two distinct mechanisms have been elucidated for the systemic antigen-specific immune suppression associated with oral tolerance. Providing a strong T cell-receptor signal to circulating T cells by feeding high doses of antigen induces either anergy or apoptosis of antigen-specific cells. By contrast, feeding multiple low doses of antigen induces regulatory T cells that mediate suppression by producing the cytokines IL-4 and TGF-β1.[10,11] Specifically, T-cell clones isolated from mice orally tolerized with MBP were structurally identical to Th1 encephalitogenic CD4+ clones in T-cell receptor usage, major histocompatibility complex (MHC) class II restriction, and epitope recognition; while secreting IL-4, IL-10, and TGF-β1, these clones suppressed ongoing MBP- or PLP-induced EAE. This indicates that these regulatory T cells migrate to the target organ and suppress the ongoing inflammatory reactions.[12]

These investigations in experimental models have led to a series of phase I-II double-blind clinical trials in subjects with multiple sclerosis and rheumatoid arthritis. We reported previously that 30 relapsing-remitting MS patients receiving daily capsules of bovine myelin showed no toxicity or side effects. The frequency of T cells reactive with MBP from myelin-treated MS individuals were reduced as compared to nonmyelin-treated control MS individuals. Clinically, there was a tendency for the treated group to have fewer exacerbations, which may have occurred in the subgroup of DR2 males.[1] A statistically significant effect using oral tolerization to type II collagen has been shown in subjects with rheumatoid arthritis.[13] The clinical efficacy of oral myelin tolerization in subjects with MS is presently under phase III investigation in a multicenter, randomized double-blind clinical trial with more than 500 patients.

Based on the identification of antigen-reactive TGF-β1-secreting T cells in mice with oral tolerization to MBP antigen, the purpose of this study was to examine whether the oral administration of myelin in MS patients alters the frequency or cytokine-secretion patterns of MBP- or PLP-reactive T cells.

METHODOLOGY

Patients

Seventeen relapsing-remitting MS patients from the continuation phase of the phase I-II oral myelin trial were examined.[1] These patients were fed 300 mg bovine myelin daily for at least two years. Bovine myelin was supplied to patients by AutoImmune, Inc. (Lexington, MA). Seventeen relapsing-remitting MS patients who did not receive bovine myelin were examined as controls. MS patients were not treated with any immunosuppressive drug during the study. Steroids were intermittently used during flare-ups in both myelin-treated and nontreated groups. Thus, blood samples were not obtained within three months of steroid usage in either group.

Antigens

Human MBP was purified from the white matter of the human brain by the method previously described and was provided by AutoImmune, Inc. (Lexington, MA).[14] Bovine PLP was purified, as previously described. Tetanus toxoid (TT) was obtained in purified form from the Massachusetts Public Health Laboratory (Boston, MA).

Antigen-specific T-cell Lines

Peripheral blood mononuclear cells (PBMC) were isolated from heparinized venous blood by Ficoll-Hypaque density gradient, washed twice with Hanks' balanced salts solution, counted, and resuspended in media containing 10% autologous serum (collected from each patient and heat-inactivated; [this serum is used throughout the experiment for each patient]) in RPMI 1640, 10 mM Hepes buffer, 2 mM L-glutamine, and 100 U/100 μg per mL penicillin/streptomycin. All media and components were purchased from BioWhittaker (Walkersville, MD). PBMC from each patient were frozen in 10% dimethyl sulfoxide/fetal bovine serum (from Sigma Co., St. Louis, MO and BioWhittaker, respectively) at −70°C and were used as antigen-presenting cells for the remainder of the assay.

PBMC from each patient were pulsed with antigen; 1.2×10^7 cells in 1.2 mL were pulsed with antigen, either MBP (50 μg/mL), PLP (bovine proteolipid protein) (50 μg/mL), or TT (12 Lf/mL) for 2 hours at 37°C, washed in media twice with 10% autologous serum, and then seeded in 96-well U-bottom plates (CoStar, Cambridge, MA) at 2×10^5 cells/well (total volume = 200 μL/well). On day 7, each well was restimulated with the primary antigen, as used at day 0. Autologous PBMC were pulsed with antigen by incubating 10^7 PBMC in 1 mL of media with antigen at a concentration of 100 μg/mL (MBP or PLP) or 10 Lf/mL (TT) for 2 hours at 37°C, washed twice in media, and then irradiated with 5000 rad; 2×10^5 antigen-pulsed PBMC were added to each well. On day 9, 100 μL media was removed from each well, and 100 μL of media with IL-2 (T-cell supernatant derived from phytohemagglutinin-stimulated human peripheral blood lymphocytes, final concentration per well, 5% v/v) (Collaborative Biomedical Products, Bedford, MA) and rIL-4 (2.5 U/mL, final concentration/well) (Boehringer Mannheim, GmbH, Mannheim, Germany) was added to the wells.

On day 14, a split-well assay was performed. Each well was split into four wells: two received 1×10^5 autologous, antigen-pulsed, washed, and irradiated cells each; and two received 1×10^5 autologous, nonantigen-pulsed, washed, and irradiated cells each. All antigen pulsing, washing, and irradiation was performed as described above for the day-7 antigen pulse. Final well volume was 200 microliters. Supernatants were collected after 24 h for cytokine estimation (IL-4 and IFN-γ) by ELISA, and serum-free media (X-Vivo 20, BioWhittaker), 150 μL/well, were added. After another 72 h, supernatants were collected for measurement of TGF-β1. Each cell line was then pulsed with 1 μCi/well of [³H]thymidine during the last 18 h of culture and subsequently harvested by an automated cell harvester (Beta plate 1295-004, Wallac, Gaithersburg, MD). [³H]Thymidine uptake was measured in a beta scintillation counter (Beta plate 1205, Wallac).

Cytokine Assays

Cytokines produced by T-cell lines were assayed by ELISA. To measure IL-4, a capture ELISA method was employed as follows: Immulon 4 microtiter plates (Dynatech, Chantilly, Virginia) were coated with capture monoclonal antibody (mAb) (Pharmingen, San Diego, CA) at 1 μg/mL diluted in 0.1 M NaHCO₃ (pH 8.2) and incubated at 4°C overnight. Plates were then blocked with 3% BSA (KPL, Gaithersburg, MD) in PBS for 2 h at RT (room temperature), and supernatant (90 μL of culture supernatant) and standards of IL-4 (R&D Systems, Gaithersburg, MD) (21-1667 pg/mL) were added and incubated at 4°C overnight. Plates were washed, and detecting biotinylated mAb (Pharmingen) was added to plates at 0.5 μg/mL and incubated for 1 h at RT. After washing, the plates were incubated for 45 min with avidin-peroxidase (Sigma) at a 1 : 2,000 dilution. Then plates were developed with 3, 3′, 5, 5′-tetramethybenzidine (TMB) one-component peroxidase substrate (KPL), and reactions were stopped by TMB one-component stop solution (KPL). Absorbance was measured using an ELISA reader (Bio-Rad, Melville, NY) at 450 nm. The standard curve for each assay was generated, and cytokine production from each line was calculated. IFN-γ was measured employing a mouse monoclonal anti-human IFN-γ at 1 μg/mL as coating antibody, a rabbit anti-human IFN-γ polyclonal antibody at 1 μg/mL for secondary antibody (both from Endogen, Cambridge, MA), followed by a goat anti-rabbit-immunoglobulin-horseradish peroxidase-labeled antibody at 1 : 20,000 (Biosource International, Camarillo, CA). IFN-γ standard was purchased from Gibco BRL (Gaithersberg, MD). An ELISA assay was completed as described above. Human TGF-β1 was measured by a TGF-β1 ELISA kit (Promega, Madison, WI), and manufacture's instructions were followed exactly. Cytokine production from each line was calculated by subtracting antigen-negative cytokine production from antigen-positive cytokine production. We considered a line positive if the antigen-specific cytokine secretion was more than 50 pg/mL of IL-4 and more than 100 pg/mL of IFN-γ or TGF-β1.

Statistics analyses

Two tailed-Student's *t* test analyses were used to examine differences between groups of numbers.

TABLE 1. Frequency of Antigen-specific T-cell Lines[a]

Group	Antigen Used for Stimulation	Frequency of Antigen-specific T-cell Lines[b]
Fed	MBP (n = 17)	1.3 ± 0.5
	PLP (n = 17)	3.7 ± 1.0
	TT (n = 8)	23.3 ± 9.0
Nonfed	MBP (n = 17)	3.4 ± 2.5
	PLP (n = 13)	7.6 ± 3.6
	TT (n = 5)	19.0 ± 8.9

[a] T-cell lines are generated, as described in METHODOLOGY. Cultures were pulsed with 1 μCi/well [³H]thymidine 90 hours after the last antigen stimulation and harvested 18 hours later. A line was considered positive if the stimulation index was >3 (antigen-stimulated cpm/no-antigen-stimulated cpm) and had a Δcpm >500. The results are expressed as the mean ± SE.

[b] The value is expressed as a percentage of antigen-reactive lines out of total generated lines.

RESULTS

Frequency of Antigen-specific T-cell Lines

The frequency of antigen-reactive T-cell lines from myelin-fed and nonmyelin-fed MS patients' PBMC was determined by [³H]thymidine incorporation. A T-cell line was considered positive when the stimulation index was greater than 3.0 and the delta cpm was greater than 500. The mean frequency of each group in response to each antigen is shown (TABLE 1). Though there was a difference between the myelin-fed group and the nonmyelin-fed group in response to MBP and PLP, it did not reach statistical significance. The frequency of TT-reactive lines showed similar frequency in both myelin-fed and nonmyelin-fed groups.

Because we wished to examine antigen-reactive T-cell lines for cytokine secretion, we screened several hundred lines (both negative and positive for antigen-induced [³H]thymidine incorporation) for secretion of IL-4, IFN-γ, and TGF-β1 by ELISA. Although a correlation between thymidine uptake and IFN-γ secretion was found (data not shown), there was no correlation between stimulation index and other cytokine secretion. Thus, we then measured cytokine secretion from every T-cell line following antigen stimulation.

Frequency of Cytokine-secreting Lines

The frequency of cytokine-secreting lines in response to MBP, PLP, and TT in T-cell lines from fed and nonfed patients was calculated for each individual subject, and the average for each group was calculated. There was a marked increase in TGF-β1-secreting lines against MBP in myelin-fed as compared to nonmyelin-fed patients (TABLE 2). A similar effect was observed in IL-4 secretion, but this did not reach statistical significance. By contrast, no difference in IFN-γ production was observed. In response to PLP, there was also a highly significant increase in the frequency of TGF-β1-secreting T-cell lines in the myelin-fed group, whereas, here, no difference was observed in IL-4. There was

TABLE 2. MBP-specific Cytokine Production with Oral Myelin[a]

| Ag | Treatment | Percent of Cytokine-producing Lines | | |
		IFN-γ	IL-4	TGF-β1
MBP	Fed (n = 17)	5.0 ± 2.5	6.5 ± 2.7	9.9 ± 2.0[b]
	Nonfed (n = 17)	6.4 ± 1.8	1.3 ± 0.7	1.3 ± 0.5

[a] Cultures were done as described in TABLE 1. Values presented are the mean percentage of antigen-specific cytokine-secreting lines from all patients. The results are expressed as the mean ± SE.
[b] $p < 0.001$.

TABLE 3. PLP-specific Cytokine Production with Oral Myelin[a]

| Ag | Treatment | Percent of Cytokine-producing Lines | | |
		IFN-γ	IL-4	TGF-β1
PLP	Fed (n = 17)	6.1 ± 2.5	3.1 ± 1.9	9.5 ± 2.2[b]
	Nonfed (n = 17)	13.7 ± 7.4	2.0 ± 1.6	1.1 ± 0.7

[a] Cultures were done as described in TABLE 1. The values shown are the mean percentage of antigen-specific cytokine-secreting lines from all patients. The results are expressed as the mean ± SE.
[b] $p < 0.003$.

TABLE 4. Tetanus Toxoid–specific Cytokine Production with Oral Myelin[a]

| Ag | Treatment | Percent of Cytokine-producing Lines | | |
		IFN-γ	IL-4	TGF-β1
TT	Fed (n = 8)	39.8 ± 12.1	1.0 ± 0.5	1.9 ± 1.2
	Nonfed (n = 5)	65.8 ± 6.3[b]	0 ± 0	2.0 ± 1.2

[a] Cultures were done as described in TABLE 1. The values shown are the mean percentage of antigen-specific cytokine-secreting lines from all patients. The results are expressed as the mean ± SE.
[b] There was not a statistically significant difference between these groups.

a trend for lower IFN-γ secretion from the myelin-fed group in response to PLP, but this was not statistically significant (TABLE 3).

To examine whether the frequency of TGF-β1-secreting lines from the myelin-fed group was specific for myelin antigens, we measured cytokine secretion from T-cell lines using TT as an antigen. Both myelin-fed and nonmyelin-fed groups showed similar frequencies of TGF-β1-, IL-4-, and IFN-γ-secreting cell lines in response to TT in both myelin-fed and nonmyelin-fed groups. The frequency of TGF-β1-secreting lines from TT is shown (TABLE 4).

Th1- or Th2-like Cytokine Secretion

We analyzed each individual T-cell line to determine whether specific cytokine-secreting subsets could be elucidated. T-cell lines from both myelin-fed and nonfed MS patients exhibited both Th1- (IFN-γ secreting) and Th2- (IL-4 secreting) like cytokine patterns. Two out of thirteen myelin-fed MS patients showed a high IL-4-, low IFN-γ-, and high TGF-β1-producing pattern in response to MBP (2/13, 15.4%), but this cytokine-producing pattern was not seen in response to PLP from the myelin-fed group and not in the nonmyelin-fed group in response to MBP and PLP antigenic stimulation. However, several nonmyelin-fed MS patients showed a low IL-4-, high IFN-γ-, and low TGF-β1-producing pattern in response to MBP (3/9, 33.3%) and PLP (2/7, 28.6%). By contrast, fewer myelin-fed MS patients showed this pattern in response to MBP (1/13, 7.7%) and PLP (2/13, 15.4%) (data not shown).

DISCUSSION

Based on the identification of antigen-reactive TGF-β1-secreting T cells in mice with oral tolerization to MBP antigen, we examined whether the oral administration of myelin in MS patients alters the frequency or cytokine-secretion patterns of MBP- or PLP-reactive T cells. We observed a marked increase in the frequency of MBP- and PLP-reactive TGF-β1-secreting T-cell lines in myelin-fed MS patients, as compared to nonmyelin-fed MS patients. These data provide the first demonstration of antigen-specific cytokine deviation in subjects with autoimmune disease.

We reported previously that the frequency of MBP-reactive T cells pre- versus postoral tolerization in MS patients was reduced, whereas no such trend was observed in the nonmyelin-fed MS patients.[1] A similar trend was observed in this cross-sectional study, but this did not reach statistical significance. A longitudinal study in patients where the frequency and cytokine-secretion patterns of MS patients is studied will begin shortly.

Myelin basic protein and PLP are the most abundant proteins in the central nervous system and may represent major targets of the putative cell-mediated autoimmune response. Antigen-specific cytokine secretion against other antigens, such as myelin-associated glycoprotein (MAG), MOG, β-crystalline, or S100β, which are also candidates for antigen to induce effector T cells, will be investigated in future studies.

Feeding a single high dose of antigen induces anergy of antigen-specific Th1 cells or clonal deletion, whereas multiple low doses of antigen induce regulatory T cells that mediate disease by producing immunosuppressive cytokines along with other factors. In this study, MS patients were fed 300 mg of bovine myelin daily, and bovine myelin contains not only MBP and PLP, but other proteins in small amounts. As mentioned above, a longitudinal dosing trial will begin shortly to determine whether the dose of myelin used in the present investigation represents a high or low dose of antigen in humans.

SUMMARY

Multiple sclerosis is a presumed autoimmune disease, associated with inflammation in the CNS white matter, mediated by autoreactive T cells. We previously reported that oral myelin tolerization of relapsing-remitting MS patients resulted in fewer attacks, as compared to a placebo-fed group.[1] Here, we examined whether oral tolerization with bovine myelin resulted in altered autoreactive T-cell populations or altered T-cell function.

We generated 4,620 T-cell lines from 34 relapsing-remitting MS patients (17 were fed bovine myelin daily), and each line was examined for proliferation to MBP, PLP, and TT and for secretion of IL-4, IFN-γ, and TGF-β1. The frequency of TGF-β1-secreting T-cell lines after MBP and PLP stimulation in fed patients was greater than that of nonfed patients. These experiments demonstrate that oral tolerization with autoantigen results in altered cytokine secretion in a human autoimmune disease with the generation of TGF-β1-secreting T cells that may regulate the inflammatory response at the site of the demyelinating lesions in multiple sclerosis. These data provide the first evidence of antigen-specific modification of cytokine secretion in a human autoimmune disease.

REFERENCES

1. WEINER, H. L., G. A. MACKIN, M. MATSUI, E. J. ORAV, S. J. KHOURY, D. M. DAWSON & D. A. HAFLER. 1993. Double-blind pilot trial of oral tolerization with myelin antigens in multiple sclerosis. Science **259:** 1321-1324.
2. MCFARLIN, D. E. & H. F. MCFARLAND. 1982. Multiple sclerosis. N. Engl. J. Med. **307:** 1183-1188.
3. HAFLER, D. A. & H. L. WEINER. 1995. Immunologic mechanisms and therapy in multiple sclerosis. Immunol. Rev. **144:** 75-107.
4. LININGTON, C., T. BERGER, L. PERRY, S. WEERTH, D. HINZE-SELCH, Y. ZHANG, H. C. LU, H. LASSMANN & H. WEKERLE. 1993. T cells specific for the myelin oligodendrocyte glycoprotein mediate an unusual autoimmune inflammatory response in the central nervous system. Eur. J. Immunol. **23:** 1364-1372.
5. KHOURY, S. J., W. W. HANCOCK & H. L. WEINER. 1992. Oral tolerance to myelin basic protein and natural recovery from experimental autoimmune encephalomyelitis are associated with downregulation of inflammatory cytokines and differential upregulation of TGF-β, IL-4 and PGE expression in the brain. J. Exp. Med. **176:** 1355-1364.
6. CHASE, M. W. 1946. Inhibition of experimental drug allergy by prior feeding of the sensitizing agent. Proc. Soc. Exp. Biol. Med. **61:** 257-259.
7. THOMPSON, H. S. G. & N. A. STAINES. 1985. Suppression of collagen-induced arthritis with pregastrically or intravenously administered type II collagen. Agents Actions **19:** 318-319.
8. THOMPSON, H. S. G. & N. A. STAINES. 1985. Gastric administration of type II collagen delays the onset and severity of collagen-induced arthritis in rats. Clin. Exp. Immunol. **64:** 581-586.
9. NAGLER-ANDERSON, C., L. A. BOBER, M. E. ROBINSON, G. W. SISKIND & G. J. THORBEKE. 1986. Suppression of type II collagen-induced arthritis by intragastric administration of soluble type II collagen. Proc. Natl. Acad. Sci. USA **83:** 7443-7446.
10. FRIEDMAN, A. & H. L. WEINER. 1994. Induction of anergy or active suppression following oral tolerance is determined by frequency of feeding and antigen dosage. Proc. Natl. Acad. Sci. USA **91:** 6688-6692.
11. WHITACRE, C. C., I. E. GIENAPP, C. G. OROSZ & D. M. BITAR. 1991. Oral tolerance in experimental autoimmune encephalomyelitis. III. Evidence for clonal anergy. J. Immunol. **147:** 2155-2163.
12. CHEN, Y., V. K. KUCHROO, J-I. INOBE, D. A. HAFLER & H. L. WEINER. 1994. Regulatory T-cell clones induced by oral tolerance: Suppression of autoimmune encephalomyelitis. Science **265:** 1237-1240.
13. TRENTHAM, D. E., R. A. DYNESIUS-TRENTHAM, E. J. ORAV, D. COMBITCHI, C. LORENZO, K. L. SEWELL, D. A. HAFLER & H. L. WEINER. 1993. Effects of oral administration of type II collagen on rheumatoid arthritis. Science **261:** 1727-1730.
14. OTA, K., M. MATSUI, E. L. MILFORD, G. A. MACKIN, H. L. WEINER & D. A. HALFER. 1990. T-cell recognition of an immunodominant myelin basic protein epitope in multiple sclerosis. Nature **346:** 183-187.

Oral Tolerance in Myasthenia Gravis[a]

DANIEL B. DRACHMAN, SEIICHI OKUMURA,[b]
ROBERT N. ADAMS, AND KEVIN R. McINTOSH

Department of Neurology
Johns Hopkins University, School of Medicine
600 North Wolfe Street
Baltimore, Maryland 21287-7519

ORAL TOLERANCE IN MYASTHENIA GRAVIS

Myasthenia gravis (MG) differs from the other autoimmune diseases discussed at this volume in at least three respects: (1) the pathogenetic mechanisms of MG are antibody mediated, rather than cell mediated; (2) the sole antigen, and target of the autoimmune attack, that is, the acetylcholine receptor (AChR) at the neuromuscular junction, is known, and has been precisely defined, in molecular and biological terms; (3) AChR is an extremely immunogenic autoantigen. Studies of MG can therefore provide important information about the use of the oral tolerance strategy in antibody-mediated autoimmune disorders. Experimental results to date indicate that oral administration of AChR can effectively prevent clinical and immunological manifestations of MG in the experimental animal model of MG (EAMG).[1,2] The use of oral antigen to treat ongoing EAMG, though encouraging, will require modifications so as to bias the immune system effectively towards unresponsiveness to AChR, while avoiding stimulation of the autoimmune response.

MYASTHENIA GRAVIS

MG is an autoimmune disease that is manifested clinically by weakness and fatigability of skeletal muscles. The distribution of muscle weakness typically follows a characteristic pattern.[3] The cranial muscles, particularly the extraocular muscles and elevators of the eyelids are often involved early, giving rise to diplopia (double vision) and ptosis. Facial weakness and weakness of the muscles involved in speech, chewing, and swallowing are common early features. In about 85% of patients, the weakness becomes generalized,[4] usually affecting proximal more than distal muscles of the limbs. Impairment of respiration or swallowing may be so severe as to require respiratory assistance or intubation. Prior to the modern era of effective immunosuppressive treatment, this occurred commonly,[5] giving rise to the adjective "gravis."

The underlying defect in MG is a decrease in the number of available AChRs at neuromuscular junctions,[6,7] due to an antibody-mediated autoimmune attack. The deficit

[a]This work was supported in part by a Grant from the NIH (1RO1 NS23719); a Fellowship sponsored by the Japanese government (S. Okumura); and gifts from the Baltimore Relief Foundation, and the Anergen Corporation.

[b]Present address: Department of Neurology, Kanazawa University, Kanazawa, Japan.

of junctional AChRs limits the effectiveness of transmission of acetylcholine to muscle cells, resulting in skeletal muscle weakness and fatigability that are characteristic of MG.

Nicotinic AChR, the target of the autoimmune attack in MG, has been extensively studied, and the molecular structures of AChRs of many species have been analyzed in detail.[8–10] The richest natural sources of AChR are the electric organs of the electric ray (*Torpedo*) and the electric eel (*Electrophorus*), which consist of arrays of neuromuscular junction-like structures capable of producing powerful electrical discharges.[11] AChR is a glycoprotein of approximately 250 kDa, composed of five subunits that are arranged like barrel staves around a central ligand-gated ion channel.[8,12] The genes for all the receptor subunits of many species, including humans, rodents, and electric rays, have been sequenced and cloned.[8–10,13] Through genetic-engineering technology, it is now possible to produce recombinant proteins consisting of large stretches or entire subunits of the AChR.[10,13,14] Recombinant AChR or variants of the natural molecules produced by modern biotechnology are likely to be extremely important in the oral immunotherapy of MG.

The development of EAMG, induced by immunization with purified *Torpedo* AChR,[15] provided support for the concept that an autoimmune response directed against AChR could account for the features of MG.[15–17] Although the mode of induction of EAMG (i.e., by injection of foreign AChR, usually in Freund's adjuvant) obviously differs from the origin of the spontaneously occurring disease in humans, there are many similarities in the pathophysiology of EAMG in animals and MG in humans. This experimental model, most commonly induced in Lewis rats, has been particularly useful for testing new therapeutic strategies,[18] as in the oral tolerance experiments described here.

The key role of autoantibodies in the pathogenesis of MG was first demonstrated by experiments involving the passive transfer of serum immunoglobulin from humans to animals. Repeated injections of IgG from myasthenic patients into mice reproduced the loss of AChRs and physiological features characteristic of MG in the recipient animals.[19] Moreover, removal of autoantibodies from myasthenic patients by plasma exchange produced improvement in MG.[20–22] The pathogenic effects of the autoantibodies in reducing the number of available AChRs have been shown to be attributable to at least three different antibody-mediated mechanisms: (1) cross-linking of the AChRs by the antibodies, resulting in accelerated endocytosis and degradation of the receptors within the muscle cells; (2) functional blockade of acetylcholine-binding sites of AChRs; and (3) complement-mediated damage to AChRs and postsynaptic membranes of neuromuscular junctions.[23–25]

Treatment of MG commonly involves the use of immunosuppressive drugs.[26] Although generally effective, these agents must be used continuously, and may produce adverse side effects, including generalized suppression of the immune system.[27,28] Ideally, therapy of MG should eliminate the autoimmune response to the known antigen, AChR, without affecting the remainder of the immune system.[29,30] Treatment should be nontoxic, and its effect should be long-lasting or permanent.

One method of inducing specific immune unresponsiveness involves the oral administration of the autoantigen, as discussed extensively in the present volume. This strategy has been shown to prevent or treat a variety of cell-mediated experimental autoimmune diseases, including experimental allergic encephalomyelitis (EAE), uveitis (EAU), and collagen-induced arthritis (CIA)[31–36] (reviewed in ref. 37). Oral antigen therapy is currently undergoing trials in the human counterparts of these conditions (refs. 37–39, and this volume). The application of the oral tolerance strategy to an antibody-mediated autoimmune disease, such as MG, presents a special challenge because of the greater difficulty in inducing tolerance of antibody responses, as contrasted with cellular responses.[10,40] This paper reviews the results of studies of prevention of EAMG and reports treatment of ongoing EAMG by the oral administration of AChR.

TABLE 1. Experimental Protocol: Prevention of EAMG

A. Experimental design
  1. Feed antigen (gavage)
     1 dose every 3 days × 5
  2. Immunize 3 days after last dose
  3. Follow through 8 weeks
     Clinical effect (weakness, weight loss)
     Antibody levels
     Cellular responses (terminal):
     Proliferation
     IL-2 production
     AChR-antibody production

B. Oral antigens

Torpedo AChR:	0.25 mg × 5, low dose
Affinity purified	1.0 mg × 5, high dose
"Unpurified"	0.5 mg × 5, low dose
	2.5 mg × 5, very high dose
Ovalbumin (control)	0.25 mg × 5, low dose
	1.0 mg × 5, high dose
	2.5 mg × 5, very high dose

ORAL TOLERANCE IN EAMG: PREVENTION

In order to evaluate the effects of oral administration of AChR in preventing the clinical and immunological manifestations of EAMG, we carried out a series of experiments in which Lewis rats were first fed various doses of affinity-purified AChR, or an unrelated control antigen, ovalbumin (OVA), and then immunized with either AChR or OVA.[1] Because of the labor-intensive procedure required for affinity purification of AChR, we also tested the effects of feeding "unpurified" AChR, consisting of solubilized, but not affinity-purified AChR, in the same vehicle as the purified AChR. The amount of AChR in each preparation was determined by a method of [^{125}I]α-bungarotoxin labeling and immunoprecipitation.[41]

The animals were examined clinically[42] and weighed throughout a period of eight weeks. During that time, they were bled at intervals for determination of anti-AChR or anti-OVA antibodies. At the end of the experimental period, the animals were killed, and lymph node cells were studied in culture for antigen-specific responses. The experimental design is outlined in TABLE 1.

Clinically, oral administration of AChR protected rats from the subsequent development of EAMG, as shown in TABLE 2. Seventy percent of control rats (*i.e.,* those that were not fed AChR) developed signs of EAMG within eight weeks after immunization with AChR. By contrast, none of the rats fed purified AChR, and only 9% of the rats fed "unpurified" AChR, developed EAMG. Similarly, the control animals that were not fed AChR lost weight after AChR immunization, whereas the AChR-fed rats gained weight despite immunization with AChR. This beneficial clinical effect was antigen specific, inasmuch as oral administration of the control antigen OVA had no effect on the induction of EAMG.

TABLE 2. Clinical Effects of Feeding AChR

Feeding[a]	Immunization	Weight from 4–8 Wk[b] (gm ± SEM)	Rats with EAMG[b] (no. affected/total in group)
Control vehicle	AChR	−22.9 ± 11.3	6/7
Low-dose pure AChR	AChR	+4.0 ± 2.8	0/6[d]
High-dose pure AChR	AChR	+13.0 ± 1.2[c]	0/8[d]
Control vehicle	AChR	−19.8 ± 18.7	3/6
Low-dose unpurified AChR	AChR	+8.0 ± 9.2	2/5
Very high-dose unpurified AChR	AChR	+6.2 ± 3.6	0/6[d]
High-dose OVA	AChR	−17.5 − 13.6	5/6
Control vehicle	AChR	−3.14 ± 9.5	4/7

[a] Rats were fed pure AChR, unpurified AChR, OVA, or control vehicle, according to the dosage schedules in TABLE 1. All groups were then immunized with AChR (50 μg in complete Freund's adjuvant).

[b] Rats were weighed and observed clinically at weekly intervals.

[c] Significantly different from control-fed rats (p <0.05).

[d] Significantly different from control-fed rats (p <0.01).

Antibody Responses

AChR antibody production was markedly and specifically inhibited by prior feeding of AChR. Rats that were fed purified AChR, either at low or high doses, produced lower antibody responses to *Torpedo* AChR at eight weeks after challenge, compared with controls (FIG. 1). Paradoxically, the initial effect of oral AChR was a mild positive immune response, with low levels of AChR antibody detectable in sera of many of the rats fed AChR. Further, antibody responses measured at early times after immunization (2 to 4 weeks) were higher in the AChR-fed rats than in the controls. However, by six weeks, the antibody levels of rats fed high-dose AChR were lower than those of controls, and by eight weeks, the AChR-antibody levels were lower in both high- and low-dose-fed animals than in controls (FIG. 1). Feeding *Torpedo* AChR induced tolerance to autologous (rat) AChR as well as to the immunizing *Torpedo* antigen. These anti-rat autoantibodies are responsible for the pathogenesis of EAMG, although they represent only a small fraction of the overall AChR-antibody population. At eight weeks after immunization, the mean anti-rat AChR-antibody level was inhibited by 81% in the fed rats, as compared with controls (measured by RIA, p < 0.05; see ref. 1 for details).

Of considerable interest, feeding unpurified extract containing *Torpedo* AChR resulted in much less marked inhibition of AChR-antibody production (only 25% inhibition at eight weeks), even though the total dose of unpurified AChR was 2.5 times that of the high-dose pure AChR feeding.[1]

The effect of oral administration of OVA on production of antibodies to OVA was more prompt and more pronounced than the corresponding effect of AChR feeding. In contrast to AChR, oral administration of OVA did not induce an initial positive antibody response in any of the animals. The antibody response to OVA was markedly inhibited from zero through eight weeks after immunization with OVA. At eight weeks, rats fed

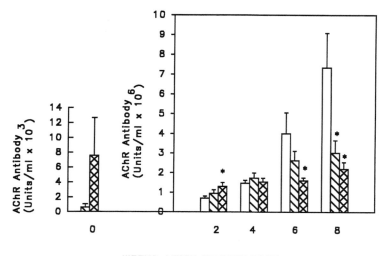

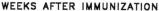

WEEKS AFTER IMMUNIZATION

FIGURE 1. Effect of oral administration of purified AChR on antibody response to *Torpedo* AChR. Rats were fed 5 times at 3-day intervals with control vehicle (phosphate-buffered saline/ 0.2% cholate; 1 mL/feeding [open bars]), low-dose AChR (0.25 mg/feeding [hatched bars]), or high-dose AChR (1.0 mg/feeding [cross-hatched bars]). Three days after the last feeding, the animals were immunized intradermally with 50 μg AChR in complete Freund's adjuvant (day 0). AChR-antibody levels were determined by kinetic ELISA assay. Results shown are mean units ± SEM. Note the significant inhibition of AChR antibodies in AChR-fed rats at 6- and 8-weeks. High-dose AChR feeding resulted in early priming, evident after feeding prior to immunization (note separate scale) and at 2 weeks after immunization. *Significantly different from controls (p < 0.05). (Okumura et al.[1] With permission from the *Annals of Neurology*.)

low-, high-, or very-high-dose OVA showed approximately 90% inhibition of antibody responses to OVA (data not shown; see ref. 1).

Lymphocyte Responses

Antigen-specific T-cell responses, including [³H]thymidine incorporation and interleu-kin-2 (IL-2) production, were determined in lymph node cells harvested from rats eight weeks after immunization. T cells from animals fed purified AChR were significantly inhibited in their ability to proliferate and to produce IL-2 in response to AChR stimulation. Proliferation was reduced by 53% to 83%, and IL-2 production was reduced by 63% to 82% in rats fed high-dose purified AChR (FIG. 2). Feeding of OVA resulted in even more marked inhibition of OVA-specific cellular responses: proliferation was reduced by 91% to 96%, and IL-2 production was reduced by 85% to 94% (data not shown). Thus, oral administration of antigens resulted in pronounced inhibition of antigen-specific cellular responses, comparable to the inhibition of antibody production.

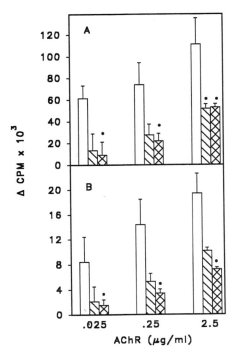

FIGURE 2. Responses of lymph node cells from rats fed purified AChR. As in Fig. 1, rats were fed control vehicle (open bars), low-dose AChR (hatched bars), or high-dose AChR (cross-hatched bars). Eight weeks after AChR immunization, they were killed and their isolated lymph node cells were restimulated *in vitro* with 0.025, 0.25, or 2.5 μg/mL AChR. **A:** Proliferative responses expressed as [³H]thymidine incorporation (mean Δcpm ± SEM). **B:** IL-2 production expressed as [³H]thymidine incorporation of an IL-2-dependent CTLL cell line (mean Δcpm ± SEM). Note the inhibition of cellular responses in AChR-fed rats. *Significantly different from controls (p < 0.05). (Okumura *et al.*[1] With permission from the *Annals of Neurology.*)

Specificity of Tolerance

To test for specificity of tolerance induced by oral antigen, we fed OVA to two groups of rats, and two control groups received saline feedings. Groups of OVA and saline-fed rats were then immunized with either AChR or OVA. The results showed that OVA feeding had no effect on antibody or cellular responses to AChR but profoundly inhibited both antibody and cellular responses to OVA (TABLE 3). Thus, the tolerogenic effects of oral administration of OVA were antigen specific.

Mechanism of Tolerance: Suppressor Cells?

Suppressor T cells (Ts) have been reported to play an important role in oral tolerance.[43–46] To determine the role of Ts in our system, rats were fed AChR (1 mg × 5) or OVA (5 mg × 5), and controls were fed vehicle alone. Seven to nine days after the last feeding (at the time reported to show maximum suppression in the EAE model),[45] the animals were killed, and their spleen cells or purified splenic T cells were evaluated for suppressor activity by their ability to inhibit proliferative activity of antigen-specific responder lymphocytes, as described previously.[47] The results showed that splenic suppressor-cell activity from rats fed AChR was weak, and generally nonspecific. Suppression was detectable only at high suppressor : responder ratios (5 : 1). Unfractionated spleen cells and purified splenic T cells from these rats produced variable suppression of AChR responses, which was not significantly greater than their suppression of unrelated OVA

TABLE 3. Specificity of Tolerance Induced by Antigen Feeding[a]

Feeding	Immunization	AChR Ab (units/mL × 10^6)[b]	Proliferation to AChR (Δcpm)[c]	AChR Ab in vitro (units/ mL × 10^3)[d]
OVA (1 mg × 5)	AChR	2.23 ± .27	215,385 ± 31,666	108.5 ± 10.2
Vehicle (1 mL × 5)	AChR	1.93 ± .10	157,859 ± 9,817	108.9 ± 13.5
		OVA Ab (units/mL × 10^6)[b]	Proliferation to OVA (Δcpm)[c]	OVA Ab in vitro (units/ mL × 10^3)[d]
OVA (1 mg × 5)	OVA	.844 ± .14[e]	2,420 ± 1,152[f]	2.4 ± 1.4[f]
Vehicle (1 mL × 5)	OVA	3.17 ± 1.04	32,530 ± 5,737	158.2 ± 64.5

[a] Rats were fed OVA or control vehicle. Groups of rats were immunized with AChR or OVA, as indicated. Note that OVA feeding inhibited antibody and cellular responses to OVA but not to AChR.

[b] Serum antibody (Ab) levels at 8 weeks after immunization.

[c] [³H]Thymidine incorporation by lymph node cells (LNC) stimulated in vitro with optimal concentration of antigen (2.5 μg/mL AChR or 40 μg/mL OVA).

[d] Antibody production in vitro by LNC stimulated with optimal concentration of antigen (0.025 μg/mL AChR or 10 μg/mL OVA).

[e] Significantly different from control, $p < 0.05$.

[f] Significantly different from control, $p < 0.01$.

or keyhole-limpet hemocyanin (KLH) responses. The suppressive activity of splenic lymphocytes from rats fed OVA was more pronounced, but also nonspecific, with no significant difference in the suppression of OVA, AChR, or KLH responses. Purified T cells from OVA-fed rats were essentially as suppressive as unfractionated spleen cells from these rats, indicating that the suppressive cells were T cells.

ORAL TOLERANCE IN ONGOING EAMG?

Therapy of human autoimmune diseases, such as MG, involves treatment during an ongoing pathological immune response. In order to test the effect of oral administration of AChR in ongoing EAMG, we first immunized Lewis rats with purified AChR. Two weeks later, after the immune response was well established, but before the development of signs of EAMG, groups of rats were fed either pure AChR (1 mg every 3 days × 5) or control vehicle (0.2% cholate) on the same schedule. The rats were examined clinically and weighed throughout a seven-week period after immunization. Blood was drawn, at intervals, for measurement of antibodies to Torpedo AChR and rat AChR. We also measured the functional ability of serum AChR antibodies to induce accelerated endocytosis and degradation of AChRs in a muscle cell-culture system, using a modification of a method previously described.[23] At the end of the experiment, the rats were killed, and draining lymph nodes were removed for in vitro study of cellular responses to AChR stimulation.

WEIGHT LOSS, 4–7 WEEKS

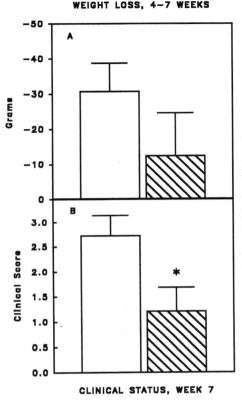

CLINICAL STATUS, WEEK 7

FIGURE 3. Clinical effects of feeding AChR in ongoing EAMG. Lewis rats were immunized intradermally with 50 μg *Torpedo* AChR in complete Freund's adjuvant. Two weeks later they were fed pure AChR (1 mg every 3 days × 5) (hatched bars), or control vehicle (open bars). They were evaluated clinically and weighed weekly. A: Mean weight loss from week 4-7 ± SEM. B: Mean clinical grade at week 7 ± SEM. *Different from control (p < 0.05).

Clinically, the AChR-fed rats fared better than the control rats (FIG. 3). The mean clinical grade of the AChR-fed rats was significantly lower than that of the controls at four, six, and seven weeks after immunization (i.e., two, three, and four weeks after completion of feeding). None of the seven AChR-fed rats died of EAMG, compared with three of the nine controls. Weight loss was more marked and consistent in the control rats, compared with the AChR-fed animals: eight of nine controls lost weight, whereas only three of seven AChR-fed rats lost weight by the end of the experiment.

In contrast to the clinical findings, anti-AChR antibody titers were actually higher in the AChR-fed rats than in the controls (FIG. 4). In the fed rats, antibodies to *Torpedo* AChR reached levels nearly four-fold those of the controls, and antibodies to rat AChR were almost two-fold those of the controls. Studies of the functional effects of serum from all the AChR-immunized rats showed marked acceleration of loss of AChRs (>60% decrease in AChRs, compared to cultures treated with normal rat serum). However, there was no significant difference in the effects of sera from AChR-fed and control rats (data not shown). Similarly, AChR-stimulated cellular responses were not significantly different in the lymph node cells from the AChR-fed and control rats (FIG. 5).

We also carried out a second set of experiments in ongoing EAMG that differed only in the procedure of oral AChR administration: that is, these rats were deprived of all food

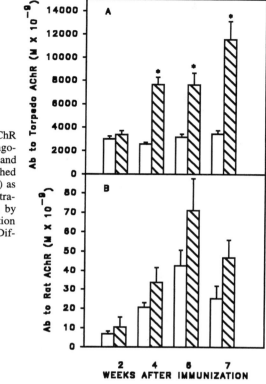

FIGURE 4. Effects of feeding AChR on AChR-antibody responses in ongoing EAMG. Rats were immunized and subsequently fed either AChR (hatched bars) or control vehicle (open bars) as in FIG. 3. A: Mean antibody concentration to *Torpedo* AChR, measured by RIA. B: Mean antibody concentration to rat AChR, measured by RIA. *Different from control (p < 0.05).

for 18 hours before antigen feeding in the hope of improving absorption from the GI tract, whereas the groups of rats in the first experiment (above) had been fed without previously removing their food supply. In this set of experiments, the clinical benefit was much less marked, with only slowing of development of EAMG and no significant difference in weights between AChR-fed and control rats. The AChR-antibody responses were only moderately affected in these animals. The maximum increase in mean anti-*Torpedo* AChR-antibody levels in the fed rats as compared to controls was only 1.95-fold, and the anti-rat AChR-antibody levels were virtually identical at all times (data not shown). We surmised that prolonged food withdrawal prior to oral administration of AChR led to greater proteolysis of the AChR within the gastrointestinal tract and thereby altered the outcome of these experiments.

DISCUSSION

The results of the studies described here clearly demonstrate that oral administration of AChR effectively prevents the development of clinical features of experimental MG, as well as antibody and cellular immune responses to the antigen. Similar findings have also been reported by the Karolinska group.[2,48] We now present preliminary evidence that

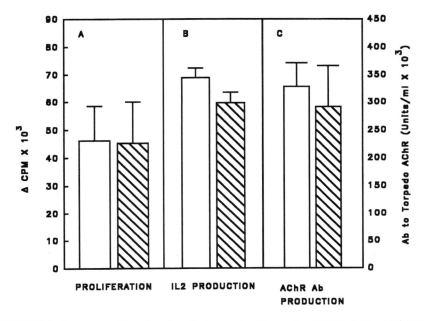

FIGURE 5. Responses of lymph node cells from rats with ongoing EAMG. Rats were immunized with AChR and subsequently fed either AChR (hatched bars) or control vehicle (open bars), as in Fig. 3. Lymphocytes were obtained from draining lymph nodes at 7 weeks after immunization. They were stimulated *in vitro* with optimal concentrations of AChR. **A:** Proliferative responses expressed as [^{3}H]thymidine incorporation (mean Δcpm $\pm$ SEM). **B:** IL-2 production expressed as [^{3}H]thymidine incorporation of an IL-2-dependent CTLL cell line (mean Δcpm $\pm$ SEM). **C:** Anti-AChR antibody (*Torpedo*) produced *in vitro*, expressed as ELISA units/mL (mean $\pm$ SEM).

AChR feeding may modify the clinical manifestations of EAMG during the course of an ongoing immune response to AChR, depending on the method of administration. These observations have important implications for the strategy of treating antibody-mediated autoimmune disorders by the oral route.

Our findings suggest that there are multiple factors that may contribute to the outcome in an antibody-mediated autoimmune disease after oral administration of antigen.

Immunogenic Property of the Antigen

As noted above, AChR feeding resulted in initial priming, which has been reported occasionally after oral administration of antigen,[49,50] but did not occur with OVA feeding in our experiments. OVA was more tolerogenic than AChR, and tolerance developed promptly after administration. It is likely that the inherent immunogenic potency of AChR in its native state is greater than that of OVA, and that this property can bias the balance between stimulatory and inhibitory immune responses. This observation suggests that an altered form of AChR might be more appropriate for oral therapy.

Dose and Purity of the Antigen

The inhibitory effects of AChR were dose dependent. The higher the dose, the more marked was the inhibition of cellular and humoral responses, and prevention of clinical manifestations of EAMG. The influence of purity of the antigen was unexpected. Although the amounts of unpurified AChR fed in these experiments were accurately determined by immunoassay, and the volume of each feeding and concentration of vehicle were the same as for pure AChR, the unpurified preparation was much less potent than pure AChR in inducing tolerance. This is similar to the reduced tolerogenic effects noted when multiple antigens were fed at short intervals,[51] or introduced simultaneously, such as at the time of weaning.[52] If this finding is reproduced for other antigens, it would suggest that antigens used for oral tolerization should be administered in purified form.

Tolerogenic Effects on Cellular and Humoral Immune Responses

Our results show that oral administration of AChR produced inhibition of both cellular and humoral immune responses. The degree of inhibition of proliferative and IL-2 responses of lymphocytes from AChR-fed rats was closely similar to the degree of inhibition of circulating antibody levels. Similarly, oral administration of OVA resulted in inhibition of lymphocyte responses and antibody levels to OVA that were closely comparable to each other. These findings demonstrate that antibody responses, including antibody responses to autoantigens, can be profoundly modified by antigen feeding. It is generally agreed that T cells are rendered unresponsive by antigen feeding, whereas B cells remain potentially reactive.[40,53] This implies that only antibody responses that are T-cell dependent can be inhibited by the oral route. Production of both AChR and OVA antibodies is T-cell dependent.[54,55] In the present study, the inhibition of T-cell function most likely accounts for the effects on antibodies.

Mechanism of Oral Tolerance

The mechanism of orally induced tolerance is complex and probably involves multiple immunoregulatory pathways. There is evidence that mechanisms of both active suppression and anergy may be involved, and that the contribution of each may depend in part on the dose of antigen given. It has been suggested that relatively low doses predispose to suppression, whereas high doses favor anergy.[46] In the present studies, cellular responses to the fed antigens were greatly reduced. Moreover, inhibition of antibody production occurred several weeks after AChR feeding, suggesting the gradual development of a suppressive mechanism, rather than anergy. However, our results demonstrated only a modest degree of suppression that was not antigen specific. Wang et al. found an increase in T cells that expressed mRNA for TGFβ, when stimulated with AChR.[48] These cells, which increased up to 2.5-fold, relatively late after immunization, could represent a suppressor-cell population. Thus, the mechanism of oral tolerance induced by AChR is not yet clear.

Inhibition of Ongoing EAMG

Oral administration of antigens has previously been reported to enhance preexisting immune responses in some instances,[56–58] although in others, tolerance, or at least no increase in immune responses, has been the result.[38,39] Our findings present a somewhat conflicting picture: On the one hand, feeding native *Torpedo* AChR after prior immunization inhibited the clinical manifestations of EAMG. On the other hand, it markedly increased the circulating anti-AChR levels. Further, a change in the AChR-feeding protocol eliminated the beneficial clinical effect and also resulted in a much less pronounced rise in AChR antibodies, suggesting a paradoxical inverse relationship between feeding-induced increase in the antibody level and clinical benefit. Based on our knowledge of the antibody-mediated pathogenesis of MG, one would anticipate that an increase in AChR antibodies should result in exacerbation of the disease process. It is possible that the extra antibodies produced were not pathogenic. Consistent with this hypothesis, testing of their functional effects on muscle cultures did not show a greater increase in the rate of AChR degradation by sera from AChR-fed rats, as compared with control sera. As yet, the effects of oral administration of AChR in ongoing EAMG are not clear. Our findings suggest that treatment of ongoing disease may require a modified molecule with less immunogenic potential than native AChR. Our current studies are designed to determine whether modified natural or recombinant AChR will prove more effective in the oral treatment of ongoing myasthenia gravis.

SUMMARY AND CONCLUSIONS

Because of the antibody-mediated pathogenesis of MG, it is of particular interest to understand the effects of oral administration of the autoantigen AChR on the disease process. It is now clear that feeding AChR prior to immunization can prevent clinical manifestation of EAMG. It initially primed, then inhibited, antibody responses to foreign (*Torpedo*) AChR and self (rat) AChR, with a delayed onset. Cellular responses to AChR, evaluated by lymphocyte proliferation and IL-2 production, were markedly inhibited. The effects were dependent on the dose and purity of the fed antigen. Tolerance to an orally administered unrelated antigen, OVA, was more prompt in development and more profound, illustrating the influence of the nature of the antigen on tolerance. The tolerance induced was antigen specific. Oral administration of AChR after immunization resulted in inhibition of the clinical manifestation of EAMG, concomitant with a paradoxical enhancement of the AChR-antibody responses. Both the clinical benefit and the antibody response appear to be dependent on the feeding protocol. These findings suggest that a molecule with less immunogenic potential than native AChR may be required for safe and effective oral treatment of ongoing disease.

REFERENCES

1. OKUMURA, S., K. McINTOSH & D. B. DRACHMAN. 1994. Oral administration of acetylcholine receptor: Effects on experimental myasthenia gravis. Ann. Neurol. **36:** 704–713.
2. WANG, Z-Y., J. QIAO & H. LINK. 1993. Suppression of experimental autoimmune myasthenia gravis by oral administration of acetylcholine receptor. J. Neuroimmunol. **44:** 209–214.
3. DRACHMAN, D. B. 1994. Myasthenia gravis. Medical Progress. N. Engl. J. Med. **330:** 1797–1810.
4. GROB, D., E. L. ARSURA, N. G. BRUNNER & T. NAMBA. 1987. The course of myasthenia gravis and therapies affecting outcome. Ann. N.Y. Acad. Sci. **505:** 472–499.
5. GROB, D., N. G. BRUNNER & T. NAMBA. 1981. The natural course of myasthenia gravis and effect of therapeutic measures. Ann. N.Y. Acad. Sci. **377:** 652–669.
6. FAMBROUGH, D. M., D. B. DRACHMAN & S. SATYAMURTI. 1973. Neuromuscular junction in myasthenia gravis: Decreased acetylcholine receptors. Science **182:** 293–5.

7. PESTRONK, A., D. B. DRACHMAN & S. SELF. 1985. Measurement of junctional acetylcholine receptors in myasthenia gravis: Clinical correlates. Muscle & Nerve **8:** 245-51.
8. CHANGEUX, J. P. 1990. Functional architecture and dynamics of the nicotinic acetylcholine receptor: An allosteric ligand-gated ion channel. *In* Fidia Research Foundation Neuroscience Award Lectures. **4:** 21-168. Raven. New York.
9. NODA, M., Y. FURUTANI, H. TAKAHASHI *et al.* 1983. Cloning and sequence analysis of calf cDNA and human genomic DNA encoding α-subunit precursor of muscle acetylcholine receptor. Nature **305:** 818-823.
10. BEESON, D., M. BRYDWON, H. WOOD, A. VINCENT & J. NEWSOM-DAVIS. 1989. Human muscle acetylcholine receptor: Cloning and expression in *Escherichia coli* of cDNA for the alpha-subunit. Biochem. Soc. Trans. **17:** 219-20.
11. COHEN, J. B. & J-P. CHANGEUX. 1975. The cholinergic receptor protein in its membrane environment. Annu. Rev. Pharmacol. **15:** 83-103.
12. UNWIN, N. 1995. Acetylcholine receptor channel imaged in the open state. Nature **373:** 37-43.
13. TALIB, S., K. R. LEIBY & T. B. OKARMA. 1991. Cloning and expression in *Escherichia coli* of a synthetic gene encoding the extracellular domain of the human muscle acetylcholine receptor alpha-subunit. Gene **98:** 289-93.
14. MISHINA, M., T. KUROSAKI, T. TOBIMATSU *et al.* 1984. Expression of functional acetylcholine receptor from cloned cDNAS. Nature **307:** 604-608.
15. PATRICK, J. & J. LINDSTROM. 1973. Autoimmune response to acetylcholine receptor. Science **180:** 871-72.
16. ENGEL, A. G., M. T. TSUJIHATA, E. H. LAMBERT, J. M. LINDSTROM & V. A. LENNON. 1976. Experimental autoimmune myasthenia gravis: A sequential and quantitative study of the neuromuscular junction ultrastructure and electrophysiologic correlation. J. Neuropathol. Exp. Neurol. **35:** 569-587.
17. PENN, A. S., H. W. CHANG, R. E. LOVELACE, W. NIEMI & A. MIRANDA. 1976. Antibodies to acetylcholine receptors in rabbits: Immunological and electrophysiological studies. Ann. N.Y. Acad. Sci. **274:** 354-76.
18. DRACHMAN, D. B., K. R. McINTOSH, J. REIM & L. BALCER. 1993. Strategies for treatment of myasthenia gravis. Ann. N.Y. Acad. Sci. **681:** 515-528.
19. TOYKA, K. V., D. B. DRACHMAN, D. E. GRIFFIN *et al.* 1977. Myasthenia gravis: Study of humoral immune mechanisms by passive transfer to mice. N. Engl. J. Med. **296:** 125-31.
20. PINCHING, A. J., D. K. PETERS & J. N. NEWSOM-DAVIS. 1976. Remission of myasthenia gravis following plasma exchange. Lancet **2:** 1373-1376.
21. KEESEY, J., D. BUFFKIN, D. KEBO, W. HO & C. HERRMANN JR. 1981. Plasma exchange alone as therapy for myasthenia gravis. Ann. N.Y. Acad. Sci. **377:**729-743.
22. DAU, P. C., J. M. LINDSTROM, C. K. CASSEL, E. H. DENYS, E. E. SHEV & L. E. SPITLER. 1977. Plasmapheresis and immunosuppressive drug therapy in myasthenia gravis. N. Engl. J. Med. **297:** 1134-1140.
23. KAO, I. & D. B. DRACHMAN. 1977. Myasthenic immunoglobulin accelerates acetylcholine receptor degradation. Science **196:** 527-9.
24. DRACHMAN, D. B., R. N. ADAMS, L. F. JOSIFEK & S. G. SELF. 1982. Functional activities of autoantibodies to acetylcholine receptors and the clinical severity of myasthenia gravis. N. Engl. J. Med. **307:** 769-75.
25. ENGEL, A. G. & K. ARAHATA. 1987. The membrane attack complex of complement at the endplate in myasthenia gravis. Ann. N.Y. Acad. Sci. **505:** 326-32.
26. DRACHMAN, D. B. 1992. Myasthenia gravis. *In* Current Therapy in Neurologic Disease. R. Johnson & J. W. Griffin, Eds. B. C. Decker. St. Louis.
27. JOHNS, T. R. 1987. Long-term corticosteroid treatment of myasthenia gravis. Ann. N.Y. Acad. Sci. **505:** 568-583.
28. MICHELS, M., R. HOHLFELD, H-P. HARTUNG, K. HEININGER, U. A. BESINGER & K. V. TOYKA. 1988. Myasthenia gravis: discontinuation of long-term azathioprine. Ann. Neurol. **24:** 798.

29. NOSSAL, G. J. V. 1987. Possible strategies for the treatment of myasthenia gravis and other autoimmune diseases. Ann. N.Y. Acad. Sci. **505:** 610-618.

30. DRACHMAN, D. B. & R. W. KUNCL. 1994. Myasthenia gravis. *In* Immunology of Neuromuscular Diseases. R. Hohlfeld, Eds.: Chapter 7: 165-207. Kluwer Academic Publishers. Dordrecht, Boston, London.

31. HIGGINS, P. J. & H. L. WEINER. 1988. Suppression of experimental autoimmune encephalomyelitis by oral administration of myelin basic protein and its fragments. J. Immunol. **140:** 440-445.

32. BITAR, D. M. & C. C. WHITACRE. 1988. Suppression of experimental autoimmune encephalomyelitis by the oral administration of myelin basic protein. Cell. Immunol. **112:** 364-370.

33. NUSSENBLATT, R. B., R. P. CASPI, R. MAHDI *et al.* 1990. Inhibition of S-antigen induced experimental autoimmune uveoretinitis by oral induction of tolerance with S-antigen. J. Immunol. **144:** 1689-1695.

34. SINGH, V. K., H. K. KALRA, K. YAMAKI & T. SHINOHARA. 1992. Suppression of experimental autoimmune uveitis in rats by the oral administration of the uveitopathogenic S-antigen fragment or a cross-reactive homologous peptide. Cell. Immunol. **139:** 81-90.

35. NAGLER-ANDERSON, C., L. A. BOBER, M. E. ROBINSON *et al.* 1986. Suppression of type II collagen-induced arthritis by intragastric administration of soluble type II collagen. Proc. Natl. Acad. Sci. USA **83:** 7443-7446.

36. THOMPSON, H. S. G. & N. A. STAINES. 1989. Suppression of collagen-induced arthritis with pergastrically or intravenously administered type II collagen. Agents Actions **19:** 318-319.

37. WEINER, H. L., A. FRIEDMAN, A. MILLER *et al.* 1994. Oral tolerance: Immunologic mechanisms and treatment of animal and human organ-specific autoimmunity diseases by oral administration of autoantigens. Annu. Rev. Immunol. **12:** 809-837.

38. WEINER, H. C., G. A. MACKIN, M. MATSUI *et al.* 1993. Double-blind pilot trial of ral tolerization with myelin antigens in multiple sclerosis. Science **259:** 1321-1324.

39. TRENTHAM, D. E., A. DYNESIUM-TRENTHAM, E. J. ORAV *et al.* 1993. Effects of oral administration of type II collagen on rheumatoid arthritis. Science **261:** 1727-1730.

40. HUSBY, S., J. MESTECKY, Z. MALDOVEANU, S. HOLLAND & C. O. ELSON. 1994. Oral tolerance in humans. J. Immunol. **152:** 4663-4670.

41. BRAY, J. J. & D. B. DRACHMAN. 1982. Binding affinities of anti-acetylcholine receptor autoantibodies in myasthenia gravis. J. Immunol. **128:** 105-110.

42. LENNON, V. A., J. M. LINSTROM & M. E. SEYBOLD. 1975. Experimental autoimmune myasthenia: A model of myasthenia gravis in rats and guinea pigs. J. Exp. Med. **141:** 1365-1375.

43. RICHMAN, L. K., J. M. CHILLER, W. R. BROWN *et al.* 1978. Enterically induced immunological tolerance. I. Induction of suppressor lymphocytes by intragastric administration of soluble proteins. J. Immunol. **121:** 2429-2434.

44. MATTINGLY, J. & B. WAKSMAN. 1978. Immunologic suppression after oral administration of antigen. I. Specific suppressor cells found in rat Peyer's patches after oral administration of sheep erythrocytes, and their systemic migration. J. Immunol. **121:** 1878-1883.

45. LIDER, O., L. M. B. SANTOS & C. S. Y. LEE. 1989. Suppression of experimental autoimmune encephalomyelitis by oral administration of myelin basic protein. J. Immunol. **142:** 748-752.

46. FRIEDMAN, A. & H. L. WEINER. 1994. Induction of anergy or active suppression following oral tolerance is determined by antigen dosage. Proc. Natl. Acad. Sci. USA **91:** 6688-6692.

47. MCINTOSH, K. R., D. B. DRACHMAN & R. W. KUNCL. 1989. Antigen-specific suppressor macrophages induced by culture with cyclosporin A plus acetylcholine receptor. J. Neuroimmunol. **25:** 75-89.

48. WANG, Z-Y., H. LINK, A. LJUNGDAHL et al. 1994. Induction of interferon γ, interleukin 4 and transforming growth factor-β in rats orally tolerized against experimental autoimmune myasthenia gravis. Cell. Immunol. **157:** 353-368.

49. HEPPEL, L. M. J. & P. J. KILSHAW. 1982. Immune responses of guinea pigs to dietary protein. Int. Arch. Allergy. Appl. Immunol. **68:** 54-59.

50. GAUTAM, S. C., N. F. CHIKKALA & J. R. BATTISTO. 1990. Oral administration of the contact sensitizer trinitrochlorobenzene: Initial sensitization and subsequent appearance of a suppressor population. Cell. Immunol. **125:** 437-448.

51. STOKES, C. R., T. J. NEWBY & F. J. BOURNE. 1983. The influence of oral immunization on local and systemic immune responses to heterologous antigens. Clin. Exp. Immunol. **52:** 399-406.

52. MOWAT, A. McI. 1987. The regulation of immune responses to dietary protein antigens. Immunol. Today **8:** 93-98.

53. WEINER, H. L. 1994. Oral tolerance. Proc. Natl. Acad. Sci. USA **91:** 10762-10765.

54. LENNON, V. A., J. M. LINDSTROM & M. E. SEYBOLD. 1976. Experimental autoimmune myasthenia gravis: Cellular and humoral immune responses. Ann. N.Y. Acad. Sci. **274:** 283-299.

55. HOHLFELD, R., K. V. TOYKA, M. MICHELS, K. HEININGER, B. CONTI-TRONCONI & S. J. TZARTOS. 1987. Acetylcholine receptor-specific human T-lymphocyte lines. Ann. N.Y. Acad. Sci. **505:** 27-38.

56. TITUS, R. G. & J. M. CHILLER. 1981. Orally induced tolerance. Int. Arch Allergy Appl. Immunol. **65:** 323-338.

57. HANSON, D. G., N. M. VAZ, D. A. RAWLINGS et al. 1979. Inhibition of specific immune responses by feeding protein antigens. II. Effects of prior passive and active immunization. J. Immunol. **122:** 2261-2266.

58. LENS, J. W., B. VAN DEN BERG, L. B. A. VAN DI PUTTE & L. VEN DEN BERSSELAAR. 1984. Flare-up of antigen-induced arthritis in mice after challenge with oral antigen. Clin. Exp. Immunol. **58:** 364-371.

Mucosal Tolerance to Experimental Autoimmune Myasthenia Gravis Is Associated with Down-regulation of AChR-specific IFN-γ-expressing Th1-like Cells and Up-regulation of TGF-β mRNA in Mononuclear Cells

CUN-GEN MA, GUANG-XIAN ZHANG
BAO-GUO XIAO, ZENG-YU WANG, JOANNE LINK,
TOMAS OLSSON, AND HANS LINK

Division of Neurology
Karolinska Institute
Huddinge University Hospital
S-141 86 Huddinge, Sweden

INTRODUCTION

Experimental autoimmune myasthenia gravis (EAMG), induced by immunizing animals with acetylcholine receptor (AChR) in complete Freund's adjuvant (CFA), is a model for human myasthenia gravis (MG). It is believed that both MG and EAMG are autoimmune diseases mediated by antibodies against the nicotinic AChR of neuromuscular junctions, and that these antibodies cause an accelerated internalization and degradation of functional AChR, complement-mediated destruction of the postsynaptic membrane, and a direct functional blockade of AChR channels.[1,2] The production of anti-AChR antibodies is regulated by AChR-specific CD4+ T-helper (Th) cells that recognize AChR in the context of class II major histocompatibility complex (MHC) molecules.[3]

Nonspecific immunosuppressive drugs show a remarkable efficacy in suppressing abnormal autoimmune responses but with potential risks of drug toxicity and global immunosuppression.[4] An ideal therapeutic approach would be the targeting of the specific immunologic reactivity that leads to the disease by eliminating and/or inhibiting the function of disease-inducing lymphocytes.[5] Oral feeding of organ-specific autoantigens suppresses diseases in other autoimmune disease models, including experimental autoimmune encephalomyelitis (EAE), experimental autoimmune uveitis (EAU), collagen and adjuvant arthritis, and diabetes.[6] Tolerance may also be induced through the respiratory tract by mechanisms similar to those after oral tolerization.[7] In this report, we demonstrate that *Torpedo* AChR administered orally in milligram doses or nasally in macrogram doses to Lewis rats prior to immunization with AChR and CFA prevented clinical signs of EAMG and suppressed AChR-specific B and T cell-mediated immune responses. Furthermore, the development of tolerance was related to suppression of interferon-γ (IFN-γ) and interleukin-4 (IL-4), but strong augmentation of TGF-β mRNA expression, implying that active

273

TABLE 1. Clinical Picture in Rats Subjected to Oral Tolerance[a]

| Feeding Regimen | Immunization | Incidence of Muscle Weakness | | Severity |
		Early	Late	
Unfed	CFA	0/10	0/10	0
Unfed	AChR + CFA	6/12	8/8	2.6 ± 0.5
STI	AChR + CFA	7/15	11/11	2.7 ± 0.3
AChR + STI	AChR + CFA	0/12	0/8	0

[a] Severity refers to maximum mean clinical scores ± SD.

suppression could be the main mechanism involved in oral and nasal tolerance in our animal models.

RESULTS

Effect on Clinical Muscular Weakness

Female Lewis rats, 6-8 weeks of age, were originally obtained from ALAB, Stockholm, Sweden. To induce oral tolerance to EAMG, rats were deprived of food, but not water, for 18 h prior to each feeding. Torpedo AChR and soybean trypsin inhibitor (STI) were suspended in 0.15 M sodium bicarbonate buffer. At each feeding, rats were gently anesthetized with ether and received 0.5 mL (10 mg) STI alone or STI followed by 1 mL of a solution containing 1.25 mg of AChR. Four feedings were administrated over an eight-day period. To induce nasal tolerance to EAMG, rats received into each nostril 30 μL PBS containing Torpedo AChR at a concentration of 100 μg/mL (group I), 150 μg/mL (group II), and 200 μg/mL (group III) using a micropipette. Among them, group I is most effective. Nontolerized controls received PBS alone. At each administration, rats were gently anesthetized with ether. The administrations were performed daily and for 10 days before induction of EAMG.

Nontolerized control rats exhibited mild (1.0) or moderately severe (2.0), transient early signs of muscular weakness 6-10 days postimmunization (p.i.) with AChR plus CFA. All nontolerized control rats developed late and progressive muscular weakness (all of them reached a clinical score of 2.5-3.0). By contrast, none of 12 rats fed with AChR and STI exhibited early or late signs of muscular weakness during observation periods up to 7-8 week p.i. with AChR (TABLE 1). Of the rats nasally tolerized with AChR, only three developed mild or moderately severe signs (clinical scores were 0.5-2.0) of muscular weakness late p.i. with AChR and CFA, and these signs disappeared within one week. In the rats belonging to group I, there were no signs of late clinical muscular weakness exhibited (FIG. 1).

Serum Anti-AChR Antibodies

Higher levels of anti-AChR antibodies were measured in serum from nontolerized EAMG control rats by both RIA (FIG. 2) for orally tolerized rats and ELISA (FIG. 3) for nasally tolerized rats. Conversely, serum anti-AChR antibodies measured in orally or nasally tolerized rats were much lower and seemed to stabilize at a constant low level over the whole observation time. The differences between nontolerized EAMG control rats and tolerized rats were significant (p <0.05 or p <0.01) on days 14, 21, 28, 35, and 42 p.i. There was no significant correlation between severity of EAMG and serum antibody levels.

Anti-AChR IgG Antibody-secreting Cells in Different Lymphoid Organs

Popliteal and inguinal lymph nodes (PILN), and spleen and thymus from nontolerized EAMG control rats contained higher numbers of anti-AChR IgG antibody-secreting cells compared to rats orally or nasally tolerized with different concentrations of AChR prior to immunization (TABLES 2 and 3). In nontolerized rats the mean numbers of anti-AChR IgG antibody-secreting cells were highest in PILN. By contrast, tolerized rats had much lower mean numbers of anti-AChR IgG antibody-secreting cells, particularly in PILN, but also in spleen and thymus.

Organ Distribution of AChR-reactive IFN-γ, IL-4, and TGF-β mRNA-expressing Cells

In situ hybridization was performed as described.[8] Briefly, aliquots of 200 μL of cell suspensions containing 4×10^5 mononuclear cells (MNC) were added into round-bottomed microtiter plates in triplicate. Separate cultures received no antigen, 10 μL aliquots of Con A, AChR, or myelin basic protein (MBP). After culture for 24 h, the cells were washed, counted, and dried onto restricted areas of ProbeOn slides. Synthetic oligonucleotide were labeled using [^{35}S]deoxyadenosine-5'-α-(thio)-triphosphate with terminal deoxynucleotidyl transferase. The oligonucleotide sequences were obtained from GenBank using the MacVector System. Cells were hybridized without pretreatment for 18 h at 42°C with 10^6 cpm of labeled probe per 100 μL of hybridization mixture. After emulsion autoradiography, development, and fixation, the coded slides were examined by dark field microscopy at 10× magnification for positive cells containing more than 15 grains per cell in a star-like distribution and checked by light microscopy. The data were expressed as numbers of cells per 10^5 cultured MNC. Numbers of cells expressing cytokine mRNA after culture without antigen added, which are considered as cells spontaneously expressing cytokine mRNA, were subtracted from the values obtained after antigen exposure.

The lymph nodes, spleen, and thymus from nontolerized control rats immunized with AChR and CFA, which all developed EAMG, contained higher numbers of AChR-reactive IFN-γ, IL-4, and TGF-β mRNA-expressing cells in most lymphoid organs studied, when compared with CFA-injected control rats (TABLE 4).

Rats orally or nasally tolerized to EAMG with different concentrations of AChR had lower mean numbers of AChR-reactive IFN-γ and IL-4-expressing cells in different lymphoid organs, whereas the mean numbers of TGF-β mRNA-expressing cells were higher when compared to nontolerized EAMG control rats (FIG. 4 and TABLE 4). By contrast, considering the IFN-γ, IL-4, and TGF-β mRNA-expressing cells recognizing the control antigen MBP, only low numbers were detected both in the tolerized and in nontolerized rats without statistical differences between the lymphoid organs under study (TABLE 4). Studies of relationships between different cytokines revealed significant negative correlations between TGF-β and IFN-γ, as well as between TGF-β and IL-4 mRNA-expressing cells in PILN.

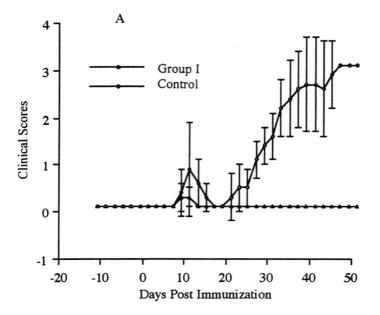

FIGURE 1A.

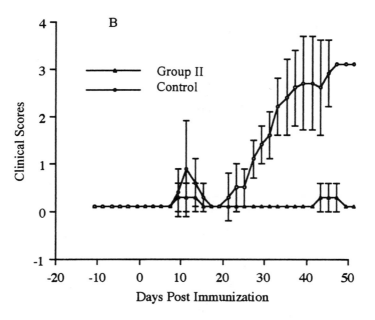

FIGURE 1B.

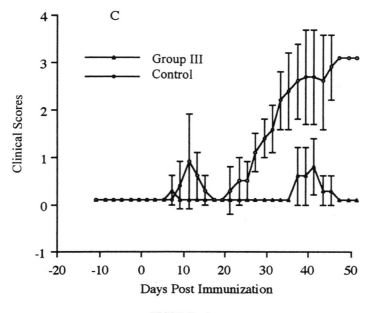

FIGURE 1C.

FIGURE 1. Clinical course of EAMG in nontolerized control rats (n = 7) and rats tolerized before immunization by nasal administration of AChR at concentrations of 100 μg/mL (group I), 150 μg/mL (group II), and 200 μg/mL (group III) (n = 4 in each group). Symbols = mean; bars = SD.

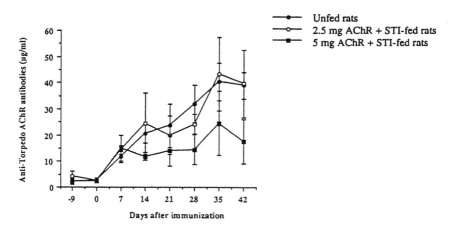

FIGURE 2. Effect of AChR feeding on serum anti-AChR antibody responses at different times postimmunization. Serum specimens from rats fed AChR at doses of 2.5 mg and 5 mg, and unfed control rats were measured by RIA. Symbols refer to mean values, bars to SD.

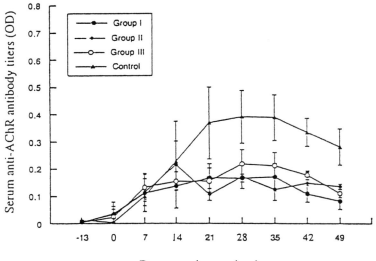

Days post immunization

FIGURE 3. Effect of nasal administration of AChR on serum anti-AChR antibody titers at different times postimmunization. Controls consisted of nontolerized rats (n = 7) with EAMG. Symbols = mean; bars = SD.

Amount of Muscle AChR Loss in Rats Tolerized to EAMG

The losses of muscle AChR in rats studied after oral or nasal administration of different concentrations of AChR were significantly lower than in nontolerized EAMG control rats (FIG. 5). Correlation analysis revealed significant negative correlations between TGF-β mRNA-expressing cells from PILN or spleen and muscle AChR losses (r values were −0.637 and −0.675, respectively, p < 0.01).

DISCUSSION

The immune system receives many external antigens through mucosal surfaces of the digestive or respiratory system, which may induce either sensitization or tolerance when the individuals subsequently experience the same antigen.[6] We observed in the present study that oral or nasal administration of *Torpedo* AChR prior to immunization with the same antigen, which has been long considered as the target for aggressive autoimmunity in both human MG and EAMG, is an effective means of suppressing EAMG. Oral or nasal tolerization not only markedly diminished the incidence and severity of clinical muscular weakness, but also significantly suppressed AChR-specific B- and T-cell responses in both peripheral blood and different lymphoid organs.

The exact mechanisms behind the induction of tolerance after oral or nasal administration of antigen are unknown. From the study of EAE and other experimental autoimmune diseases, it has been deduced that tolerance obtained by the oral administration of antigens is mediated by either active suppression by way of specific activation of CD8+ T cells or

TABLE 2. Mean Numbers of Cells Secreting IgG Antibodies to AChR and to the Control Antigen MBP per 10^5 Mononuclear Cells Isolated from the Popliteal and Inguinal Lymph Nodes, Mesenteric Lymph Nodes, Spleen and Thymus of Unfed Rats, Rats Fed with STI, and Rats Fed with AChR + STI Postimmunization with AChR plus CPA[a]

Feeding Regimen	Popliteal and Inguinal Lymph Nodes		Mesenteric Lymph Nodes		Spleen		Thymus	
	AChR	MBP	AChR	MBP	AChR	MBP	AChR	MBP
Unfed								
m (SD)	33.5 (6.0)	0.8 (0.4)	1.9 (0.8)	0.6 (0.5)	7.8 (1.9)	1.2 (0.5)	1.6 (0.9)	0.5 (0.4)
p*	<0.001	NS	<0.05	NS	<0.001	NS	<0.01	NS
STI fed								
m (SD)	32.3 (11.1)	0.8 (0.5)	2.4 (1.3)	0.5 (0.4)	8.1 (2.5)	1.0 (0.4)	1.7 (0.9)	0.5 (0.5)
p*	<0.001	NS	<0.05·	NS	<0.001	NS	<0.01	NS
p**	NS	NS	NS	NS	NS	NS	NS	NS
AChR + STI fed								
m (SD)	8.1 (1.7)	0.6 (0.4)	1.8 (1.0)	0.5 (0.5)	3.1 (1.0)	1.0 (0.5)	0.6 (0.6)	0.3 (0.3)
p*	<0.001	NS	<0.05	NS	<0.001	NS	NS	NS
p**	<0.001	NS	NS	NS	<0.001	NS	<0.01	NS
CPA injected								
m (SD)	1.0 (0.4)	0.8 (0.4)	1.0 (0.3)	0.8 (0.3)	1.6 (0.5)	1.1 (0.5)	0.8 (0.6)	0.4 (0.3)

[a] Control rats were injected with CFA only. Rats were killed 3, 5, and 7–8 weeks postimmunization. m refers to mean and SD to standard deviation. p* values refer to comparisons between unfed, STI-fed, or AChR + STI-fed rats that all were immunized with AChR plus CFA, and control rats injected with CFA only. p** values refer to comparisons between STI-fed or AChR + STI-fed rats and unfed rats. NS, not significant.

TABLE 3. Mean Numbers of anti-AChR IgG Antibody-secreting Cells per 10^5 MNC from Different Lymphoid Organs of Nasally Tolerized Rats and Nontolerized EAMG Control Rats

Groups		PILN	Spleen	Thymus
Tolerized				
Group I	Mean (SD)	6.9 (3.5)**	0.8 (0.6)*	0.5 (0.4)*
Group II	Mean (SD)	10.5 (9.7)**	1.5 (0.7)	0.9 (0.3)
Group III	Mean (SD)	20.9 (14.9)*	2.4 (1.1)	2.4 (3.2)
Nontolerized	Mean (SD)	45.6 (8.3)	3.0 (1.6)	1.6 (0.6)

*p < 0.05; **p < 0.01.

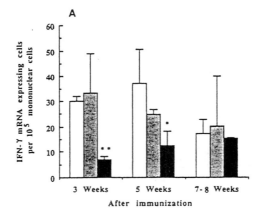

FIGURE 4. Numbers of AChR-reactive IFN-γ (A), IL-4 (B), and TGF-β (C) mRNA-expressing cells per 10^5 MNC in popliteal and inguinal lymph nodes of different animal groups. Rats were killed 3, 5, and 7-8 weeks postimmunization. Symbols refer to mean values, and bars refer to SD. Asterisks refer to p values; p < 0.05(*) or p < 0.01(**). □ unfed rats; ▨, STI-fed rats; ■, AchR + STI-fed rats.

through clonal anergy.[6] The CD8+ T cells in active suppression are generated after being triggered by the oral tolerogen and suppress the activities of other immune cells both *in vitro* and *in vivo* through secretion of the immunosuppressive cytokine TGF-β.[9] The up-regulation of AChR-reactive TGF-β mRNA-expressing cells in lymphoid organs of rats orally or nasally tolerized to EAMG are in line with those observations. Our method of suppressing EAMG by means of oral or nasal administration of AChR will allow further studies of the underlying B- and T-cell responses in this model of tolerance against EAMG, in particular the cytokines produced by T and non-T cells.

This study demonstrates that EAMG in Lewis rats is associated with elevated levels of cells in lymphoid organs expressing IFN-γ, IL-4, and TGF-β mRNA in response to the disease-related autoantigen AChR when compared with CFA-injected control rats, showing that both Th1- and Th2-like cells producing IFN-γ and IL-4, respectively, are

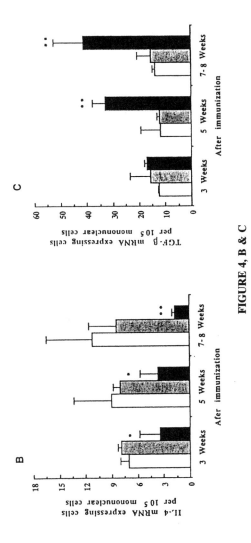

FIGURE 4, B & C

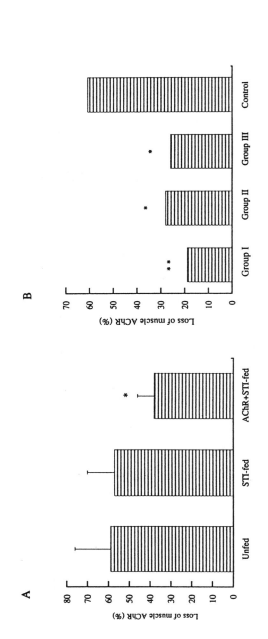

FIGURE 5. Loss of rat muscle AChR contents. The muscle carcasses from orally (**A**) and nasally (**B**) tolerized and control EAMG rats were examined for AChR content by RIA. Symbols refer to mean values. Asterisks refer to p values < 0.05 (*) or < 0.01 (**).

most probably involved in the induction of EAMG. Even though EAMG is also associated with elevated numbers of AChR-reactive TGF-β-mRNA expressing cells, oral or nasal tolerization with different concentrations of AChR induced a further increase in the levels of cells expressing this cytokine, whereas the numbers of cells expressing IFN-γ and IL-4 were reduced. Moreover, correlation analyses revealed that the suppression of IFN-γ and IL-4 as well as the decreased amount of muscle AChR loss in rats orally or nasally tolerant to EAMG was related to the up-regulation of TGF-β.

It has been implicated that IFN-γ secreted at the target for autoaggressive immunity is important for the pathogenesis of the tissue damage in EAE, which can be induced in susceptible animal species and strains by immunization with myelin proteins, like myelin basic protein (MBP) together with CFA, and which represents an animal model for multiple sclerosis.[10,11] Even human MG is related to high levels of AChR-reactive IFN-γ-secreting cells and AChR-reactive IFN-γ mRNA-expressing cells in peripheral blood.[8,12] Injections of recombinant IFN-γ into the eye and spinal cord cause a transient inflammatory response,[10,13] and patients undergoing therapy with IFN-γ may develop various autoimmune syndromes and an exacerbation of previously latent autoimmunity.[14] Gu *et al.* recently reported that ε-IFN-γ-transgenic mice, which produce IFN-γ within the neuromuscular junction, exhibited clinical muscle weakness and functional disruption of the neuromuscular junction. The results suggested that expression of IFN-γ at motor end plates provokes an autoimmune humoral response, thus linking the expression of IFN-γ with the development of EAMG.[15] IFN-γ has multiple effects, such as the induction of MHC class II antigen expression,[16] B-cell maturation,[17] and up-regulation of other cytokines like tumor necrosis factor-α (TNF-α) and interleukin-1 (IL-1).[18] Even though only low numbers of MNC have been found in association with neuromuscular junctions in striated muscles from MG patients,[19] such MNC may still be important for the induction of damage of AChR by the local secretion of IFN-γ and other cytokines. The high levels of AChR-reactive IFN-γ mRNA-expressing cells noticed in lymphoid organs in EAMG clearly implicate that AChR-responsive Th1-like cells have relevance for the development of EAMG. By contrast, orally and nasally tolerized rats showed a significant suppression of this Th1-like cell response to AChR in some lymphoid organs. This decrease of target antigen-reactive Th1-like cells producing and secreting IFN-γ could be pivotal for the suppression of EAMG.

It is well known that anti-AChR antibodies play an important role in the pathogenesis of MG and EAMG. The Th2-related IL-4 is necessary for antibody synthesis and class switches.[20] Our nontolerized EAMG rats had high levels of AChR-reactive IL-4 mRNA-expressing cells in certain lymphoid organs, compared to CFA-injected control rats. This observation is consistent with findings in human MG of elevated numbers of AChR-reactive IL-4 mRNA expressing MNC in peripheral blood[8,21] and implicates that IL-4 is involved in the development of both EAMG and MG. Here we report that the levels of AChR-reactive IL-4 mRNA-expressing cells were lower in some lymphoid organs of rats orally and nasally tolerized to EAMG when compared to nontolerized EAMG rats. This complies with the decreased concentrations of anti-AChR antibodies in serum from orally and nasally tolerized rats. These observations imply that induction of tolerance to EAMG by oral or nasal administration with AChR might partly be a result of down-regulation of AChR-reactive IL-4 producing TH2 cells.

TGF-β is an important endogenous immunoregulatory, mainly immunosuppressive cytokine[22] that suppresses B-cell proliferation and immunoglobulin (IgG and IgM) secretion,[23] down-regulates production of IFN-γ and IL-4,[24] antagonizes TNF-α function,[25] inhibits the development of autoantigen-specific T cells,[26] down-regulates MHC class II molecule expression and further counteracts the up-regulatory effects on MHC molecules by other cytokines,[27] and interferes with the adhesion of lymphoid cells to blood-vessel endothelia.[28] MG patients treated with thymectomy to induce disease remission showed

TABLE 4. Mean Numbers of AChR-reactive IFN-γ, IL-4, and TGF-β mRNA-expressing Cells per 10^5 MNC Isolated from Different Lymphoid Organs of Rats Tolerized to EAMG by Nasal Administration of Different Concentrations (Group I, II, and III) of AChR, from Nontolerized EAMG Control Postimmunization Rats with AChR plus CFA, and from Nontolerized Control Rats Receiving PBS Nasally and Injected with CFA Only

| Lymphoid Organs | | Rats Nasally Tolerized to EAMG and Immunized with AChR plus CFA | | | | | | | | | Nontolerized EAMG Control Rats | | | Nontolerized Control Rats Receiving PBS Nasally and Injected with CFA Only | | |
| | | Group I | | | Group II | | | Group III | | | | | | | | |
		IFN-γ	IL-4	TGF-β	IFN-γ	IL-4	TGF-β	IFN-γ	IL-4	TGF-β	IFN-γ	IL-4	TGF-β	IFN-γ	IL-4	TGF-β
PILN	Mean	7.5*	2.5*	23.0*	7.3*	5.0	19.0*	7.5*	5.0	19.3	16.4	7.6	8.4	3.2	2.8	4.0
	SD	3.4	1.7	7.4	2.9	2.9	5.9	4.4	2.9	12.1	5.9	2.7	4.2	2.3	3.0	2.4
Spleen	Mean	8.3	4.0	14.8*	4.3*	3.5	11.0*	4.8*	4.3	13.8	11.2	4.4	6.0	3.5	2.2	3.6
	SD	4.3	2.9	5.4	2.6	2.4	3.4	3.1	2.7	6.7	5.1	3.5	2.6	3.0	2.1	2.0
Thymus	Mean	4.8	3.4	11.8	6.9	2.5	8.0	6.1	3.1	10.5	6.6	3.8	4.6	2.4	2.6	1.8
	SD	3.1	2.5	3.3	3.6	2.4	4.1	2.5	2.6	4.8	3.9	3.4	3.8	0.6	1.3	2.0
SCLN	Mean	6.6	6.9	18.0*	5.4	6.4	12.8	6.5	4.1	15.2	5.5	5.6	7.3	5.3	2.1	4.5
	SD	4.6	3.5	6.1	3.1	2.9	4.4	5.1	2.1	7.7	3.2	3.8	3.0	3.9	2.1	3.1

[a] Asterisk refers to p values < 0.05 when results between nasally tolerized rats and nontolerized EAMG control rats were compared. PILN, popliteal and inguinal lymph nodes. SCLN, superficial cervical lymph nodes. SD, standard deviation.

higher numbers of AChR-reactive TGF-β mRNA expressing MNC in peripheral blood,[29] whereas recombinant TGF-β at a concentration of 1 femtogram/200 μL of blood MNC culture suppressed AChR-reactive mRNA expression for the proinflammatory cytokines IFN-γ, IL-4, IL-6, TNF-α, TNF-β, and perforin but not for the endogenously produced immunosuppressive cytokine IL-10 or for TGF-β itself.[30] In the present study, levels of AChR-reactive TGF-β mRNA-expressing cells in certain lymphoid organs were higher in orally and nasally tolerized rats than in nontolerized rats, and the losses of muscle AChR were lower in mucosally tolerized rats and correlated negatively with the numbers of TGF-β mRNA-expressing cells in some lymphoid organs. Taken together, these results clearly point to an important role for TGF-β in determining the outcome of EAMG and MG. It seems appropriate to assume that the down-regulation of IFN-γ and IL-4 as well as the decreased muscle AChR losses are the result of the up-regulation of TGF-β. As in oral tolerance to EAE, active suppression could be the main mechanism for oral and nasal tolerance to EAMG achieved with different concentrations of AChR in our animal models.

The profile of cytokines involved in an immune response can be assumed to determine the clinical outcome of autoimmune diseases. When transferring the observations from oral and nasal tolerance induction against EAMG to human MG, it is obvious that both IFN-γ and IL-4 have a central role in the development of disease, whereas TGF-β most probably down-regulates both EAMG and MG. Specific immunotherapies based on autoantigen immunodominance and restricted T cell-receptor usage become, for many reasons, increasingly less promising as future treatments of human autoimmune diseases. Instead, new therapeutic measures should be possible to identify, based on their influence of the relationship between proinflammatory and immunosuppressive cytokines, as shown here for nasal tolerance against EAMG.

Induction of tolerance is a highly attractive therapy because of its natural and powerful immunosuppression. Compared with oral tolerance, nasal tolerance against EAMG has advantages in the sense that it requires much smaller doses of AChR, is more convenient to induce, and does not require STI, which is used to inhibit the degradation of AChR in the gastrointestinal tract. Pilot clinical trials of oral tolerance in multiple sclerosis, rheumatoid arthritis, and uveoretinitis have demonstrated positive clinical effects with no apparent toxicity and with accompaning decreases in T-cell autoreactivity.[6] These two approaches should also be feasible in MG, and the nasal administration of the autoantigen could be advantageous.

SUMMARY

Oral and nasal administration of nicotinic acetylcholine receptor (AChR) to Lewis rats prior to myasthenogenic immunization with AChR and complete Freund's adjuvant (CFA) resulted in prevention or marked decrease of the severity of experimental autoimmune myasthenia gravis (EAMG) and suppression of AChR-specific B-cell responses and of AChR-reactive T-cell function. To examine the involvement of immunoregulatory cytokines and the underlying mechanisms involved in tolerance induction, *in situ* hybridization with radiolabeled cDNA oligonucleotide probes was adopted to enumerate mononuclear cells (MNC) expressing mRNA for the proinflammatory cytokine interferon-γ (IFN-γ), the B cell-stimulating interleukin-4 (IL-4), and the immunosuppressive transforming growth factor-β (TGF-β). Popliteal and inguinal lymph nodes from EAMG rats contained elevated numbers of AChR-reactive IFN-γ, IL-4, and TGF-β mRNA-expressing cells, compared to control rats receiving PBS orally or nasally and injected with CFA only. Oral and nasal tolerance was accompanied by decreased numbers of AChR-reactive IFN-γ and IL-4 mRNA-expressing cells and strong up-regulation of TGF-β mRNA-positive cells in lymphoid organs when compared to nontolerized EAMG control rats. The results suggest that IFN-γ and IL-4 are central effector molecules in the development of EAMG and that TGF-β plays an important role in tolerance induction to EAMG.

REFERENCES

1. LINDSTROM, J., D. SHELTON & Y. FUJII. 1988. Myasthenia gravis. Adv. Immunol. **42:** 233.
2. DRACHMAN, D. B. 1994. Myasthenia gravis. N. Engl. J. Med. **330:** 1797.
3. HOHLFELD, R., I. KALIES, B. KOHLEISEN, K. HEININGER, B. CONTI-TRONCONI & K. V. TOYKA. 1986. Myasthenia gravis: stimulation of antireceptor autoantibodies by autoreactive T cell lines. Neurology **36:** 618.
4. BACH, J. F. 1993. Immunosuppressive therapy of autoimmune diseases. Immunol. Today **14:** 322.
5. DRACHMAN, D. B., K. R. McINTOSH, S. DE SILVA, R. W. KUNCL & C. KAHN. 1988. Strategies for the treatment of myasthenia gravis. Ann. N.Y. Acad. Sci. **540:** 176-186.
6. WEINER, H. L., A. FRIEDMAN, A. MILLER, S. J. KHOURY, A. AL-SABBAGH, L. SANTOS, M. SAYEGH, R. B. NUSSENBLATT, D. A. TRENTHAM & D. A. HAFLER. 1994. Oral tolerance: Immunologic mechanisms and treatment of murine and human organ specific autoimmune diseases by oral administration of autoantigens. Annu. Rev. Immunol. **12:** 809.
7. DICK, A. D., Y. F. CHENG, A. McKINNON, J. LIVERSIDGE & J. V. FORRESTER. 1993. Nasal administration of retinal antigens suppresses the inflammatory response in experimental allergic uveoretinitis. A preliminary report of intranasal induction of tolerance with retinal antigens. Br. J. Ophthalmol. **77:** 171.
8. LINK, J., M. SÖDERSTRÖM, A. LJUNGDAHL, B. HÖJEBERG, T. OLSSON, Z. XU, S. FREDRIKSON, Z. Y. WANG & H. LINK. 1994. Organ-specific autoantigans induce IFN-γ and IL-4 mRNA expression in mononuclear cells in multiple sclerosis and myasthenia gravis. Neurology **44:** 728.
9. MILLER, A., O. LIDER, A. B. ROBERTS, M. B. SPRON & H. L. WEINER. 1992. Suppressor T cells generated by oral tolerization to myelin basic protein suppress both *in vitro* and *in vivo* immune responses by the release of transforming growth factor β following antigen-specific triggering. Proc. Natl. Acad. Sci. USA **89:** 421.
10. SIMMONS, R. D. & D. O. WILLENBORG. 1990. Direct injection of cytokines into the spinal cord causes autoimmune encephalomyelitis-like inflammation. J. Neurol. Sci. **100:** 37.
11. MUSTAFA, M. I., P. DIENER, B. HÖJEBERG, P. VAN DER MEIDE & T. OLSSON. 1991. T cell immunity and interferon-γ secretion during experimental allergic encephalomyelitis in Lewis rats. J. Neuroimmunol. **31:** 165.
12. LINK, H., O. OLSSON, J. B. SUN, W. Z. WANG, G. ANDERSSON, H. P. EKRE, T. BRENNER, O. ABRAMSKY & T. OLSSON. 1991. Acetylcholine receptor-reactive T and B cells in myasthenia gravis and controls. J. Clin. Invest. **87:** 2191.
13. HAMEL, C. P., B. DETRICK & J. J. HOOKS. 1990. Evaluation of Ia expression in rat ovular tissues following inoculation with interferon-gamma. Exp. Eye Res. **50:** 173.
14. SCHATTNER, A. 1994. Lymphokines in autoimmunity—a critical review. Clin. Immunol. Immunopathol. **70:** 177.
15. GU, D., L. WOGENSEN, N. A. CALCUTT, G. XIA, S. ZHU, J. P. MERLIE, H. S. FOX, J. LINDSTROM, H. C. POWELL & N. SARVETNICK. 1995. Myasthenia gravis-like syndrome induced by expression of interferon γ in the neuromuscular junction. J. Exp. Med. **181:** 547.
16. SKOSKIEWICZ, M. H., R. B. CALLIN, E. E. STERNBERGER & P. S. RUSSEL. 1985. Widespread and selective induction of major histocompatibility complex determined antigens *in vivo* by γ interferon. J. Exp. Med. **162:** 1645.
17. SIDMAN, C. L., J. D. MAXWELL, L. D. SCHULTZ, W. P. GRAY & H. M. JOHNSON. 1984. γ-Interferon is one of several direct B cell-maturing lymphokines. Nature **309:** 801.
18. COLLART, M. A., J. BELIN, D. VASSALLI, S. DE KOSSODO & P. VASSALLI. 1986. Gamma-interferon enhances macrophage transcription of the tumor necrosis factor/cachectin,

interleukin-1, and urokinase genes, which are controlled by short-lived repressors. J. Exp. Med. **164:** 2113.

19. NAKANO, S. & A. G. ENGEL. 1993. Myasthenia gravis: quantitative immunocytochemical analysis of inflammatory cells and detection of complement membrane attack complex at the end-plate in 30 patients. Neurology **43:** 1167.
20. FINKELMAN, F. D. & J. HOLMES. 1990. Lymphokine control of *in vivo* immunoglobulin isotype selection. Annu. Rev. Immunol. **8:** 303.
21. LINK, J., V. NAVIKAS, M. YU, S. FREDRIKSON, P. O. OSTERMAN & H. LINK. 1994. Augmented interferon-γ, interleukin-4 and transforming growth factor-β mRNA expression in blood mononuclear cells in myasthenia gravis. J. Neuroimmunol. **51:** 185.
22. SASAKI, H., R. B. POLLARD, D. SCHMITT & F. SUZUKI. 1992. Transforming growth factor-β in the regulation of the immune response. Clin. Immunol. Immunopathol. **65:** 1.
23. KEHRL, J. H., C. THEVENIN, P. RIECKMANN & A. S. FAUCI. 1991. Transforming growth factor-β suppresses human B lymphocyte Ig production by inhibiting synthesis and the switch from the membrane form to the secreted form of Ig mRNA. J. Immunol. **146:** 4016.
24. KEHRL, J. H., L. D. WAKEFIELD, A. B. ROBERTS, S. JAKOWLEW, M. ALVAREZ-MON, R. DERYNCK, M. B. SPORN & A. S. FAUCI. 986. Production of transforming growth factor β by human T lymphocytes and its potential role in the regulation of T cell growth. J. Exp. Med. **163:** 1037.
25. STEVENS, D. B., K. E. GOULD & R. H. SWANBORG. 1994. Transforming growth factor-β1 inhibits tumor necrosis factor-α/lymphotoxin production and adoptive transfer of disease by effector cells of autoimmune encephalomyelitis. J. Neuroimmunol. **51:** 77.
26. KIM, K. J., J. ABRAMS & M. ALPHONSO. 1990. Role of endogenously produced interleukin-6 as a second signal in murine thymocyte proliferation induced by multiple cytokines: regulatory effects of transforming growth factor-β1. Cell. Immunol. **131:** 261.
27. CZARNIECKI, C. W., H. H. CHIU, G. W. WONG, S. M. McCABE & M. A. PALLADINO. 1988. Transforming growth factor-β1 modulates the expression of class II histocompatibility antigens on human cells. J. Immunol. **140:** 4217.
28. GAMBLE, J. R. & M. A. VADAS. 1991. Endothelial cell adhesiveness for human T lymphocytes is inhibited by transforming growth factor-β. J. Immunol. **146:** 1149.
29. LINK, J., S. FREDRIKSON, M. SÖDERSTRÖM, T. OLSSON, B. HÖJEBERG, Å. LJUNGDAHL & H. LINK. 1994. Organ-specific autoantigens induce transforming growth factor-β mRNA expression in mononuclear cells in multiple sclerosis and myasthenia gravis. Ann. Neurol. **35:** 197.
30. LINK, J., B. HE, V. NAVIKAS, W. PALASIK, S. FREDRISKON, M. SÖDERSTRÖM & H. LINK. 1995. TGF-β1 suppresses autoantigen-induced expression of proinflammatory cytokines but not IL-10 in multiple sclerosis and myasthenia gravis. J. Neuroimmunol. **58:** 21.

Antigen-presenting Function of the Mouse CD1 Molecule[a]

SHABNAM TANGRI,[b] HILDA R. HOLCOMBE,[b]
A. RAUL CASTAÑO,[c] JEFFREY E. MILLER,[d]
MICHAEL TEITELL,[e] WILLIAM E. HUSE,[d]
PER A. PETERSON,[c] AND
MITCHELL KRONENBERG [b]

[b]Department of Microbiology and Immunology
and
Molecular Biology Institute
University of California, Los Angeles
405 Hilgard Avenue
Los Angeles, California 90095-1570

[c]R. W. Johnson Research Institute
La Jolla, California 92037

[d]Ixsys Corporation
La Jolla, California 92037

[e]Department of Pathology
Brigham and Women's Hospital
Boston, Massachusetts 02215

INTRODUCTION

CD1 molecules were first identified as cell-surface molecules expressed by human thymocytes.[1] Like the thymus-leukemia (TL) antigen expressed by mouse thymocytes, CD1 molecules were found to be coexpressed with β2 microglobulin (β2m) and to be relatively nonpolymorphic. It was therefore speculated that CD1 might be the homologue of the mouse TL antigen. In 1986, the group of Cesar Milstein reported the first isolation of a gene encoding a CD1 molecule.[2] The translated nucleotide sequence revealed that unlike the TL antigen, CD1 is only distantly related to classical class I molecules with no statistically significant sequence similarity in the α1 and α2 domains that encode the peptide antigen-binding site. Therefore, although the TL antigen and human CD1 might be functional homologues, they clearly are not structural homologues.

CD1 genes and molecules have been discovered subsequently in a number of species including mice, rats, and rabbits.[3] In humans there are five closely linked CD1 genes encoded on chromosome 1, unlinked to the major histocompatibility complex (MHC). Four of these genes, CD1a, CD1b, CD1c, and CD1d, are known to encode cell-surface

[a]This work was supported by NIH Grants R01 CA52511 (M. Kronenberg), K11 AI01213 (H. R. Holcombe), and T32 GM 08042 (M. Teitell); Grants from the Jonsson Cancer Center Foundation and the Jaye Haddad Foundation (S. Tangri); and by a Fellowship from the Ministeno de Educacion y Ciencia of Spain (A. R. Castaño)

proteins.[4] Although all of the human CD1 genes share distinct sequence features that distinguish them from other class I genes, they are not particularly closely related to one another. For example, the human CD1d protein, which is the most divergent human CD1 molecule, shares no more than 37-40% sequence similarity in the $\alpha1$ and $\alpha2$ domains to the other human CD1 molecules. In addition, each human CD1 molecule has a distinct pattern of expression. As a group, CD1 molecules are expressed on a limited number of cell types that seem to have an antigen-presenting function. CD1a is expressed by Langerhans' cells in the skin,[5] and CD1d is expressed by intestinal epithelial cells.[6]

The mouse has two closely related CD1 genes, CD1.1 and CD1.2. These two are most similar in sequence to human CD1d.[2,3] As in the human, the mouse CD1 (mCD1) genes are encoded outside of the MHC located on mouse chromosome 3. The two CD1 genes in mice are closely linked and are presumed to have derived from a relatively recent gene duplication. mCD1 molecules are expressed by both small and large intestine epithelial cells.[6] Using immunohistochemistry, some mCD1 expression also is detectable in lymph node and thymus. As in the mouse, the only known rat CD1 gene is CD1d-like,[7] and the rat CD1 mRNA also is expressed in the intestine.[7] Similarly, one of the two known rabbit CD1 genes, CtrbCD1, is a CD1d homologue.[8] CD1d, therefore, is the only nonclassical class I molecule known to have been conserved throughout much of mammalian evolution.

It is thought that CD1 molecules are likely to have a specialized antigen-presenting function. Despite this, prior to the work reported in reference 9 and in this manuscript, there was no evidence for antigen presentation by mCD1. By contrast, T cells reactive to each of the four human CD1 molecules have been reported.[10-13] Evidence from several laboratories indicates that antigen presentation by CD1 is distinct from MHC-encoded molecules. First, most of the T cells reactive with human CD1 are CD4, CD8 double negative,[10] although there are some exceptions.[14] The CD1-reactive T cells express either $\alpha\beta$ or $\gamma\delta$ T-cell antigen receptors (TCRs). Second, CD1b transfectants of T2 cells can present a mycobacterial antigen to reactive T cells.[10] Because T2 cells are defective for both TAP (transporter associated with antigen processing) subunits and the LMP2 and LMP7 proteins, which are MHC-encoded subunits of the proteosome, this demonstrates that the pathway for antigen processing and presentation by human CD1b is distinct from that of MHC class I. Consistent with this, CD1b-mediated presentation of the mycobacterial antigen was inhibitable by chloroquine,[10] suggesting that endosomal acidification is necessary for presentation. The processing and presentation pathway must also be different from the MHC class II pathway, as T2 cells lack the DM molecule that is required for efficient peptide loading of class II molecules.[15] Third, Beckman and co-workers[16] have recently demonstrated that the mycobacterial antigen presented to a CD1b-restricted T-cell clone is mycolic acid, a bacterial lipid.

There are several reasons why the antigen-presenting function of CD1 molecules might be relevant for investigators interested in oral tolerance. First, CD1 molecules are expressed in a TAP-independent fashion,[17] and they may traffic to an endosomal compartment. If this were true, they might be capable of "sampling" antigens from the lumen of the gut. Third, because they are not polymorphic, they could prove to be useful targets for any specific immunotherapy directed to an antigen-presenting molecule. In this chapter, we present our recent data demonstrating that mCD1 also has a distinct non-class I, non-class II antigen-presenting function. We define one type of antigen that can bind to mCD1, and we characterize the first peptide-specific and mCD1-restricted T cells.

DEFINITION OF PEPTIDES THAT BIND TO mCD1

We initially made stable mCD1 transfectants in TAP-deficient RMA-S cells, in the hope that these transfectants would prove to be useful in the definition of mCD1-binding peptides. Classical class I molecules, which are not loaded with peptide in RMA-S cells, can reach the cell surface when these TAP-deficient cells are cultured at 23°C. When the culture temperature is raised to 37°C, however, the empty molecules become unstable and they denature.[18] If peptide capable of binding the class I molecule is added prior to the shift to 37°C, the class I molecules are stabilized. A heat stabilization assay, therefore, can be used to screen for peptides capable of class I binding. When mCD1 transfectants of RMA-S were tested in this way, however, we were surprised to find that equally high levels of surface expression of mCD1 were obtained in 23°C and 37°C cultures.[19] We also tested *Drosophila melanogaster* cells, which are presumed to have a broader defect in peptide loading than the TAP-2-deficient RMA-S cells. Transfected *D. melanogaster* cells synthesize empty classical class I molecules that are thermally unstable.[19] Stable mCD1 transfectants of *D. melanogaster* embryo cells showed equal levels of mCD1 surface expression when cultured at the normal temperature of 23°C or following a two-hour shift to either 33°C or 37°C. We, therefore, conclude that the mCD1 surface expression is TAP independent.

In an attempt to identify the possible peptide-binding ability of mCD1, recombinant soluble CD1-β2m complexes produced in *D. melanogaster* cells were used to screen a random peptide phage-display library (RPPDL). The phage-display library was generated by cloning oligonucleotides encoding random 22 amino acid sequences into the mature NH2 terminus of the gene VIII coat protein. When this library was screened with soluble and presumably empty mCD1 molecules derived from insect cells, 47 different clones were selected by mCD1 binding. Alignment of the amino-terminal sequences encoded by these phages shows a well-defined core motif consisting of an aromatic Phe or Trp amino acid at position one (100% of the clones), an amino acid with a long, aliphatic side chain at position four (38/47), and a Trp at position seven (35/47). Therefore, mCD1 seems to select phages with a hydrophobic binding motif, preferring aromatic residues at positions one and seven and aliphatic residues at position four. The sequence motifs obtained by screening RPPDL with classical class I molecules are characterized by an anchor amino acid in fixed positions relative to the N terminus,[20] consistent with the binding of the N terminus buried in a conserved pocket.[21] This is not, however, a characteristic shared by the mCD1 motif; the N terminus of the mCD1-selected peptides is at a variable distance from the anchor binding motif, suggesting that mCD1, like class II molecules, is capable of binding peptides with extended N and C termini. The K_d determined for peptide binding to mCD1 is in the range of an intermediate to good binder for class I molecules and in the range of naturally processed peptides copurified with class II molecules.[21]

It was possible that the synthetic peptides bind to some portion of the mCD1 molecule other than the putative peptide binding groove formed by the α1 and α2 domains. To begin to assess the immunologic relevance of the biochemical data on peptide binding, we raised several peptide-specific and mCD1-restricted T-cell lines. Most of these mCD1-reactive T-cell lines were generated from lymph nodes of mice immunized with mCD1 transfectants of the RMA-S cell line that had been preloaded with peptide p99a-2.12 (EHF̲HH̲IR̲EWGNHWK); the putative anchor amino acids for mCD1 binding are underlined. The reactive T cells require both mCD1 and peptide for stimulation, as measured by γ-interferon synthesis, as shown in TABLE 1. Three different mCD1 transfectants, RMA-S T cells, L-cell fibroblasts, and J774 macrophages stimulated the T cells in the presence of peptide, indicating independence of any other MHC molecule for T-cell stimulation.

Using a variety of synthetic peptides, we found that there was a reasonably good correlation between the ability of a synthetic peptide to bind to soluble mCD1 and its ability to stimulate mCD1-restricted T cells *in vitro,* confirming the importance of the putative anchor amino acids and their relevance for antigen presentation. For example, single substitutions of each of the anchor residues with alanine reduced the peptide binding

TABLE 1. Peptide plus CD1 Are Recognized by T Cells as Assayed by IFNγ Production[a]

Interferon-γ Production (U/mL)	
(a) RMAS CD1[+] and peptide	25.2
(b) J774 CD1[+] and peptide	17.4
(c) J774 (no peptide)	1.1

[a] Table shows IFNγ produced by T cells when stimulated with either RMAS CD1[+] cells pulsed with peptide (a), J774 CD1[+] cells pulsed with peptide (b), or with peptide alone (c).

to mCD1 drastically, and these peptides could not effectively stimulate the peptide-specific, mCD1-restricted T cells. To rule out the possibility that stabilization of the mCD1 molecule by peptide is responsible for T-cell stimulation, we tested two peptides that had the same anchor amino acids for binding to mCD1 but differed in the probable T-cell binding sites. Even though these two peptides had the same binding constant to mCD1 as the original peptide, both of them were unable to stimulate the T cells. These data argue against the possibility that any mCD1-binding peptide causes a conformational change in mCD1 that can be sensed by the reactive TCR. Instead, they are most consistent with a more conventional model in which some amino acid side chains contribute to mCD1 binding, and others side chains point towards the TCR for recognition by specific clones.

Because we have shown that peptides up to 22 amino acids long, or longer, might bind to mCD1 *in vitro*, it was necessary to show that no further trimming of these peptides to the more typical 8-9 amino acid size was occurring. In order to do this, we used purified mCD1 molecules to eliminate the possibility of any intracellular peptide-antigen processing or trimming. Plates were coated with soluble mCD1 on 96-well plates. Some of the wells were incubated with appropriate antigenic peptide, mCD1-reactive cells were added to the cultures, and the production of γ-interferon was measured by ELISA. We demonstrated that the cell-free mCD1-stimulation system was reasonably effective when the correct peptide was present; plates coated with mCD1 molecules in the absence of peptide did not stimulate γ-interferon release. Studies using serum-free medium showed that proteases in serum are not required for extracellular processing of long peptides that are presented by mCD1.

We have carried out a preliminary phenotypic characterization of the T cells reactive to mCD1. Flow-cytometric analysis of the T cells in a line raised to the peptide p99a.-2.12 demonstrated that nearly all the cells express an αβ TCR and the CD8 molecule (FIGURES 1A and 1B). These data demonstrate that the mCD1-reactive T cells can have a conventional phenotype for class I-reactive cells from the lymph node, in contrast to the CD1-reactive cells from the human peripheral blood that tend to be either TCR αβ[+] and double negative, or TCR γδ[+].

A MODEL FOR INTRACELLULAR TRAFFICKING OF mCD1

We propose a model for intracellular trafficking of mCD1 based on the following. (1) Expression of mouse and human CD1 molecules is TAP independent.[11,19] (2) mCD1 molecules, as well as some CD1 molecules in other species, have an endosomal localization signal in their intracytoplasmic tail.[22] For example, mCD1 has the sequence YQDI in its

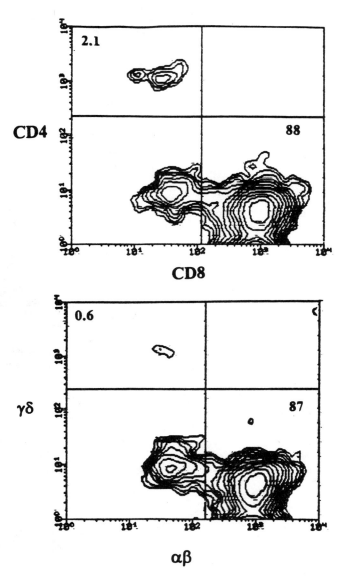

FIGURE 1. Flow cytometric analysis of a CD1-reactive T-cell line. Top: Staining of the cells with anti-CD4 (phycoerythrin, PE) and anti-CD8 (fluorescein isothiocyanate, FITC) antibodies. Bottom: Staining of the T-cell line with anti-γδ TCR (PE) and anti-αβ TCR (FITC).

intracytoplasmic domain. (3) Preliminary data indicate that the mCD1 molecules produced by *D. melanogaster* cells are free of peptide. (4) Mycobacterial antigen presentation by CD1b requires acidified endosomes.[11] Based on these facts, we hypothesize that assembly of CD1-class heavy chain and β_2m is sufficient to release the complex from binding to calnexin or any similar chaperons, and that the heavy-chain/β_2m complex makes its way to an acidified vesicular compartment where it will contact antigens present in this compartment.

DISCUSSION

The results described above clearly establish that mCD1 can present a distinct set of peptides to CD8+, cytotoxic T cells. A number of important questions remain unanswered. First, what are the natural ligands presented by mCD1? A search of protein-sequence databases indicates that the mCD1-binding motif is present in a great variety of proteins of both microbial and nonmicrobial origin. From this search, there is nothing to suggest why an antigen-presenting molecule that presents peptides with a WXXLXXW sequence motif, or similar sequences consistent with the motif, might be conserved through evolution. Because all CD1 molecules are related to one another, the finding of peptide binding by mCD1 and lipid binding by human CD1b is puzzling. There are several possibilities. First, all CD1 molecules might naturally be lipid binding, and peptides were obtained for mCD1 only because a peptide display library was screened. The attractive feature of this model is that it can help to explain the relative lack of CD1 polymorphism.

Because lipids are the end product of a complex biosynthetic pathway, they may be presumed to change more slowly in evolution than the amino acids of antigenic peptides, many of which are likely to be nonessential from the viewpoint of function of that protein. In addition, bacterial lipids are distinct from those in eukaryotic cells, thereby allowing CD1 molecules to carry out a basic form of self/nonself description. Despite this conceptual appeal, the model requires that the hydrophobic mCD1 peptide-binding motif obtained from the bacteria phage display library is essentially a mimic for the natural lipid ligand. It is not known how the anchor amino acid side chains and the mycobacterial fatty acids would be capable of binding to the same peptide groove. A second model holds that CD1 molecules are selected primarily for their ability to traffic to a highly acidic late endosomal or lysosomal compartment where they might be capable of binding to hydrophobic ligands that are generated by antigen-processing enzymes there. These ligands could be either hydrophobic peptides, lipids, lipoproteins, or glycolipids. A third possibility is that there are at least two different categories of CD1 molecules. According to this view, CD1d-like molecules, which are distantly related to the others, present hydrophobic peptides, whereas molecules such as CD1b, which are not present in rodents, present lipids. It is interesting to note that the $\alpha 1$ and $\alpha 2$ domains of CD1b apparently are the most divergent in the CD1 family.[8]

A second major issue concerns the diversity and distribution of CD1-reactive T cells. It is unlikely that the synthetic peptide sequence p99.a-2.12 is uniquely capable of stimulating the generation of mCD1-restricted cells, although this remains to be formally proven by generating T lymphocytes specific for other mCD1-binding peptides. How might a diverse repertoire of mCD1-restricted T cells be generated? Are these cells thymus dependent? Do they require positive selection by mCD1, or by cross-reaction? Are they positively selected with another class I molecule? Are they all CD8 positive? Most important, from the point of view of this volume, what is the frequency and specificity of mCD1-restricted T cells in the intestine? In future experiments, we intend to determine if mCD1-restricted and peptide-reactive T lymphocytes can be detected in lamina propria and among intraepithelial lymphocytes following *in vivo* priming. If such cells exist in lamina propria, and if they are capable of recirculating from that site, then mCD1-restricted cells sensitized in the gut could, in part, be responsible for the induction of systemic oral tolerance. Finally, it is possible that mCD1 can acquire long peptides in the lumen of the gut for further processing to 9 amino acids and presentation by classical class I molecules. This would require escape from the endosome into a classical class I peptide-loading pathway, a process that is known to occur for some bacterial proteins.[23]

SUMMARY

CD1 molecules are distantly related to major histocompatibility complex (MHC)-encoded class I molecules, and they are coexpressed with β2 microglobulin (β2m). In the mouse, CD1 is expressed by intestinal epithelial cells and also by some cells in spleen and lymph node. We have shown that surface expression of mouse CD1 (mCD1) is not dependent upon a functional transporter associated with antigen processing (TAP). This, and other data, suggest that mCD1 may acquire peptides in an intracellular compartment other than the endoplasmic reticulum, where classical class I molecules bind peptide. mCD1 molecules also are distinct from classical class I molecules with regard to the types of peptides that they bind. We have demonstrated that mCD1 molecules preferentially bind peptides much longer than the 8-9 amino acids typical of the peptides that bind to classical class I molecules. The sequence motif for mCD1 peptide binding is characterized by the presence of bulky and hydrophobic amino acid side chains. We have generated mCD1-restricted and peptide-specific T-cell lines, thereby demonstrating the immunologic relevance of peptide binding to mCD1. The reactive T cells are TCR αβ+ and CD8+, a phenotype typical of many lymphocytes in both lymph node and intestinal mucosae. We speculate that mCD1 molecules may be capable of sampling peptides from the gut lumen and presenting them to mucosal T lymphocytes. In this way, they may function in the maintenance of normal mucosal immune homeostasis, and perhaps also in the induction of systemic tolerance to antigens delivered by the oral route.

In summary, CD1 molecules are a novel category of antigen-presenting molecules that have features in common with class I molecules, features in common with class II, and properties distinct from either subset of antigen-presenting molecules. Further studies of the antigen-presenting function of these molecules are certain to yield new insight into immune regulation and perhaps also into the mechanism of oral tolerance.

ACKNOWLEDGMENTS

We thank Mr. David Ng for help with preparation of the manuscript and the Jonsson Cancer Center Flow Cytometry Core Facility for assistance with flow cytometric analysis.

REFERENCES

1. McMichael, A. J., J. R. Pilch, G. Galfre, D. Y. Mason, J. W. Fabre & C. Milstein. 1979. A human thymocyte antigen defined by a hybrid myeloma monoclonal antibody. Eur. J. Immunol. 9: 205-210.
2. Calabi, F. & C. Milstein. 1986. A novel family of human major histocompatibility complex-related genes not mapping to chromosome 6. Nature 323: 540-543.
3. Bradbury, A., K. T. Belt, T. M. Neri, C. Milstein & F. Calabi. 1988. Mouse CD1 is distinct from and co-exists with TL in the same thymus. EMBO J. 7: 3081-3086.

4. BALK, S. P., P. A. BLEICHER & C. TERHORST. 1989. Isolation and characterization of a cDNA and gene coding for a fourth CD1 molecule. Proc. Natl. Acad. Sci. USA **86:** 252-256.

5. FITHIAN, E., P. KUNG, G. GOLDSTEIN, M. RUBENFELD, C. FENOGLIO & R. EDELSON. 1981. Reactivity of Langerhans cells with hybridoma antibody. Proc. Natl. Acad. Sci. USA **78:** 2541-2544.

6. BLEICHER, P. A., S. P. BALK, S. J. HAGEN, R. S. BLUMBERG, T. J. FLOTTE & C. TERHORST. 1990. Expression of murine CD1 on gastrointestinal epithelium. Science **250:** 679-682.

7. ICHIMIYA, S., K. KIKUCHI & A. MATSUURA. 1994. Structural analysis of the rat homologue of CD1. Evidence for evolutionary conservation of the CD1D class and widespread transcription by rat cells. J. Immunol. **153:** 1112-1123.

8. HUGHES, A. L. 1991. Evolutionary origin and diversification of the mammalian CD1 antigen genes. Mol. Biol. Evol. **8:** 185-201.

9. CASTAÑO, A. R., S. TANGRI, J. E. W. MILLER, H. HOLCOMBE, M. R. JACKSON, B. HUSE, M. KRONENBERG & P. A. PETERSON. 1995. Mouse CD1 is an antigen presenting molecule with novel peptide binding properties. Science. **269:** 223-226.

10. PORCELLI, S., C. T. MORITA & M. B. BRENNER. 1992. CD1b restricts the response of human CD4⁻8⁻ T lymphocytes to a microbial antigen. Nature **360:** 593-597.

11. PORCELLI, S., M. B. BRENNER, J. L. GREENSTEIN, S. P. BALK, C. TERHORST & P. A. BLEICHER. 1989. Recognition of cluster of differentiation 1 antigens by human CD4⁻CD8⁻ cytolytic T lymphocytes. Nature **341:** 447-450.

12. BALK, S. P., E. C. EBERT, R. L. BLUMENTHAL, F. V. MCDERMOTT, K. W. WUCHERPFENNIG, S. B. LANDAU & R. S. BLUMBERG. 1991. Oligoclonal expansion and CD1 recognition by human intestinal intraepithelial lymphocytes. Science **253:** 1411-1415.

13. FAURE, F., S. JITSUKAWA, C. MIOSSEC & T. HERCEND. 1990. CD1c as a target recognition structure for human T lymphocytes: analysis with peripheral blood gamma/delta cells. Eur. J. Immunol. **20:** 703-706.

14. PANJA, A., R. S. BLUMBERG, S. P. BALK & L. MAYER. 1993. CD1d is involved in T cell-intestinal epithelial cell interactions. J. Exp. Med. **178:** 1115-1119.

15. MORRIS, P., J. SHAMAN, M. ATTAYA, M. AMAYA, S. GOODMAN, C. BERGMAN, J. J. MONACO & E. MELLINS. 1992. An essential role for HLA-DM in antigen presentation by class II major histocompatibility molecules. Nature **360:** 593-597.

16. BECKMAN, E. M., S. A. PORCELLI, C. T. MORITA, S. M. BEHAR, S. T. FURLONG & M. B. BRENNER. 1994. Recognition of a lipid antigen by CD1-restricted alpha beta⁺ T cells. Nature **372:** 691-694.

17. HANAU, D., D. FRICKER, T. BIEBER, M. E. ESPOSITO-FARESE, H. BAUSINGER, J. P. CAZENAVE, L. DONATO, M. M. TONGIO & H. DE LA SALLE. 1994. CD1 expression is not affected by human peptide transporter deficiency. Hum. Immunol. **41:** 61-68.

18. LJUNGGREN, H. G., N. J. STAM, C. OHLEN, J. J. NEEFJES, P. HOGLUND, M. T. HEEMELS, J. BASTIN, T. N. SCHUMACHER, A. TOWNSEND & K. KARRE. 1990. Empty MHC class I molecules come out in the cold. Nature **346:** 476-480.

19. TEITELL, M., H. R. HOLCOMBE, M. J. JACKSON, L. POND, S. P. BALK, C. TERHORST & M. KRONENBERG. Nonclassical behavior on the mouse CD1 class I-like molecule. Submitted for publication.

20. MADDEN, D. R., J. C. GORGA, J. L. STROMINGER & D. C. WILEY. 1991. The structure of HLA-B27 reveals nonamer self-peptides bound in an extended conformation. Nature **353:** 321-325.

21. CHICZ, R. M., R. G. URBAN, W. S. LANE, J. C. GORGA, L. J. STERN, D. A. VIGNALI & J. L. STROMINGER. 1992. Predominant naturally processed peptides bound to HLA-

DR1 are derived from MHC-related molecules and are heterogeneous in size. Nature **358:** 764-768.

22. SANDOVAL, I. V. & O. BAKKE. 1994. Targeting of membrane proteins to endosomes and lysosomes. Trends Cell Biol. **4:** 292-296.

23. PFEIFER, J. D., M. J. WICK, R. L. ROBERTS, K. FINDLAY, S. J. NORMARK & C. V. HARDING. 1995. Phagocytic processing of bacterial antigens for class I MHC presentation to T cells. Nature **361:** 359-362.

Arthritis: Animal Models of Oral Tolerance[a]

N. A. STAINES, N. HARPER, F. J. WARD,
H. S. G. THOMPSON,[c] AND S. BANSAL[b]

Infection and Immunity Research Group
Division of Life Sciences
King's College London
Campden Hill Road
London W8 7AH, United Kingdom

[b]*Department of Pharmacy*
Division of Health Sciences
King's College London
Manresa Road, London W6, United Kingdom

INTRODUCTION

Four experimental arthritides have been investigated through the study of induced mucosal tolerance for the control of autoimmunity. The first report of the successful control of an autoimmune disease concerned a study from the author's group of collagen-induced arthritis (CIA) in rats in which the prior oral dosing with soluble-type II collagen (CII) suppressed the subsequent development of arthritis that would normally have followed from immunization with CII,[1] and similar results were published shortly afterwards by Thorbecke's group on the suppression of CIA in the mouse.[2] These experiments were done against a background of speculation that dietary antigens might influence the initiation or progression of autoimmune diseases.[3] However, until that time the speculation had not been matched by experiment. In common with the many other diseases discussed in this volume, CIA has been shown to be modified in many of its aspects by oral dosing with specific antigen (CII in this case); the parallel modification of disease symptoms and immune parameters has underlined the link between the modification of immunity through transmucosal encounter with antigen and the amelioration of inflammatory autoimmune lesions. The history of the subject, of course, established that mucosal immunization had systemic effects distinct from those that ensue from parenteral immunization, and more recent approaches, also described elsewhere in this book, have led to attempts to modify human autoimmune conditions by induced mucosal tolerance.

Aside from CIA in the rat and the mouse, it has been shown that adjuvant arthritis (AA) in the rat[4] and Pristane-induced arthritis (PIA) in the mouse[5] can be prevented by oral dosing with CII. These diseases have pathologies that bear some comparison to human rheumatoid arthritis (RA), but the extent to which they model RA itself is not so much the question that matters here. Rather, the question is, To what extent does their modification by oral dosing with CII predict what will happen in humans? Here we will review briefly

[a]We express our gratitude to the Arthritis and Rheumatism Council of Great Britain for their support of this work.

[c]Current address: Cantab Pharmaceuticals Research Ltd, Milton Road, Cambridge CB4 4GN, UK.

the studies of these diseases and will present new studies on the use of collagen peptides delivered nasally as a means to prevent CIA.

ON THE SUPPRESSION OF EXPERIMENTAL ARTHRITIS BY ORAL TOLERANCE

The common features of disease suppression in CIA, PIA, and AA are that inflammatory joint destruction is restrained by oral tolerance to CII.[1,2,4,5] The affected features that have been reported to be reduced include synovial hyperplasia, mononuclear infiltration, pannus formation, and cartilage and bone erosions. Immunologically, reduced proliferative T-cell responses to CII *in vitro* are the central feature that can account for the changes in joint pathology, known from many studies to be a function of T cells, and in antibody production, which, although not consistently affected, can show changes in the profile of anti-CII antibodies of different IgG subclasses, consistent with increased activation of Th2-type CD4+ cells and the relative suppression of Th1-type cells.[1,2,6] Thus in understanding the way in which oral tolerance can be applied to control arthritis, there is an emphasis on suppression of pathogenic Th1-CD4+ cells. Whether B cells are affected directly is uncertain, and the effects upon antibody responses could be ascribed to changes secondary to the modification of T-cell function in tolerant animals.

The induction of CIA in rats depends upon the dose of CII,[1,6] and in the WA/KIR/kcl rat (a Wistar Rt-1^u strain uniquely held in our laboratories) between 0.5 and 1.0 mg CII solubilized from pig laryngeal or bovine nasal septal cartilages will consistently induce disease in more than 95% of animals when injected in Freund's incomplete adjuvant (FIA) (FIG. 1a). The amount of CII required depends to some extent upon the batch of CII, but our experience of testing many different CII preparations, not all solubilized to precisely the same protocol, shows a remarkable consistency in arthritogenicity. In these studies, and in others that use CII to ameliorate arthritis,[2,3,5] one must question whether the CII preparations are not active because they are contaminated with arthritogenic minor collagens that are potential contaminants of CII prepared by acid-enzyme solubilization and fractional salt precipitation. Proteoglycans can be arthritogens and are unlikely to be contaminants because of the way CII is prepared.

THE U-SHAPED CURVE OF SUPPRESSION IN ORAL TOLERANCE TO COLLAGEN TYPE II

The tolerizing effects of CII given orally are also dose dependent (FIG. 1b), but a remarkable feature of CIA in both rats[1,6] and mice,[2] and of AA,[4] is that the optimum dose of CII can easily be exceeded, such that high doses do not protect at all against arthritis, although they may modify immune responsiveness in a way that might be expected to lead to reduced pathology (FIG. 2). Thus in CIA in rats, the best effects are obtained when five daily doses of around 0.25 μg/g body weight are given immediately preceding immunization with CII in FIA. It is relevant, because of the method of induction of AA, to note that complete adjuvant (FCA) is not used to induce CIA in the rat: in the mouse, however, it is, but this species generally is rather resistant to mycobacteria-induced AA.[7] The comparative data, to the extent that different dosing schedules can be compared, for the three diseases are summarized in FIGURE 2. The "U"-shaped response curve seen in AA has not been recorded in CIA, but clearly more analysis is needed to reach any firm conclusion. The results show that different response mechanisms are evoked according to the dose used for oral dosing. In no case has it been possible to prevent disease appearing

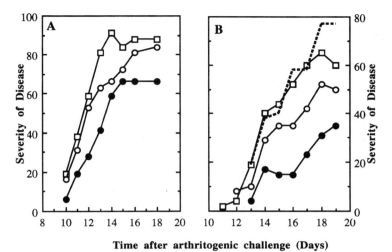

Time after arthritogenic challenge (Days)

FIGURE 1. Immune activity of CII in inducing and suppressing CIA through oral tolerance. **A:** WA/KIR/kcl male rats were immunized with (●) 0.25 mg, (○) 0.5 mg, or (□) 1.0 mg bovine CII in FIA, and the severity of clinical disease was determined by established methods.[1,6] **B:** Rats were given CII in 0.1 M acetic acid by direct gavage into the stomach in the total amount of (●) 0.3 mg, (○) 1.3 mg, or (□) 3.1 mg, divided as five daily doses (with acetic acid as a control vehicle, broken line) on consecutive days, immediately preceding immunization[1,6] with 0.25 mg CII in FIA as in panel **A.**

in all treated animals, and this distinguishes the oral tolerance effects in the arthritides from those in other diseases, such as experimental allergic encephalomyelitis (EAE).[8] The most obvious common feature is that the clinical or histological severity of each of these arthritides can be reduced by oral dosing with CII.

Thus the inverse relationship (as a part of the dose-response curve) between dose of CII given orally and the extent of the protection it affords against arthritis presents a problem in the design of rational clinical therapies. Only in AA has a dose-ranging experiment revealed the expected positive relationship, but in this case there is only a narrow window of dose within which an optimum effect can be achieved (FIG. 2). In PIA a direct relationship was seen between dose and protection over the range of 5 to 500 μg total CII given orally.[5] Clearly, more experimentation is needed to determine if high doses of CII are ineffective in all arthritides: we assume that very low doses must be ineffective in all diseases. The fact that four experimental arthritic diseases of different etiology in different hosts can each be modified by CII given orally implies that they converge sufficiently at some point in their etiopathogenesis to allow a single antigen to be effective in their control. This is consistent with CII working through a bystander suppression effect.[9] However, this has been studied only in rat CIA and then only under limited conditions of antigen dosing. Thus, we have found that tolerant spleen cells from rats that had been gavaged daily for five days with 1.0 μg CII/gram body weight could suppress the proliferative responses of anti-CII lymph node cells from arthritic rats[6] (TABLE 1). This shows that at the doses of CII used, tolerance is an active peripheral phenomenon. However, it is to be expected that different mechanisms operate at different doses of CII. The lack of protective effect of high doses of CII given orally may be modeled by the

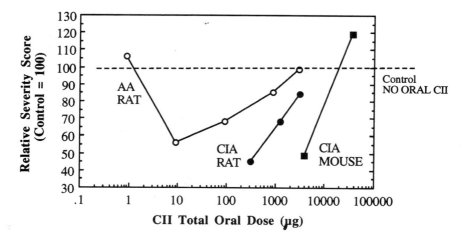

FIGURE 2. The U-shaped dose-response curve for oral tolerance induced by CII in collagen-induced arthritis (CIA) in the DBA/1 mouse and WA/KIR/kcl rat, and adjuvant arthritis (AA) in the Lewis rat. Data are derived from FIGURE 1 for CIA in the rat and from published work on CIA in the mouse[2] and AA in the rat.[4] In each case, the best estimate of protection has been expressed as a percent of the severity of disease in vehicle-treated controls and related to the total dose of CII given orally before immunization: different dosing schedules were used in each study.

TABLE 1. The Suppressive Effect of Spleen Cells from Orally Tolerized Rats on Antigen-specific Lymphocyte Proliferation Is Overcome at High Doses of Antigen, Indicating a Mechanism of Active Suppression[a]

Modulator: Responder ratio	Proliferation to CII in MTT Assay Mean ± SD ($A_{570}-A_{650}$ × 1000)		
	No CII	CII 9 µg/mL	CII 90 µg/mL
No modulators	191 ± 32	421 ± 66	529 ± 64
1:1	183 ± 20	365 ± 28	547 ± 49
2:1	195 ± 17	216 ± 16	540 ± 91
4:1	253 ± 19	216 ± 9	344 ± 62

[a] Modulator cells were taken after 11 days from spleens of rats gavaged with CII, and responder cells were from brachial and axillary lymph nodes of rats injected 11 days earlier with CII in FIA (as in FIG. 1). The total number of cells in each culture well was kept constant at different ratios of modulator:responder cells by addition of filler cells from normal rat spleen. Responder cells were at 10^5/well in all cases.[6]

in vitro suppression just mentioned: in a coculture system, an increase in the concentration of CII could overcome the modulating effects of tolerant spleen cells.

The demonstration that the active suppression associated with oral tolerance can be overcome by relatively high concentrations of antigen may be important for interpretation of the oral tolerance effect *in vivo*. In the first place, the ineffectiveness of high doses of CII given orally may be because they involve the absorption of sufficient antigen to activate Th1 cells in the face of suppressive cytokines made by the activated Th2 cells. One implication is that the threshold for activation of Th2 cells is at a lower dose of mucosally absorbed antigen than that for activation of Th1 cells. In support of this model, it has been shown that antigen absorbed through Peyer's patches selectively activates Th2 cells in the mouse.[10] Second, the CII injected intradermally in adjuvant provides a depot of antigen that can be released at concentrations sufficient to activate Th1 cells, even though modulatory Th2 cells have been also activated by mucosal encounter with antigen. In human disease, it may be that even inflamed joints do not provide such a quantitatively strong stimulus for Th1 cells, and so oral tolerance may be more effective. This is aside from considerations that antigen is processed in some way by passage through the mucosal epithelium and its associated lymphoid tissue to make it peculiarly tolerogenic.[11]

COLLAGEN PEPTIDES DELIVERED NASALLY SUPPRESS ARTHRITIS

Although the mechanisms of induced oral tolerance vary according to dose of antigen, it is reasonable to assume that the dose dictates which cells are involved and also that different lymphocyte types are differentially susceptible to activation, anergy, or deletion at the hands of antigen. It is also logical that different epitopes of the same antigen molecule stimulate different lymphocyte types. The phenomenon of bystander suppression also predicts that suppressive cells activated to one epitope will suppress, by this mechanism, responses to other epitopes of the same antigen and also responses to different antigens. Accordingly, antigenic peptides may offer a means to selectively activate suppressive cells. The experimental evidence supports this and suggests that there is no inherent limitation on pathogenic cells being able to recognize the antigen peptide, but that rather it is the mucosal route of immunization that favors the activation of Th2 over Th1 cells. We have used synthetic nested peptides of the sequences of the CB11 fragment of the bovine $\alpha 1(\text{II})$ chain to map the epitopes recognized by proliferating (assumed Th1) T cells in arthritic rats. The immunodominant epitope is included in the bovine CB11.61-75 sequence, and a synthetic peptide of this (made by solid-phase Fmoc peptide synthesis) has been found to be tolerogenic for CIA in rats.[12]

The immunological interconnection of the mucosal tissues is revealed by the findings that nasal delivery of CII can, like oral delivery, prevent the progression of arthritis. Although full dose-ranging experiments have not been done, a total dose of 1500 μg CII, given nasally to the same schedule of five daily doses preceding the induction of disease that was used to induce oral tolerance, halved disease severity (arthritic index of 23% at day 21 compared to 43% for saline-treated controls). This is as effective as CII given orally (illustrated in FIG. 1B), but in this case a smaller total dose of 120 μg CII was not protective.[12] This direct dose-response relationship contrasts with the U-shaped curve for oral dosing, but without full-dose ranging and pharmacokinetic studies, a firm conclusion that the two routes have fundamentally different immunological consequences is not justified.

The nasal delivery of the immunodominant bCB11.61-75 peptide in a total dose of 250 μg divided over the same regimen gave comparable protection against disease. This represents a 29-fold molar excess over the amount of CII giving the same protection.

These amounts of peptide are in accord with those used to induce mucosal tolerance in other studies, such as the Ac1-11 peptide of myelin basic protein used by Metzler and Wraith to suppress EAE in the mouse.[13] The 61-75 collagen II peptide is not itself arthritogenic, but T cells from peptide-immunized rats respond to both the peptide and to the intact CII molecule as antigen in an *in vivo* proliferative T-cell assay. The immunogenicity of the peptide is enhanced if it is amino acetylated, which is in accord with other studies of MHC class II-restricted antipeptide responses.

The nasal route may offer advantages over the oral route for the induction of tolerance, especially to peptides. Ease of administration and a less proteolytic environment are two advantages, but the direct drainage to the cervical lymph nodes from the nasal cavity may deliver antigen to the immune system in a way not found with oral dosing.[14] In any event, the immunological effects and the consequences for CIA development are similar with the two routes. Thus, we have found that anti-CII antibodies of the IgG1 isotype are elevated, and those of the IgG2b isotype reduced after nasal dosing with CII or bCB11.61-75 peptide. In both cases we interpret these changes in antibody isotype to result from a selective activation of Th2 CD4 cells by mucosal delivery of CII or peptide. This is consistent also with the suppression of proliferating anti-CII T cells in a coculture system using spleen cells from orally tolerant rats (TABLE 1).

EPITOPE SPREADING IN THE COLLAGEN RESPONSE

One feature of the developing T-cell response against CII is epitope spreading. Thus, analysis of epitopes recognized by cells taken at 2, 3, and 4 weeks shows spreading to be maximum at 3 weeks, and responses to all epitopes (peptides) to be reduced naturally by 4 weeks, although there may still be active arthritis at this time. The response to the 61-75 epitope dominates at all stages, but four subdominant epitopes represented by residues 28-42, 97-111, 136-150, and 208-222 are also recognized, and it is significant that all but the last are also active autoantigenic epitopes in the corresponding sequence of CII in the rat. The 28-42 and 97-111 sequences also include B-cell epitopes of which there are four in the CB11 fragment, at least as far as the Rt-1^u rat is concerned. This identifies a likely role for B cells in collagen antigen presentation to T cells in CIA. We have noted that the (total Ig) antibody response to the B-cell epitopes defined by linear 8mer overlapping peptides were not significantly depressed in rats orally tolerized with CII (unpublished experiments with Dr. K. Morgan, Manchester).

PREVENTION AND CURE OF EXPERIMENTAL ARTHRITIS

The timing of oral dosing with CII has not been examined extensively. In accord with other studies on induced mucosal tolerance, the experimental arthritides have been prevented by induced oral tolerance but have not been shown conclusively to be cured. In a range of experiments, we have found that dosing orally with CII in the week before disease induction has been the most protective, and an example is illustrated in FIGURE 3. Dosing with the same amount at earlier times has not affected the subsequent progression of disease, nor did dosing over a five-day period up to four weeks after induction. However, there was clear evidence of immunological changes following dosing before or after disease induction: for example, IgG1 anti-CII antibodies were elevated after dosing one, two, or three weeks beforehand or in the first week after induction; IgG2b antibodies, on the other hand, were depressed by prior dosing and tended to be elevated by dosing after induction. This we interpret as evidence that Th1 cells primed by the intradermal injection

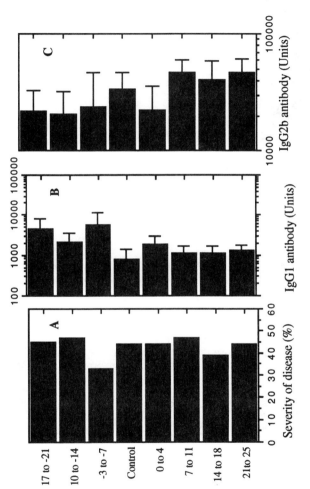

FIGURE 3. Time of oral dosing on the induction of tolerance that protects against CIA in the rat and modifies immune reactivity. WA/KIR/kcl rats were treated orally with a standard dose of bovine CII at times indicated relative to injection with CII (1.5 mg) in FIA to induce arthritis, and control animals received acetic acid gavage on days −5 to −1 (details in Fig. 1). **A:** Disease severity (at 21 days) is given as a cumulative arthritic score. **B:** IgG1 isotype anti-CII antibodies and (**C**) IgG2b isotype anti-CII antibodies were determined by ELISA (at day 14, but comparable results were obtained at day 21) and are expressed as arbitrary units of activity.[6] In this series, disease was only reduced when CII was given orally in the days immediately preceding immunization; on the other hand, depression of IgG2b and elevation of IgG1 antibodies were seen with all preimmunization dosing schedules and with dosing immediately after immunization.

of CII in FIA cannot be easily suppressed by subsequent activation of Th2 cells, which are in turn those preferentially activated by mucosal dosing in the normal rat. These experiments also show that changes in antibody isotypes can be dissociated from disease. We have found before that the suppression of IgG2b antibodies is more strongly associated with protection from disease than the elevation of IgG1 antibodies.[6] Thus the memory of oral tolerance in adults that protects against arthritis does not last as long as that which modifies the isotype balance of the antibody response.

Without a relapsing-remitting arthritic disease to manipulate, it is not possible to predict with any certainty that established disease cannot be ameliorated by oral tolerance to CII. What has not been examined, and what may hold the key, is the dose-response relationship between oral dosing and effect at different times in relation to disease onset or induction. One can predict, however, that there will be a complex relationship between the optimum dose of antigen to tolerize and the immune status and genetic makeup of the host.

ACKNOWLEDGMENTS

The studies of B cell-epitope mapping of CII referred to here (to be published in detail elsewhere) were conducted in collaboration with Dr. Keith Morgan of Manchester, UK, who died during the preparation of this manuscript: we dedicate this to his memory as a small token of our friendship.

REFERENCES

1. THOMPSON, H. S. G. & N. A. STAINES. 1986. Gastric administration of type II collagen delays the onset and severity of collagen-induced arthritis in rats. Clin. Exp. Immunol. **64:** 581-586.
2. NAGLER-ANDERSON, C., L. A. BOBER, M. E. ROBINSON, G. W. SISKIND & G. J. THORBECKE. 1986. Suppression of type II collagen-induced arthritis by intragastric administration of soluble type II collagen. Proc. Natl. Acad. Sci. USA **83:** 7443-7446.
3. KAGNOFF, M. F. 1982. Oral tolerance. Ann. N.Y. Acad. Sci. **392:** 248-265.
4. ZHANG, Z. J., C. S. Y. LEE, O. LIDER & H. L. WEINER. 1990. Suppression of adjuvant arthritis in Lewis rats by oral administration of type II collagen. J. Immunol. **145:** 2489-2493.
5. THOMPSON, S. J., H. S. G. THOMPSON, N. HARPER, M. J. DAY, A. J. COAD, C. J. ELSON & N. A. STAINES. 1993. Prevention of pristane-induced arthritis by oral administration of type II collagen. Immunology **79:** 152-157.
6. THOMPSON, H. S. G., N. HARPER, D. J. BEVAN & N. A. STAINES. 1993. Suppression of collagen induced arthritis by oral administration of type II collagen: Changes in immune and arthritic responses mediated by active peripheral suppression. Autoimmunity **16:** 189-199.
7. KNIGHT, B., D. R. KATZ, D. A. ISENBERG, M. A. IBRAHIM, S. LE PAGE, P. HUTCHINGS, R. S. SCHWARTZ & A. COOKE. 1992. Induction of adjuvant arthritis in mice. Clin. Exp. Immunol. **90:** 459-465.
8. HIGGINS, P. J. & H. L. WEINER. 1988. Suppression of experimental autoimmune encephalomyelitis by oral administration of myelin basic protein and its fragments. J. Immunol. **140:** 440-445.
9. MILLER, A., O. LIDER & H. L. WEINER. 1991. Antigen-driven bystander suppression after oral administration of antigens. J. Exp. Med. **174:** 791-798.
10. ASHERSON, G. L., M. ZEMBALA, M. A. A. C. PERERA, B. MAYHEW & W. R. THOMAS. 1977. Production of immunity and unresponsiveness in the mouse by feeding contact

sensitizing agents and the role of suppressor cells in Peyer's patch, mesenteric lymph nodes and other lymphoid tissues. Cell. Immunol. **33:** 145-151.

11. FURRIE, E., M. W. TURNER & S. STROBEL. 1994. Failure of SCID mice to generate an oral tolerogen after a feed of ovalbumin: a role for a functioning gut-associated lymphoid system. Immunology **83:** 562-567.

12. STAINES, N. A., N. HARPER, F. J. WARD, V. MALISSEN, R. HOLMDAHL & S. BANSAL. 1995. Mucosal tolerance induced by nasal inhalation of a synthetic peptide of type II collagen: Immune changes and suppression of collagen arthritis. Clin. Exp. Immunol. In press.

13. METZLER, B. & D. C. WRAITH. 1993. Inhibition of experimental autoimmune encephalomyelitis by inhalation but not oral administration of the encephalitogenic peptide: influence of MHC binding affinity. Int. Immunol. **5:** 1159-1165.

14. KUPER, C. F., P. J. KOORNSTRA, D. M. H. HAMELEERS, J. BIEWENGA, B. J. SPIT, A. M. DUIJVESTIJN, P. J. C. VAN BREDA VRIESMAN & T. SMINIA. 1992. The role of nasopharyngeal lymphoid tissue. Immunol. Today **13:** 219-224.

Evidence That Type II Collagen Feeding Can Induce a Durable Therapeutic Response in Some Patients with Rheumatoid Arthritis

DAVID E. TRENTHAM

Division of Rheumatology
Beth Israel Hospital
and
Harvard Medical School
330 Brookline Avenue
Boston, Massachusetts 02115

Rheumatoid arthritis (RA) is a common disease caused by a chronic inflammatory reaction in the synovial membrane of diarthroidial joints. It proceeds in a pattern of both overgrowth (in the synovial membrane) and destruction of adjoining structures (cartilage and bone). In some patients, it assumes a relatively mild course, but in others it follows a devastating degradative path.

PROBLEMS WITH RA

With RA, three major problems exist. First, its etiology is unknown. Accordingly, there is no intellectual basis for attempting to formulate a way to prevent the disease. Second, although rheumatologists are loathe to admit it, RA is poorly responsive to all current therapies. Treatments only partially alleviate the symptoms of RA (pain, stiffness, and fatigue); they do not demonstrably retard the apparent natural history of RA in most patients. Third, every treatment for RA carries a risk for the patient, in terms of a potential for adverse side effects. Fortunately, presently used drugs have a sufficient track record to make the degree of risk accurately calculable. On the debit side is the liability imposed by stronger or more effective drugs being intrinsically more hazardous. An additional toll on the patient is imposed by psychological factors. Methotrexate is a modern mainstay of RA treatment but is also used as a cancer chemotherapy. Perhaps it is not inappropriate to consider RA as a localized malignancy of joints, but cajoling a patient to accept methotrexate treatment exacts a psychic cost as well. The fact that methotrexate is actually fairly safe does not solve this problem. The situation is analogous to flying, which is safe statistically but still can be nerve-racking.

PATHOGENESIS OF RA

All evidence points to RA being an autoimmune disease that is T-cell mediated.[1] What breaks self-tolerance is unknown. An infectious insult as the trigger for this breakdown continues to be a popular conjecture. T-cell mediation is shown by the ability of T cell-specific interventions to palliate RA. The initial demonstration, that is, thoracic duct drainage, has been substantiated by trials of total lymphoid irradiation, antithymocyte globulin, cyclosporin, anti-CD4 monoclonal antibodies, and an immunotoxin directed at cells expressing the high-affinity interleukin-2 (IL-2) receptor. Pathologic appraisals show that the synovial lesion (termed pannus) in RA resembles a delayed-type hypersensitivity reaction. In addition, there seems to be an incompatibility between AIDs and RA. When profound CD4 lymphopenia, attributable to HIV infection, has been reached, either RA does not develop or, if previously present, enters a stage of remarkable quiescence.

T cells appear to propagate RA through the release of cytokines.[2] Probably a variety of other cells join T cells in generating these soluble factors. Cytokines produced by cells of the Th-1 subset are probably the most provocative. These include IL-2 and interferon-γ. T cell-derived cytokines may help to stimulate monokine production. Tumor necrosis factor-α (TNF-α) is, primarily, a monocyte product that may be particularly important in the pathogenesis of RA, as evidenced by recent clinical trials aimed at blocking TNF-α activity.[3]

By phenotypic identification, large numbers of cells termed mature memory T cells reside in the rheumatoid synovium. The presence and normal functioning of these cells could account for the biochemical milieu of the RA joint; that is, they proliferate poorly, and release little IL-2, but vigorously promote monokine and immunoglobulin production. These recruited factors could furnish important contributory pathways in rheumatoid arthritis.

Memory T cells imply previous exposure to antigen and suggest that this earlier encounter occurred locally.[1] If true, it would form the basis for envisioning RA as being a result of T cells reacting to antigen within the joint. If the antigen were host derived, that is, an autoantigen, it would explain, in a unifying fashion, the disease. Most importantly, such a concept would predict that antigen-specific immunosuppression would be an effective therapeutic maneuver, if the offending autoantigen could be identified.

Several candidate antigens have been proposed. Some, such as mycoplasma and heat-shock protein, are of bacterial origin. Others, such as IgG (which is the target for rheumatoid factor) and collagen, are of host origin. Over 10 biochemically distinct collagens have been isolated, but the most abundant species are types I and II. The former protein is ubiquitously distributed through a variety of tissues and organ parenchyma. In sharp contrast, type II collagen is restricted physically and provides support for only cartilage and the vitreous of the eye. Immunizing animals with type II collagen creates an inflammatory arthritis that morphologically resembles RA. Thus, type II collagen is an arthritogen. By placing an arthritis-inducing protein in the center of a joint, has nature permitted a horrendous mistake to occur?

TYPE II COLLAGEN AS A CANDIDATE AUTOANTIGEN FOR RA

Slowly, evidence favoring an autoantigenic role for type II collagen in RA has become more persuasive. Some strains of rats immunized and boosted to induce collagen arthritis have developed anterior uveitis as well. Thus, as a composite, collagen arthritis can closely resemble the clinical situation in juvenile rheumatoid arthritis (JRA), where both arthritis and uveitis are frequently dominant. Additional species have been found to be susceptible to collagen arthritis. Certain strains of mice were the first identified, but perhaps the most provocative observation is in nonhuman primates. Collagen arthritis is easily inducible in both squirrel and rhesus monkeys, which are genomically close to the human. Collagen arthritis remains the sole primate model for RA. Autoimmunity to type II collagen is a component shared by many inducible models of RA. It clearly exists in rat adjuvant arthritis, which is created by immunization with mycobacterial particles found in complete

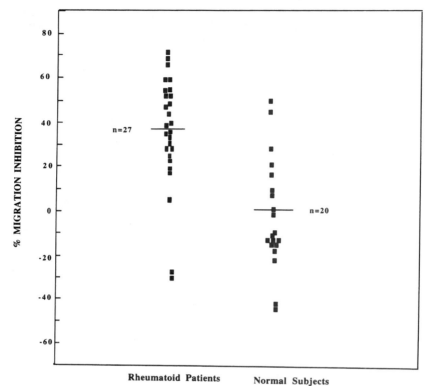

FIGURE 1. Comparison of leukocyte inhibitory factor (LIF) responses to native type II collagen, assessed functionally in a migration inhibition assay, using purified human polymorphonuclear indicator cells, by patients with RA versus normal controls. Data excerpted from a previously published study.[6]

Freund's adjuvant. Pristane-induced arthritis in mice, a recently recognized system, is another morphologic counterpart of RA in which concurrent collagen autoimmunity has been detected.

Likewise humoral and cellular immunity to type II collagen is present in many patients with RA. Initial demonstrations, using functional cytokine assays (FIG 1), appeared definitive,[4-6] but the results became controversial when it was widely recognized that native type II collagen elicited only minimal proliferative responses.[4] The explanation for this paradox remains unknown. When cloning techniques were perfected, successful isolation of type II collagen-reactive T-cell clones, established from the synovium of a patient with RA, was reported,[7] but much effort seeking to verify this finding in other patients has ended in failure. To resolve this dilemma, perhaps it is best to recall that autoantibodies to type II collagen are clearly present in the serum of a sizable proportion of patients with active, established RA.[8] Because collagen is a T cell-dependent antigen in animals, it is highly likely that collagen antibody production is under T-cell control in RA as well. *A priori* collagen-sensitized T cells should exist. Probably other immunoregulatory cells are also present and prevent T-cell reactivity to collagen from being readily detected *in vitro.*

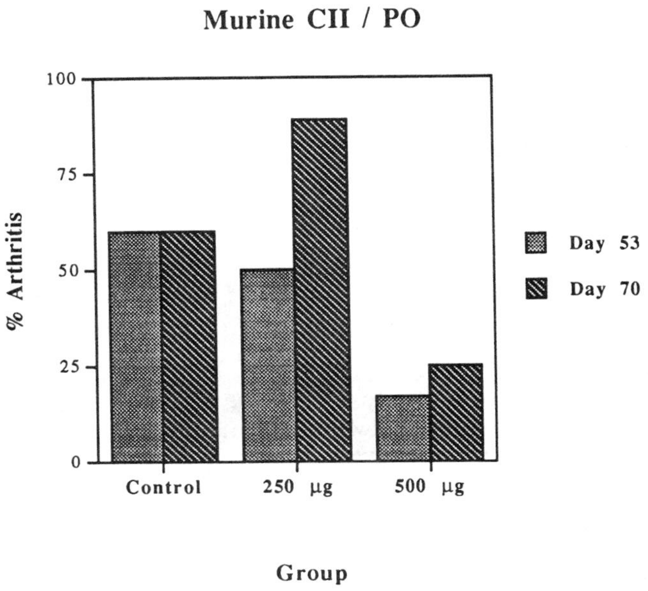

Murine CII / PO

FIGURE 2. Use of the Nagler-Anderson et al.[11] protocol (12 oral feedings of native type II collagen) to suppress collagen arthritis in groups of male DBA/1 mice. Experiments performed by Carlos Lorenzo, Dawton Torigoe, and Daniel Combitchi in the author's laboratory.

Another recently conducted study seems insightful. In an experiment designed to analyze the intrasynovial B-cell repertoire in RA, particularly that involved with the fine specificities of rheumatoid factor production, an unanticipated shift was encountered.[9] In 13 of the 14 patients studied, the vast majority of B cells isolated were vigorously involved, not with rheumatoid factor production, but with the generation of appreciable quantities of immunoglobulin with specificity for type II collagen. This finding suggests that intrasynovial sequestered autoreactivity to collagen is a hallmark of RA. In summary, these cellular and humoral data can elicit judgments ranging from a disbelief in the presence of autoimmunity to type II collagen in RA to, at the other extreme, an acknowledgment that they are virtually integral processes.

A final thought while grappling with the collagen-RA conundrum. The MHC makeup, which seems to influence RA and governs susceptibility to collagen arthritis in mice, appears to be indistinguishable. Thus, at the most scientifically elegant level, collagen immunity and the pathogenesis of RA must continue to be considered seriously.

SUPPRESSION OF EXPERIMENTAL ARTHRITIS BY COLLAGEN FEEDING

Autonomous studies, using rats in London[10] and mice in New York,[11] showed almost 10 years ago that collagen arthritis could be suppressed by oral tolerance approaches using native type II collagen. FIGURE 2 depicts use of the Nagler-Anderson et al.[11] protocol

TABLE 1. Complete Resolution

1. No swollen or tender joints.
2. No AM stiffness or PM fatigue.
3. "Absent arthritis" (patient and physician global assessment).[a]
4. Functional class I.
5. Normal ESR[b] (< 28).
6. 1–5 off prednisone.

[a] See TABLE 2.
[b] Erythrocyte sedimentation rate.

in the author's laboratory to suppress collagen arthritis in DAB-1 mice as further corroboration. The most detailed dissection of the clinical and immunologic effects of type II collagen feeding in experimental arthritis was conducted by Zhang *et al.*[12] Several important observations emerged from this study in rats with adjuvant arthritis. Most importantly it was effective and was a nontoxic approach. A well-defined dose-response pattern was found whereby lower but not higher doses were active. Collagen feeding was shown to be T-cell immunospecific, in that suppression of delayed hypersensitivity to collagen but not mycobacteria (present in the adjuvant inoculum) occurred. Finally it was disease specific; that is, adjuvant arthritis could not be modified by feeding of irrelevant autoantigen, such as myelin basic protein, which induces experimental autoimmune encephalomyelitis (EAE) and, when fed, is capable of suppressing this model of multiple sclerosis. Close observation of these evolving data was a powerful impetus to try to achieve oral tolerance in RA patients. By consensus, type II collagen would be the initial antigen investigated.

IMPROVEMENT IN RA BY COLLAGEN FEEDING: REFLECTIONS ON THE FIRST TWO TRIALS

In the first trial, 10 patients were selected to receive solubilized native-chick type II collagen in an open format of 3 months' duration.[8] The doses of collagen selected, 0.1 mg daily for one month and then 0.5 mg daily for the remainder of the study, represented an attempt, based on the low doses found to be effective in rats with adjuvant arthritis,[12] to simulate the animal work. In this trial, patients seemed to either respond markedly to collagen treatment or be totally refractory to the intervention. The degree of response observed in some cases was sufficiently impressive to prompt reformulating the original American Rheumatism Association remission criteria for RA into a more rigorous set of rules designated "complete resolution"[8] (TABLE 1). An impetus for prospectively revamping these criteria was their projected use in the subsequent 60-patient double-blind, placebo-controlled effort.[8] FIGURE 3 shows the mean group responses in the placebo and active-treatment limbs in this trial. When the groups are considered as a whole, statistically significant improvement with collagen feeding was evident by one to two months after initiating treatment. Four of the 28 patients randomized to collagen fulfilled the newly proposed criteria for complete resolution after three months of treatment.

This study has been criticized due to the lack of a washout period interposed between discontinuation of disease-modifying drug (DMARD) (chiefly methotrexate) and beginning study medication. This omission was intentional, reflected a desire to conduct the trial in an expeditious manner as possible, and was considered appropriate because of its

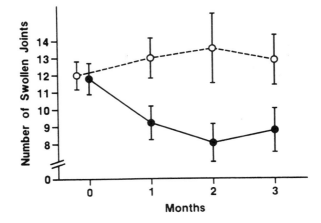

FIGURE 3. Average number of swollen joints ± one standard error at entry and each monthly follow-up for the collagen- (●) and placebo- (o) treated patients. A significant difference (p = 0.026) between collagen and placebo patients is demonstrated by repeated measures of variance.

extremely preliminary nature. Because many patients treated with collagen were able to show improvement, relative to baseline (when methotrexate had just been discontinued), the findings were encouraging. Also promising was the lack of side effects encountered with collagen treatment.

At the end of these phase I (open label) and phase II (placebo-controlled) trials, three major questions remained unanswered. First, there was no explanation of why some patients responded to collagen and others did not. The presence of serum antibodies to collagen and human leukocyte antigen (HLA) haplotype did not define responsiveness and did not relate to disease chronicity or severity. Second, the mechanism for the improvement with collagen feeding was not addressed in this study. Although its design was founded on the induction of oral tolerance to collagen in animals, whether this occurred in RA is unclear. No effect on collagen antibody titers was noted at the end of this trial, but three months after initiating therapy may be an insufficient period for detecting changes. Finally, the dose used, although somewhat of an extrapolation from animals, was arbitrary, and the optimum dose for the treatment of RA is unknown. In particular, whether higher doses would be more effective or would lead to the paralysis of oral tolerance (as in animals) is entirely unclear.

ADDITIONAL EVIDENCE THAT COLLAGEN FEEDING CAN PALLIATE SOME CASES OF RA

At present, two additional, albeit unblinded, appraisals suggest that collagen feeding can improve some cases of RA. Immediately after the data had been analyzed in the phase II trial,[3,8] three months of type II collagen treatment (one month at 0.1 mg daily and then escalating to a 0.5-mg daily dose) were offered to the 31 patients that had been randomized to placebo. The primary purpose of this extension was a compassionate-use gesture for participants in the study. Because 39 of the 60 patients in the phase II study resided outside Boston, often in quite geographically distant sites, there was no obligation, only a request, to voluntarily return for follow-up. DMARD, prednisone, and NSAID usage were as described in the phase II trial. The number of swollen and painful/tender joints was ascertained immediately prior to and at the end of the treatment period. Reductions of greater than 50% were designated "substantial" responses, whereas changes of less than 30% were regarded as "unchanged."[8] Of the 31 patients, including 4 dropouts, 17 elected to participate. Three patients dropped out prior to completing three months of collagen therapy. Three completers failed to return for follow-up at three months. This left 11 subjects as fully evaluable at baseline and three months. As judged by the number of swollen joints, 5 patients exhibited a substantial response. According to the number of painful/tender joints, 6 patients had a substantial response. The other patients were regarded as having no change at three months. As in the phase I and II trials, no side effects were observed. The percentage of patients responding to collagen in this open-label compassionate-use trial was 35–40%, inasmuch as the 3 dropouts were unlikely to have received benefit from collagen therapy. In addition, the uncontrolled nature of the study did not permit the improvement to be attributed to a biologic effect of collagen, because placebo effects could explain the results. Nonetheless, these additional data also suggest that oral collagen can be an effective treatment for some patients with severe RA and is notable for its freedom from side effects.

One further open label assessment provides evidence that collagen treatment can lead to a lengthy therapeutic response in some patients with RA. When all patients that had received collagen in the phase I or II trials had reached a point of at least two years after starting their initial treatment, a follow-up inquiry was sent by mail. A total of 60 were selected, based on compliance with the study protocol in the past. One collagen-treated patient had died of a myocardial infarction more than two years posttherapy, and another had been lost to follow-up. Of the 60, 43 (72%) returned the questionnaire. Time since collagen treatment began ranged from two to four years. Prior to mailing the questionnaire, criteria to establish sustained improvement with collagen treatment (including additional three-month treatment periods) were formulated. There was an attempt to base this judgment on maximally objective and clinically relevant parameters. It was decided to use the term "durably better." For a patient to achieve this ranking, there had to be no DMARD exposure since beginning collagen treatment, and the patient's self-assessment had to indicate improvement with collagen treatment (and retreatment). Of the 43 patients that returned their questionnaires, 9 (21%) were found to be durably better. TABLE 2 depicts additional data found in the nine patients who most definitively reflected a collagen treatment-improved subgroup.

Three findings in TABLE 2 may be of particular interest. First, the number of DMARDs a patients with RA has received in the past generally connotes the severity of the disease process. There was no correlation between the degree of prior DMARD exposure and capacity to respond long term to collagen. By inference, these findings suggest that collagen may also help patients with severe and long-standing RA. Second, in many patients, only one or two three-month, treatment courses provided some degree of relief for up to two to four years. If one assumes that oral tolerance was achieved, then T-cell anergy rather than active Th-2 cytokine-mediated bystander suppression[13] would be more likely to explain this long-lasting phenomenon. Finally, collagen treatment seems to be highly popular with some patients, because all 9 patients would prefer it to DMARD readministration in the future. Clearly these patients perceive it to be an effective nontoxic therapy. Unfortunately they seem to be a minority of collagen-treated patients.

ASPECTS FOR THE FUTURE

Currently a large multicenter dose-ranging trial is well underway in the United States. Controlled trials at institutions other than our own are also either planned or beginning.

TABLE 2. Collagen Treatment-improved Subgroup

Total	9
Female	6
Age	
Average	48
Range	24-68
Number of DMARDs in past	
None	1
One	2
Two	2
Three	4
Time since first treatment began	
Average	36 months
Range	24-49
Number of three-month treatment courses	
One	5
Two	3
Three	1
Patient global[a]	
Absent	2
Mild	4
Moderate	1
Severe	1
Very severe[b]	1
If required, would prefer collagen retreatment	9

[a] Current patient:global assessment of status.
[b] Patient flaring and reinitiating collagen treatment.

Soon additional information to judge the usefulness of the collagen approach should be available. Until that time, certain limitations regarding the work accomplished to date should be appreciated. Most importantly, the number of patients treated remains extremely small. Sometimes identical protocols give different outcomes in RA trials. This could be the case with collagen. RA trials are notoriously susceptible to the placebo phenomenon, even when the trial is quite long in nature.[14] Placebo-like effects could contaminate the outcome in patients receiving collagen. An additional deficiency is the inability to identify and thus monitor a laboratory parameter reflecting an oral collagen-induced biologic response. Reliance on clinical appraisal is a notoriously subjective way to grade RA disease activity.

Nonetheless, the findings in RA are encouraging. Although few conclusions can be drawn from the clinical trials, in the past therapeutic screening in animal models has been quite predictive of a drug's subsequent outcome in RA.[15] Clearly collagen feeding is effective in collagen and adjuvant arthritis. It would therefore be highly surprising if it did not work in humans as well.

ACKNOWLEDGMENT

The author wishes to gratefully acknowledge the assistance of Roselynn Dynesius-Trentham in the preparation of the questionnaires and manuscript.

REFERENCES

1. SEWELL, K. L. & D. E. TRENTHAM. 1993. Pathogenesis of rheumatoid arthritis. Lancet **341:** 283–286.
2. KOCH, A. E., S. L. KUNKEL & R. M. STRIETER. 1995. Cytokines in rheumatoid arthritis. J. Invest. Med. **43:** 28–38.
3. ELLIOTT, M. J., R. N. MAINI, M. FELDMANN, A. LONG-FOX, P. CHARLES, P. KATSIKIS, F. M. BRENNAN, J. WALKER, H. BIJL, J. GHRAYEB & J. N. WOODY. 1993. Treatment of rheumatoid arthritis with chimeric monoclonal antibodies to tumor necrosis factor α. Arthritis Rheum. **36:** 1681–1690.
4. TRENTHAM, D. E., R. A. DYNESIUS, R. E. ROCKLIN & J. R. DAVID. 1978. Cellular sensitivity to collagen in rheumatoid arthritis. N. Engl. J. Med. **299:** 327–332.
5. STUART, J. M., A. E. POSTLETHWAITE, A. H. KANG & A. S. TOWNES. 1980. Cell-mediated immunity to collagen in rheumatoid arthritis and other rheumatic diseases. Am. J. Med. **69:** 13–18.
6. TRENTHAM, D. E., G. M. KAMMER, W. J. McCUNE & J. R. DAVID. 1981. Autoimmunity to collagen: A shared feature of psoriatic and rheumatoid arthritis. Arthritis Rheum. **24:** 1363–1369.
7. LONDEI, M., C. M. SAVILLE, A. VERHOEF & M. FELDMANN. 1989. Persistence of collagen type II-specific T-cell clones in the synovial membrane of a patient with rheumatoid arthritis. Proc. Natl. Acad. Sci. USA **86:** 636–640.
8. TRENTHAM, D. E., R. A. DYNESIUS-TRENTHAM, E. J. ORAV, D. COMBITCHI, C. LORENZO, K. L. SEWELL, D. A. HAFLER & H. L. WEINER. 1993. Effects of type II collagen on rheumatoid arthritis. Science **261:** 1727–1730.
9. TARKOWSKI, A., L. KLARESKOG, H. CARLSTEN, P. HERBERTS & W. J. KOOPMAN. 1989. Secretion of antibodies to type I and type II collagen by synovial tissue cells in patients with rheumatoid arthritis. Arthritis Rheum. **32:** 1087–1092.
10. THOMPSON, H. S. G. & N. A. STAINES. 1986. Gastric administration of type II collagen delays the onset and severity of collagen-induced arthritis in rats. Clin. Exp. Immunol. **64:** 581–586.
11. NAGLER-ANDERSON, C., L. A. BOBER, M. E. ROBINSON, G. W. SISKIND & G. L. THORBECKE. 1986. Suppression of type II collagen-induced arthritis by intragastric administration of soluble type II collagen. Proc. Natl. Acad. Sci. USA **83:** 7443–7446.
12. ZHANG, J. A., C. S. Y. LEE, O. LIDER & H. L. WEINER. 1990. Suppression of adjuvant arthritis in Lewis rats by oral administration of type II collagen. J. Immunol. **145:** 2489–2493.
13. WEINER, H. L., A. FRIEDMAN, A. MILLER, S. J. KHOURY, A. AL-SABBAGH, R. B. NUSSEN-BLATT, D. E. TRENTHAM & D. A. HAFLER. 1994. Oral tolerance: Immunologic mechanisms and treatment of animal and human-specific autoimmune disease by oral administration of autoantigens. Annu. Rev. Immunol. **12:** 809–837.
14. TILLEY, B. C., G. S. ALARCON, S. P. HEYSE, D. E. TRENTHAM, R. NEUNER, D. A. KAPLAN, D. O. CLEGG, J. C. C. LEISEN, L. BUCKLEY, S. M. COOPER, H. DUNCAN, S. R. PILLEMER, M. TUTTLEMAN & S. E. FOWLER for the MIRA TRIAL GROUP. 1995. Minocycline in rheumatoid arthritis: A 48 week double-blind, placebo-controlled trial. Ann. Intern. Med. **122:** 81–89.
15. TRENTHAM, D. E. & R. A. DYNESIUS-TRENTHAM. 1995. Collagen-induced arthritis *In* Mechanisms and Models in Rheumatoid Arthritis. B. Henderson & J. Edwards, Eds. 447–456. Academic Press. London.

Cytokine-dependent Modulation of Oral Tolerance in a Murine Model of Autoimmune Uveitis

RACHEL R. CASPI,[a] LESLIE R. STIFF,[a,d]
R. MORAWETZ,[c] NANCY E. MILLER-RIVERO,[a]
CHI-CHAO CHAN,[a] BARBARA WIGGERT,[b]
ROBERT B. NUSSENBLATT,[a]
HERBERT C. MORSE III,[c] AND LUIZ V. RIZZO [a]

[a]Laboratory of Immunology

[b]Laboratory of Cell and Molecular Biology
National Eye Institute

[c]National Institute of Allergy and Infectious Diseases
9000 Rockville Pike
Building 10, Room 10N222
10 Center Drive, MSC 1858
Bethesda, Maryland 20892

THE EAU MODEL IN MICE

Experimental autoimmune uveoretinitis (EAU) is induced in mice by immunization with the interphotoreceptor retinoid-binding protein (IRBP) or its peptides, or by CD4[+] T-cell lines specific to these antigens, and serves as a model for human posterior uveitis. The target tissue in murine EAU, as in EAU in other species, is the neural retina. The EAU model in mice was first established by us in 1988 and has since yielded useful information on immunological and immunogenetic mechanisms of ocular autoimmunity.[1-3] The EAU model in mice has some characteristics that distinguish it from the better-studied Lewis rat EAU model. Disease in the mouse is typically chronic (except at the highest immunization doses), there is a need for a more intense immunization protocol that includes an obligatory dose of pertussis toxin, and the preferred uveitogen is (bovine) IRBP. Unlike in the rat, bovine S-antigen was found to be poorly uveitogenic in mice. The salient features of the mouse model of EAU are summarized in TABLE 1. Unless stated otherwise, in all the experiments described in this report, we used the B10.A strain of mice, and the immunization protocol used to elicit EAU consisted of a subcutaneous injection of 50 μg of IRBP in complete Freund's adjuvant (CFA) that had been supplemented with *Mycobacterium tuberculosis* strain H37RA to 2.5 mg/mL and a dose of 0.5 μg *Bordetella pertussis* toxin (PTX) injected intraperitoneally (ip) at the same time. A full description of the EAU model, including quantitative disease scoring criteria (scale of 0 to 4), has been published.[4]

[d]L. R. Stiff is supported by the Howard Hughes Medical Institute Scholars Program.

TABLE 1. Characteristics of the Mouse EAU Model[1,3,11-13]

Feature	Characteristics
Disease course	Usually chronic. Symptoms first start 12-14 days after immunization, followed by remissions and relapses.
Histopathology	Focal to diffuse.
Eliciting antigen	IRBP and IRBP peptides.
Immunization	Pertussis toxin needed as adjuvant (in addition to CFA).
Susceptibility	MHC: $H-2^r > H-2^k > H-2^b$.
	Background: B10 > A > AKR.

ORAL TOLERANCE IN THE MOUSE EAU MODEL

It was shown previously that oral tolerance to retinal proteins and peptides can be reproducibly induced in Lewis rats.[5-7] Depending on the dose of the antigen fed, both active suppression and anergy-mediated mechanisms can act in a nonmutually exclusive fashion to induce protection from disease.[5] The EAU model in mice resembles some types of human uveitic conditions better than the rat EAU model. In addition, the mouse has some obvious advantages over the rat for immunological research. For these reasons we set out to test whether oral tolerance can be induced in mice.

B10.A mice were fed with different doses of IRBP or with PBS, either 3 or 5 times, using the regimens depicted in FIGURE 1. All mice were subsequently immunized with a uveitogenic dose of IRBP to induce EAU. Retinal histopathology performed 21 days after immunization showed that, across the dose range of 0.05 mg, 0.2 mg, or 0.5 mg IRBP per feeding, three feedings were not protective, whereas five feedings protected from EAU (FIG. 2). The "intermediate" 0.2 mg feeding dose was chosen for further study and is the dose employed in all the experiments described below.

The antiinflammatory cytokines IL-4, IL-10, and TGF-β were assayed by ELISA or by bioassay in supernatants of IRBP-stimulated lymph node and Peyer's patch (PP) cells of the protected (5× fed) and unprotected (3× fed) mice given the 0.2 mg feeding dose.[6] The titers of these cytokines were minimal to undetectable in both feeding groups. Thus, there was no evidence for active suppression as a major mechanism of tolerance in the

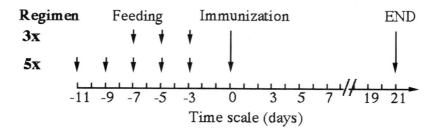

FIGURE 1. Preimmunization feeding regimens. Mice were fed and challenged with IRBP for EAU induction on the indicated days.

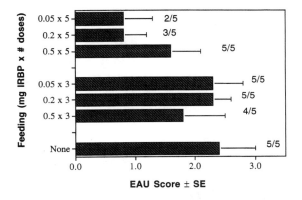

FIGURE 2. Feeding IRBP 5 times, but not 3 times, protects mice from a subsequent EAU challenge. B10.A mice were fed the indicated doses of IRBP either by the 5× or the 3× protocol. All were subsequently immunized with 50 μg of IRBP in CFA and 0.5 μg PTX, as described.[6] EAU was scored by histopathology 21 days after immunization.

protective 5× feeding regimen. We hypothesize, therefore, that protection from EAU elicited by the 5× regimen is due to "silencing" of the pathogenic cells by a mechanism of anergy or deletion. Although direct proof of this hypothesis awaits the results of suppression-transfer experiments (currently in progress), this interpretation is supported by the observation that under some circumstances protection from EAU can be accompanied by antigen-specific production of antiinflammatory cytokines by immunocompetent cells of protected mice (see ahead).

An important question from the clinical point of view is whether feeding of IRBP, commenced after priming of the uveitogenic CD4[+] effector cells has already occurred, can also be protective. To answer that question, a multiple-dose regimen of 0.2 mg IRBP per feeding was administered to mice every other day, beginning 7 days after immunization. The disease was scored after 21 days. The results indicated that such delayed feeding could ameliorate the expression of EAU, as judged by histopathology (FIG. 3). The

FIGURE 3. Feeding IRBP can protect already primed mice from EAU. B10.A mice were immunized with 50 μg IRBP in CFA and were given 0.5 μg PTX. Starting 7 days after immunization, some mice were fed 0.2 mg IRBP every other day (fed), and some were given PBS (unfed). EAU was scored by histopathology 21 days after immunization.

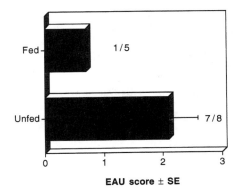

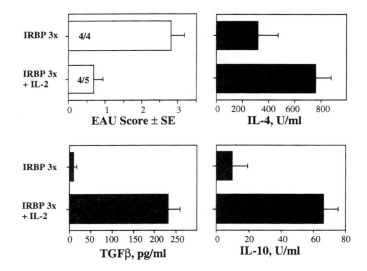

FIGURE 4. Protection from EAU in IRBP-fed and IL-2-treated mice correlates with production of Th2-type cytokines. Mice were fed with 0.2 mg IRBP 3 times, as depicted in FIGURE 1, and received 1000 IU IL-2 ip at the time of immunization. Eyes and Peyer's patch cells were collected at 21 days. Shown is EAU by histopathology and cytokine production in IRBP-stimulated supernatants of PP cells of unprotected mice fed 3 times with IRBP, and protected mice fed 3x + IL-2. The histopathology scores and cytokine production of unfed mice were essentially identical to the 3x-fed animals. Cytokines were assayed as described.[6]

mechanism of tolerance (anergy or suppression) that is responsible for the protection afforded by delayed feeding of IRBP remains to be elucidated.

EFFECT OF IL-2 ON INDUCTION OF ORAL TOLERANCE

The balance between the two known major mechanisms responsible for oral tolerance, anergy and suppression, is affected by the dose and the frequency of antigen feeding. The antigens involved in human disease are unknown, so that it is the latter mechanism, with its potential for eliciting bystander suppression, that is probably the more desirable one from the perspective of clinical therapy. Because it is likely that anergy and suppression are induced in parallel, we hypothesized that an appropriately timed administration of the T-cell growth factor IL-2 might enhance putative regulatory cells elicited by IRBP feeding and skew the balance in favor of active suppression.[8] Indeed, mice fed three times with 0.2 mg/feeding of IRBP and injected intraperitoneally with IL-2 at the time of immunization were protected from EAU by histopathological evaluation on day 21 after a uveitogenic immunization with IRBP. Furthermore, unlike the situation with mice protected from EAU by the 5x feeding regimen, PP cells that were obtained from the 3x + IL-2-fed mice produced copious amounts of antiinflammatory T helper 2 (Th2)-type cytokines when stimulated *in vitro* with IRBP (FIG. 4, and ref. 6). Lymph node cells of these mice produced IL-4, but little or no IL-10 and TGF-β were seen in stimulated lymph node cell supernatants (not shown).

TABLE 2. Effect of Timing and Dose of IL-2 Administration[a]

Feeding and Treatment		EAU	Incidence
Antigen	IL-2 (U); Day	(score ± SE)	(positive/total)
IRBP	1,000; 0	0.7 ± 0.3	4/5
IRBP	30,000; 0	<u>1.0 ± 0.3</u>	5/5
IRBP	30,000; −7, −5, −3	<u>0.75 ± 0.5</u>	4/5
IRBP	30,000; +3	1.9 ± 0.6	4/5
IRBP	30,000; +7	1.7 ± 0.6	4/5
IRBP	1,000; +7	1.8 ± 0.7	5/5
IRBP	None	2.8 ± 0.4	4/4
OVA	None	2.7 ± 0.4	5/5

[a] IRBP was fed 3 times as in FIG. 1, at 0.2 mg/dose. The uveitogenic challenge was 50 μg IRBP in CFA and PTX on day 0. EAU was scored by histopathology on day 21. The underlined scores are significantly different from controls ($p < 0.05$) by Snedecor and Cochran's test for Linear Trend in Proportions.

The tolerance-promoting effect was maintained across a wide range of IL-2 doses, as long as the timing of IL-2 administration was before or at the time of immunization (TABLE 2). IL-2 administered three or seven days after immunization was not protective. Furthermore, IL-2 administered repeatedly after immunization, together with multiple feedings of IRBP, was not protective. In fact, the treated mice were as sick as unfed (and untreated) control mice that received only the uveitogenic immunization (data not shown). Analysis of the cytokines produced by PP of the various groups shown in TABLE 1 revealed that, across the board, groups that were significantly protected from EAU produced large amounts of TGF-β, IL-4, and IL-10, whereas the unprotected groups did not.

The finding that protection from EAU elicited by the 3× + IL-2 regimen correlates strictly with production of antiinflammatory cytokines raises the possibility that oral tolerance elicited by this regimen is, at least in part, effected by regulatory (Th2 type?) cells. A role for such cells in oral tolerance to myelin basic protein (MBP) has been proposed on the basis of the ability of Th2-like cells, cloned from mesenteric lymph nodes of MBP-fed mice, to protect from MBP-induced EAE.[7] If indeed Th2-like regulatory cells are evoked by the 3× + IL-2 feeding regimen and participate in effecting protection from EAU, we would predict that appropriately timed administration of the Th2-type cytokines IL-4 and IL-10 should potentiate the induction of oral tolerance, whereas their neutralization should impede it. The following experiments were designed to test this prediction.

EFFECT OF IL-4 AND IL-10; CAN THEY SUBSTITUTE FOR IL-2 IN PROMOTING TOLERANCE?

Il-4 and IL-10 promote differentiation of Th2-type cells.[8] On the assumption that such cells are in fact induced by feeding, B10.A mice were fed three times with IRBP and on the day of each feeding were injected intraperitoneally with recombinant mouse IL-4 or with recombinant mouse IL-10 (kindly provided by Dr. S. Narula, Schering-Plough Research Institute, Kenilworth, NJ). All mice were immunized with a uveitogenic dose of IRBP on day 0. The delayed hypersensitivity (DH) response to IRBP and the disease severity

TABLE 3. Effect of IL-4 or IL-10, Administered at the Time of Feeding, on Induction of Oral Tolerance to IRBP[a]

Feeding Regimen	DH (micrometers)	EAU (score ± SE)	Incidence (positive/total)
3× fed + 1× IL-2 at immunization	11 ± 5	0.25 ± 0.1	2/5
3× fed + 3× IL-2 at feeding	25 ± 4	1.7 ± 0.2	4/4
3× fed + 3× IL-4 at feeding	11 ± 3	1.55 ± 0.3	5/5
3× fed + 3× IL-10 at feeding	20 ± 6	1.3 ± 0.3	5/5
3× fed (no cytokine)	40 ± 7	2.0 ± 0.7	4/4
Unfed (no cytokine)	38 ± 4	2.6 ± 0.4	5/5

[a] B10.A mice were fed with 0.2 mg IRBP or were not fed. The indicated groups were injected ip with 15 μg of IL-4 (three divided doses), 15 μg of IL-10, or 10,000 U of IL-2, at the time of feeding, or with a single dose of 10,000 IU of IL-2 at the time of immunization. All mice were immunized with 50 μg IRBP in CFA + PTX on day 0. DH was determined by ear assay, as previously described,[14] and is expressed as specific increment in ear thickness in μm, 24 h after challenge with IRBP, compared to PBS. EAU was scored by histopathology.

were assayed on day 21 in comparison to positive controls of mice fed similarly but treated with IL-2, either at the time of feeding or at the time of immunization, and to cytokine-untreated control groups (TABLE 3). The results showed that the DH responses of mice given IL-4 or IL-10 at the time of feeding were reduced in comparison to cytokine-untreated controls. The reduction in DH was similar to, or better than, that of positive-control mice given IL-2 at the time of feeding. None of the three cytokines administered at feeding afforded much protection from EAU, which was, however, effectively ameliorated by IL-2 administered at the time of immunization. These data suggest that Th2-type cytokines are capable of promoting oral tolerance, and variations of the protocol that might result in better protection from EAU should be explored, such as timing and the dose of administration, as well as possible combination with IL-2.

ROLE OF ENDOGENOUSLY PRODUCED IL-4 AND IL-10 IN ORAL TOLERANCE

The question whether IL-4 and IL-10 are required for oral tolerance in the EAU model was examined on two levels: the ability of mice genetically deficient in IL-4 or in IL-10 to develop oral tolerance, and the effect on oral tolerance of treatment with neutralizing anticytokine antibodies.

IL-4 and IL-10 "knockout" (KO) mice, in which the cytokine gene in question was disrupted in the germline by gene targeting,[9,10] were backcrossed onto the C57BL/6 background for eight or more generations. Phenotypically normal wild-type +/+ and +/− littermates served as controls. The immunization protocol for IRBP induction was adjusted in order to accommodate the special requirements of these mice, namely, the IRBP and PTX doses were increased, whereas the *M. tuberculosis* in the CFA was reduced. This was done because, on the one hand, the IL-4 and IL-10 KO mice tend to develop hyperacute inflammatory responses that can result in lethality, and, on the other hand, because C57BL/6 mice (H-2[b]) are only moderately susceptible to EAU and require a comparatively intense immunization. The results showed that both the IL-4 KO and the IL-10 KO mice

TABLE 4. IL-4 and IL-10 Knockout Mice Are Deficient in Developing Oral Tolerance by the 3× + IL-2 Feeding Regimen, but Not by the 5× Feeding Regimen[a]

Genotype	Feeding	EAU (score ± SE)	Incidence (positive/total)
Wild type	control	1.9 ± 0.5	13/14
	3× + IL-2	0.4 ± 0.2	5/12
	5×	0.2 ± 0.1	2/4
IL-4 KO	control	1.9 ± 1.3	2/2
	3× + IL-2	1.5 ± 0.5	5/6
	5×	0	0/2
IL-10 KO	control	0.9 ± 0.6	3/3
	3× + IL-2	1.4 ± 0.5	5/6
	5×	0	0/2

[a] Mice were fed with 0.2 mg of IRBP 3× + IL-2 or 5×, as indicated. Controls were fed with OVA (3× + IL-2). All mice were immunized with 100 μg IRBP in CFA containing 1 μg/mL *M. tuberculosis* and were given 2 μg PTX. EAU was scored by histopathology on a scale of 0 to 4, 16–19 days after immunization. Results are a composite of 5 experiments.

are deficient in developing oral tolerance by the 3× + IL-2 feeding regimen (TABLE 4). Assays of supernatants from IRBP-stimulated cultures of PP cells, splenocytes, and lymph node cells of the KO mice showed that whereas they were deficient in production of the disrupted cytokine, most fed individuals produced normal or even elevated levels of the reciprocal cytokine compared to wild-type controls (data not shown). These results suggest that tolerance involving putative regulatory cells requires the ability to produce both cytokines, and even elevated levels of one cytokine cannot substitute for a lack of the other. Interestingly, neither the IL-4 nor the IL-10 knockout mice were deficient in developing tolerance by the 5× regimen, which suggests that tolerance with a major component of anergy can be induced in the absence of at least one of these cytokines (TABLE 4). FIGURE 5 depicts the EAU histopathology in IL-10 KO mice fed by the different regimens. Essentially identical features were seen in parallel groups of IL-4 KO mice.

It is important to mention that the IL-10 KO mice typically develop an inflammatory bowel disease that is fatal by 8–9 weeks of age.[9] We have found that these mice do not have identifiable PP by the time that the experiments are harvested, 16–19 days after immunization. Thus, we had to consider the possibility that reasons other than the lack of IL-10 might impede normal development of oral tolerance in response to the 3× + IL-2 regimen in these mice. This possibility was addressed by experiments in which (phenotypically normal) B10.A mice were fed with IRBP by the 3× + IL-2 regimen and were treated with monoclonal antibodies to IL-10 at the time of feeding. These mice, similarly to the IL-10 KO mice, were deficient in developing oral tolerance as assessed by protection from EAU (TABLE 5), supporting the interpretation that IL-10 is needed for induction of putative regulatory cells involved in this form of oral tolerance.

SUMMARY AND CONCLUSIONS

In summary, our data suggest that oral tolerance in the mouse EAU model may occur by anergy/deletion or by suppression, depending on the feeding regimen. Tolerance

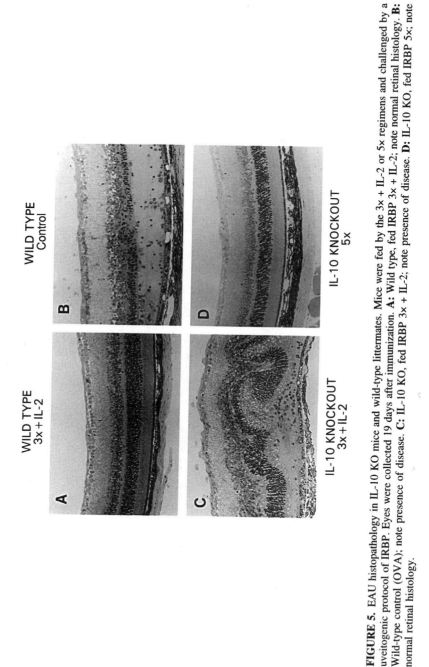

FIGURE 5. EAU histopathology in IL-10 KO mice and wild-type littermates. Mice were fed by the 3x + IL-2 or 5x regimens and challenged by a uveitogenic protocol of IRBP. Eyes were collected 19 days after immunization. **A:** Wild type, fed IRBP 3x + IL-2; note normal retinal histology. **B:** Wild-type control (OVA); note presence of disease. **C:** IL-10 KO, fed IRBP 3x + IL-2; note presence of disease. **D:** IL-10 KO, fed IRBP 5x; note normal retinal histology.

TABLE 5. Treatment with Neutralizing Monoclonals to IL-10 Inhibits Oral Tolerance[a]

Feeding	Monoclonal Antigen	EAU (score $\pm$ SE)	Incidence (positive/ total)
PBS	None	2 ± 0.2	11/11
3× IRBP + IL-2	None	0.9 ± 0.2	4/4
3× IRBP + IL-2	Anti-IL-10	1.5 ± 0.2	10/10

[a] Mice were treated with 1 mg of the JES5-2A5 anti-IL-10 monoclonal antibody at the time of each feeding (total dose: 3 mg) and received 10,000 of IL-2 at the time of immunization with IRBP on day 0. EAU was scored by histopathology on a scale of 0 to 4, 21 days after immunization.

involving putative regulatory cells appears to require the ability to produce both Il-4 and IL-10, whereas induction of tolerance involving anergy may not require the presence of IL-4 and IL-10. We propose that regulatory cells induced by three feedings of IRBP can be selectively enhanced through the use of cytokines. From the point of view of clinical therapy, it would be worthwhile to explore postimmunization feeding regimens involving administration of IL-4 and IL-10.

REFERENCES

1. CASPI, R. R., C. C. CHAN, B. WIGGERT & G. J. CHADER. 1990. The mouse as a model of experimental autoimmune uveoretinitis (EAU). Curr. Eye. Res. **9**(suppl.): 169-174.
2. CASPI, R. R. 1992. Immunogenetic aspects of clinical and experimental uveitis. Reg. Immunol. **4**: 321-330.
3. CASPI, R. R., F. G. ROBERGE, C. C. CHAN, B. WIGGERT, G. J. CHADER, L. A. ROZENSZAJN, Z. LANDO & R. B. NUSSENBLATT. 1988. A new model of autoimmune disease. Experimental autoimmune uveoretinitis induced in mice with two different retinal antigens. J. Immunol. **140**: 1490-1495.
4. CASPI, R. R. 1994. Experimental Autoimmune Uveoretinitis—Rat and Mouse. *In* Autoimmune Disease Models: A Guidebook. I. Cohen & A. Miller, Eds.: 51-81. Academic Press. New York.
5. GREGERSON, D. S., W. F. OBRITSCH & L. A. DONOSO. 1993. Oral tolerance in experimental autoimmune uveoretinitis. Distinct mechanisms of resistance are induced by low dose vs. high dose feeding protocols. J. Immunol. **151**: 5751-5761.
6. RIZZO, L. V., N. E. MILLER-RIVERO, C. C. CHAN, B. WIGGERT, R. B. NUSSENBLATT & R. R. CASPI. 1994. Interleukin-2 treatment potentiates induction of oral tolerance in a murine model of autoimmunity. J. Clin. Invest. **94**: 1668-1672.
7. CHEN, Y., V. K. KUCHROO, J. INOBE, D. A. HAFLER & H. L. WEINER. 1994. Regulatory T cell clones induced by oral tolerance: Suppression of autoimmune encephalomyelitis. Science **265**: 1237-1240.
8. SEDER, R. A. & W. E. PAUL. 1994. Acquisition of lymphokine-producing phenotype by CD4+ T cells. Annu. Rev. Immunol. **12**: 635-673.
9. KUHN, R., J. LOHLER, D. RENNICK, K. RAJEWSKY & W. MULLER. 1993. Interleukin-10-deficient mice develop chronic enterocolitis. Cell **75**: 263-274.
10. KOPF, M., G. LE GROS, M. BACHMANN, M. C. LAMERS, H. BLUETHMANN & G. KOHLER. 1993. Disruption of the murine Il-4 gene blocks Th2 cytokine responses. Nature **362**: 245-248.

11. CASPI, R. R., C. C. CHAN, W. C. LEAKE, M. HIGUCHI, B. WIGGERT & G. J. CHADER. 1990. Experimental autoimmune uveoretinitis in mice. Induction by a single eliciting event and dependence on quantitative parameters of immunization. J. Autoimmunity **3:** 237-246.
12. CASPI, R. R., B. G. GRUBBS, C. C. CHAN, G. J. CHADER & B. WIGGERT. 1992. Genetic control of susceptibility to experimental autoimmune uveoretinitis in the mouse model: Concomitant regulation by MHC and non-MHC genes. J. Immunol. **148:** 2384-2389.
13. CHAN, C. C., R. R. CASPI, M. NI, W. C. LEAKE, B. WIGGERT, G. J. CHADER & R. B. NUSSENBLATT. 1990. Pathology of experimental autoimmune uveoretinitis in mice. J. Autoimmunity **3:** 247-255.
14. SILVER, P. B., L. V. RIZZO, C. C. CHAN, L. A. DONOSO, B. WIGGERT & R. R. CASPI. 1995. Identification of a major pathogenic epitope in the human IRBP molecule recognized by mice of the H-2^r haplotype. Invest. Ophthalmol. Vis. Sci. **36:** 946-954.

Intraocular Inflammatory Disease (Uveitis) and the Use of Oral Tolerance

A Status Report

ROBERT B. NUSSENBLATT, SCOTT M. WHITCUP,
MARC D. DE SMET, RACHEL R. CASPI,
ALEXANDER T. KOZHICH, HOWARD L. WEINER,[a]
BARBARA VISTICA, AND IGAL GERY

Laboratory of Immunology
National Eye Institute
Building 10, Room 10N202
10 Center Drive
National Institutes of Health
Bethesda, Maryland 20892

[a]*Department of Neurology*
Harvard Medical School Center for Neurologic Diseases
Brigham and Women's Hospital
Boston, Massachusetts

INTRODUCTION

Intraocular inflammatory disease or uveitis is a common disorder that ophthalmologists must deal with in their everyday practice. The term uveitis is an old one, harking back to the last century. Though at one time indicating where the nidus of the inflammatory response was thought to reside, that is, the uvea, the term today has taken on a generic characteristic and indicates only that there is an inflammatory response inside the eye. Therefore disorders, such as sympathetic ophthalmia, which primarily affects the choroid of the eye, and Behçet's disease, which primarily affects the retina, are both termed uveitis. Further, an infectious process, such as toxoplasmosis and cytomegalovirus, both of which have a propensity for the retina, and candidiasis, which begins in the choroid, are also considered one of the many uveitides. It is the cause of about 10% of the severe visual handicap in the United States.

The mechanism of action of intraocular inflammatory disease has been debated over the years. Initially, most physicians caring for patients with this problem considered that the uveitis was a reflection of systemic infections. In one study performed at the Wilmer Eye Institute in the 1940s, essentially all the patients examined with granulomatous uveitis were diagnosed as having either tuberculosis or syphilis.[1] Over the years, these diagnoses simply could not explain what was observed in the eye. Additionally, immunologic theories and laboratory techniques permitted a more in-depth evaluation of pathologic processes. The presence of circulating immune complexes, as well as in the eye, were described in patients with uveitis.[2,3] Because of these observations, it was suggested that the mechanism of uveitis was a type III hypersensitivity reaction. Therapeutic strategies were initially based on these concepts. Subsequent studies have suggested that uveitis patients with immune complexes have better visual outcomes than those without immune complexes.[4] An explanation offered has been that immune complexes are present as a way to more rapidly clear debris and potentially toxic materials from the eye or circulation, and therefore help as well to limit the inflammatory process.

The development of an animal model for intraocular inflammatory disease altered immeasurably our ability to study the underlying mechanisms of this disorder. Several uveitogenic antigens have been isolated and purified.[5] The first and certainly one of the best characterized is the retinal S-antigen (S-Ag), which is found in the photoreceptor region of the retina. Isolated and purified by Wacker et al.[6] and Faure et al.,[7] immunization of genetically susceptible lower mammals with this 55 kDa protein will result in a bilateral uveitis several weeks later. S-Ag is also found in the pineal, and a pinealitis accompanies the ocular inflammatory response. A second uveitogenic antigen that has been extensively used as a model for human uveitis is IRBP, the interphotoreceptor retinoid-binding protein. This antigen, about thrice as large as the S-Ag (140 kDa), produces an inflammatory response that is similar to that of the S-antigen. Although both the S-Ag and IRBP are capable of inducing a uveitis in genetically prone rats, mice appear to be much more susceptible to IRBP-induced experimental autoimmune uveitis.[8]

Experimental autoimmune uveitis (EAU) can be induced not only in lower mammals but in nonhuman primates as well.[5] The disorder induced has many characteristics of severe human uveitis. Studies investigating the underlying mechanism of this model have repeatedly shown the importance of T cells. The disease cannot be induced in athymic rats, nor will a transfer of anti-S-Ag antibody to naive immunocompetent hosts result in disease. However, the transfer of T cells to naive hosts will result in disease. T-cell lines are efficient in transferring disease.[9] These lines bear large numbers of IL-2 receptors on their cell surface and have a cytokine profile that would define them as TH1 cells. Recent work would suggest that as the disorder progresses, TH2 cells appear in the eye, apparently in an attempt to down-regulate the inflammatory response.

Because the animal model for uveitis effectively mimics the human situation, we used this model to evaluate various immunomodulatory approaches. This practice began with the use of cyclosporine (CsA).[10] The results demonstrated that CsA very effectively prevented the expression of EAU in Lewis rats. The response was dose dependent. Therapy could be initiated even seven days after immunization, a point at which uveitogenic cells can be found in the draining lymph nodes of S-Ag-immunized rats. The inhibition of disease was obtained also when lines of uveitogenic T cells were transferred to naive hosts. CsA treatment did not, in our hands, induce a long-standing tolerance, because the disease would appear if therapy was stopped, whereas S-Ag was still present at the immunization site. On the basis of these observations, CsA has been used in the treatment of uveitis in patients (see below).

EAU has become a template for the evaluation of various immunomodulatory approaches. To date, almost all new immunomodulatory agents destined for the treatment of severe intraocular inflammatory disease have been tested in this model. FK-506, with a mechanism of action thought to be virtually identical to CsA, was shown to be effective in inhibiting EAU both in rodents as well as in nonhuman primates.[11,12] Other agents, such as rapamycin and mycophenolate mofetil (CellCept), have been used and found to inhibit disease.[13,14] Other immunomodulatory approaches, such as T-cell vaccination[15] and the recombinantly produced material, IL-2PE40, have been tried and found useful in treating the disorder.[16]

With new approaches to therapy constantly being evaluated in the animal model for human uveitis, it would be helpful to put into perspective what is presently used to treat patients. The initial drug of choice is corticosteroid. This drug can be used systemically, in periocular injections or topically. For most serious sight-threatening uveitides, most patients have posterior pole involvement, invariably necessitating the use of systemic corticosteroid. Long-term use is problematic, particularly so because the initial dosages needed to effect a positive therapeutic response are relatively high, 1 to 1.5 mg/kg, as are the doses needed to maintain this effect, usually 20-40 mg of prednisone per day. Alternative approaches would include cyclosporine, as well as cytotoxic and antimetabolic agents. Cyclosporine has begun to be used widely as a second line agent or as a steroid-sparing agent. In cases of Behçet's disease, it may be used as an initial treatment. The use of cytotoxic agents has become less popular because of their long-term potential side effects. They, at least anecdotally, appear to be helpful in the treatment of uveitis, and, if used for fairly short periods of time at low doses, in certain cases may have an acceptable risk of secondary effects. Antimetabolites, particularly Imuran and methotrexate, have undergone a resurgence of use, at lower dosages than previously used, and often as a steroid or CsA-sparing agent.

Clearly there is a practical need for the development of less toxic and, we hope, more specific therapies for uveitis. Oral tolerance, with its effect shown in experimental autoimmune encephalomyelitis and reports of positive therapeutic effects in two clinical studies, would be an obvious choice. We report here in summary the results of some of the animal work, using EAU as a model to evaluate various aspects of oral tolerance and the status of studies in humans.

MATERIAL AND METHODS

Studies with Rats

Six- to ten-week-old Lewis rats were gavage fed with S-Ag or a nonspecific protein (keyhole limpet hemocyanin (KLH) or bovine serum albumin (BSA)) at a dose of 1 mg/feeding on specific intermittent days relative to immunization. In other experiments, rats were fed bovine IRBP peptide 1179-1191, LPS, GMDP (an analogue of muramyl dipeptide), or combinations of the peptide and either LPS or GMDP. Rats were immunized with either S-Ag (20 μg) or IRPB peptide 1179-1191 (1 nmol), depending on the experiment. Animals were examined regularly for evidence of ocular inflammatory disease and then sacrificed at various points after immunization. The histological changes in their eyes were examined and their immune responses evaluated.

In one set of experiments, some Lewis rats were splenectomized prior to feeding, whereas control rats received sham operations.

In another set of experiments, female Lewis rats were treated intraperitoneally with the anti-CD8 antibody, OX8 (9 mg total), and control animals received PBS or an isotype-matched irrelevant antibody. The rats were fed either S-Ag or BSA, as above, at specific points during the injection schedule, then subsequently immunized with S-Ag (20 μg). Evidence for disease was evaluated for three weeks; then the rats were sacrificed and their immune responses measured.

Studies with Mice

Six- to twelve-week-old mice, deficient in CD8 lymphocytes [β2m (−/−)], and immunologically intact 129/J control mice were fed intermittently with either ovalbumin (OVA) or myosin prior to immunization with OVA (20 μg). Cellular immune responses were measured by the lymphocyte proliferation assay two weeks after immunization.

In Vitro *Human Studies*

Two × 10^5 cells isolated from the blood of the patient were placed into microtiter wells. At the initiation of the cultures, each well was pulsed with 20 μg/well of purified bovine retinal S-antigen. Cultures were performed in sextuplicate and harvested on day five. Sixteen hours before the termination of the culture, [^{3}H]thymidine was added to the wells. The results are expressed as a stimulation index, which is obtained by dividing the counts per minute obtained in the wells pulsed with retinal S-Ag by those counts obtained in the control wells that just received culture medium. A stimulation index of 2 or more is considered as evidence of an anamnestic response to the retinal S-Ag (indicated by the dashed line).

RESULTS

Feeding S-Antigen before the Immunization with S-Antigen[17]

Feeding S-Ag three times (−7, −5, −3) before immunization with S-Ag resulted in abrogation of the disease. The observation appeared to be dose dependent, with animals receiving 1 mg at each feeding being essentially totally protected. Lower doses resulted in an attenuated form of the disease, when measured by a masked observer approximately two weeks after immunization. Proliferative responses of T cells taken from the draining lymph nodes to the immunizing antigen were decreased as compared to those animals fed as a control antigen.

Feeding Antigen after Immunization

The effect of oral tolerance as a means of inhibiting disease after immunization has been evaluated as well. Animals fed S-Ag 3, 5, and 7 days after immunization were noted to have either no disease or a disease process that was far less severe than control animals.

Role of the Spleen in Oral Tolerance

The effect of splenectomy on oral tolerance was also evaluated.[18] It was noted that animals that were splenectomized soon after birth developed severe uveitis, even if fed with S-Ag at a dose that was capable of protecting animals who had received sham operations. This would suggest that an intact gut-spleen-ocular axis is important for the development of oral tolerance.

Effects of Bacterial Products on Oral Tolerance

Interest has been raised as to whether oral tolerance could be enhanced if bacterial products are fed at the same time as the uveitogenic antigens. Lewis rats immunized with an immunodominant fragment of IRBP, peptide 1179-1191, developed disease in all cases. The development of EAU could be exacerbated by feeding the rats with lipopolysaccharide (LPS) or GMDP prior to immunization. By contrast, the disease was markedly diminished when these bacterial products were fed along with the IRBP peptide used later for immunization.[19]

Role of CD8 Cells in Oral Tolerance

Rats that received injections of the anti-CD8 antibody OX8 and were fed S-Ag prior to immunization with S-Ag responded similarly to their controls. As can be seen in FIGURE 1, the use of the antibody did not affect the induction of oral tolerance, as compared to treatment with PBS. As well, FIGURE 2 shows that the proliferative responses from the draining lymph nodes of S-Ag immunization gave identical proliferative responses.

Mice

Cellular immune responses from CD8-deficient mice [β2m (–/–)] and their 129/J controls were very similar; feeding with OVA markedly reduced the cellular response against this antigen (FIG. 3).[20]

Animal Studies: Discussion

Oral tolerance appears to be a mode of immunosuppression that protects against EAU. The effect is dose dependent and can be induced when feeding begins before or even after immunization. Although fragments have been reported to be effective in preventing the expression of EAU, we have not seen a particularly remarkable effect with fragments of the retinal S-Ag. The immunodominant fragment of the retinal S-Ag in human disease is not clear inasmuch as patients' cells will respond to several fragments when tested *in vitro*. Additionally, usually these fragments are not those to which rat lymphocytes respond.[21] Experiments not shown here have not been overwhelmingly convincing in demonstrating a bystander suppression effect, such as has been reported in other animal models. It may be that doses of the antigen used in our experiments induced anergy and therefore no bystander suppression was induced. As well, experiments would suggest that CD8+ cells are not necessary for the induction of oral tolerance. This finding needs to be discussed in the context of an earlier finding that the addition of anti-CD8 antibody to cultures of splenically derived lymphocytes from S-Ag-fed rats reversed the down-regulation noted in proliferation assays.[17] We have seen, as well, the importance of the ocular splenic axis in our system. This mimics other immunosuppressive mechanisms involving the eye, most notably ACAID (anterior chamber associated immune deviation).[22] Of interest was the finding that CD8-positive cells were not needed for the induction of oral tolerance.

Based on the observations that the EAU model would be a good "predictor" of an effect in human disease, a pilot study involving two patients was initiated.

Human Studies

Two patients were included in a pilot study initiated about two and one-half years ago. The first patient is a 28-year-old man with pars planitis (a common form of intermediate uveitis), who had been taking prednisone orally. This medication controlled his ocular inflammatory activity with maintenance of good visual acuity. However, he would suffer a recurrence of his uveitis with any significant decrease in his prednisone dosage. The second patient is a 42-year-old woman with over a 12-year history of Behçet's disease.[23] She was begun on cyclosporine in 1983 and has required this medication, as well as a low dosage of prednisone, in order to maintain remission of her ocular disease. In 1986

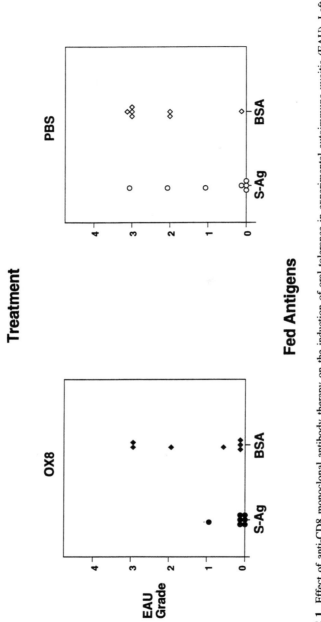

FIGURE 1. Effect of anti-CD8 monoclonal antibody therapy on the induction of oral tolerance in experimental autoimmune uveitis (EAU). Left panel: animals received OX8 (anti-CD8) therapy and then were fed either S-Ag or BSA. Right panel: the results after PBS therapy are shown. The monoclonal antibody therapy did not abrogate the effect of oral S-Ag therapy.

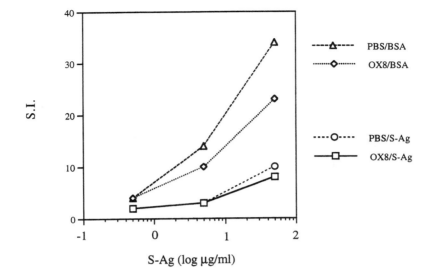

FIGURE 2. Panel shows the proliferative responses of cells from draining lymph nodes of the S-Ag immunization site. Some animals were treated with the anti-CD8 antibody systemically, and others received only PBS. Those fed S-Ag had significantly lower stimulation indices than those fed BSA, whether they were treated beforehand with antibody or not.

she received a trial of Leukeran, but this resulted in multiple ocular attacks, necessitating a return to cyclosporine therapy. These patients were chosen because of the documented recurrences of their ocular disease that occurred with dosage reduction, and because they manifested *in vitro* cell-mediated proliferative responses to the retinal S-antigen.

Both patients in this pilot phase of the study initially received 30 mg of bovine-derived retinal S-Ag, given orally, three times a week with a subsequent decrease in S-Ag dosing to once a week; their subsequent course can be seen on FIGURES 4 and 5. The FIGURES also show the results of *in vitro* proliferative assays to the retinal S-Ag performed over time.

The patient with Behçet's disease (FIG. 4) had a minor inflammatory episode as the decrease of her cyclosporine therapy began, but this problem stabilized, and she remained free of activity for over two years. She suffered a recurrence at this point, necessitating a short-term course of cyclosporine and prednisone that then was stopped. She was placed on a maintenance of 50 mg of Imuran and continued to be fed with S-Ag. Of interest in both cases was the fact that the stimulation indices for the S-Ag in the main appeared to elevate, with decreases in immunosuppressive or dosing before an attack.

FIGURE 5 summarizes the clinical course of the patient with pars planitis. As one can see, there was an initial high stimulation index of about nine. After three weeks of S-Ag therapy, the stimulation index fell to below two. With the discontinuation of prednisone therapy and, as well, a decrease in the frequency of S-Ag administration, an increase of the stimulation index back to the original level was noted, but no change in the clinical status of the patient was seen. With time, a decrease in the stimulation index was noted, but again this increased as the S-Ag feeding was stopped, which was done in an attempt to see if long-term immunologic tolerance had been permanently induced. The patient remained off all medication from week 24 until week 62, when he returned because of

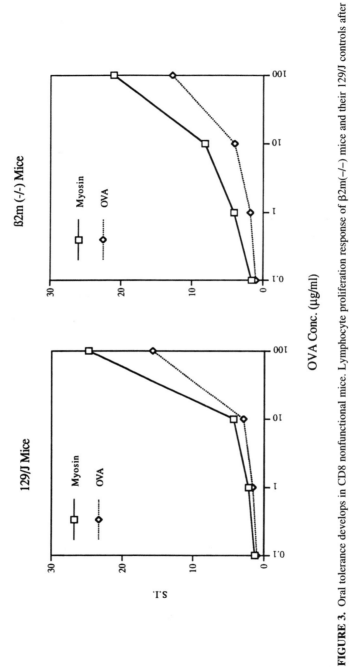

FIGURE 3. Oral tolerance develops in CD8 nonfunctional mice. Lymphocyte proliferation response of β2m(−/−) mice and their 129/J controls after three feedings with either 0.3 mg OVA or a control antigen (myosin).

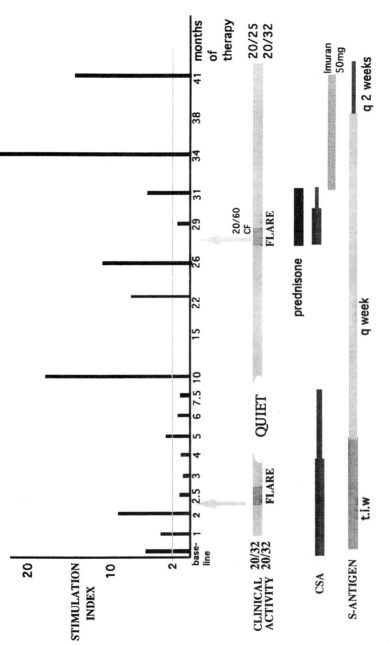
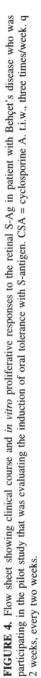

FIGURE 4. Flow sheet showing clinical course and *in vitro* proliferative responses to the retinal S-Ag in patient with Behçet's disease who was participating in the pilot study that was evaluating the induction of oral tolerance with S-antigen. CSA = cyclosporine A. t.i.w., three times/week. q 2 weeks, every two weeks.

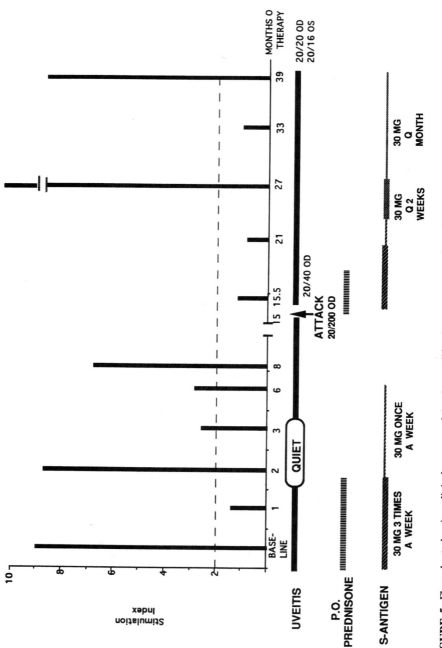

FIGURE 5. Flow sheet showing clinical course and *in vitro* proliferative responses to the retinal S-Ag in a patient with pars planitis who was participating in the pilot study that was evaluating the induction of oral tolerance with S-antigen.

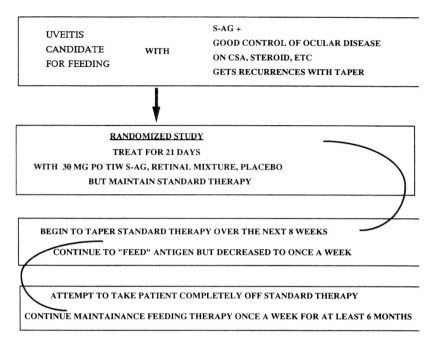

FIGURE 6. Modulation of human uveitis with ocular antigens. Outline of double-masked study protocol evaluating the use of orally administered retinal antigens and the induction of oral tolerance.

an ocular inflammatory attack. He was treated with prednisone, and feeding of the retinal S-Ag (three times a week) was reinstituted. Tested two weeks after the initiation of therapy, the stimulation index had once again fallen to well below two. He had a mild drop in vision in one eye, with his local physician giving him a periocular injection, but has not required systemic immunosuppression; he has continued to take S-Ag and has excellent vision in both eyes.

The results of these two pilot study patients were most helpful. Although, of course, not proving the potential universal therapeutic efficacy of this approach, it did give us an indication that such an approach could be useful, inasmuch as neither clinical course would have been expected, based on the natural history of either patient's disease. Both have retained good vision for the past two and one-half years. The stimulation indices appear to be a sensitive indicator of either a change in immunosuppression or of an impending attack. Because of these positive therapeutic responses in these two patients, a randomized double-masked study has begun, where the efficacy, not only of the retinal S-Ag but also of a retinal mixture made up of soluble retinal antigens at low concentrations, is being tested (FIG. 6). Patients with intermediate or posterior uveitis of a noninfectious cause necessitating systemic immunosuppressive therapy are potential candidates. Their circulating lymphocytes are tested for evidence of responsiveness to the retinal S-antigen. If they are positive, patients are randomized either to placebo, a retinal mixture, S-Ag (bovine source), or a combination of the retinal mixture and S-antigen. Once fed one of these combinations for three weeks, while maintaining their immunosuppressive therapy necessary to maintain good vision, they are tapered off from their therapeutic regimen over 10 weeks, while continuing the feeding of the retinal materials or placebo. The intent is to induce a tolerogenic state with the feeding, therefore obviating the need for further immunosuppressive therapy (or at a lower dose). The end point of the study is timed to recurrence of disease and the dosage of immunosuppressive agents used at the time of recurrence.

SUMMARY

Intraocular inflammatory disease, or uveitis, is a disorder that mostly affects children and young adults. It is the cause of about 10% of the severe visual handicap in the United States. Many of the severe, sight-threatening uveitic conditions are thought to be driven by putative autoimmune mechanisms, often with high-dose oral prednisone use as treatment, along with cytotoxic agents, antimetabolites, and cyclosporine adjunctively. The feeding of the uveitogenic retinal S-Ag to rats immunized with the same antigen resulted in clinical protection. A pilot study in which two patients, one with pars planitis and the other with Behçet's disease, were fed with the retinal S-Ag resulted in these patients' immunosuppressive medication being decreased and/or stopped. The trial also provided us with information concerning dosage and expected immune responses. A randomized, masked study looking at the effect of feeding retinal antigens to uveitis patients is ongoing.

REFERENCES

1. SCHLAEGEL, T. F. JR. 1969. Essentials of Uveitis. p. 27. Little Brown & Co. Boston.
2. CHAR, D. H., P. STEIN, R. MASI et al. 1979. Immune complexes in uveitis. Am. J. Ophthalmol. **87:** 678-681.
3. DERNOUCHAMPS, J. P., J. P. VAERMAN, J. MICHIELS et al. 1977. Immune complexes in the aqueous humor and serum. Am. J. Ophthalmol. **84:** 24-31.
4. KASP, E., E. GRAHAM, M. R. STANFORD et al. 1989. A point prevalence study of 150 patients with idiopathic retinal vasculitis. 2. Clinical relevance of antiretinal autoimmunity and circulating immune complexes. Br. J. Ophthalmol. **73:** 722-730.
5. CASPI, R. R. 1994. Experimental Autoimmune Uveoretinitis—Rat and Mouse. In Autoimmune Disease Models: A Guidebook. I. Cohen & A. Miller, Eds. Chapter 5: 57-81. San Diego. Academic Press.
6. WACKER, W. B., L. A. DONOSO, C. M. KALSOW et al. 1977. Experimental allergic uveitis. Isolation, characterization, and localization of a soluble uveitopathogenic antigen from bovine retina. J. Immunol. **119:** 1949-1958.
7. FAURE, J. P. 1980. Autoimmunity and the retina. Curr. Top. Eye Res. **2:** 215-302.
8. CASPI, R. R., F. G. ROBERGE, C. C. CAHN, B. WIGGERT, G. J. CHADER, L. A. ROZENSZAJN, Z. LANDO & R. B. NUSSENBLATT. 1988. A new model of autoimmune disease. Experimental autoimmune uveoretinitis induced in mice with two different retinal antigens. J. Immunol. **140:** 1490-1495.
9. CASPI, R. R., F. G. ROBERGE, C. G. MCALLISTER, M. EL-SAIED, T. KUWABARA, I. GERY, E. HANNA & R. B. NUSSENBLATT. 1986. T-cell lines mediating experimental autoimmune uveoretinitis (EAU) in the rat. J. Immunol. **136:** 928-933.
10. NUSSENBLATT, R. B., M. M. RODRIGUES, W. B. WACKER, S. J. CEVARIO, M. C. SALINAS-CARMONA & I. GERY. 1981. Cyclosporin A: Inhibition of experimental autoimmune uveitis in Lewis rats. J. Clin. Invest. **67:** 1228-1231.
11. KAWASHIMA, H., Y. FUJINO & M. MOCHIZUKI. 1988. Effects of a new immunosuppressive agent, FK506, on experimental autoimmune uveoretinitis in rats. Invest. Ophthalmol. Vis. Sci. **29**(8): 1265-71.

12. Fujino, Y., C. C. Chan, M. D. de Smet, N. Hikita, I. Gery, M. Mochizuki & R. B. Nussenblatt. 1991. FK506 treatment of experimental autoimmune uveoretinitis in primates Transplant. Proc. **23**(6): 3335-8.

13. Roberge, F. G., D. Xu, C. C. Chan, M. D. de Smet, R. B. Nussenblatt & H. Chen. 1993. Treatment of autoimmune uveoretinitis in the rat with rapamycin, an inhibitor of lymphocyte growth factor signal transduction. Curr. Eye Res. **12**: 191-196.

14. Chanaud III, N. P., B. P. Vistica, E. Eugui, R. B. Nussenblatt, A. C. Allision & I. Gery. 1995. Inhibition of experimental autoimmune uveoretinitis by mycophenolate mofetil, an inhibitor of purine metabolism. Exp. Eye Res. **61**: 429-434.

15. Beraud, E., S. Kotake, R. R. Caspi, S. M. Oddo, C. C. Chan, I. Gery & R. B. Nussenblatt 1992. Control of experimental autoimmune uveoretinitis by low dose T cell vaccination. Cell. Immunol. **140**: 112-122.

16. Roberge, F. G., H. Lorberboum-Galski, P. Le Hoang, M. de Smet, C. C. Chan, D. Fitzgerald & I. Pastan. 1989. Selective immunosuppression of activated T cells with the chimeric toxin IL-2-PE40. Inhibition of experimental autoimmune uveoretinitis. J. Immunol. **143**(11): 3498-502.

17. Nussenblatt, R. B., R. Caspi, R. Mahdi, C. C. Cahn, F. Roberge, O. Lider & H. L. Weiner. 1990. Inhibition of S-antigen induced experimental autoimmune uveoretinitis by oral induction of tolerance with S-antigen. J. Immunol. **144**(5): 1689-1695.

18. Suh, E. D. W., B. Vistica, C. C. Chan, I. Gery & R. B. Nussenblatt. 1993. Splenectomy abrogates the induction of oral tolerance in experimental autoimmune uveoretinitis. Curr. Eye Res. **12**: 833-839.

19. Kozhich, A. T., R. B. Nussenblatt & I. Gery. 1994. Enhancement of oral tolerance by bacterial products. *In* Advances in Ocular Immunology. Proceedings of the 6th International Symposium on the Immunology and Immunopathology of the Eye, Bethesda. R. B. Nussenblatt, S. M. Whitcup, R. R. Caspi & I. Gery, Eds.: 217-220. Elsevier. Amsterdam.

20. Chanaud, III, N. P., N. J. Felix, P. B. Silver, L. V. Rizzo, R. R. Caspi, R. B. Nussenblatt & I. Gery. 1994. Induction of oral tolerance in CD8 cell deficient mice. *In* Advances in Ocular Immunology. Proceedings of the 6th International Symposium on the Immunology and Immunopathology of the Eye, Bethesda. R. B. Nussenblatt, S. M. Whitcup, R. R. Caspi & I. Gery, Eds.: 213-216. Elsevier. Amsterdam.

21. de Smet, M. D., J. H. Yamamoto, M. Mochizuki, I. Gery, V. K. Singh, T. Shinohara, B. Wiggert, G. J. Chader & R. B. Nussenblatt. 1990. Cellular immune responses of patients with uveitis to retinal antigens and their fragments. Am. J. Ophthalmol. **110**: 135-142.

22. Gery, I. & J. W. Streilein. 1994. Autoimmunity in the eye and its regulation. Curr. Opinion Ophthalmol. **6**: 938-945.

23. Nussenblatt, R. B., M. D. de Smet, H. L. Weiner & I. Gery. The treatment of the ocular complications of Behçet's disease with oral tolerization. The International Congress on Behçet's disease. Paris, France. June 1993.

Mechanisms of Oral Tolerance by MHC Peptides

MOHAMED H. SAYEGH,[a] SAMIA J. KHOURY,[b]
WAYNE W. HANCOCK,[c] HOWARD L. WEINER,[b] AND
CHARLES B. CARPENTER [a]

[a]Laboratory of Immunogenetics and Transplantation
and
[b]Center for Neurologic Diseases
Brigham and Women's Hospital
75 Francis Street
Harvard Medical School
Boston, Massachusetts 02115

[c]Department of Pathology
Deaconess Hospital
Harvard Medical School
Boston, Massachusetts

MECHANISMS OF ALLORECOGNITION

The principal targets of the immune response to allografts are the major histocompatibility complex (MHC) molecules, and T-cell recognition of allo-MHC is the primary and central event that initiates allograft rejection.[1] It is now clear that there are two pathways of allorecognition (FIG. 1).[2,3] In the so-called direct pathway, T cells recognize intact allo-MHC molecules on the surface of donor or stimulator cells. Peptides, derived from endogenous proteins, including MHC molecules, bound into the groove of the MHC, appear to play an important role in this mode of allorecognition. In the so-called indirect pathway, T cells recognize processed alloantigen presented as allopeptides by self-antigen-presenting cells (APCs). These allopeptides are derived from allo-MHC molecules or from minor histocompatibility or tissue-specific antigens. Mounting evidence indicates that this indirect pathway, analogous to self-restricted T-cell recognition of nominal antigens, occurs during allograft rejection[4-7] and plays an important role in the rejection process.[8-11] Indirect allorecognition leads to activation of CD4+ T-helper cells that secrete cytokines and provide the necessary signals for the growth and maturation of effector mechanisms responsible for graft destruction, namely activation of CD4+ T cells and macrophages mediating delayed-type hypersensitivity (DTH) responses, cytotoxic CD8+ T lymphocytes, and B lymphocytes.[12] Direct and indirect allorecognition need not be mutually exclusive pathways, as each is mediated by different sets of T-cell clones and may both contribute to the rejection process simultaneously. It has been suggested that early acute allograft rejection is predominantly mediated by the direct pathway, because the graft contains a significant number of donor-derived passenger APCs (particularly dendritic cells) that are capable of providing the necessary costimulatory signals for full T-cell activation. Liu et al.[13] showed, by limiting dilution analysis, that the frequency of self-restricted T cells that recognize processed allo-MHC is approximately 100-fold lower than that of T cells recognizing intact allo-MHC, and suggested that the indirect pathway of allorecognition may play a minor role in acute allograft rejection but possibly a major

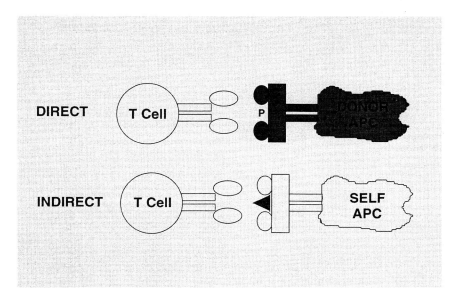

FIGURE 1. Mechanisms of allorecognition. Schematic diagram showing the two pathways by which T cells recognize alloantigens. In the direct pathway, T cells recognize intact allo-MHC on the surface of donor cells with an array of endogenous peptides bound in the groove of the MHC. In the indirect pathway, T cells recognize processed alloantigen in the form of allopeptides presented by self-(recipient) APCs.[2,3]

role in chronic allograft rejection. Braun *et al.*[14] showed that adoptive transfer of a rat CD4+ T-cell line/clone primed by the direct pathway could effect early acute rejection of normal kidney grafts, but could not initiate rejection of passenger cell-depleted kidney allografts. They concluded that T cells primed by the direct pathway play a dominant role in acute or early allograft rejection, but not in chronic allograft rejection, suggesting that T cells primed by the indirect pathway may play the dominant role in chronic rejection. At this time, the relative contribution of either pathway to acute versus chronic rejection is unknown, and formal studies are required to address this issue.

ORAL TOLERANCE TO ALLOANTIGENS

In an initial series of experiments, we studied the effects of oral administration of allogeneic splenocytes on the alloimmune response in the rat.[15,16] Lymphocytes harvested from inbred LEW (RT1^l) rats that were prefed allogeneic WF (RT1^u) splenocytes or their lysates exhibited significant antigen-specific reduction of the mixed lymphocyte response (MLR) *in vitro* and DTH responses *in vivo*, when compared to unfed controls. In an accelerated allograft rejection model, LEW rats were presensitized with BN (RT1^n) skin allografts seven days before challenging them with (LEWxBN)F1 or BN-vascularized cardiac allografts. Although sensitized control animals hyperacutely reject their cardiac allografts within two days, animals prefed with BN splenocytes maintained cardiac allograft survival to seven days, a time similar to that observed in unsensitized control recipients.

This phenomenon was antigen specific, as third-party WF grafts were rejected within two days. Immunohistologic examination of cardiac allografts harvested on day 2 from the fed animals had markedly reduced deposition of IgG, IgM, C3, and fibrin, in addition to significantly less cellular infiltrates of total white blood cells, neutrophils, macrophages, T cells, IL-2 receptor-positive T cells, and mononuclear cells, with positive staining for the Th1 cytokines IL-2 and IFN-γ. Staining for the Th2 cytokine, IL-4, however, was significantly increased in these allografts. These initial observations indicate that oral administration of allogeneic splenocytes down-regulates the systemic cell-mediated alloimmune response *in vitro* and *in vivo*. These phenomena appear to be mediated by selective inhibition of Th1 cell function and sparing of Th2 cell function in the target organ.

We then studied the tolerogenicity of orally administered synthetic class II MHC allopeptides in the rat model.[17] Inbred LEW (RT1[1]) rats, used as responders, were immunized in the foot pad with a mixture of 8 class II synthetic 25mer MHC allopeptides emulsified in complete Freund's adjuvant (CFA). These sequences represent the full-length hypervariable domain of RT1.B[u] (DQ or I-A like, 4 peptides) and RT1.D[u] (DR or I-E like, 4 peptides) β chains of the WF rat. *In vitro,* responder lymphocytes harvested from the draining lymph nodes of immunized animals exhibited significant proliferation to the MHC allopeptides. *In vivo,* when compared to controls, these animals had significant DTH responses to the allopeptide mixture, and to allogeneic WF splenocytes, but not to syngeneic LEW splenocytes or to third-party allogeneic BN splenocytes. Not all polymorphic peptides were immunogenic. In LEW responders, only 2 RT1.B (residues 1-25 and 20-44) and 2 RT1.D (residues 1-25 and 20-44) peptides were immunogenic, as determined by *in vitro* proliferation as well as by *in vivo* DTH responses. Oral administration of the allopeptide mixture to LEW responder rats daily for five days before immunization effected significant reduction of DTH responses both to the allopeptide mixture and to allogeneic splenocytes. This reduction was antigen specific, because there was no reduction of DTH responses to *Mycobacterium tuberculosis*, the antigen present in CFA. Interestingly, only the immunogenic peptides (2 RT1.B and 2 RT1.D) were tolerogenic, when administered orally.

We recently extended the above observations and examined the tolerogenic effect of orally administered synthetic MHC allopeptides on the MLR and cytotoxic T lymphocyte (CTL) generation *in vitro*. Based on dose-response studies with single MHC peptides, preliminary studies showed that oral administration of the class II peptide mixture to inbred LEW rats (1 mg daily for 15 days) effected significant reduction of proliferation of LEW responder lymphocytes to allogeneic WF stimulator, but not third-party BN (RT1[n]) stimulator cells, as compared to naive unfed controls. Oral administration of either RT1.D[u] or RT1.B[u] peptides alone resulted in significant, yet less-marked, MLR suppression, as compared to the RT1.D[u] plus RT1.B[u] mixture. In addition, when we compared the tolerogenicity of the immunogenic versus the nonimmunogenic peptides, MLR suppression was significantly higher with the immunogenic peptides. Similarly, we could detect significant reduction of CTL generation in fed animals, as compared to controls, and the effect appeared to be mediated predominantly by the immunogenic peptides. Currently, studies are focused on studying the effect of oral administration of polymorphic class I MHC allopeptides and studying oral tolerance by MHC peptides in models of primary vascularized allografts.[18] Specific questions that will be addressed include effect of oral tolerance on acute versus chronic rejection, and effect of immunosuppressive drugs on oral tolerance.

MECHANISMS OF ORAL TOLERANCE BY MHC PEPTIDES

The "effector" mechanisms of oral tolerance have been extensively studied in autoimmune models, particularly the experimental autoimmune encephalomyelitis model. These mechanisms appear to be determined primarily by the dose of antigen fed.[19] Low doses of antigen favor the generation of regulatory cells that suppress the specific immune response in the target organ, whereas high doses of antigen induce an antigen-specific anergic/deletional state in the peripheral immune system, although these mechanisms need not be mutually exclusive.[20] Low doses of orally administered antigen are taken up by gut-associated antigen-presenting cells. These cells, through complex cellular interactions, which are not completely understood, preferentially induce regulatory T cells, which, upon recognition of antigen in the target organ, secrete suppressive cytokines, such as TGFβ, IL-4, and IL-10.[19,21,22] One of the most interesting findings related to the generation of regulatory cells is that it is not necessary to feed the exact antigen that ultimately is responsible for the induction of the immune response and the disease process. This phenomenon is known as antigen-driven bystander suppression,[23] that is, any antigen that is expressed in the target organ could potentially be used to induce specific oral tolerance. High doses of orally administered antigen, on the other hand, appear to pass through the gut and enter the systemic circulation, either as intact or processed protein, thus inducing unresponsiveness of T-cell function primarily through clonal anergy/deletion. High doses of orally administered antigen are also specific for the fed antigen.[19]

We investigated the mechanisms of oral tolerance to alloantigens induced by oral administration of synthetic polymorphic class II MHC allopeptides by performing detailed immunopathological evaluation of DTH skin lesions from orally tolerized animals. These studies showed that oral therapy decreased T-cell and macrophage infiltration in the DTH skin lesions, as compared with large perivascular dermal mononuclear cell collections in lesions of control rats. In addition, there was marked reduction in staining for activation markers and inflammatory cytokines. Furthermore, there was significant reduction of staining for the Th1 cytokines IL-2 and IFN-γ, associated with increased staining of the TH2 cytokine IL-4 (Fig. 2) and preservation of staining for TGF-β. We conclude that the mechanisms of unresponsiveness induced by oral synthetic MHC allopeptides may be mediated by a state of immune deviation to a predominance of Th2 cell function in the target organ,[24] similar to what has been observed in the autoimmune models.[9]

The exact cellular interactions in the gut immune system that lead to the ''induction'' of oral tolerance are not well understood. Intestinal epithelial cells express surface class I and class II MHC molecules and present protein antigens to primed T cells *in vitro*. They are the first group of cells to encounter ingested antigens. We studied the potential role of intestinal epithelial cells in antigen presentation of ingested MHC allopeptides.[25] Small intestinal epithelial cells from naive LEW (RT1¹) rats, pulsed *in vitro* with a synthetic immunogenic MHC allopeptide RT1.D^{u}β20-44, induced specific proliferation of RT1.D^{u}β20-44-primed LEW T cells *in vitro*. Intestinal epithelial cells isolated from LEW rats that received a single oral dose of RT1.D^{u}β20-44 18 hours earlier also induced proliferation of RT1.D^{u}β20-44-primed LEW T cells, as compared to naive or LEW rats that received oral RT1.B^{u}β20-44 specificity-control peptide. Furthermore, epithelial cells harvested from LEW rats that received WF (RT1^u) splenocytes orally 18 hours earlier also induced proliferation of RT1.D^{u}β20-44-primed LEW T cells, as compared to LEW rats that received syngeneic LEW or third-party BN (RT1^n) splenocytes. These data indicate that intestinal epithelial cells are capable of taking up processed alloantigen *in vitro* and *in vivo* for presentation as peptides to primed T cells. Whether presentation of ingested MHC peptides by intestinal epithelial cells or other gut APCs lead to preferential activation of regulatory Th2 cells remains to be established.[19]

ORAL TOLERANCE BY NONPOLYMORPHIC MHC PEPTIDES

Krensky and Clayberger[26] studied the immunomodulatory effects of peptides derived from the alpha helices of the HLA class I molecule. Synthetic peptides corresponding to

IL-2   IFN-γ

CONTROL   ORAL   CONTROL   ORAL

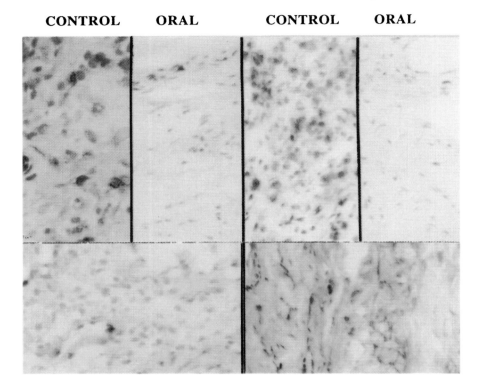

CONTROL   ORAL
                  IL-4

FIGURE 2. Immunohistology of DTH skin lesions in control LEW rats and in LEW rats tolerized by oral administration of polymorphic class II MHC allopeptides.[17] Staining for Th1 cytokines, IL-2 and IFN-γ, is markedly decreased in the orally tolerized animals, whereas staining for the Th2 cytokine, IL-4, is significantly increased in the orally tolerized animals, as compared to controls.[24]

the α1 alpha helix that inhibited CTL function were tested in a rat heterotopic LEW into an ACI heart transplant model. Oral or intravenous administration of high doses (10-20 mg/kg) of class I MHC peptide with subtherapeutic doses of cyclosporine effected long-term allograft survival in 75% of animals. Long-term surviving animals were specifically tolerant, inasmuch as they accepted a second heart or skin transplant from the same donor strain but rejected third-party allografts. Studies on the mechanisms of tolerance indicated that the subtherapeutic doses of cyclosporine A and peptide resulted in specific T-cell anergy.[27] Subsequent studies on the cellular and molecular mechanisms of action of these class I MHC peptides indicate that they bind to a T-cell receptor (or possibly heat shock protein (hsp) 70) and induce calcium flux resulting in T-cell anergy.[28] We are currently studying the immunomodulatory effects of class II MHC peptides derived from highly conserved regions on the alloimmune response *in vitro* and *in vivo*.[29]

CONCLUSION

There is ample evidence that MHC peptides play an important role in T-cell recognition of alloantigen, and potent degrees of allotolerance can be induced by oral administration of MHC peptides. Oral tolerance induced by polymorphic class II MHC allopeptides appears to be associated with a state of immune deviation towards a predominance of Th2 cell function in the target organ, and the hypothesis is that Th2 regulatory cells may mediate the unresponsive state. The gut immune system appears to play an important part in the induction of oral tolerance, and studies focused at delineating the exact cellular interactions leading to peripheral tolerance are underway. Peptides derived from highly conserved regions of MHC class I and class II molecules immunomodulate the alloimmune response, and oral administration of high doses of class I peptide is tolerogenic. The mechanisms of tolerance in these circumstances appear to be related to T-cell anergy, although the exact cellular and molecular mechanisms of how this occurs need further evaluation. Oral administration of MHC peptides may provide a novel approach to immunomodulate the immune response and induce systemic tolerance in human autoimmune diseases as well as in organ transplantation.[28,30]

SUMMARY

Recent evidence indicates that MHC peptides play an important role in T-cell recognition of alloantigen. We studied the tolerogenicity of orally administered synthetic MHC allopeptides in the rat model. Initially, we demonstrated that oral administration of synthetic class II MHC allopeptides significantly inhibited the DTH response to the peptides as well as to donor-derived cells. The tolerogenic effect was antigen specific and was induced by immunogenic, but not by nonimmunogenic, allopeptides. Immunohistological studies of DTH skin lesions showed that oral tolerance is associated with a state of "immune deviation" to a predominance of Th2 cell function in the lesions. We recently extended the above observations and examined the tolerogenic effect of orally administered synthetic MHC allopeptides on MLR and CTL generation. We found that oral administration of the class II allopeptides effected significant reduction of MLR proliferation and CTL generation, which was antigen specific. In addition, similar to the DTH results when we compared the tolerogenicity of the immunogenic versus the nonimmunogenic peptides, MLR and CTL suppression was significantly higher with the immunogenic peptides. The gut immune system plays an important role in oral tolerance by MHC peptides. Initial experiments showed that intestinal epithelial cells pulsed *in vitro* with immunogenic MHC allopeptides, or *in vivo* by oral administration of immunogenic peptides, were capable of presenting these peptides to primed T cells *in vitro*. Whether such presentation by intestinal epithelial cells or other gut antigen-presenting cells leads to preferential activation of Th2 regulatory cells, which ultimately suppress Th1 alloimmune responses, remains to be determined.

REFERENCES

1. KRENSKY, A. M., A. WEISS, G. CRABTREE, M. M. DAVIS & P. PARHAM. 1990. T-lymphocyte-antigen interactions in transplant rejection. N. Engl. J. Med. **322:** 510-517.

2. SHOSKES, D. A. & K. J. WOOD. 1994. Indirect presentation of MHC antigens in transplantation. Immunol. Today **15:** 32-38.
3. SAYEGH, M. H., B. WATSCHINGER & C. B. CARPENTER. 1994. Mechanisms of T cell recognition of alloantigen: the role of peptides. Transplantation **57:** 1295-1302.
4. BENICHOU, G., A. P. TAKIZAWA, A. C. OLSON, M. MCMILLAN & E. E. SERCARZ. 1992. Donor major histocompatibility complex (MHC) peptides are presented by recipient MHC molecules during graft rejection. J. Exp. Med. **175:** 305-308.
5. FANGMANN, J., R. DALCHAU, G. J. SAWYER, C. A. PRIESTLY & J. W. FABRE. 1992. T cell recognition of donor major histocompatibility complex class I peptides during allograft rejection. Eur. J. Immunol. **22:** 1525-1530.
6. WATSCHINGER, B., L. GALLON, C. B. CARPENTER & M. H. SAYEGH. 1994. Mechanisms of allorecognition: Recognition by *in vivo* primed T-cells of specific major histocompatibility complex polymorphisms presented as peptides by responder antigen-presenting cells. Transplantation **57:** 572-577.
7. GALLON, L., B. WATSCHINGER, B. MURPHY, E. AKALIN, M. H. SAYEGH & C. B. CARPENTER. 1995. Indirect pathway of allorecognition: The occurrence of self-restricted T cell recognition of allo-MHC peptides early in acute allograft rejection and its inhibition by conventional immunosuppression. Transplantation **59:** 612-616.
8. FANGMANN, J., R. DALCHAU & J. W. FABRE. 1992. Rejection of skin allografts by indirect allorecognition of donor class I major histocompatibility complex peptides. J. Exp. Med. **175:** 1521-1529.
9. AUCHINCLOSS, H. J., R. LEE, S. SHEA, J. S. MARKOWITZ, M. J. GRUSBY & L. H. GLIMCHER. 1993. The role of "indirect" recognition in initiating rejection of skin grafts from major histocompatibility complex class II-deficient mice. Proc. Natl. Acad. Sci. USA **90:** 3373-3377.
10. LEE, R. S., M. L. GRUSBY, L. H. GLIMSHER, H. J. WINN & H. J. AUCHINCLOSS. 1994. Indirect recognition by helper cells can induce donor-specific cytotoxic T lymphocytes *in vivo.* J. Exp. Med. **179:** 865-872.
11. BENHAM, A. M., G. J. SAWYER & J. W. FABRE. 1995. Indirect T cell allorecognition of donor antigens contributes to the rejection of vascularized kidney allografts. Transplantation **59:** 1028-1032.
12. SAYEGH, M. H. & M. H. CARPENTER. 1995. Role of indirect allorecognition in allograft rejection. Int. Rev. Immunol. In press.
13. LIU, Z., Y. SUN, Y. XI, A. MAFFEI, E. REED, P. HARRIS & N. SUCIU-FOCA. 1993. Contribution of direct and indirect recognition pathways to T cell alloreactivity. J. Exp. Med. **177:** 1643-1650.
14. BRAUN, Y. M., A. MCCORMACK, G. WEBB & R. J. BATCHELOR. 1993. Mediation of acute but not chronic rejection of MHC-incompatible rat kidney grafts by alloreactive CD4 T cells activated by the direct pathway of sensitization. Transplantation **55:** 117-182.
15. SAYEGH, M. H., Z. J. ZHANG, W. W. HANCOCK, C. A. KWOK, C. B. CARPENTER & H. L. WEINER. 1992. Down-regulation of the immune response to histocompatibility antigens and prevention of sensitization by skin allografts by orally administered alloantigen. Transplantation **53:** 163-166.
16. HANCOCK, W. W., M. H. SAYEGH, C. A. KWOK, H. L. WEINER & C. B. CARPENTER. 1993. Oral but not intravenous alloantigen prevents accelerated allograft rejection by selective intragraft Th2 cell activation. Transplantation **55:** 1112-1118.
17. SAYEGH, M. H., S. K. KHOURY, W. W. HANCOCK, H. L. WEINER & C. B. CARPENTER. 1992. Induction of immunity and oral tolerance with polymorphic class II MHC allopeptides in the rat. Proc. Natl. Acad. Sci. USA **89:** 7762-7766.
18. SAYEGH, M. H., H. L. WEINER & C. B. CARPENTER. 1994. Oral Tolerance. *In* Pancreatic Islet Transplantation. Volume II: Immunomodulation of Pancreatic Islets. R. P. Lanza & W. L. Chick, Eds.: 153-159. R. G. Landes. Austin, TX.
19. WEINER, H. L., A. FRIEDMAN, A. MILLER, S. J. KHOURY, A. AL-SABBAGH, L. SANTOS, M. H. SAYEGH, R. B. NUSSENBLATT, D. E. TRENTHAM & D. A. HAFLER. 1994. Oral

tolerance: Immunologic mechanisms and treatment of murine and human organ specific autoimmune diseases by oral administration of autoantigens. Annu. Rev. Immunol. **12:** 809-837.

20. FRIEDMAN, A. & H. L. WEINER. 1994. Induction of anergy or active suppression following oral tolerance is determined by antigen dosage. Proc. Natl. Acad. Sci. USA **91:** 6688-92.

21. KHOURY, S. J., W. W. HANCOCK & H. L. WEINER. 1992. Oral tolerance to myelin basic protein and natural recovery from experimental autoimmune encephalomyelitis are associated with downregulation of inflammatory cytokines and differential upregulation of transforming growth factor-β and prostaglandin E expression in the brain. J. Exp. Med. **176:** 1355-1364.

22. CHEN, Y., V. K. KUCHROO, J.-I. INOBE, D. A. HAFLER & H. L. WEINER. 1994. Regulatory T cell clones induced by oral tolerance: Suppression of autoimmune encephalomyelitis. Science **265:** 1237-1240.

23. MILLER, A., O. LIDER & H. L. WEINER. 1991. Antigen-driven bystander suppression following oral administration of antigens. J. Exp. Med. **174:** 791.

24. HANCOCK, W. W., S. J. KHOURY, C. B. CARPENTER & M. H. SAYEGH.1994. Differential effects of oral versus intrathymic administration of polymorphic MHC class II peptides on mononuclear and endothelial cell activation and cytokine expression during a delayed-type hypersensitivity response. Am. J. Pathol. **144:** 1149-1158.

25. BRANDEIS, J. M., M. H. SAYEGH, L. GALLON, R. S. BLUMBERG & C. B. CARPENTER. 1994. Rat intestinal epithelial cells present major histocompatibility complex allopeptides to primed T cells. Gastroenterology **107:** 1537-1542.

26. KRENSKY, A. M. & C. CLAYBERGER. 1994. The induction of tolerance to alloantigens using HLA based synthetic peptides. Curr. Opinion Immunol. **6:** 791-796.

27. NISCO, S., P. VRIENS, G. HOYT, S.-C. LYU, F. FARFAN, P. POULETTY, K. A. M. & C. CLAYBERGER. 1994. Induction of allograft tolerance in rats by an HLA class I derived peptide and cyclosporine A. J. Immunol. **152:** 3786-3792.

28. SAYEGH, M. H. & A. M. KRENSKY. 1995. Novel immunotherapeutic strategies using MHC derived peptides. Kidney Int. In press.

29. MURPHY, B., E. AKALIN, B. WATSCHINGER, C. B. CARPENTER & M. H. SAYEGH. 1995. Inhibition of the alloimmune response with synthetic non-polymorphic class II MHC peptides. Transplant. Proc. **27:** 409-410.

30. SAYEGH, M. H., L. GALLON & C. B. CARPENTER. 1994. Immunomodulating the alloimmune response with synthetic peptides. *In* New Immunosuppressive Modalities and Antirejection Approaches in Organ Transplantation. J. W. Kupiec-Weglinski, Ed.: 155-168. R. G. Landes. Austin, TX.

Oral Tolerance to Insulin and the Insulin B-Chain

Cell Lines and Cytokine Patterns

RUTH MARON,[a] NANCY S. BLOGG,[a]
MALU POLANSKI,[a] WAYNE HANCOCK,[b] AND
HOWARD L. WEINER [a]

[a]Center for Neurologic Diseases
Brigham and Women's Hospital and Harvard Medical School
Boston, Massachusetts 02115

[b]Department of Pathology and Sandoz Center for Immunobiology
New England Deaconess Hospital
and
Harvard Medical School
Boston, Massachusetts 02115

INTRODUCTION

Type 1 diabetes or insulin-dependent diabetes mellitus (IDDM) is thought to be an autoimmune disease in humans.[1,2] The nonobese diabetic (NOD) mouse spontaneously develops IDDM that has many immunological and pathological similarities to human type 1 diabetes.[3] The autoimmune nature of the disease is suggested by the lymphocytic infiltration of the islets of Langerhans, which precedes the destruction of insulin-producing beta cells. As such, the NOD mouse has served as one of the primary models for IDDM and a model in which a major focus of research has been the investigation of immunological mechanisms to suppress the disease process and of new approaches for immunotherapy.[4] A variety of immunomodulatory treatments have been studied in the NOD mouse. In general, treatments that affect T-cell function or are immunosuppressive have been effective.[5,6] A major goal of such studies has been to develop approaches that may be used to treat human type 1 diabetes. In the last few years, it has been shown in a number of systems that oral administration of an autoantigen can down-regulate experimental autoimmune diseases.[7-9] The gut-associated lymphoid tissue is unique as it favors the induction of cells that secrete suppressive and regulatory cytokines, such as TGF-β or IL-4/IL-10.[10,11] Because the regulatory cells induced by feeding act by way of secretion of antigen nonspecific cytokines, the phenomenon of bystander suppression occurs.[12] Bystander suppression solves a major problem related to therapy for inflammatory autoimmune diseases, such as diabetes, in which multiple autoantigens exist in the target tissue.[13] Thus one need not know the specific antigen that is the target of an autoimmune response, but only feed the antigen capable of inducing regulatory cells that will migrate to the target tissue and suppress inflammation. Thus, an orally administered pancreatic autoantigen theoretically represents an ideal therapeutic intervention for IDDM. In NOD mice, Th1 cells that secrete IL-2, IFN-γ, and TNF-α and support cell-mediated immunity have been implicated in the pathogenesis of diabetes.[14] Autoantigens such as glutamate decarboxylase (GAD) induce the production of large amounts of IFN-γ in NOD,[15,16] and anti-IFN-γ antibodies can prevent the development of diabetes in NOD mice.[17] Similarly, Th2 cells can serve a protective role in IDDM.[14] Systemic administration of IL-4 prevents diabetes in NOD,[18] and CFA vaccination, which protects against diabetes, is associated with more IL-4 production than IFN-γ in the islets.[19]

This study describes the cytokine patterns in the islets of orally tolerized animals. It also describes the cell type and cytokine expression associated with the development of diabetes in NOD mice and contrasts it with findings in mice following oral antigen exposure. To characterize regulatory cells generated by the oral administration of antigen, T-cell lines were developed and tested for proliferation and cytokine production.

MATERIAL AND METHODS

Animals

NOD mice were purchased from Taconic Farms (Germantown, NY) and housed in a viral antibody-free (VAF) facility. Female NOD mice developed diabetes at 12–15 weeks, and by 26 weeks 80% of the mice were diabetic. Diabetes was confirmed by showing hyperglycemia (> 250 mg/dL) for two consecutive testing days. Antigen was administered with a ball-type feeding needle in a 0.2 mL volume.

Chemicals

Insulin, insulin B-chain, and ovalbumin were purchased from Sigma (St. Louis, MO). GAD 35 (524–543) was synthesized (Biopolymers Facilities, Howard Hughs Medical Institute, Harvard Medical School). Incomplete Freund's adjuvant and *Mycobacterium tuberculosis* were purchased from Difco (Detroit, MI).

Cell Culture

Spleens or popliteal lymph nodes within each group were pooled. Cells were cultured in minimum essential medium, supplemented with 10 mM HEPES, 4 mM glutamine, 10 mM nonessential amino acids, 1 mM sodium pyruvate, 5×10^{-5} M 2-mercaptoethanol, 50 μ/mL penicillin, 50 μ/mL streptomycin, and either 1% syngeneic serum or 10% fetal calf serum. When serum-free cultures were required, X-VIVO 20 was substituted for DMEM. All cell-culture reagents were purchased from Bio Whitticaker (Walkersville, MD).

Isolation and Propagation of Antigen-specific T-cell Lines

A single cell suspension was prepared from pooled lymph nodes removed from mice injected 10 days earlier with antigen in CFA. The cells (5×10^6/mL) were suspended in culture medium with antigen (25–50 μg/mL). After 72 hours in culture, the cells were reseeded in propagation medium (culture medium + 10% T-cell growth factor (TCGF)) with medium change or splitting. For enrichment of antigen-specific cells, the cultures are restimulated with antigen after two weeks of *in vitro* propagation. Lymphoblasts (2×10^5/mL) and irradiated syngeneic normal spleen cells (5×10^6/mL) are restimulated in culture medium with antigen for 72 hours.

Feeding and Immunization Procedures

NOD mice were fed insulin B-chain (600 μg/mL × 5 feedings). Two days after the last feeding, fed and nonfed mice were immunized in the foot pad with 100 μg insulin B-chain in 50 μg CFA per mouse.

Adoptive Transfer

The adoptive-transfer experiments were carried out as previously described,[20] with slight modification. Donor splenocytes were prepared from diabetic female NOD mice and injected intravenously (10^7 cells/mouse) into 5- to 7-week-old male NOD mice, which were irradiated with 600 R from a (^{137}cesium) source four hours prior to the transfer. The recipients were injected with diabetic cells alone or in conjunction with 10^7 splenocytes from tolerized donors or line cells. Beginning at 10 days posttransfer, recipients were monitored for diabetes.

Proliferation and Cytokine Assays

For proliferation assays, 5×10^5 cells/well were cultured in 96-well plates with 25–50 μg/mL antigen for 72 hours. [^{3}H] thymidine (1 μCi/well) was added for the last seven hours of culture. For cell-line proliferation, 5×10^4 cells per well were used in the presence of 5×10^5 syngeneic irradiated spleen cells, serving as antigen-presenting cells. Incorporation of [^{3}H] thymidine was measured using the LKB Betaplate liquid scintillation counter following harvesting on a Tomtec harvester. The proliferation response was measured as Δ cpm (cpm test minus cpm control without antigen) or stimulation index (s.i.), namely cpm test divided by cpm control. Cytokines (IL-2, IL-4, IFN-γ, IL-10, and TGF-β) were quantified according to our published methods.[7] Briefly, Maxisorp plates (Nunc, Naperville, IL) were coated with capture monoclonal antibodies (1–5 μg/mL, 4 °C overnight); plates were washed and standards and samples added for another overnight incubation at 4 °C. Wells were washed and cytokine levels determined by monoclonal antibodies and a peroxidase visualization system. Antibodies and reagents used in the assays were purchased from Pharmingen (San Diego, CA). Avidin-peroxidase was purchased from Sigma. For the TGF-β assay, chicken anti-TGF-β was obtained from R and D systems (Minneapolis, MN) and murine anti-TGF-β from Celtrix. Peroxidase-labeled goat anti-mouse IgG was purchased from Kirdegaard and Perry Inc. (Gathersburg, MD). IL-2 and IL-4 were analyzed after 24 hours of incubation with antigen, IL-10, and IFN-γ after 40 hours, and TGF-β after 72 hours.

Immunohistology and Sample Evaluation

Tissues were quick frozen in liquid nitrogen and stored at −70 °C. Cryostat sections were fixed in paraformaldehyde-lysine-periodate for demonstration of leukocyte and activation antigens, or in acetone for localization of cytokines. Detailed methods and antibodies used for tissue staining are described by Hancock et al.[21]

TABLE 1. Suppression of Insulitis in NOD Mice Fed with Insulin Is Associated with Selective Expression of IL-4, IL-10, TGF-β, and PGE[a]

Feature	Insulin Fed	Ovalbumin Fed
Histology	Mild to Moderate Periislet	Dense Periislet and Intraislet MNC[b] Infiltrates
T cells	>75% MNC+	>75% MNC+
CD4+ subset	>75% MNC+	>75% MNC+
CD8+ subset	Few cells/section	~5% periislet cells
Macrophages	Few adventitial and periislet MNC	5-10% of MNC (intra- and periislet cells)
IL-2R	Few cells/section	5-10% MNC+
IL-2	Negative	5-10% MNC+
IFN-γ	Negative	>50% intra- and periislet MNC
IFN-α	Negative	>50% intra- and periislet MNC
IL-4	5-10% intra- and periislet MNC	Negative
IL-10	5-10% intra- and periislet MNC	Negative
TGF-β	10-20% intra- and periislet MNC	Negative
PGE	10-20% intra- and periislet MNC	Negative

[a] n = 3 animals/groups. Histology, cells, and cytokines at week 10 in pancreata of NOD mice fed insulin or ovalbumin. Equine insulin or ovalbumin was given twice weekly to NOD mice, beginning at week 5, for a total of 5 weeks. Immunohistochemistry was performed at 10 weeks (3 mice/group).[21]

[b] MNC, mononuclear cells.

RESULTS AND DISCUSSION

Selective Modulation of Cellular Activation and Cytokine Expression, in the Target Organ, Associated with Oral Antigen Exposure

The purpose of this study was to analyze the cell types and cytokine expression associated with development of diabetes in NOD mice and to contrast it with the findings in mice fed with insulin.[21] Animals were fed 1 mg of control antigen (ovalbumin) or equine insulin, twice a week, for five weeks beginning at five weeks of age. Histological features and the results of semiquantitative analysis of cytokines within pancreatic tissues from control NOD mice or mice fed with equine insulin are summarized in TABLE 1. At 10 weeks of age, control NOD mice or mice fed with ovalbumin showed dense infiltration of mononuclear cells (MNC) consisting mainly of CD4+ T cells within pancreatic tissues. The MNC were associated with dense expression of IFN-γ and TNF-α, as well as focal IL-2 and IL-2R expression, but lacked labeling for IL-4, IL-10, TGF-β, or prostaglandin-E (PGE). In contrast to control NOD mice, or those fed ovalbumin, oral equine insulin administration markedly altered the extend of insulitis and this type of cytokine expression. Oral insulin not only decreased the overall incidence of insulitis but suppressed to background levels the extend of IL-2R expression and eliminated production of IL-2, IFN-γ, or TNF-α. However, the effects of oral insulin were not only inhibitory; NOD mice fed with insulin showed labeling for IL-4, IL-10, TGF-β, and PGE (FIG. 1). These data support

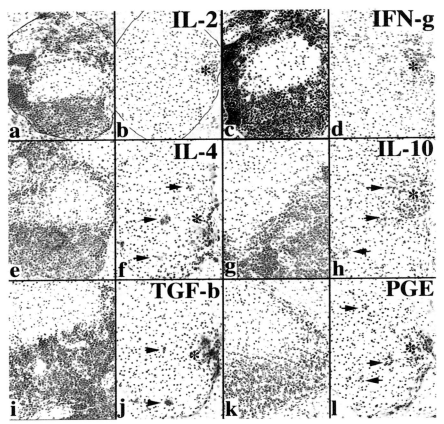

FIGURE 1. Immunoperoxidase staining of pancreatic sections from NOD mice fed ovalbumin or insulin (week 10). Representative photomicrographs of the contrasting patterns of labeling for key cytokines and PGE in these animals are shown; for each antigen, the left panel is from an animal fed ovalbumin, and the paired right panel shows the effects of insulin feeding. At the magnification used here to adequately document discrete cells (**a** and **b**), IL-2 labeling of small numbers of intraislet MNC was detected in the ovalbumin-fed group, whereas residual MNC (*) associated with the mild isletitis of the insulin-fed group were unstained. Similarly, labeling for IFN-γ (**c** and **d**) was confined to the ovalbumin-fed group; diffuse staining over MNC infiltrating an islet is seen. No labeling of residual MNC in the insulin group (*) was observed. In contrast to the results for IL-2 and IFN-γ, labeling for IL-4 (**e** and **f**), IL-10 (**g** and **h**), TGF-β (**i** and **j**), and PGE (**k** and **l**) was essentially confined to scattered intraislet MNC (arrows) plus the residual collection of MNC (*) within the axial stalk of the islet in the insulin-fed group (right), whereas these proteins were absent from the albumin-fed group (left). (For cryostat sections and hematoxylin counterstain, all magnifications × 250; reduced here by 29%).

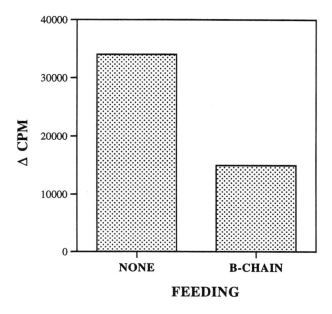

FIGURE 2. Proliferation profile of popliteal lymph node cells (PLN) from NOD mice immunized and stimulated *in vitro* with insulin B-chain. Primary proliferative responses of PLN pooled from nonfed mice or mice fed with insulin B-chain; both groups were immunized and stimulated *in vitro* with insulin B-chain. Results are the means of triplicate cultures of cells pooled from 3 animals. Data are representative of 5 experiments.

the concept[22] that oral administration of insulin affects the development of diabetes in NOD mice through the generation of cells that regulates cytokines within the target organ and shifts the balance from that of a Th1 to a Th2 pattern of cytokine expression. These Th2 cells are antigen specific and preferentially localize to the islets where insulin is expressed, inasmuch as sections of liver and kidney from the insulin-fed mice do not show Th2 cells or Th2 related cytokines.

Characterization of Regulatory Cell Lines Generated by Oral Administration of Target Antigens in Diabetes

The results presented in the previous section analyzed the cell type and cytokine expression associated with development of diabetes in NOD mice and contrasted it with the findings in insulin-fed mice. It appears that modulation of the immune response toward a Th2 type pattern has an ameliorating effect on diabetes in the NOD mouse. Our next goal was to characterize the regulatory cells generated by the oral administration of antigen and test their effect on suppressing diabetes. In addition, we wanted to determine if a Th1 type cell generated by conventional immunization would be able to induce diabetes. Immunization of NOD mice with either insulin B-chain or GAD peptide 35 in CFA raised a clear proliferative response, *in vitro,* when the draining lymph node cells were stimulated with the immunizing antigen. However, the proliferation was suppressed if the mice were fed with the antigen prior to immunization (FIGURES 2 and 3).

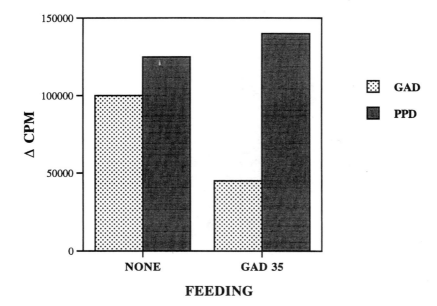

FIGURE 3. Proliferation profile of PLN from NOD mice immunized and stimulated *in vitro* with GAD 35 (524–543). Primary proliferation response of PLN pooled from nonfed mice or mice fed with the GAD peptide 524–543. Both groups were immunized with the GAD peptide in CFA and stimulated *in vitro* with either the GAD peptide or PPD.

As can be seen in FIGURE 3 the response to PPD was not affected by feeding, so the suppressed proliferation is only to the fed antigen and not to the adjuvant antigen. FIGURE 4 shows the cytokine pattern of the lymphocytes, generated from the nonfed and insulin B-chain-fed mice. The T-cell lymphocytes from nonfed NOD mice produce about 4 ng/mL IFN-γ, which decreases to 1 mg/mL upon feeding. The reverse picture is seen if one analyzes the response to TGF-β. In T cells from NOD mice immunized with insulin B-chain, there is no TGF-β production, whereas if the mice are fed prior to immunization, a moderate TGF-β level (200 pg/mL) is seen. The cytokine profile shown in the pancreas, the target organ, and the proliferation and cytokine pattern shown in the popliteal draining lymph node cells, support the concept that oral administration of an islet-cell autoantigen, such as insulin or GAD, results in the activation of Th2 type T cells and subsequent suppression of Th1 mediated autoimmune responses. These Th2 cells are antigen specific and preferentially localize to the inflamed target, either the islets or the draining lymph nodes.

Our next goal was to determine if we could generate Th1 and Th2 cell lines from the nonfed and fed NOD mice, keeping them under the same conditions *in vitro*. In FIGURE 5 the proliferation pattern of the lines generated from the nonfed and fed mice is depicted. The cell line from nonfed immunized mice proliferates much better than the cells isolated from fed mice. The response is specific to insulin B-chain as the T-cell line does not respond to PPD. FIGURE 6 shows the cytokine pattern of the two lines. Nontolerized animals secreted IL-2 and IFN-γ in response to *in vitro* insulin B-chain stimulation, whereas orally tolerized animals secreted IL-4 and IL-10.

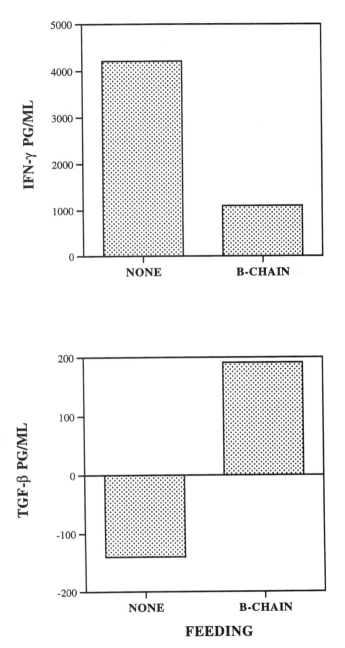

FIGURE 4. IFN-γ and TGF-β production in PLN from NOD mice immunized and stimulated *in vitro* with insulin B-chain. Cells identical to those in Fɪɢ. 2 were cultured with 50 μg/mL of antigen. Supernatants were collected, cleared by centrifugation, and assayed or kept frozen at −70 °C until assayed. Results are averages from duplicate cultures. Data are representative of 5 experiments, levels of TGF-β (pg/mL) present in 72-hour supernatant, and levels of IFN-γ (ng/mL) present in 40-hour supernatant.

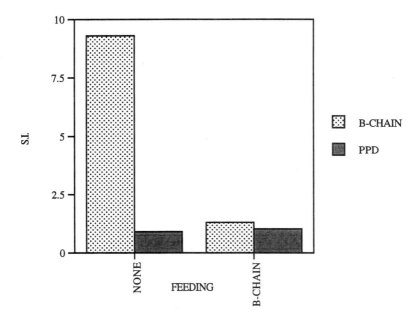

FIGURE 5. Proliferation profile of T-cell lines from NOD mice stimulated *in vitro* with insulin B-chain (6th stimulation). The cells described in Fig. 2 were kept in propagation medium after the primary stimulation and every 2-3 weeks were restimulated with APC and insulin B-chain for 72 hours. The lines that were established to insulin B-chain did not respond to PPD contrary to the primary culture. However, the response to insulin B-chain showed the same profile as the primary culture. The line from the nonfed mice proliferated nicely, whereas the line from the fed mice kept a low proliferation level.

In preliminary experiments, we investigated whether the Th1 and Th2 cell lines were able to induce or protect mice adoptively transferred with diabetic cells. The recipients, NOD-irradiated males, received 10^7 conconavalin A-activated line cells or 10^7 spleen cells from diabetic mice together with 10^7 activated line cells. TABLE 2 summarizes initial results of using T-cell lines as modulators. Mice receiving diabetic cells only developed diabetes at day 30, whereas mice receiving diabetic cells together with the Th2 cell line had a delay in the onset of disease to day 108. Seventy-five percent of NOD mice injected with the Th1 line only developed diabetes with a slight delay, compared to the no-modulator group, whereas mice receiving the Th2 T-cell line did not develop diabetes at all. It must be emphasized that these experiments are preliminary and the number of mice in each group is small; however, a T-cell line generated from insulin B-chain-fed and immunized animals, which produces Th2-type cytokines, appears able to serve as a modulator in delaying diabetes onset. Recently Cooke *et al.*[23,24] reported the generation of Th1 and Th2 lines from spleens of diabetic NOD mice that were able to transfer diabetes, and Th2 cells that caused nondestructive insulitis.

In summary, oral administration of insulin or insulin B-chain can delay and suppress the development of insulitis and diabetes in NOD mice by a T cell-dependent mechanism, as shown by adoptive transfer experiments.[20] It appears that CD4$^+$ cells play a primary role in this system.[25] We also have preliminary data that suggests that CD4$^+$ cells are

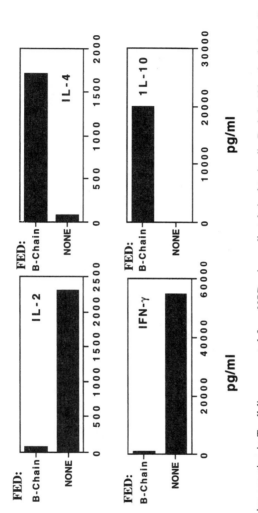
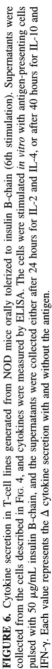

FIGURE 6. Cytokine secretion in T-cell lines generated from NOD mice orally tolerized to insulin B-chain (6th stimulation). Supernatants were collected from the cells described in Fig. 4, and cytokines were measured by ELISA. The cells were stimulated *in vitro* with antigen-presenting cells pulsed with 50 μg/mL insulin B-chain, and the supernatants were collected either after 24 hours for IL-2 and IL-4, or after 40 hours for IL-10 and IFN-γ. Each value represents the Δ cytokine secretion with and without the antigen.

TABLE 2. Adoptive Transfer of Diabetes: T-cell Lines as Modulators[a]

Cells	Number of Diabetic Mice	Day of Onset
Diabetic cells	4/5	30
Insulin B chain Th1 cell line	3/4	65
Insulin B chain Th2 cell line	0/2	—
Insulin B chain Th2 cell line + diabetic cells	2/3	108

[a] Irradiated NOD male recipients received 10^7 splenocytes from female diabetic donors intravenously, either alone or in combination with 10^7 activated T cell-line cells. Some groups received activated T-cell lines without diabetic cells. The T-cell lines described in FIG. 4 are the lines used for the adoptive transfer experiment. The mice were checked twice a week, starting 10 days after the transfer for diabetes onset.

important in mediating active suppression to oral insulin. Following oral administration of insulin, a selective expansion of TH2 cells is occurring that localizes to the pancreatic beta cells.[21] T-cell lines generated from NOD mice fed and immunized with insulin B-chain secrete IL-4 and IL-10 cytokines and are able to delay diabetes onset.

REFERENCES

1. CASTANO, L. & G. S. EISENBARTH. 1990. Type-1 diabetes: A chronic autoimmune disease of human, mouse and rat. Annu. Rev. Immunol., **8:** 647-679.
2. BACH, J.-F. 1994. Insulin-dependent diabetes mellitus as an autoimmune disease. Endocr. Rev. **15**(4): 516-542.
3. LEITER, E. H., D. V. SERREZE & K. A. M. PROCHAZ. 1990. The epidemiology of diabetes in NOD mice. Immunol. Today **11:** 147-149.
4. SHIZURU, A., C. EDWARDS-TAYLOR, B. A. BANKS, A. K. GREGORY & C. G. FATHMAN. 1988. Immunotherapy of the NOD mouse: Treatment with an antibody to T-helper lymphocytes. Science **240:** 659-662.
5. MORI, Y., M. SUKO, H. OKUDIARA, I. MATSUBA, S. TSURUOKA, A. SASAKI, H. YOKOYAMA, T. TANASE, T. SHIDA, M. NISHIMURA, E. TERADA & Y. IKEDA. 1986. Preventive effects of cyclosporin on diabetes in NOD mice. Diabetologia **29:** 244-247.
6. OGAWA, M., T. MARUYAMA, T. HASEGAWA, T. KANAYA, F. KUBAYASHI, Y. TOCHINO & H. UDA. 1985. The inhibitory effect of neonatal thymectomy on the incidence of insulitis in non-obese diabetes (NOD) mice. Biomed. Res. **6:** 103-105.
7. CHEN, Y., V. K. KUCHROO, J.-I. INOBE, D. A. HAFLER & H. L. WEINER. 1994. Regulatory T cell clones induced by oral tolerance: Suppression of autoimmune encephalomyelitis. Science **265:** 1237-1240.
8. ZHANG, Z. J., C. S. Y. LEE, O. LIDER & H. L. WEINER. 1990. Suppression of adjuvant arthritis in Lewis rats by oral administration of type II collagen. J. Immunol. **145:** 2489-2493.
9. WEINER, H. L., A. FRIEDMAN, A. MILLER, S. J. KHOURY, A. AL-SABBAGH, L. M. B. SANTOS, M. SAYEGH, R. B. NUSSENBLATT, D. E. TRENTHAM & D. A. HAFLER. 1994. Oral tolerance: Immunologic mechanisms and treatment of animal and human organ-specific autoimmune diseases by oral administration of autoantigens. Annu. Rev. Immunol. **12:** 809-837.
10. DAYNES, R., B. ARANEO, T. DOWELL, K. HUANG & D. DUDLEY. 1990. Regulation of murine lymphokine production *in vivo*. III. The lymphoid tissue microenvironment exerts regulatory influences over T helper cell function. J. Exp. Med. **171:** 979-996.

11. COFFMAN, R., D. LEBMAN & B. SHRADER. 1989. Transforming growth factor beta (TGFb) specifically enhances IgA production by lipopolysaccharide-stimulated murine B lymphocytes. J. Exp. Med. **169:** 170-177.

12. MILLER, A., O. LIDER & H. L. WEINER. 1991. Antigen-driven bystander suppression after oral administration of antigens. J. Exp. Med. **174:** 791-798.

13. ATKINSON, M. A. & N. K. MACLAREN. 1993. Islet cell autoantigens in insulin-dependent diabetes. J. Clin. Invest. **92:** 1608-1616.

14. LIBLAU, R. S., S. M. SINGER & H. O. MCDEVITT. 1995. Th1 and Th2 CD4⁺ T cells in the pathogenesis of organ-specific autoimmune diseases. Immunol. Today **16:** 34-38.

15. KAUFMAN, D. L., M. CLARE-SALZLER, J. TIAN, T. FORSTHUBER, G. S. P. TING, P. ROBINSON, M. A. ATKINSON, E. E. SERCARZ, A. J. TOBIN & P. V. LEHMANN. 1993. Spontaneous loss of T-cell tolerance to glutamate decarboxylase in murine insulin-dependent diabetes. Nature **366:** 69-72.

16. TISCH, R., X.-D. YANG, S. M. SINGER, R. S. LIBLAU, L. FUGGER & H. O. MCDEVITT. 1993. Immune response to glutamic acid decarboxylase correlates with insulitis in non-obese diabetic mice. Nature. **366:** 72-75.

17. DEBRAY-SACHS, M., C. CARNAUD, H. BOITARD, H. COHEN, P. GRESSER, P. BEDOSSA & J.-F. BACH. 1991. Prevention of diabetes in NOD mice treated with antibody to murine INF-γ. J. Autoimmunity **4:** 237-248.

18. RAPOPORT, M. J., A. JARAMILLO, D. ZIPRIS, A. H. LAZARUS, D. V. SERREZE, E. H. LEITER, P. CYOPICK, J. S. DANSKA & T. L. DELOVITCH. 1993. Interleukin 4 reverses T cell proliferative unresponsiveness and prevents the onset of diabetes in non obese diabetic mice. J. Exp. Med., **178:** 87-99.

19. SHEHADEH, N. N., F. LAROSA & K. J. LAFFERTY. 1993. Altered cytokine activity in adjuvant inhibition of autoimmune diabetes. J. Autoimmunity **6:** 291-300.

20. ZHANG, Z. J. A., L. DAVIDSON, G. EISENBARTH & H. L. WEINER. 1991. Suppression of diabetes in NOD mice by oral administration of porcine insulin. Proc. Natl. Acad. Sci. USA **88:** 10252-10256.

21. HANCOCK, W. W., M. POLANSKI, Z. J. ZHANG, N. BLOGG & H. L. WEINER. 1995. Suppression of insulitis in NOD mice by oral insulin administration is associated with selective expression of IL-4, IL-10, TGF-β and prostaglandin-E. Am. J. Path. **147:** 1193-1199.

22. RABINOVITCH, A. 1994. Immunoregulatory and cytokine imbalances in the pathogenesis of IDDM. Diabetes **43:** 613-622.

23. KATZ, J. D., C. BENOIST & D. MATHIS. 1995. T helper cell subsets in insulin-dependent diabetes. Science **268:** 1185-1188.

24. HEALEY, D., P. OZEGBE, S. ARDEN, P. CHANDLER, J. HUTTON & A. COOKE. 1995. *In vivo* activity and *in vitro* specificity of CD4⁺ Th1 and Th2 cells derived from the spleens of diabetic NOD mice. J. Clin. Invest. **95:** 2979-2985.

25. BERGEROT, I., N. FABIEN, V. MAGUER & C. THIVOLET. 1994. Oral administration of human insulin to NOD mice generates CD4⁺ T cells that suppress adoptive transfer of diabetes. J. Autoimmunity **7:** 655-663.

Local and Systemic Immune Responses in SJL/J Mice during Prolonged Oral Myelin Basic Protein Administration

YEVGENYA AKSELBAND, THERESA L. HOFFER,
PATRICIA A. NELSON, PATRICIA A. GONNELLA,[a]
AND HOWARD L. WEINER [a]

AutoImmune Inc.
128 Spring Street
Lexington, Massachusetts 02173-7802

[a]*Center for Neurologic Disease*
Brigham and Women's Hospital
Boston, Massachusetts 02115

Antigen-driven tolerance is an effective method of suppressing cell-mediated immune responses. It has been shown that oral administration of myelin antigens reduces the incidence and severity of experimental autoimmune encephalomyelitis (EAE) in rats and mice, an animal model of human multiple sclerosis.[1,2] The major protective and therapeutic effects are believed to be the result of induced specific oral tolerance after antigen feeding. The main mechanism is the generation of regulatory cells, which modulate an immune response of antigen-specific lymphocytes by producing preferentially TGF_β- and Th_2-type cytokines.[3-5] In the present study, local mucosal and systemic immune activity of lymphoid cells during prolonged low-dose oral treatment with gpMBP with or without subsequent intraperitoneal (ip) immunization with gpMBP/CFA have been investigated.

gpMBP (250 μg) was given orally to SJL/J mice, eight weeks old (two times a week for one to five weeks), and then the animals were immunized ip with 100 μg of gpMBP in 0.25 mL of PBS emulsified in an equal (0.25 mL) volume of CFA (400 μg/mL of dried MT $H_{37}Ra$). Two weeks after immunization, a DTH test was performed by injection of 100 μg of gpMBP in 50 μL of PBS in a footpad. Injection of 50 μL of PBS in the other footpad was used as a control. Footpad thickness was measured in 48 hours by a Digimatic Indicator (Mitutoyo, Japan), and results were calculated after subtraction of background (footpad thickness before DTH test). Four days after the DTH test, the animals were sacrificed. Spleen, mLN, and PP cells were isolated and tested for *in vitro* activity ([^{3}H]thymidine incorporation and cytokine production analysis).

Results of the *in vivo* DTH test showed significant decrease in gpMBP-specific reactivity in mice treated orally with the antigen prior to immunization, compared with only immunized animals. Intensity of the local immune reaction after boosting correlated with the number of previous oral administrations of the antigen. Swelling decreased proportionally during the first three weeks of treatment, remaining suppressed until the end of the experiment (FIG. 1).

The *in vitro* proliferative response of the cells in the presence of orally administered antigen showed initial sensitization at the beginning of the treatment regimen (after one week of oral administration of the antigen). This response was decreased in a dose-

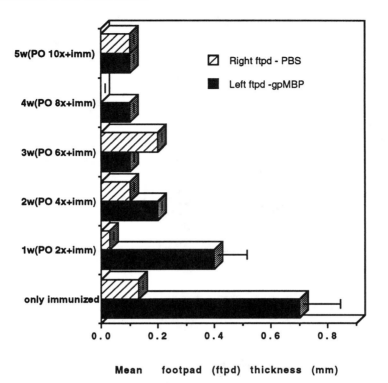

FIGURE 1. Clinical data of DTH response (48 h) in SJL/J mice treated orally with gpMBP and immunized ip with gpMBP/CFA.

dependent manner only in the orally treated and immunized group of animals. After 5 weeks (10 oral administrations of the antigen), it was very close to that seen in naive animals (FIG. 2).

For cytokine detection in cell culture supernatants, functional assays with CTLL-2 cells (IL-2), CT-4S cells (IL-4), and CLL-64 cells (TGFβ) were used. It was shown that in mice treated only with oral administration of gpMBP for 1 and 3 weeks, spontaneous (no antigens *in vitro*) IL-2 production by spleen, mLN, and PP cells was < 2000 pg/mL. The level of detected IL-2 in this group of animals increased after five weeks of oral treatment. However, antigen-specific inhibition of IL-2 production was seen in spleen and mLN cell cultures. The highest inhibition was found after five weeks of oral treatment. During the experiment, steady low levels of IL-2 (150–700 pg/mL) were detected in cell supernatants from mice immunized with gpMBP after oral treatment, regardless of the continuation of the treatment. Higher levels of IL-4 production by all tested types of cells were found in the group of mice only treated with oral administration of gpMBP compared with animals immunized with the same antigen after the same treatment. Moreover, increased spontaneous production of this cytokine in cell supernatants from only orally treated animals as well as antigen-specific increase in the orally treated and immunized group correlated with the frequency of oral administrations of gpMBP. The antigen-

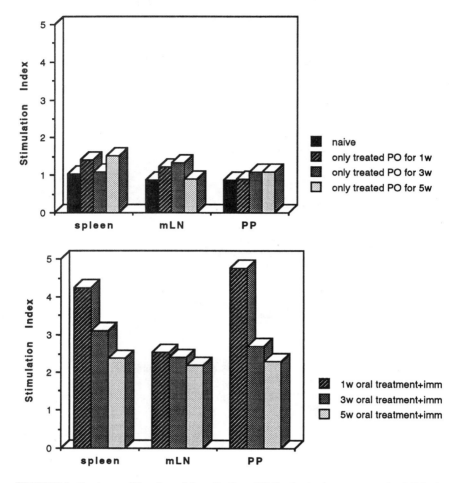

FIGURE 2. *In vitro* proliferation of the cells from SJL/J mice in the presence of gpMBP (25 μg/mL).

specific increase in TGF_β production by the cells from both groups of mice (with and without ip immunization) was always seen in cell supernatants, but this increase did not correlate with the number of oral administrations of gpMBP.

These observations show that prolonged oral administration of a low dose of gpMBP to mice results in induction of hyporesponsiveness of cells to this antigen in mucosal and peripheral sites of the immune system, demonstrated by a decreased DTH response and inhibition of gpMBP-induced proliferation. A cytokine production profile seen *in vitro* was predominantly of the Th_2 type. Initial sensitization seen in the antigen-induced proliferative response of lymphoid cells *in vitro* after one to three weeks of oral treatment with gpMBP was abrogated when the treatment regimen lasted for five weeks (10 oral administrations) before immunization. Presented results demonstrate that prolonged oral administration of a low dose of an antigen has an immunomodulatory effect on host reactivity and can be used as a therapeutic method in treatment of different kinds of immunological disorders, including autoimmune diseases.

REFERENCES

1. HIGGINS, P. J. & H. L. WEINER. 1988. J. Immunol. **140**(2): 440-445.
2. LIDER, O., L. M. B. SANTOS, C. S. Y. LEE, P. J. HIGGINS & H. L. WEINER. 1989. J. Immunol. **142**(3): 748-752.
3. MILLER, A., O. LIDER, A. B. ROBERTS, M. B. SPORN & H. L. WEINER. 1992. Proc. Natl. Acad. Sci. USA **89**: 421-425.
4. KHOURY, S. J., W. W. HANCOCK & H. L. WEINER. 1992. J. Exp. Med. **176**: 1355-1364.
5. CHEN, Y., V. K. KUCHROO, J. INOBE, D. A. HAFLER & H. L. WEINER. 1994. Science **265**: 1237-1240.

Active Suppression of Diabetes after Oral Administration of Insulin Is Determined by Antigen Dosage

I. BERGEROT, N. FABIEN, A. MAYER, AND
C. THIVOLET

INSERM U. 197
Faculté de Médecine Alexis Carrel
rue G. Paradin
69372 Lyon Cedex 08, France

INTRODUCTION

Oral administration of autoantigens or specific peptides of autoantigen has been shown to suppress several experimental autoimmune diseases (reviewed in ref. 1). Type 1 (insulin-dependent) diabetes mellitus is an autoimmune form of diabetes associated with insulitis and selective destruction of beta cells, which is thought to be T cell mediated.[2] The nonobese diabetic (NOD) mouse is a spontaneous model of diabetes that offers a unique opportunity to study the autoreactive T cells involved in the process of beta-cell destruction[3] and to settle preventive strategies before clinical onset of the disease. The number of committed T cells in the spleen of diabetic animals can be evaluated *in vivo* during adoptive T-cell transfer into nondiabetic syngeneic animals.[4] Oral insulin administration has been shown to delay the onset and the incidence of diabetes in NOD mice over a one-year period of administration.[5] We have previously demonstrated that oral administration of human insulin can trigger an active mechanism of protection, depending on CD4+ regulatory T cells.[6] The aims of the present study were to determine the effects of antigen dosage on this active mechanism of protection.

MATERIAL AND METHODS

Mice

NOD mice were bred under standard conditions in our own facilities. The incidence of spontaneous diabetes in our colony reached 80% in females by 30 weeks, whereas diabetes occurred in only 20% of males at the same period. Diagnosis of diabetes was characterized by polydipsia, weight loss, glycosuria (Urine Chemstrips, Ames-Bayer, Germany), and persistent hyperglycemia (Blood Glucose Chemstrips, Lifescan, USA). Diabetic NOD females served as donors of autoreactive T cells.

Oral Insulin Administration

For insulin-dosage experiments, young NOD females were fed at six weeks of age with 400 μL of a solution containing either 10 units (group A), 20 units (group B), or 40 units (group C) of recombinant human insulin (NovoNordisk Laboratories, Baegsvaerd,

Denmark) or PBS alone by gastric intubation with an 18-gauge stainless steel feeding needle. Mice were fed at intervals of 2–3 days for 15 days before transfer experiments.

Cell Preparation and Adoptive Transfers

Splenocytes from diabetic mice were isolated in Hanks' balanced salt solution (HBSS) by pressing the spleens through a stainless steel mesh, and enriched T-cell populations were obtained by filtration through nylon wool columns eluting 20 to 25% of the initial cell preparation. More than 90% of the final cell suspension was from the Thy1,2[+] phenotype during flow cytometry analysis. After numeration and viability evaluation, 5 × 10[6] T cells from treated mice were mixed with 5 × 10[6] T cells originating from the spleens of diabetic NOD females and intravenously (iv) injected into 8- to 10-week-old irradiated NOD males (750 rads), as previously described.[4] In order to determine whether the timing of cell interactions was critical to obtain the protective effects, 5 × 10[6] T lymphocytes obtained from the spleens of mice fed with 20 units of human insulin every 2–3 days for 15 days were iv injected immediately with diabetogenic T cells or during two occasions at day 7 and day 14 after the adoptive cell transfer.

Histologic Procedures

All mice were killed by cervical dislocation. Pancreatic glands were excised and processed for conventional histological studies after fixation in Bouin's alcoholic solution. Five-micron sections were stained with hematoxylin-eosin, as described previously.[7] The severity of insulitis was scored on at least 25 islets for each specimen as 0, when islet cells had no visible sign of inflammation, 1, when islets had lymphocytes at the periphery or peri-insulitis, 2, when islets were mildly infiltrated (< 40%), and 3, when islets were completely infiltrated. The percentages of islets of each category were compared between the different groups of mice.

Statistical Analysis

The effects of treatment on diabetes transfer were analyzed using a two-tailed Wilcoxon rank sum test and chi-square analysis. Scores of insulitis were compared using the Student's *t* test for unpaired samples.

RESULTS

Effects of Antigen Dosage on the Induction of Active Suppression of Adoptive Transfer of Diabetes

The capacity of oral administration of human insulin to generate active suppression during cotransfer experiments has been analyzed using three different concentrations

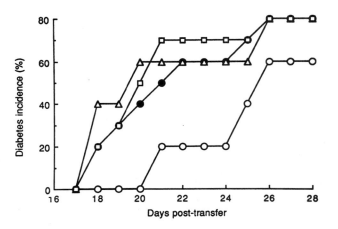

FIGURE 1. Incidence of successful transfers in mice receiving 5×10^6 T cells from diabetic females in addition to 5×10^6 T cells from mice that were administrated orally human insulin every 2–3 days for 15 days: 10 units (open triangles), 20 units (open circles), 40 units (open squares), or PBS (closed circles) for 30 days.

during the 15 days of treatment. As shown in FIGURE 1, only T cells from mice fed 6 times with 20 units of insulin were able to delay significantly the capacity of autoreactive T cells to transfer the disease (p = 0.002), in comparison to T lymphocytes from PBS-fed animals. However, the final incidence of successful transfers was not significantly different (X2 = 0.47; p = 0.75). By contrast, no effect was seen for T lymphocytes obtained from mice fed each time with 10 units or 40 units. The severity of insulitis was quantified and compared between experimental groups of mice. As shown in FIGURE 2, mice cotrans-

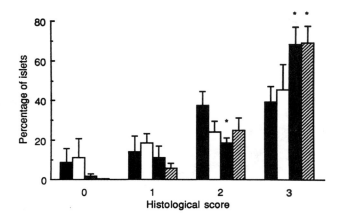

FIGURE 2. Severity of islet-cell infiltration in recipient mice transferred with 5×10^6 T cells from diabetic females and 5×10^6 T cells from saline-fed mice (dark bars), or mice fed with 20 units (open bars), 10 units (dotted bars), or 40 units (hatched bars) of insulin. The asterisk indicates statistical significance, with the p value below 0.05.

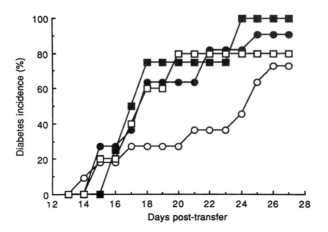

FIGURE 3. Incidence of successful transfers in mice receiving 5×10^6 T cells from diabetic females in addition to 5×10^6 T cells from insulin-fed mice (open symbols) or PBS-fed mice (closed symbols) injected immediately after cell transfer (circles) or at two occasions, day 7 and day 14, after cell transfer (squares).

ferred with autoreactive T cells and T cells from insulin-fed animals had similar lesions of insulitis as in control mice. However, it is important to note during the analysis of severely infiltrated islets that mice that received T lymphocytes from mice fed with 20 units every 2–3 days for 15 days had a significantly lower percentage of islets with severe insulitis (group B, n = 5, 39.4 ± 8%), in comparison to the group fed with 40 units (group C, n = 5, 69.2±8%, p = 0.03) or 10 units (group A, n = 5, 68.4±8%, p = 0.04). Although the percentages of normal islets were comparable between mice from group B and control mice, the percentages of islets with peri-insulitis was significantly higher in group B than in group C (18.8±4% vs. 5.7±2%, p = 0.04), in concordance with the differences observed in the incidences of diabetes transfer.

Effects of Repeated Cell Injections after the Adoptive Cell Transfer

To determine whether regulatory T cells may still induce a protective effect at the distance of the adoptive cell transfer, groups of animals receiving diabetogenic T cells and T lymphocytes from insulin-fed animals were compared according to the time of injection of regulatory T cells at day 0 or at day 7 and day 14. As shown in FIGURE 3, only regulatory T cells coinjected with diabetogenic T cells were able to delay diabetes onset in the recipients (p < 0.001), whereas injections of the same cells at the distance of the adoptive cell transfer did not change the incidence curve of diabetes (p = 0.07).

DISCUSSION

In the present study, we have found that T cells mediate active suppression of the adoptive transfer of diabetes in the NOD mouse after oral administration of insulin and that this protection was dictated by antigen dosage. A similar dose-related effect has been previously reported in the model of experimental autoimmune encephalomyelitis,[8] where different antigen dosages produce either cytokine-mediated active suppression or anergy. Only one dosage of insulin was found to be able to generate a regulatory T-cell response. Surprisingly, T lymphocytes from the low-dose fed animals did not have the capacity to reduce the incidence of diabetes. This is contrast with other experimental models where minute amounts of antigen induced active suppression.[9] From the histological findings, the islets of mice cotransferred with T lymphocytes from low-dose fed mice were more severely infiltrated. These data indicate that, in the absence of regulatory T cells, NOD recipients probably received higher amounts of committed T cells that accelerated both insulitis and diabetes and probably did not reflect an accentuation of the autoimmune process.

Insulin is a major constituant of the beta cells and is involved in both B-[10] and T-cell[11] responses during the early events of beta-cell aggression. Although insulin is probably not the major autoantigen, oral administration of insulin induced regulatory T cells that may reach the islets and prevent beta-cell destruction. From previous experiments in other animal models, it is hypothesized that these regulatory T cells have Th2-type responses[1,12] and release locally antiinflammatory cytokines like IL-4 and TGF-β. Feeding insulin to diabetes-prone animals does not prevent islet-cell infiltration. The discordance between the development of insulitis and diabetes onset is also illustrated in NOD mice by differences in disease incidence between males and females, despite similar islet-cell infiltration. In addition, mice treated with complete Freund's adjuvant are protected from diabetes despite the development of insulitis.[13] From these observations, it can be concluded that insulitis by itself is not sufficient for the development of clinical disease and that differences may occur in the composition of islet-cell infiltrates between destructive and nondestructive lesions.

During the adoptive-cell transfer model, we have recently demonstrated that pancreatic lymph nodes harbor autoreactive T cells prior to islet-cell invasion beginning at day 4.[14] These observations may explain the absence of suppression when regulatory T cells are injected later in the disease process because the delay for T-cell homing to the pancreas may be too long to produce any clinical benefits.

SUMMARY

We have previously demonstrated that feeding six-week-old female mice with 20 units of human insulin every 2-3 days for 15 or 30 days induced an active mechanism of suppression through the generation of regulatory T cells that reduced the number of successful diabetic transfers in irradiated NOD recipients. In the present study, we analyzed the effects of antigen dosage and the critical period of cell injection to obtain protection. The effects of the dose of insulin feeding were therefore compared during cotransfer experiments of 5×10^6 T cells from diabetic mice and 5×10^6 T cells from the spleen of mice receiving 10 units, 20 units, or 40 units of insulin or saline every 2-3 days for 15 days. Only T lymphocytes from mice fed with 20 units conferred active cellular protection during adoptive transfer with a significant delay in diabetes onset ($p = 0.002$). No significant difference was noticed during histological analysis of pancreatic glands, indicating that insulitis was not prevented. However, mice receiving T lymphocytes from the 20 units of insulin-fed animals had a milder form of inflammation, with a significantly lower percentage of severely infiltrated islets. Injecting regulatory T cells 7 days and 14 days after iv injection of diabetogenic T cells did not modify the incidence curves of diabetes in the recipients, suggesting that cellular interactions and delay in cell trafficking were determinants. These results may have important clinical implications in humans.

In conclusion, this study indicates the importance but also the limits of antigen therapy in type I diabetes. Antigen dosage is a critical element for active suppression. Such analysis is important to perform in humans before the initiation of a large-scale prevention trial in prediabetic individuals.

ACKNOWLEDGMENTS

We thank A. Durand and A. Steffanutti for excellent technical assistance.

REFERENCES

1. WEINER, H. L., A. FRIEDMAN, A. MILLER, S. J. KHOURY, A. AL-SABBAGH, L. SANTOS, M. SAYEGH, R. B. NUSSENBLATT, D. E. TRENTHAM & D. A. HAFLER. 1994. Oral tolerance: Immunologic mechanisms and treatment of animal and human organ specific autoimmune diseases by oral administration of autoantigens. Annu. Rev. Immunol. **12:** 809-837.
2. MAKINO, S., K. KUNIMOTO, Y. MUREOKA, Y. MIZUSHIMA, X. KATAGIRI & Y. TOCHINO. 1980. Breeding of a non-obese diabetic strain of mice. Exp. Anim. **29:** 1-13.
3. CASTANO, L. & G. S. ESENBARTH. 1990. Type 1 diabetes: a chronic autoimmune disease of human, mouse and rat. Annu. Rev. Immunol. **8:** 647-679.
4. THIVOLET, C. H., A. BENDELAC, P. BEDOSSA, J. F. BACH & C. CARNAUD. 1991. CD8⁺ T-cell homing to the pancreas in the non-obese diabetic mouse is CD4⁺ T-cell- dependent. J. Immunol. **146:** 85-88.
5. ZHANG, Z. J., L. DAVIDSON, G. EISENBARTH & H. L. WEINER. 1991. Suppression of diabetes in nonobese diabetic mice by oral administration of porcine insulin. Proc. Natl. Acad. Sci. USA **88:** 10252-10256.
6. BERGEROT, I., N. FABIEN, V. MAGUER & C. THIVOLET. 1994. Oral administration of human insulin to NOD mice generates CD4⁺ T cells that suppress adoptive cell transfer of diabetes. J. Autoimmunity **7:** 655-663.
7. THIVOLET, C. H., E. GOILLOT, P. BEDOSSA, A. DURAND, M. BONNARD & J. ORGIAZZI. 1991. Insulin prevents adoptive cell transfer of diabetes in the autoimmune non-obese diabetic mouse. Diabetologia **34:** 314-319.
8. FRIEDMAN, A. & H. L. WEINER. 1994. Induction of anergy or active suppression following oral tolerance is determined by antigen dosage. Proc. Natl. Acad. Sci. USA **91:** 6688-6692.
9. ZHANG, J. Z., C. S. Y. LEE, O. LIDER & H. L. WEINER. 1990. Suppression of adjuvant arthritis in Lewis rats by oral administration of type II collagen. J. Immunol. **145:** 2489-2493.
10. PALMER, J. P., C. M. ASPLIN, P. CLEMONS, K. LYEN, O. TATPATI, P. K. RAGHU & T. L. PACQUETTE. 1983. Insulin antibodies in insulin dependent diabetics before insulin treatment. Science **222:** 1337-1339.
11. KELLER, R. J. 1990. Cellular immunity to human insulin in individuals at high risk for the development of type I diabetes mellitus. J. Autoimmunity **3:** 321-327.
12. MOSMANN, T. R., H. CHERWINSKI, M. W. BOND, M. A. GIEDLIN & R. L. COFFAMN. 1986. Two types of murine helper T cell clone. I. Definition according to profiles of lymphokine activities and secreted proteins. J. Immunol. **136:** 2348-2357.
13. SHEHADEH, N. N., F. LAROSA & K. LAFFERTY. 1993. Altered cytokine activity in adjuvant inhibition of autoimmune diabetes. J. Autoimmunity **6:** 291-300.
14. FABIEN, N., I. BERGEROT, V. MAGUER-SATTA, J. ORGIAZZI & C. THIVOLET. 1995. Pancreatic lymph nodes are early targets of T cells during adoptive cell transfer of diabetes in NOD mice. J. Autoimmunity **8:** 323-334.

Induction of Transplantation Tolerance by Feeding or Portal Vein Injection Pretreatment of Recipient with Donor Cells

RONALD I. CARR, JUAN ZHOU,
DONNA LEDINGHAM, CATHERINE MALONEY,
VIVIAN McALISTER, MICHEL SAMSON,
HINRICK BITTER-SUERMANN, AND
TIMOTHY D. G. LEE

Departments of Medicine, Microbiology/Immunology, and Surgery
Transplantation and Immunology Research Laboratory
10 A-D, Tupper Building
Dalhousie University
Halifax, Nova Scotia, Canada B3H-4H7

Oral tolerance appears to be most effective in inducing suppression if activated prior to the primary antigen exposure. Thus kidney or other organ and tissue transplantation would be likely candidates for this approach to antigen-specific immunosuppression. The prospective donor is commonly identifiable sufficiently prior to transplantation, and the recipient could therefore receive donor cells (or even isolated specific determinants), using an oral tolerance–inducing protocol to obtain specific immunosuppression. We have begun to examine two potential routes of mucosal exposure. The first is gastric intubation (the usual way of inducing oral tolerance), and the second is direct portal vein (PV) injection, a method based on Cantor and Dumont's paper in 1967,[1] which indicated that feeding dinitrochlorobenzene did not induce tolerance in an animal whose liver had been bypassed by a portacaval shunt. This raised the possibility that the liver played a significant role in oral tolerance. Although conflicting reports have appeared with respect to the liver's role in "classic" oral tolerance, there is a growing transplantation literature in which this route of tolerance induction has been assessed.[2-7] We decided to examine both classic oral tolerance and portal tolerance in concert, both to assess the potential value of these approaches for transplantation, and then to examine the mechanism(s) involved in each, to clarify whether portal tolerance is simply a variant of oral tolerance, or if the two phenomena involve different mechanisms. It may be that one approach is better than the other, and/or that combining them might be the optimal approach. Our initial studies were carried out in mice. We examined the feeding or PV injection of BALB/c mice with C3H spleen cells, measuring the suppression of BALB/c mixed-lymphocyte reactions (MLRs) against C3H spleen cells *in vitro*. Naive BALB/c mice received (1) no pretreatment, (2) an intragastric feeding of 10^7 C3H cells daily for 5 days, or (3) one portal vein injection of 10^7 C3H cells on the same day as the fifth feeding day for group 2. All mice were then challenged by being given 10^7 C3H spleen cells subcutaneously 14 days after the pretreatment, and tolerance induction was assessed by performing the MLRs 14 days later. As shown in TABLE 1, both feeding and PV injection induced a marked suppression of the MLR.

TABLE 1. Results of the MLR Assays (BALB/c Responders vs. C3H Stimulators)

Pretreatment	MLR (cpm [³H]Thymidine Incorporated)
None	28,101
Five intragastric feedings of 10⁷ C3H spleen cells	9,073
One portal vein injection of 10⁷ C3H spleen cells	5,892

TABLE 2. Results of the Kidney Transplantation Experiments

Pretreatment	Survival (Days)	Mean Survival (Days)	
None	8, 10, 11, 6, 9	8.8 ± 1.9	
Five intragastric feedings of 10⁸ BN spleen cells	14, 17, 15, 23, 21, >35	20.8 ± 7.8	p < 0.01
One portal vein injection of 10⁸ BN spleen cells	30, 15, 46, 30, 29, 51, 34	33.6 ± 11.9	p < 0.01

We have also examined the ability of feeding and PV injection to prolong an actual kidney transplantation (in the rat). The experiments were carried out as follows: Lewis rats were fed freshly prepared 10⁸ Brown Norway (BN) splenocytes every day for five days or were given a single PV inoculation of 10⁸ BN splenocytes one week prior to transplanting (*i.e.,* the day equivalent to day 5 of feeding). One week after the last feeding or the PV injection, the recipient Lewis rats' left kidneys were removed and replaced with BN kidney grafts. Three days after the transplantation, the animal's native right kidney was removed, leaving the animals surviving on only the transplanted kidneys. As can be seen in TABLE 2, both feeding and PV injection significantly prolong kidney graft survival. In these studies we have used live cells, but we have also used hypotonically lysed cells and obtained essentially similar results (data not shown). Further studies are underway examining "antigen dose" effects, cytokine patterns, and immunohistochemistry of the grafts at various times after transplantation. Sayegh and colleagues have previously reported that prefeeding donor cells, or even synthesized MHC determinants, delays accelerated rejection, converting second-set rejection of cardiac heterografts to a primary type of rejection (at least in terms of survival times).[8–10] They have also found a shift in cytokine patterns, suggesting an activation of Th2 type cytokine secretion by the feeding, which led to the increased survival.

As described in this paper, we have found a marked prolongation of primary kidney transplant survival by prior feeding and by prior portal vein injection of intact donor cells.

REFERENCES

1. CANTOR, H. M. & A. E. DUMONT. 1967. Nature **215:** 744.
2. FUJIWARA, H., J. H. QIAN, S. SATO *et al.* 1986. J. Immunol. **136:** 2763-2768.

3. KENICK, S., R. P. LOWRY, R. D. C. FORBES *et al.* 1987. Transplant. Proc. **19:** 478-480.
4. KOKUDO, S., S. SATO, J. H. QIAN *et al.* 1988. Microbiol. Immunol. **32:** 283-292.
5. SATO, S., J. H. QIAN, S. KOKUDO *et al.* 1988. J. Immunol. **140:** 717-722.
6. SQUIERS, E. C., D. R. SALOMON, L. L. PICKARD *et al.* 1990. Transplantation **50:** 171-173.
7. KAMEI, T., M. P. CALLERY & M. W. FLYE. 1990. J. Surg. Res. **48:** 393-396.
8. SAYEGH, M. H., Z. J. ZHANG, W. W. HANCOCK *et al.* 1992. Transplantation **53:** 163-166.
9. HANCOCK, W. W., M. H. SAYEGH, C. A. KWOK *et al.* 1993. Transplantation **55:** 1112-1118.
10. SAYEGH, M. H., S. J. KHOURY, W. W. HANCOCK *et al.* 1992. Proc. Natl. Acad. Sci. USA **89:** 7762-7766.

Intranasal Administration of Insulin Peptide B : 9–23 Protects NOD Mice from Diabetes

DYLAN DANIEL[a] AND DALE R. WEGMANN [b,c]

Barbara Davis Center for Childhood Diabetes
and
[a]*Interdepartmental Program of Immunology*
[b]*Department of Immunology*
[c]*Department of Biochemistry, Biophysics, and Genetics*
University of Colorado Health Sciences Center
4200 East 9th Avenue
Box B-140
Denver, Colorado 80220

The NOD mouse develops insulin-dependent diabetes (IDDM) with many similarities to the human disease and is considered to be a good model of IDDM.[1] Type I diabetes is considered to be a T-cell mediated disease, and we have recently reported that insulin-specific T cells are a predominant component of the islet infiltrates that accumulate in NOD mice.[2] In more detailed investigations it was observed that (1) insulin-specific T cells are present in these infiltrates from the early stages of infiltration until development of diabetes, (2) TH1-like cells dominate in this response, (3) insulin-specific T-cell clones can mediate the adoptive transfer of diabetes, and (4) this spontaneous T-cell response to insulin is directed almost entirely toward a 15 residue peptide encompassing residues 9-23 of the B chain (B : 9-23).[3,4] These characteristics of the T-cell response to insulin make insulin-specific T cells ideal candidate populations toward which to target antigen-specific intervention strategies.

The reports that administration of insulin to prediabetic NOD mice leads to a decrease in the incidence of diabetes,[5–7] in conjunction with our findings concerning the prevalence of insulin-specific T cells in islet infiltrates, raises the question as to whether the protective effect of prophylactic administration of insulin is mediated by modulating the T-cell response to insulin. In this report we have addressed this issue by treating 12-week-old NOD mice with either B : 9-23 or a control peptide, TT : 830-843 (residues 830-843 of tetanus toxin) by the intranasal route, and assessing the effect of this treatment on the incidence of diabetes. This route has been reported to be effective in regulating the T-cell response of mice to experimental peptide antigens.[8]

The first experiment involved intranasal treatment of 12-week-old female littermate NODbdc mice with 40 μg per day of either B : 9-23 or TT : 830-843 for three consecutive days, dividing each litter into experimental and control groups (FIG. 1). The results of this experiment indicated that B : 9-23-treated mice had a delayed onset of diabetes (p = 0.0018 by Mann-Whitney test). We have also performed experiments in which either B : 9-23 or TT : 830-843 were administered to female NODbdc mice at four weeks of age and every four weeks thereafter. The results of this experiment (not shown) indicate that multiple treatments with B : 9-23, starting at four weeks of age, provide more complete protection from diabetes than a single treatment.

The intranasal route is minimally invasive, and the results we have obtained indicate that B : 9-23 protects NOD mice from diabetes when given by this route. This treatment

371

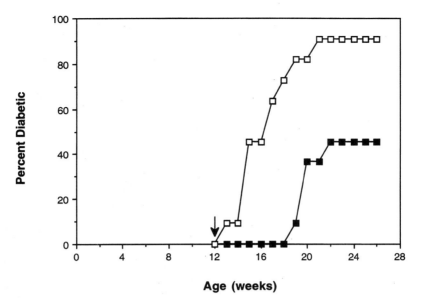

FIGURE 1. Effect of intranasal administration of insulin peptide B : 9-23 on diabetes incidence in NOD mice. Twelve-week-old female NOD mice that received intranasal B : 9-23 (n = 11) (filled squares) show delayed onset of diabetes (p = 0.0018; Mann-Whitney test) when compared to littermates that received intranasal TT : 830-843 (n = 11) (open squares). Arrow indicates time of intranasal treatment.

may therefore have clinical applications as a means of delaying the onset of diabetes in at-risk individuals.

REFERENCES

1. MAKINO, S., K. KUNIMOTO, Y. MURAOKA, Y. MIZUSHIMA, K. KATAGIRI & Y. TOCHINO. 1980. Exp. Anim. **29:** 1-13.
2. WEGMANN, D. R., M. NORBURY-GLASER & D. DANIEL. 1994. Eur. J. Immunol. **24:** 1853-1857.
3. DANIEL, D., R. G. GILL, N. SCHLOOT & D. WEGMANN. 1995. Eur. J. Immunol. **25:** 1056-1062.
4. WEGMANN, D. R., R. G. GILL, M. NORBURY-GLASER, N. SCHLOOT & D. DANIEL. 1994. Analysis of the spontaneous T cell response to insulin in NOD mice. J. Autoimmunity **7:** 833-843.
5. ZHANG, Z. J., L. DAVIDSON, G. EISENBARTH & H. L. WEINER. 1991. Proc. Natl. Acad. Sci. USA **88:** 10252-10256.
6. ATKINSON, M. A., N. K. MACLAREN & R. LUCHETTA. 1990. Diabetes **39:** 933-937.
7. MUIR, A., A. PECK, CLARE-SALZLER, Y.-H. SONG, J. CORNELIUS, R. LUCHETTA, J. KRISCHER & N. MACLAREN. 1995. J. Clin. Invest. **95:** 628-634.
8. HOYNE, G. F., R. E. O'HEHIR, D. C. WRAITH, W. R. THOMAS & J. R. LAMB. 1993. J. Exp. Med. **178:** 1783-1788.

Breaking of Oral Tolerance by an Encapsulated Antigen

MICHAEL FLANAGAN, SHILPA JAIN, AND
J. GABRIEL MICHAEL

Department of Molecular Genetics, Biochemistry, and Microbiology
College of Medicine
University of Cincinnati
Cincinnati, Ohio 45212-0524

Induction of oral tolerance is influenced by the form of antigen delivered. We showed that an intact soluble protein antigen or its enzymatic digest (antigenic fragments), when administered orally to mice, are both capable of inducing oral tolerance. However, when these two forms of antigen are administered directly into the ileum, the intact antigen becomes immunogenic, but antigenic fragments remain tolerogenic.[1] We concluded that if the digestion of the antigen *in vivo* by the proteolytic enzymes of the gastrointestinal tract is prevented, orally administered antigen will be immunogenic. To test this concept, hen egg albumin (OVA) was encapsulated by a novel technology developed in our laboratory. This technology uses an acrylic, pH-sensitive polymer, resistant to dissolution at acidic pH (< 6.0), but dissolving at higher pH. Thus, encapsulated proteins are not affected by proteolytic enzymes of the stomach and are delivered intact to the small intestine where they interact with the gut-associated lymphoid tissue.

Several antigens were encapsulated and administered orally to mice, rats, and guinea pigs. Also, in two FDA-approved studies, encapsulated allergens were given orally to humans (ragweed extract allergens to ragweed-sensitive individuals). These encapsulated antigens initiated a powerful immune response. Both primary and secondary responses were observed. These responses were characteristic of a Th2 cell dependent activation, inasmuch as IgG_1, IgA, and IgE classes of antibodies predominated. IgG_{2a} and IgG_{2b} classes of antibodies, which are Th1 dependent, were not detected. To study the T-cell activation patterns of encapsulated OVA, the number of cytokine-secreting cells were enumerated in lymphoid organs by an ELISPOT assay. Mice fed with encapsulated OVA

TABLE 1. Cytokine Secretion by Splenic T Cells following Oral Immunization with Encapsulated OVA

Form of Antigen Orally Administered	Number of OVA-specific Cytokine Secreting Cells per 10^4 Cells[a]	
	IL-4	IFN-γ
Water (control)	0	0
OVA in aqueous solution (5 mg)	330 ± 200	20 ± 20
Encapsulated OVA (5 mg)	930 ± 50	20 ± 5

[a] Spleen cells from mice harvested 14 days postimmunization cultured in the absence of antigen.

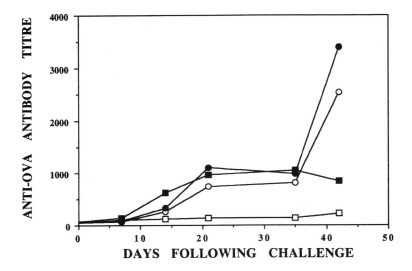

FIGURE 1. Oral administration of encapsulated OVA to mice breaks previously established oral tolerance to OVA. BDF_1 mice, 8–12 weeks old, were tolerized by the oral administration of 10 mg of OVA in water on days −14, −13, and −12 (open symbols), or were untreated (closed symbols). On days 0, 1, and 2, groups of tolerized (—O—) and nontolerized (—●—) mice were orally administered encapsulated OVA (1 mg OVA per day). On day 0, groups of tolerized (—□—) and nontolerized (—■—) mice were immunized by ip injection of 0.1 mg of OVA absorbed onto alum (0.2 mL). Serum samples were collected at weekly intervals assayed for anti-OVA antibodies by ELISA. Antibody titers were determined on pooled sera by comparison to a high titered mouse anti-OVA standard antibody.

exhibited a significant increase in the number of IL-4 secreting cells (TABLE 1). The effect of orally administered encapsulated OVA on orally tolerized mice (BDF_1 females, 8-12 weeks old) was next examined. These mice were made unresponsive to parenteral (ip) challenge both at the humoral and T-cell proliferative level by the oral administration of 10 mg soluble OVa on three consecutive days. These mice responded with an antibody response to encapsulated antigen. As shown in FIGURE 1, the immune response in tolerized mice is similar to that observed in nontolerized animals. Encapsulated proteins have the capacity to activate the T lymphocytes of the gastrointestinal tract, and, therefore, it will be of interest to determine if abrogation of oral tolerance will occur at the T-cell level. Abrogation of oral tolerance by cholera toxin to unrelated antigens has been reported.[2] This is the first report that such abrogation was demonstrated by a homologous antigen. The mechanism of this phenomenon remains unresolved at present. Conceivably, antigenic forms (fragments) responsible for the induction of oral tolerance follow a different path of delivery than the unmodified structures retained through encapsulation.[3] Thus presentation and processing of these two forms of antigen occurs at different sites, resulting in antibody formation or immunosuppression.

REFERENCES

1. MICHAEL, J. G. 1989. The role of digestive enzymes in orally induced immune tolerance. Immunol. Invest. **18**(9 & 10): 1049-1054.
2. WEINER, H. L. 1994. Oral tolerance. Proc. Natl. Acad. Sci. USA **91:** 10762-10765.
3. ZHANG, Z., R. J. APPLE, A. PESCE & J. G. MICHAEL. 1987. Peptic fragments of bovine serum albumin bind antigen-specific T suppressor cells from orally tolerized mice. Cell. Immunol. **104:** 426-433.

Effects of Cyclosporin A on the Induction of Oral Tolerance

A. FUKUSHIMA,[a,b] S. M. WHITCUP,[a]
R. B. NUSSENBLATT,[a] AND I. GERY [a]

[a]Laboratory of Immunology
National Eye Institute
Building 10, Room 10N210
Bethesda, Maryland 20892-1858

[b]AutoImmune Inc.
Lexington, Massachusetts 02173-7802

Uveitis describes a group of disorders characterized by intraocular inflammation. Many uveitic conditions are presumed to have an autoimmune etiology and are treated with immunosuppressive drugs, including cyclosporin A (CsA).[1,2] The National Eye Institute is conducting a phase II clinical trial of oral tolerance as a treatment for uveitis.[3] In this study, patients with stable disease on immunosuppressive medications are fed with retinal antigens and then have their immunosuppressive medications discontinued. Some of these patients are taking CsA when feeding of retinal antigens is begun. We therefore decided to study the effect of CsA on the induction of oral tolerance in experimental autoimmune uveitis (EAU), an animal model for human uveitis.[1]

MATERIAL AND METHODS

EAU was induced in 37 male Lewis rats by immunization with 50 μg of retinal S-antigen (S-Ag), emulsified with complete Freund's adjuvant.[4] Groups of rats were given daily intramuscular injections of CsA dissolved in olive oil (5 mg/kg/day) from 13 days to 1 day prior to immunization with S-Ag, and fed with bovine S-Ag (n = 10, 1 mg/ feeding) or PBS (n = 9) 11, 9, 7, 5, and 2 days prior to immunization. Control animals received daily intramuscular injections of olive oil instead of CsA and then were fed with bovine S-Ag (n = 9) or PBS (n = 9) as described above. Animals were examined daily for clinical ocular disease and graded on a scale of 0-4, as previously described.[4] The level of cellular immunity was determined by a lymphocyte proliferative assay,[4] using lymph node cells collected 21 or 24 days postimmunization, and humoral immunity was assessed by measuring antibody levels of sera collected at the above times by ELISA.[4]

RESULTS AND DISCUSSION

When treated with the vehicle, rats fed S-Ag had decreased clinical signs of EAU (FIG. 1A) and diminished lymphocyte proliferation (FIG. 2) when compared to animals fed with PBS. Importantly, the feeding effect was essentially abolished in rats receiving CsA. CsA-treated rats developed similar degrees of clinical disease (FIG. 1B) and immune response, (FIG. 2) whether they were fed with S-Ag or PBS. The effect of oral tolerance on antibody response was similarly abrogated by treatment with CsA (data not shown).

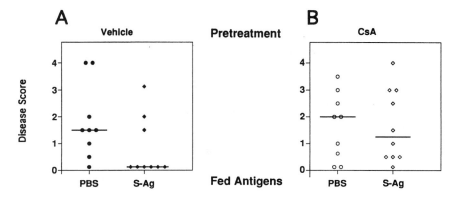

FIGURE 1. CsA treatment abrogates the oral tolerance effect on development of EAU. Clinical scores of individual rats. Horizontal bars depict the median values of each group.

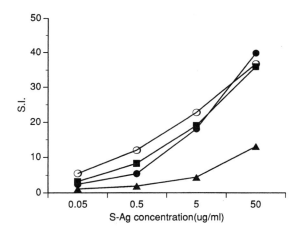

FIGURE 2. CsA abrogates the oral tolerance effect on the lymphocyte proliferative response. Responses are expressed as stimulation index (S.I.) values of cultures of pooled lymph node cells from 3 rats in each tested group. Feeding/treatment: ——●——, PBS/vehicle; ——⊖——, S-Ag/CsA; ——■——, PBS/CsA; and ——▲—— S-Ag/vehicle.

To the best of our knowledge, the present study is the first to demonstrate that treatment with CsA abrogates the induction of oral tolerance. The mode of action of CsA in this system is not clear, but it could be related to the capacity of CsA to inhibit the induction of anergy,[5] one mechanism by which oral tolerance is elicited.[6] This notion is currently under investigation. The significance of the observation recorded here is underscored by the ongoing study in patients with uveitis, in which CsA is administered in certain patients concurrently with feeding with S-antigen.[3]

REFERENCES

1. NUSSENBLATT, R. B. & A. G. PALESTINE. 1989. Uveitis. Fundamentals and Clinical Practice. Year Book Medical Publishers. Chicago.
2. WHITCUP, S. M. & R. B. NUSSENBLATT. 1993. Treatment of Autoimmune Uveitis. Ann. N.Y. Acad. Sci. **696:** 307-318.
3. NUSSENBLATT, R. B., S. M. WHITCUP, M. D. DE SMET, R. R. CASPI, A. T. KOZHICH, H. L. WEINER, B. VISTICA & I. GERY. 1996. Intraocular inflammatory disease (uveitis) and the use of oral tolerance: A status report. This volume.
4. SUH, E. D. W., B. P. VISTICA, C. C. CHAN, J. M. RABER, I. GERY & R. B. NUSSENBLATT. 1993. Curr. Eye Res. **12:** 833-839.
5. SLOAN-LANCASTER, J., B. D. EVAVOLD & P. M. ALLEN. 1993. Nature **363:** 156-159.
6. WEINER, H. L., A. FRIEDMAN, A. MILLER, S. J. KHOURY, A. AL-SABBAGH, L. SANTOS, M. SAYEGH, R. B. NUSSENBLATT, D. E. TRENTHAM & D. A. HAFLER. 1994. Annu. Rev. Immunol. **12:** 809-837.

Rheumatoid Arthritis and the Drop in Tolerance to Foods

Elimination Diets and the Reestablishment of Tolerance by Low-dose Diluted Food

P. GIANFRANCESCHI, G. FASANI, AND
A. F. SPECIANI

Associazione Di Ricerca Intolleranze Alimentari
(Association for Research into Food Intolerances)
via Brera 17
20121 Milano, Italy

INTRODUCTION

Many studies have recently confirmed the relationship between diet and some pathological features of rheumatoid arthritis (RA). The existence of a food-induced arthritis,[1] the induction of type A synoviocytes that bind exogenous food antigens,[2] has been reported. We tried to determine the effects induced by a dietary approach, reestablishing the usual tolerance to foods, on three pathological features of rheumatoid arthritis (stiffness, pain, and joint swelling). We compared two different diets on the same subject: a well-balanced normocaloric one, and a diet in which patients avoided foods suspected to interfere with their own immune system.

Twelve patients, aged 42 to 69, suffering from stable RA for an average time of 10.1 years, under drug control, entered a crossover study to evaluate the clinical effects of two different normocaloric diets. They underwent a dynamometric challenge test (DRIA test), which allows physicians to detect foods suspected of causing intolerance. Patients were randomly and blindly assigned to diet A (no suspect foods admitted) or B (well-balanced diet) for three months and then crossed over after a one-month washout.

THE DRIA TEST

The test is a dynamometric challenge test, designed to point out in a repeatable way, in standard condition, the interference induced onto muscular strength by contact between the mouth and a liquid preparation of food. An electric strength transducer sends objective electric data to a connected computer that analyzes the variations of strength. The test allows physicians to take notice of foods interfering with the whole body system, and to alert the suspect to a drop in tolerance to specific foods.

379

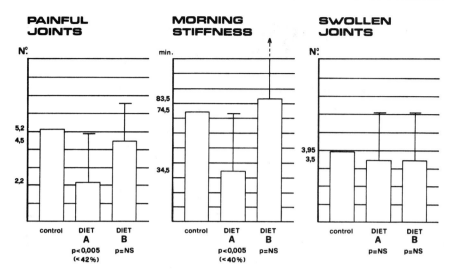

FIGURE 1. Diet A excluded all foods identified by the DRIA test. Diet B included all kinds of food. After the A diet, patients had 42% less joint pain (CI from −58% to −25%; p < 0.005). Results from the B diet were not significant. After the A diet, morning stiffness was reduced by 40% (CI from −66% to −13%; p < 0.005). Results from the B diet were not significant. Both diets slightly reduced the number of swollen joints; the results were not significant.

RESULTS

The results had been statistically analyzed with the two-tailed Wilcoxon test for ranked pairs (FIG. 1). Diet and avoidance of selected foods appear to be useful in RA management, and the DRIA test represents a practical clinical tool for establishing the best diet.[3] A drop in tolerance to foods is strictly individual. The diet for the relief of RA symptoms cannot be a standard one, but should be selected according to individual food hypersensitivities.

More recently, ten people with RA, whose food intolerances were detected with the DRIA test, which included a drop in tolerance to dairy products, underwent a study in which they could eat any amount of the suspect foods twice a week.[4] At the same time, the patients took a 1 mL solution of these foods, daily, in order to reestablish tolerance to those foods.[5] The suitable, strictly individual concentration was defined during the DRIA test. Our attempt was to take advantage of the induction of low-dose tolerance by means of low (but still considerable) dosage of antigens (*e.g.,* 0.25 mg of milk diluted in 1 mL of water), thus creating tolerance towards the responsible antigen, and in some cases, the reestablishment of a correct immune reaction to other antigens causing the symptoms.[6] Preliminary results appear to match those obtained with the elimination diet. Not only is a tolerance-inducing oral treatment suitable for relief of symptoms, but it also allows for better diet compliance.

REFERENCES

1. PANUSH, R. S. 1990. Food induced (allergic) arthritis: Clinical and serologic studies. J. Rheumatol. **17**(3): 291-4.

2. BELLON, T. *et al.* 1989. Synoviocytes type A bind exogenous antigens recognized by antibodies present in rheumatoid arthritis. Scand. J. Immunol. **30:** 563-71.
3. SPECIANI, A. F. *et al.* 1994. Significant reduction of stiffness and pain but not of swelling in patients with RA avoiding suspected food hypersensitivities. ACI News (Suppl. 2): 173.
4. MARTELLETTI, P. *et al.* 1989. Evidence for an immune mediated mechanism in food induced migraine from a study on activated T cells, IgG4 subclass, anti-IgG antibodies and circulating immune complexes. Headache **29:** 664-70.
5. WELLS, H. G. 1919. Studies on the chemistry of anaphylaxis. III. Experiments with isolated proteins especially those of the hen's egg. J. Infect. Dis. **9**(2): 147-71.
6. MARSHALL, J. S. 1992. Chronic antigen challenge alters the mast cell response to a second antigen in a dose dependent manner. J. Allergy Clin. Immunol. **89**(part 2): 222.

Oral Tolerance in Autoimmune Encephalomyelitis

In Vivo Reversal of Anergy

INGRID GIENAPP, KAREN COX, NAJMA JAVED,
AND CAROLINE WHITACRE

The Department of Medical Microbiology and Immunology
Ohio State University College of Medicine
333 West 10th Avenue, Room 2078
Columbus Ohio 43210

Experimental autoimmune encephalomyelitis (EAE) in the Lewis rat is a monophasic disease of the central nervous system that is an often used animal model for the human demyelinating disease, multiple sclerosis. We and others have shown that the oral administration of myelin basic protein (MBP) to Lewis rats prior to encephalitogenic challenge suppresses the development of EAE.[1,2] Low doses of MBP (5 mg) administered orally have been reported to suppress EAE in the rat by means of a bystander suppression mechanism in which CD8+ T cells release transforming growth factor β.[3] We have reported that feeding higher doses of MBP (20 mg) results in oral tolerance mediated by a clonal anergy mechanism.[4] Anergized T cells are characterized by their inability to proliferate or secrete IL-2, yet still possess IL-2 receptors. Recently, protocols have been reported for the successful reversal of anergy *in vivo* by the injection of large doses of IL-2 in mice.[5]

We undertook the present study to determine whether *in vivo* administration of IL-2 could reverse the oral tolerance induced by either low- or high-dose MBP. Rats were orally tolerized by feeding either 5 mg MBP (1 mg per feeding 5 times) or 20 mg (5 mg per feeding four times with soybean trypsin inhibitor). After completion of the feeding regimen, rats received four injections of recombinant human IL-2 (2000, 8,000, or 20,000 units/day) or saline. Animals were challenged by injecting MBP with adjuvant and were monitored for EAE clinical signs, lymphocyte proliferative responses to MBP, and MBP-reactive T-cell frequencies. Following encephalitogenic challenge, vehicle-fed rats exhibited severe signs of EAE, whether injected with IL-2 or not. Rats fed both low- and high-dose MBP had significantly decreased clinical signs, indicating the induction of oral tolerance. Injection of IL-2, however, caused a reversal of suppression in the low dose, but not in the high dose–fed group (FIG. 1). Rats fed low-dose MBP exhibited maximal clinical EAE after receiving even the lowest dose of IL-2 (8,000 U). Proliferative responses of lymph node cells were correlated with the clinical picture, in that proliferation to MBP was observed in the low-dose but not the high-dose group.

Limiting-dilution analyses revealed that there was a significant difference in MBP-reactive T-cell frequencies between saline-fed (1/20,227), low-dose MBP-fed (1/50,271), and high-dose MBP-fed rats (1/519,596). Injection of IL-2 resulted in an increase in the frequency of IL-2-secreting cells in both control and low dose–fed groups. High dose–fed rats exhibited dramatically low frequencies (1/691,502) at all doses of IL-2. These results suggest that there is an anergy component to low-dose oral tolerance and that deletion of MBP-reactive T cells accompanies high-dose oral tolerance.

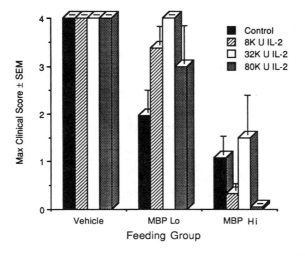

FIGURE 1. Reversal of oral tolerance with IL-2 administration *in vivo*. Feeding Lewis rats low-dose MBP (1 mg per feeding 5 times) followed by *in vivo* IL-2 injections reversed clinical signs of oral tolerance, whereas feeding high dose (20 mg per feeding 4 times) did not.

REFERENCES

1. BITAR, D. M. & C. C. WHITACRE. 1988. Suppression of experimental autoimmune encephalomyelitis by oral administration of myelin basic protein. Cell. Immunol. **112:** 364.
2. HIGGINS, P. J. & H. L. WEINER. 1988. Suppression of experimental autoimmune encephalomyelitis by the oral administration of myelin basic protein and its fragments. J. Immunol. **140:** 440.
3. MILLER, A., O. LIDER & H. L. WEINER. 1991. Antigen-driven bystander suppression after oral administration of antigens. J. Exp. Med. **174:** 791.
4. WHITACRE, C. C., D. M. BITAR, I. E. GIENAPP & C. G. OROSZ. 1991. Oral tolerance in experimental autoimmune encephalomyelitis. III. Evidence for clonal anergy. J. Immunol. **147:** 2155.
5. GUTIERREZ-RAMOS, J. C., I. MORENO DE ALBORAN & A. C. MARTINEZ. 1992. *In vivo* administration of interleukin-2 turns on anergic self-reacting T cells and leads to autoimmune disease. Eur. J. Immunol. **222:** 2867.

Protein B: An Important Human IgA-binding Reagent

M. A. GRUNDY, M. S. BLAKE, AND K. MURRAY[a]

Blake Laboratories Corporation
98 Cutter Mill Road
Suite 475N
Great Neck, New York 11021

INTRODUCTION

Protein B is an IgA receptor that is a useful new reagent for studying mucosal immunity and other immune responses involving human IgA. This protein was first described by Russell-Jones et al.[1] and is found on certain group B streptococci. It has the unique ability to bind human IgA of both subclasses.[1–3] Jacalin is a lectin that also shows some affinity to human IgA.[4] We have compared Protein B, Jacalin, and purified anti-human α chain in several assays for sensitivity and specificity.

RESULTS

The comparison between Protein B and Jacalin for binding to human IgA was made in an ELISA-based assay. The results demonstrated that Protein B was severalfold more sensitive in these assays as compared to Jacalin (FIG. 1). A small part of this increase might have been due to the fact that Protein B binds both subclasses of IgA, whereas Jacalin binds only IgA1.[4] However, IgA2 makes up only 20% of the total serum IgA. Because the difference is much greater, it suggests that Protein B has a much higher affinity for human IgA.

This higher affinity could be demonstrated in the ability of Protein B to bind human IgA in even small concentrations. Similar findings were reported by Eckrich et al. of the American Red Cross, who found Protein B superior in the binding and detection of vanishing concentrations of IgA in human sera as compared to other reagents.[5] It was found that the presence of other serum components did not interfere with this high sensitivity, suggesting that the binding of human IgA by Protein B is extremely specific.

Protein B was also compared with purified anti-human α chain antibodies in their ability to capture IgA from whole serum and to measure the amount of IgA to a specific antigen. The antigen in this case was conjugated to alkaline phosphatase as the detection system. Because Protein B binds to the Fc portion of the IgA molecule,[1] this leaves the antigen-binding portion of the IgA free to interact with specific antigens. Using Protein B as the capturing agent gave a much higher sensitivity in these assays (FIG. 2). In addition, known negative controls gave much lower backgrounds.

---

[a] Send correspondence to Dr. K. Murray, P.O. Box 2494, 52 Dragon Court, Woburn, MA 01888.

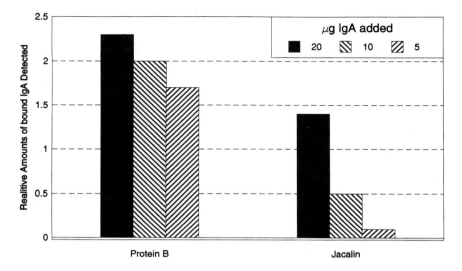

FIGURE 1. A comparison between Protein B and Jacalin in their ability to bind human IgA. Microtiter plates (Nunc-Immuno Plate IIF, Vangard International, Neptune, NJ) were sensitized by adding 0.1 mL per well of either Protein B (Blake Laboratories Corp., Great Neck, NY) or Jacalin (Pierce Chemical Co., Rockford, IL) at 2 μg/mL in 0.1 carbonate buffer, pH 9.6, with 0.02% azide. The plates were incubated overnight at 37 °C. The plates were washed five times with 0.9% NaCl, 0.05% Brij 35, 10 mM sodium acetate pH 7.0, and 0.02% azide. Human IgA was diluted in PBS with 0.5% Brij 35 to various concentrations, added to the plates, and incubated for 1 h at room temperature. The plates were again washed as before, and the secondary antibody, alkaline phosphatase–conjugated goat anti-human IgA (Tago Inc., Burlingame, CA), was diluted in PBS-Brij, added to the plates, and incubated for 1 h at room temperature. The plates were washed as before, and p-nitrophenyl phosphate (Sigma Phosphatase Substrate 104) (1 mg/mL) in 0.1 M diethanolamine, 1 mM $MgCl_2$, 0.1 mM $ZnCl_2$, and 0.02% azide pH 9.8 was added. The plates were incubated at 37 °C for 1 h, and the absorbance at 405 nm was determined using an Elisa-5 microtiter plate reader (Physica, New York, NY). Control wells lacked either the primary and/or secondary antibody.

SUMMARY

Protein B had a much higher affinity for human IgA than Jacalin, increasing the sensitivity and specificity of the measurement of total human IgA. Protein B, used as a capturing agent, greatly enhanced the measurement of antigen-specific IgA as compared to α chain–specific antibodies.

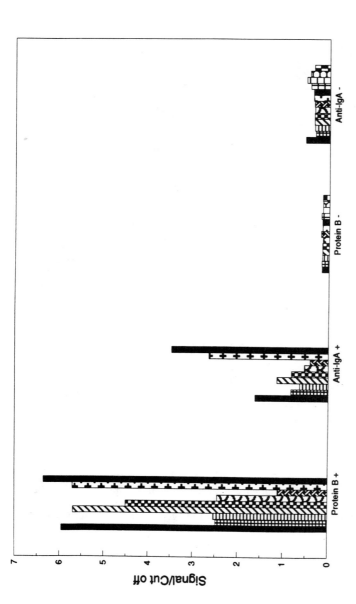

FIGURE 2. A comparison between Protein B and anti-human α chain–specific antibodies to capture and measure specific human IgA. Microtiter plates (Nunc-Immuno Plate IIF, Vangard International, Neptune, NJ) were sensitized by adding 0.1 mL per well of either Protein B (Blake Laboratories Corp., Great Neck, NY) or goat anti-human α chain–specific IgG (Tago Inc., Burlingame, CA) at 2 μg/mL in 0.1 carbonate buffer, pH 9.6, with 0.02% azide. The plates were incubated overnight at 37 °C. The plates were washed five times with 0.9% NaCl, 0.05% Brij 35, 10 mM sodium acetate pH 7.0, and 0.02% azide. Human sera known to contain either IgA antibodies to the specific antigen or completely lacking such antibodies were diluted 1 : 100 in PBS with 0.5% Brij 35 and added to the plates. The plates were incubated for 1 h at room temperature. The plates were again washed as before, and the alkaline phosphatase-conjugated antigen was diluted in PBS-Brij, added to the plates, and incubated for 1 h at room temperature. The plates were washed as before, and *p*-nitrophenyl phosphate (Sigma Phosphatase Substrate 104) (1 mg/mL) in 0.1 M diethanolamine, 1 mM MgCl₂, 0.1 mM ZnCl₂, and 0.02% azide pH 9.8 was added. The plates were incubated at 37 °C for 1 h, and the absorbance at 405 nm was determined using an Elisa-5 microtiter plate reader (Physica, New York, NY). The mean average reading of the known negative controls was calculated and doubled to determine the cutoff value in each case.

REFERENCES

1. RUSSELL-JONES, G. J., E. C. GOTSCHLICH & M. S. BLAKE. 1984. A surface receptor specific for human IgA on group B streptococci possessing the Ibc protein antigen. J. Exp. Med. **160:** 1467–1475.

2. CLEAT, P. H. & K. N. TIMMIS. 1987. Cloning and expression in *Escherichia coli* of the Ibc protein genes of group B streptococci: Binding of human immunoglobulin A to the beta antigen. Infect. Immun. **55:** 1151–1155.

3. FAULMANN, E. L., J. L. DUVALL & M. D. P. BOYLE. 1991. Protein B: A versatile bacterial Fc-binding protein selective for human IgA. Biotechniques **10:** 748–755.

4. KONDOH, H., K. KOBAYASHI, K. HAGIWARA & T. KAJII. 1986. Jacalin, a jackfruit lectin, precipitates IgA1 but not IgA2 subclass on gel diffusion reaction. J. Immunol. Methods **88:** 171–173.

5. ECKRICH, R. J., D. M. MALLORY & S. G. SANDLER. 1993. Laboratory tests to exclude IgA deficiency in the investigation of suspected anti-IgA transfusion reactions. Transfusion (Bethesda) **33:** 488–492.

Multiple Emulsions Oral Vaccine Vehicles for Inducing Immunity or Tolerance

THOMAS L. HEARN, MARGARET OLSEN, AND
ROBERT L. HUNTER

Department of Pathology and Laboratory Medicine
Woodruff Memorial Building, Room 762 Emory University
1639 Pierce Drive
Atlanta, Georgia 30322

It has been known since the 1960s that water-in-oil-in-water or multiple emulsions are effective adjuvants, but instability of available preparations precluded widespread use.[1] Our research on the adjuvant activity of nonionic block copolymers suggested that larger hydrophobic molecules would be more effective.[3,4] When such agents were synthesized, we found that they were not only excellent adjuvants but that they also effectively stabilized multiple emulsions.[2] Being insoluble in both oil and water, these amphipathic copolymers preferentially localize on and stabilize oil-water interfaces. These multiple emulsions are formed of particles ranging from 5 to 50 microns in diameter and consisting of 80% saline and 20% oil phase (squalene:span 80 at 9:1), with the copolymer in the aqueous phase. The antigen is also in the saline, which is dispersed in droplets that are smaller than the resolution of light microscopes. These particles are suspended in a second aqueous phase of arbitrary volume. Multiple emulsions can be prepared with practically any antigen with equal ease.

When fed to animals, multiple emulsions pass through the upper gastrointestinal tract to the colon intact. Emulsion particles can be seen over Peyer's patches in mice from 20 minutes, and to 8 hours after oral infusion. Most of the particles break in the colon as the feces dehydrate. Using titanium dioxide particles as a marker, it was shown that the emulsions promote particle uptake by the domes of Peyer's patches. Very few particles were taken up by Peyer's patches without copolymer in emulsion even though they are not digestible.

Multiple emulsions can be effective vehicles for inducing both serum IgG and secretory IgA antibody responses.[2] For example, ICR outbred mice were immunized orally one, two, or three times at two-week intervals with various doses of TNP_{10}-ovalbumin and were followed for a year before boosting with an identical oral immunization. The proportion of responders and titers increased with increasing dose and number of immunizations so that 100% of animals produced both intestinal secretory IgA and circulating IgG antibody responses to three infusions of 100 μg of antigen. The IgG titers persisted for one year and were boosted by a further oral immunization. Oral immunization using multiple emulsions also uniformly primed animals for an increased response following parenteral immunization (FIG. 1). We found no evidence of tolerance (defined as a reduction in response to parenteral immunization) in this model.

Recently, M. Elson reported that oral immunization with egg albumin in the same delivery system induced tolerance. We were aware of these results and tried to reproduce them. We were unable to induce tolerance with TNP_{10}-ovalbumin, even though tolerance was regularly induced with ovalbumin. These data suggest that the outcome of immuniza-

388

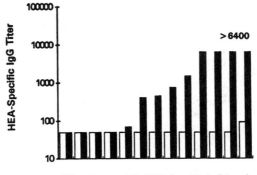

FIGURE 1. Ovalbumin-specific IgG antibody after parenteral boosting of orally immunized mice. Mice received three oral immunizations with 50 μg of TNP$_{10}$-ovalbumin on days 0, 16, and 38 followed by a subcutaneous boost with the same formulation of day 160. Antibody titers 14 days later are shown. Black bars show the titers of individual mice. White bars show the titers of mice immunized subcutaneously only. HEA, hen egg albumin.

tion (immunity or tolerance) to antigens administered orally with multiple emulsions depends upon multiple factors, including the properties of the antigen.

REFERENCES

1. HERBERT, W. J. 1978. Mineral-oil adjuvants and the immunization of laboratory animals. *In* Handbook of Experimental Immunology. D. W. Weier, Ed: A3.1-A3.14.
2. HUNTER, R. L., M. R. OLSEN & B. BENNETT. 1995. Copolymer adjuvants and TiterMax®. *In* Theory and Practical Applications of Adjuvants. D. E. S. Stewart-Tull, Ed. John Wiley & Sons. New York.
3. HUNTER, R. L., M. R. OLSEN & S. BUYNITZKY. 1991. Adjuvant activity of nonionic block copolymers. IV. Effect of molecular weight and formulation on titer and isotype of antibody. Vaccine **9:** 250-256.
4. HUNTER, R. L., F. STRICKLAND & F. KEZDY. 1981. Studies on the adjuvant activity of nonionic block polymer surfactants. I. The role of hydrophile-lipophile balance. J. Immunol. **127:** 1244-1250.

In Vivo Administration of IL-4 Induces TGF-β-producing Cells and Protects Animals from Experimental Autoimmune Encephalomyelitis

JUN-ICHI INOBE, YOUHAI CHEN, AND
HOWARD L. WEINER

Center for Neurological Diseases
Brigham and Women's Hospital
Harvard Medical School
Boston, Massachusetts 02115

INTRODUCTION

Interleukin-4 (IL-4) is a switching factor for the generation of T-helper type 2 (TH2) cells.[1] We have recently found that oral administration of myelin basic protein (MBP)

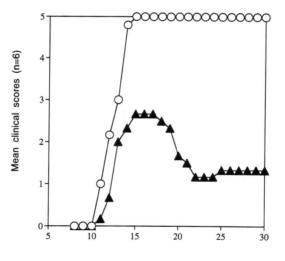

FIGURE 1. *In vivo* administration of IL-4 protects animals from EAE. Two groups of female PLJ × SJL F1 mice, 6 mice per group, were immunized for EAE with MBP in CFA. On the day of immunization, mice received an intraperitoneal (ip) injection of either recombinant mouse IL-4 (5000 U/mouse) in 0.5 mL PBS or PBS alone. The maximum clinical score and fatality of IL-4-treated animals were significantly lower than the PBS-treated group (p = 0.007 and 0.0192, respectively). ——○——, ip PBS; ——▲——, ip IL-4.

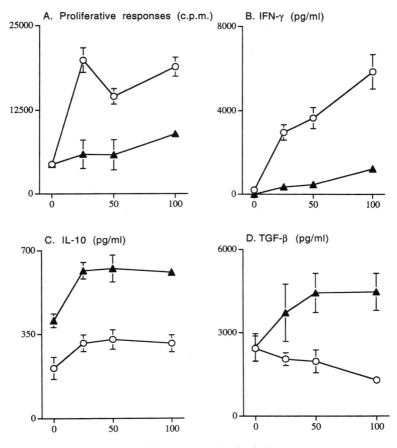

FIGURE 2. T-cell proliferation and cytokine production after *in vivo* administration of IL-4. Mice were immunized as in Fıɢ. 1. Ten days after the immunization, spleens were removed and single cell suspensions were prepared. Splenocytes, 1×10^6/well, were cultured in 0.2 mL of serum-free medium with various concentrations of MBP. For proliferation assays (**A**), 1 µCi of [³H]thymidine was added to each well 72 h later. Cells were harvested and radioactivity counted 16 h later. For cytokine assays (**B-D**), culture supernatants were collected 40 h (for IFN-γ, IL-10) or 72 h (for TGF-β) later. Cytokine concentration was determined by ELISA. ——O——, ip PBS; ——▲—— ip IL-4.

generates regulatory T cells that secrete transforming growth factor-β (TGF-β) and TH2 cytokines.[2] In this study, we investigated the role of IL-4 in the generation of TGF-β-secreting cells and in the regulation of experimental autoimmune encephalomyelitis (EAE).

MATERIAL AND METHODS

For induction of EAE, female PLJ × SJL F1 mice were injected subcutaneously, with mouse MBP (400 µg/mouse) in complete Freund's adjuvant (CFA), and intravenously with pertussis toxin (PT, 100 ng/mouse). Mice received a second injection of PT 48 h later and were scored for EAE as follows: 0, no disease; 1, tail paralysis; 2, hind-limb weakness; 3, hind-limb paralysis; 4, hind-limb plus fore-limb paralysis; 5, moribund. For *in vitro* T-cell assays, all mice were sacrificed 10 days after immunization (before the onset of the disease).

RESULTS AND DISCUSSION

As others reported with a different system,[3] we have found that *in vivo* administration of IL-4 protected mice from EAE (FIG. 1) and suppressed the proliferative responses to MBP (FIG. 2A). However, as shown in FIG. 2, the disease protection was associated with a decreased TH1 cytokine (IFN-γ) production and increased Th2 (IL-10) and TGF-β secretion. This suggests that one mechanism for IL-4, mediating *in vivo* suppression of EAE, may be by activating cells producing TGF-β and TH2 cytokines. Preliminary experiments show that oral administration of MBP in conjunction with IL-4 enhances TGF-β secretion and fecal IgA production. Thus, IL-4 may play an important role in generating TGF-β-secreting T cells *in vivo* and may function synergistically to enhance the effects of oral tolerance.

REFERENCES

1. LeGros G. *et al.* 1990. J. Exp. Med. **172:** 921.
2. Chen, Y. *et al.* 1994. Science **265:** 1237.
3. Racke, M. K. *et al.* 1994. J. Exp. Med. **180:** 1961.

Oral Tolerance in Experimental Autoimmune Encephalomyelitis

Specificity of Peptide-induced Oral Tolerance[a]

NAJMA H. JAVED, INGRID GIENAPP, KAREN COX,
AND CAROLINE C. WHITACRE

Department of Medical Microbiology and Immunology
The Ohio State University
College of Medicine
The Ohio State University
333 West 10th Avenue, Room 2078
Columbus, Ohio 43210

Experimental autoimmune encephalomyelitis (EAE) in the Lewis rat is a T cell-mediated autoimmune disease induced by the injection of myelin basic protein (MBP) and complete Freund's adjuvant. Inasmuch as EAE has been recognized as a disease model with similarities to human multiple sclerosis, much attention has been given to the strategies for treatment in order to prevent or suppress EAE. Earlier studies from our laboratory have shown that oral administration of guinea pig MBP prior to encephalitogenic challenge induces T-cell anergy and results in the suppression of clinical signs and CNS histopathologic changes of EAE.[1] By contrast, oral administration of the self-antigen rat MBP does not confer protection, suggesting that oral tolerance in EAE is specific for the fed antigen, extending to species-specific determinants on the MBP molecule.[2] A side-by-side comparison of male and female Lewis rats following feeding of MBP has revealed important differences between the two genders in terms of oral tolerance induction. In the male rat, MBP-induced oral tolerance is achieved only when soybean trypsin inhibitor (STI) is administered together with MBP. In the female, tolerance is demonstrable with or without STI. The present study was undertaken in female rats to determine the tolerogenicity of the major encephalitogenic peptide 68-88,[3] derived from guinea pig (GP) MBP and rat MBP, as well as the minor encephalitogenic MBP peptide 87-99 when administered with and without STI. The rat and GP 68-88 peptides differ by a single amino acid at position 80 (serine/threonine substitution).[4] We found that Lewis rats fed 5 mg of GP 68-88 along with STI were protected from EAE induced with GP 68-88 or rat 68-88 (FIG. 1). By contrast, feeding GP 68-88 suspended in 0.15 M sodium bicarbonate alone did not protect the animals against challenge with either peptide. Interestingly, feeding 5 mg of rat 68-88 or GP 87-99 with or without STI offered no protection (FIG. 1). This implies that tolerance is occurring at the level of T-cell recognition, because there is suggestive evidence that residue 80 within the 68-88 sequence is a T-cell receptor contact residue.[5] In control animals, feeding STI alone did not affect the induction of EAE. These findings suggest that the presence of STI or an analogous protease inhibitor is essential for demonstration of peptide-induced oral tolerance. The use of STI presumably prevents the degradation

[a] This work was supported by National Multiple Sclerosis Society Grants FG979-A-1 and RG2302-A-3, and by NIH Grants NS23561 and AI35960.

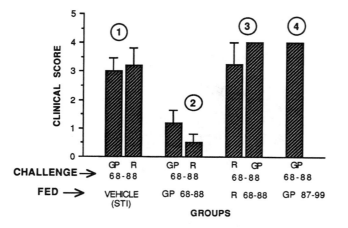

FIGURE 1. Suppression of EAE clinical signs in female Lewis rats by the oral administration of guinea pig MBP 68-88, but not rat 68-88 or GP 87-99 peptide. Values indicate mean maximum clinical score ± SEM. Numbers on each set of bars indicate the feeding groups. Results shown represent 5-6 rats per group. This experiment was repeated 3 times with comparable results.

of peptide in the gastrointestinal tract by digestive enzymes, such as pepsin. Our findings indicate the importance of the physical form of the oral antigen, the gender differences in induction of oral tolerance, and the amino acid sequence of the fed antigen, where small structural differences at the single amino acid primary sequence level can produce dramatic differences in clinical outcome. These findings have important implications for the design of multiple sclerosis clinical trials.

REFERENCES

1. WHITACRE, C. C., D. M. BITAR, I. E. GIENAPP & C. G. OROSZ. 1991. Oral tolerance in experimental autoimmune encephalomyelitis. III. Evidence for clonal anergy. J. Immunol. **147**(7): 2155-2163.
2. BITAR, D. M. & C. C. WHITACRE. 1988. Suppression of experimental autoimmune encephalomyelitis by the oral administration of myelin basic protein. Cell Immunol. **112:** 364-370.
3. CHOU, C.-HJ., F. C-H. CHOU, T. J. KOWALSKI, R. SHAPIRA & R. F. KIBLER. 1977. The major site of guinea pig myelin basic protein encephalitogenic in Lewis rat. J. Neurochem. **28:** 115-119.
4. MARTENSEN, R. E. 1984. *In* Experimental Allergic Encephalomyelitis, A Useful Model for Multiple Sclerosis. **511.** Alan R. Liss, Inc. New York.
5. MANNIE, M. D., P. Y. PATERSON, D. C. U'PRICHARD & G. FLOURET. 1989. Encephalitogenic and proliferative responses of Lewis rat lymphocytes distinguished by position 75- and 80-substituted peptides of myelin basic protein. J. Immunol. **142**(8): 2608-2616.

Mucosal Tolerance Induced by Flour Dust

M. N. KOLOPP-SARDA, M. C. BENE, N. MASSIN,
AND G. C. FAURE

Laboratoire d'Immunologie
Faculté de Médecine, BP 184
GRIP-UHP Nancy I & INRS
54500 Vandoeuvre-les-Nancy, France

INTRODUCTION

Indirect observations suggest that lowered specific immune responses may develop after oral challenge in humans, inasmuch as the induction of immune tolerance to dietary antigens has mostly been reported after oral administration of food components in animal models, after feeding or direct delivery in the gastrointestinal tract.[1,2] The mechanisms involved could depend on bystander or specific suppression, or anergy.[1] Immune tolerance is most frequently reported as the absence of peripheral antibodies specific for the orally administered antigen. Conversely, mucosal antibodies can often be evidenced in the secretions of tolerized animals.[3] Peripheral specific antibodies can sometimes be detected, but T-cell responses are universally recognized to be suppressed, and no clinical manifestations follow oral or parenteral challenge with the relevant antigen. The persistence of this tolerized state appears to rely in experimental animals on the repeated administration of relatively large doses of the tolerogen. We report a series of investigations performed in two groups of healthy individuals exposed to a common food antigen, wheat flour.[4,5] Exposure occurred either through the common daily intake of bakery products or, in addition, through the respiratory tract, in the atmosphere of mills or industrial bakeries. Although both groups of individuals were clinically healthy, their adaptation to this environmental antigen appeared to involve different types of immune responses.

SUBJECTS AND METHODS

The study involved 121 mill workers, 38 bakery workers, and a control group of 41 employees from a salt factory. All subjects completed a medical questionnaire and had an auscultation. Hypersensitivity was explored by a prick test with total saline flour extract. Anti-flour and anti-gliadin IgG, IgA, and IgM were assayed on serum and saliva samples in ELISA. Peripheral lymphocyte subsets (CD3, CD4, CD8, CD29, CD45RA, CD57, and sIg) were measured by flow cytometry.

RESULTS

The questionnaires and physical examination showed that occupational exposure to flour had no clinical consequence. Prick tests yielded mild immediate reactions in 8 millers and 4 bakers, but no DTH. Professionally exposed workers had significantly higher levels

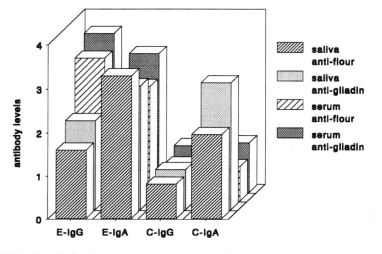

FIGURE 1. Specific antibody levels in the serum and saliva of professionally exposed individuals (E) and controls (C). Data are expressed as OD ratios.

of serum anti-flour and anti-gliadin IgG and IgA than controls (FIG. 1). Mucosal responses were also significant in exposed subjects, with high levels of salivary anti-flour and anti-gliadin IgG and IgA. In controls, only an anti-gliadin IgA response was observed in salivary samples at levels similar to exposed subjects. Classical B- and T-cell subsets were similar in both groups. CD29$^+$ (memory) T cells were significantly lower in exposed subjects, although they had slightly more CD45$^+$ (naive) T cells (FIG. 2).

DISCUSSION

This study reports on the different immune status of healthy individuals exposed to flour antigens, either orally and occasionally, or, additionally, through daily respiratory exposure to flour dust. In the first group, the most classically reported features of oral tolerance were noted, that is, the presence of mucosal-specific antibodies (IgA) and absence of peripheral-specific antibodies. The doses and routes of contact with flour antigens were larger in the group of professionally exposed workers. Yet, all appeared to be in good health upon physical examination, without any clinical history of intolerance. This could be related to the immune balance observed in professionally exposed workers, different from that of unexposed subjects. They had both mucosal and peripheral-specific antibodies but were unresponsive to skin tests. Moreover, although their peripheral lymphocyte subsets were within the normal range, they had a significant decrease of peripheral CD29$^+$ cells that could be interpreted as a decreased number of memory cells or impaired beta1-integrin-mediated recirculation. These observations suggest that mucosal tolerance successfully protected the workers studied from the possibly deleterious effect of their professional environment. From a more fundamental point of view, these data indicate that immune tolerance may develop in humans with features similar to those reported in experimental models. Finally, our observations suggest that respiratory tissues could be involved, as well as the gastrointestinal tract, in the induction of mucosal tolerance.

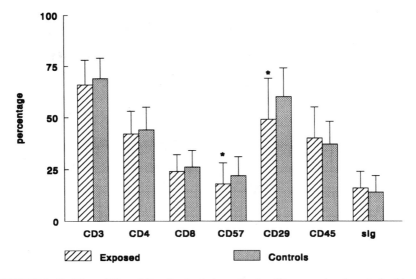

FIGURE 2. Partition of B- and T-cell subsets in professionally exposed and control subjects. Statistically significant differences (p < 0.005) are indicated by asterisks.

REFERENCES

1. MELAMED, D. & A. FRIEDMAN. 1993. Eur. J. Immunol. **23:** 935-942.
2. ENOMOTO, A., M. KONISHI, S. HACHIMURA & S. KAMINOGAWA. 1993. Clin. Immunol. Immunopathol. **66:** 136-142.
3. GUERRA, R. 1991. Braz. J. Med. Biol. Res. **24:** 107-109.
4. KOLOPP-SARDA, M. N., N. MASSIN, B. GOBERT, P. WILD, J. J. MOULIN, M. C. BÉNÉ & G. C. FAURE. 1994. Am. J. Ind. Med. **26:** 671-679.
5. KOLOPP-SARDA, M. N., M. C. BÉNÉ, N. MASSIN, P. WILD & G. C. FAURE. 1995. Am. J. Ind. Med. **28:** 497-504.

Pilot Study of Oral Tolerance to Keyhole Limpet Hemocyanin in Humans

Down-regulation of KLH-reactive Precursor-cell Frequency

MAKOTO MATSUI,[a] DAVID A. HAFLER, AND
HOWARD L. WEINER [b]

Center for Neurologic Diseases
Division of Neurology
Department of Medicine
Brigham and Women's Hospital
and
Harvard Medical School
Boston, Massachusetts 02115

Oral tolerance has long been recognized as a method of evoking antigen-specific suppression of immune responses and has recently been used to suppress autoimmune diseases in both animals and humans (reviewed in ref. 1). To determine whether the oral administration of a protein antigen could down-regulate immune responses in humans, we conducted a two-part pilot study using KLH as an antigen. In part 1, two healthy volunteers, who had not been immunized with KLH, were fed 30 mg of KLH every other day for a minimum of six weeks, and KLH-reactive precursor cell frequency was measured. In part 2, six healthy volunteers were fed KLH or OVA for four weeks and immunized by the intradermal injection of KLH. We observed substantial numbers of KLH-reactive cells in the peripheral blood of unimmunized subjects (natural immunity) and found a decrease in the cell frequency with feeding. In addition, oral KLH decreased the frequency in KLH-reactive cells in immunized subjects fed KLH versus those fed ovalbumin (OVA).

METHODS

Preparation of Antigens

KLH and OVA (Grade V) were purchased from Calbiochem (La Jolla, CA) and Sigma Chemical (St. Louis, MO), respectively. Both antigens were dialyzed against phosphate-buffered saline, passed twice through 0.45 μm membrane filter systems, and lyophilized in 50-mL polystyrene culture tubes (approximately 30 mg/tube).

---

[a] Present address: Division of Neurology, Department of Internal Medicine, Saga Medical School, Saga 849, Japan.
[b] To whom correspondence should be sent.

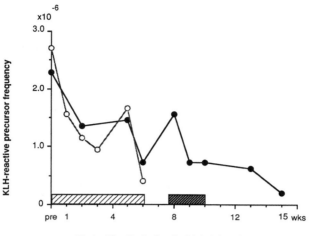

Weeks After Beginning Oral Administration of KLH

FIGURE 1. Time course of KLH-reactive precursor cell frequency. Thirty milligrams of KLH was administered orally every other day to each subject. Subject A (closed circles) took KLH for six weeks (the hatched bar) and then ceased for 10 days. Oral KLH was readministered for 18 consecutive days between the middle of the eighth week and the end of the tenth week of the study (the coarse hatched bar). Subject B (open circles) took KLH every other day for six weeks (the hatched bar).

Subjects and Administration Schedule

For part 1, two healthy male volunteers (ages 37 and 46) were fed 30 mg of KLH dissolved in water plus an equivalent amount of grapefruit juice every other day. Subject A followed this schedule for six weeks. After 10 days without receiving the antigen, that is, missing five doses, he was then given KLH for 18 consecutive days, after which he received no further LKH (10-week-course). Subject B received KLH on alternate days for the same six weeks. Both subjects were examined serially at one- or two-week intervals. For part 2 of the study, six other healthy volunteers (3 men and 3 women), whose ages ranged from 24 to 41 years, were paired into three study groups; each pair of subjects was examined concurrently. One subject in each group received 30 mg of KLH orally every other day for four weeks, and the other received 30 mg of OVA orally. At the beginning of the fifth week of the study, subjects in each group were immunized with intradermal injections of either 1 or 5 mg of KLH.

Preparation of Antigen-presenting Cells

Peripheral blood mononuclear cells, separated by Ficoll-Paque density gradient centrifugation before the administration of KLH was begun, served as antigen-presenting cells (APC) in all experiments. The APC in aliquots of 10^7 cells per tube were kept frozen at -70 °C until use.

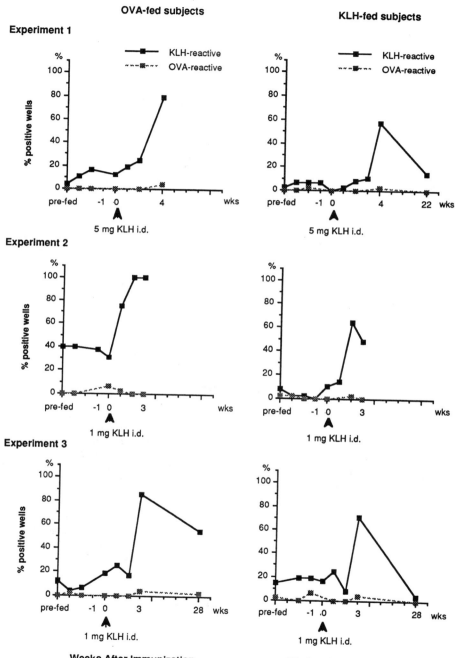

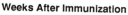

Immunological Parameters

KLH- and OVA-reactive precursor cell frequencies were measured according to a previously reported method.[2] Preliminary experiments showed that 2.5 and 5.0 μg/mL of KLH and between 10 and 50 μg/mL of OVA had the highest efficiency in generating antigen-reactive cell lines. Culture media were supplemented with 10% pooled human AB sera. The cell culture was maintained for 13 days with 5% IL-2 (ABI, Columbia, MD) and 2 U/mL of recombinant IL-4 (Genzyme, Boston, MA), which were added every 3 to 4 days. An aliquot of the cell line from each well was then checked for reactivity to the relevant antigen, that is, either KLH or OVA, by plating, in duplicate (1 to 2 × 10^4 line cells together with 1 × 10^4 APC). The APC had been preincubated with or without 100 μg/mL of the antigen for 1 hour and then irradiated (4500 rad) and washed to remove the antigen. The cells were incubated for three days, and [^{3}H]thymidine (0.63 μCi/well) was added 18 hours prior to cell harvesting. Cell lines that had a stimulation index (mean Δ cpm of wells containing antigen-pulsed APC divided by mean Δ cpm of wells containing antigen-nonpulsed APC) exceeding 3.0 and whose Δ cpm in positive wells was more than 500 were considered as being reactive to the antigen. Previous experiments performed by this method for generating cell lines have shown that cells in a positive well were derived from a single antigen-reactive cell.[2] Thus, either of the higher percentages of positive wells obtained in a total of 48 wells set up for each concentration of KLH (2.5 and 5.0 μg/mL) and OVA (10 and 50 μg/mL) was used as representative KLH- and OVA-reactive precursor cell frequencies at the time of blood sampling. For example, 10% positive wells indicated that the precursor cell frequency was $10/100/[2 × 10^5] = 0.5 × 10^{-6}$. Preliminary studies showed a difference between the lots of pooled human AB sera in terms of efficiency in generating KLH-reactive cell lines. The lot that gave less than 20% positive wells (cell frequency, $1.0 × 10^{-6}$), rather than one that gave high percentages used in part 1 of the study, was selected for part 2 of the study.

Statistical Analysis

To analyze the decrease in KLH-reactive precursor cell frequency for the two subjects in part 1 of the study, the two-way analysis of variance (two-way ANOVA) was used. The two-way ANOVA with repeated measures (repeated-measure ANOVA) was performed for analyzing the differences of immunological parameters in the KLH-fed and OVA-fed subjects in part 2 of the study.

RESULTS

Part 1

As shown in FIGURE 1, in subject A (closed circles), KLH-reactive precursor cell frequency was $2.3 × 10^{-6}$ before the oral administration of KLH; the cell frequency

FIGURE 2. Time course of the percentage of positive wells for KLH- and OVA-reactive cell lines. The percentages of positive wells for KLH and OVA are shown in solid and broken lines, respectively. KLH or OVA was administered orally for four weeks prior to the intradermal immunization with KLH. The immunization is denoted by large arrowheads. The results obtained in the subjects who received oral KLH are shown on the right side of the FIGURE, and those from the oral OVA subjects are shown on the left side.

decreased to about half the original level in two weeks and decreased further to one third, until the end of the first part of the feeding schedule (the hatched bar in FIG. 1). The frequency of KLH-reactive cells increased when oral KLH was discontinued and then decreased once again to one tenth of the original level after 18 days' consecutive intake of KLH (the coarse hatched bar). At four months and nine months after the discontinuation of KLH, KLH-reactive precursor cell frequency was found to be approximately 1.0×10^{-6}, less than one half of the original level (data not shown). Subject B (open circles) showed a rapid decrease in the cell frequency: 2.7×10^{-6} before starting KLH, and less than 0.5×10^{-6} after six weeks' oral administration of KLH (the hatched bar). The decrease in KLH-reactive precursor cell frequency during the first six weeks of KLH feeding in both subjects was statistically significant ($p = 0.0157$), when analyzed by the two-way ANOVA. The decrease in precursor cell frequency was not due to the impaired function of frozen APC, because there was no difference in the percentage of positive wells in the assay plates containing frozen APC or fresh APC.

Part 2

The intradermal injection of KLH, at concentrations of both 1 and 5 mg, elicited strong cellular immune responses to the antigen in all six subjects, as shown in FIGURE 2. KLH-reactive precursor cell frequency (solid lines) reached a peak two to four weeks after immunization, whereas OVA-reactive precursor-cell frequency (broken lines) remained at low levels. Throughout the postimmunization period, all three subjects who received KLH orally had lower numbers of KLH-reactive cells than the three paired subjects who received OVA orally. This down-regulation observed in the three KLH-fed subjects showed a positive trend but did not achieve statistical significance ($p = 0.071$) when the results prior to immunization (zero week) were compared with those obtained at the peak of KLH-reactive cell frequency by means of a repeated-measure ANOVA (FIG. 3).

DISCUSSION

In this pilot study, we found that oral administration of a protein antigen can down-regulate cell-mediated immunity to the fed antigen in humans as measured by cell frequency. The substantial numbers of KLH-reactive cells in the peripheral blood of the two nonimmunized subjects in part 1 of the study decreased with the oral administration of KLH, indicating that oral KLH suppressed preexisting or natural cellular immunity to this antigen. The presence of KLH-reactive cells in the subjects who had not been immunized with KLH is consistent with the reported detection of low levels of anti-KLH antibodies in the sera of nonimmunized human subjects.[3] Part 2 of the study showed that prior four-week oral administration of KLH showed a trend in decreasing the number of antigen-reactive cells triggered after intradermal immunization with KLH. Of note is that all three subjects fed OVA experienced moderate pruritus at the site of the KLH injection, whereas none of the three subjects who received KLH orally did.

Other investigators have studied immune responses to KLH in human subjects immunized with KLH following oral[4] or nasal[5] administration of KLH. In fed subjects, a decrease in T-cell but not B-cell responses was observed following immunization; 50 mg of KLH was fed daily for a total of 10 days. In nasally treated subjects, 100 mg KLH was administered weekly over 3 to 4 weeks. Nasal administration, alone, primed for antibody responses but suppressed both antibody and DTH responses following subcutateous immunization with KLH. In our studies, we immunized with a 10- to 50-times higher amount

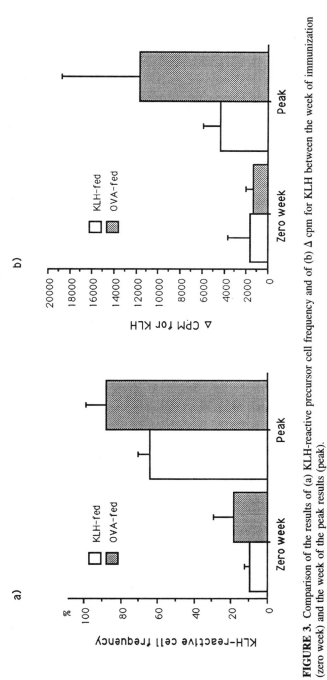

FIGURE 3. Comparison of the results of (a) KLH-reactive precursor cell frequency and of (b) Δ cpm for KLH between the week of immunization (zero week) and the week of the peak results (peak).

(1 mg or 5 mg) of KLH than the aforementioned studies. This most probably explains why we observed only a trend in the suppression of cellular immune responses as measured by reactive cell lines following immunization.

Oral tolerance is now recognized to involve multiple mechanisms, including active suppression, anergy, and deletion, depending on the dose fed.[6] Subsequent to this pilot study with KLH, we have observed the induction of antigen-specific TGF-β-secreting cells following oral administration of myelin antigens.[7] In terms of KLH, our results in this pilot study and the results of others demonstrate that mucosal administration of KLH has a clear effect in reducing cell mediated-type responses to KLH. Given our better understanding of the dose-dependent mechanisms of oral tolerance and the increase in human studies involving oral administration of autoantigens for the treatment of autoimmune diseases, further studies will help delineate the immune responses to oral antigens in humans.

ACKNOWLEDGEMENTS

The authors wish to thank Ms. Blishda Lacet for her excellent technical assistance.

REFERENCES

1. WEINER, H. L., A. FRIEDMAN, A. MILLER et al. 1994. Annu. Rev. Immunol. **12:** 809.
2. OTA, K., M. MATSUI, E. L. MILFORD, G. A. MACKIN, H. L. WEINER & D. A. HAFLER. 1990. Nature **346:** 183.
3. VOLKMAN, D. J., H. C. LANE & A. S. FAUCI. 1981. Proc. Natl. Acad. Sci. USA **78:** 2528.
4. HUSBY, S., J. MESTECKY, Z. MOLDVEANEAU, S. HOLLAND & C. O. ELSON. 1994. J. Immunol. **152:** 4663.
5. WALDO, F. B., A. W. L. VAN DEN WALL BAKE, J. MESTECKY & S. HUSBY. 1994. Clin. Immunol. Immunopathol. **72:** 30.
6. CHEN, Y., J. INOBE, R. MARKS, P. GONELLA, V. J. KUCHROO & H. L. WEINER. 1995. Nature **376:** 177.
7. FUKAURA, H., S. C. KENT, M. J. PIETRUSEWICZ, S. J. KHOURY, H. L. WEINER & D. A. HAFLER. 1996. This volume.

The Protective Role of Enteral IgA Supplementation in Neonatal Gut-origin Sepsis

R. T. MAXSON, D. D. JOHNSON, R. J. JACKSON,
AND S. D. SMITH

Department of Surgery
University of Arkansas and Arkansas Children's Hospital
800 Marshall Street
Little Rock, Arkansas 77202-3591

INTRODUCTION

A significant number of neonatal infections are thought to originate from the gastrointestinal tract. Many preterm infants in the neonatal intensive care unit are unable to tolerate normal enteral feeding and are particularly susceptible to bacterial infections of gut origin.[1,2] Little work has focused on neonates and the prevention of gut-origin sepsis. There is strong epidemiological evidence that breast feeding is important in protecting against infection,[3] and secretory IgA is found in high concentration in breast milk. We propose that secretory IgA luminally administered to a neonatal rabbit model for systemic infection will protect against gut-origin sepsis.

MATERIAL AND METHODS

Sixty New Zealand white rabbit pups were randomized to one of two groups: IgA group (n = 26) and non-IgA group (n = 34). All animals were fed twice daily by intragastric gavage. On postdelivery days 3 and 4, the IgA group received sterile human secretory IgA. The non-IgA group received an equal volume of saline. After the evening feed of postdelivery day 3, all animals were challenged with 1×10^2 cfu/mL of *E. coli* K100 (O75; K100; H5) (TABLE 1).

All animals were sacrificed 40 hours after the bacterial challenge. Peritoneal swabs were performed and cultured. All animals were positive peritoneal swabs were considered to be contaminated and were excluded from analysis. The mesenteric lymph node complex (MLN), liver, spleen, and cecum were harvested, and quantitative aerobic and anaerobic cultures obtained.

Translocation incidence to the MLN and organs was compared between groups using the Fisher's exact test. Quantity of bacteria in the ceca, MLNs, and organs was analyzed using Student's *t* test.

RESULTS

There were three positive peritoneal swabs, two in the IgA group, and one in the non-IgA group. These animals were excluded from the following results.

405

TABLE 1.

	MLN Incidence (%)	Log quantity cfu/mL	Liver Incidence (%)	Log quantity cfu/mL	Spleen Incidence (%)	Log quantity cfu/mL	Cecum Log quantity cfu/mL
IgA n = 24	7 (29)	4.1 ± .7*	6 (25)*	3.3 ± .4*	2 (8)*	3.8 ± .3*	10.1 ± 1.5
No IgA n = 33	18 (55)	5.5 ± 1.4	19 (58)	4.4 ± 1.0	15 (45)	5.6 ± 1.0	9.7 ± 1.3

* p < 0.05 for IgA group vs. no IgA.

There were no anaerobic bacteria identified in any organ, including the cecum in either the IgA or no-IgA groups. There was no significant difference in cecal colonization between groups.

The log quantity of bacteria that translocated to the MLN, liver, and spleen was significantly less in the IgA group. There was also a significant decrease in the incidence of bacterial translocation to the liver and spleen in the IgA group, whereas the MLN failed to reach statistical significance.

DISCUSSION

A significant number of newborn infections originate from the gastrointestinal tract, and the premature infant is at particular risk of developing infections because of an immature gut barrier. Studies have demonstrated that breast milk protects the neonate against pathogens in the gastrointestinal tract.[4] Secretory IgA is the principal immunoglobulin present in breast milk, which also contains lesser amounts of IgM and IgG. The protective role of secretory IgA occurs by preventing organisms from colonizing and binding to the intestinal epithelium. *In vitro* studies using the modified Ussing chamber have demonstrated that whereas secretory IgA will bind *E. coli* and prevent passage of the bacteria across rat mucosal epithelia, IgG binds the organism but does not prevent transepithelial passage.[5]

Evidence supports the contention that IgA is an important protective factor in breast milk, but its role in reducing bacterial translocation in an *in vivo* model has never been shown. Our data demonstrate that neonatal formula supplemented with human secretory IgA decreases the quantity of bacteria and incidence of bacterial translocation of *E. coli* K100 in a neonatal rabbit model. This suggests that oral supplementation of IgA would be beneficial for those neonates who are at particular risk for gut-origin sepsis.

REFERENCES

1. LEBENTHAL, E., P. C. LEE & L. A. HEITLINGER. 1983. Impact of development of the gastrointestinal tract on infant feeding. J. Pediatr. **102:** 109.
2. KEREN, D. F. 1989. Mucosal IgA elaboration. Crit. Rev. Clin. Lab. Sci. **27:** 159–176.
3. CUNNINGHAM, A. S., D. B. JELLIFFE & E. F. P. JELLIFFE. 1991. Breast-feeding and health in the 1980's. 1991. A global epidemiologic review. J. Pediatr. **118:** 659–666.

4. MIETENS, C., H. KEINHORST, H. HILPERT *et al.* 1979. Treatment of infantile *E. coli* gastroenteritis with specific bovine anti-*E. coli* milk immunoglobulins. Eur. J. Pediatr. **132:** 239–252.
5. ALBANESE, C. T., S. D. SMITH, S. WATKINS, A. KURKBASCHE, R. L. SIMMONS & M. I. ROWE. 1994. Effects of secretory IgA on transepithelial passage of bacteria across the intact ileum *in vitro.* J. Am. Coll. Surg. **179:** 679–688.

Immune Deviation during the Induction of Tolerance by way of Nasal Installation

Nasal Installation Itself Can Induce Th-2 Responses and Exacerbation of Disease[a]

M. E. F. MELO, T. J. GOLDSCHMIDT,[b]

V. BHARDWAJ, L. HO, A. MILLER, AND E. SERCARZ

Department of Microbiology and Molecular Genetics
and
[b]*Department of Microbiology and Immunology*
Molecular Sciences Building, Room 4610A
405 Hilgard Avenue
University of California, Los Angeles
Los Angeles, California 90024-1489

INTRODUCTION

In many situations to date, it has been shown that when mucosal surfaces are exposed to antigen, tolerance at the Th-1 level results. This may be part of an evolutionary process to avoid allergies to food and airborne antigens. Oral administration has also been considered in cases where immune responses at a mucosal port of entry need to be enhanced, such as in infectious immunity. Two examples of this are the vaccines to *Salmonella typhi*[1] and to poliovirus.[2] Accordingly, it is of the greatest importance to establish the mucosal mechanisms of inducing immunity and tolerance, so that they can be used with impunity in addressing an appropriate response. Of particular interest to us has been the great effectiveness of nasal installation (NI) in regulating and deviating the systemic immune response to protein antigens and peptides. Understanding the molecular and physiologic mechanisms underlying tolerance induction will not only allow better planning of successful treatment for allergy and transplantation but also may provide insights for the regulation of systemic autoimmune diseases.

ARE THE RULES OF TOLERANCE IDENTICAL FOR PARENTERAL AND MUCOSAL ACCESS TO ANTIGENIC DETERMINANTS?

Subdominant (SD) and cryptic determinants are not processed from native globular proteins by antigen-presenting cells as efficiently as immunodominant (ID) determinants. The prediction follows that autoimmune processes are directed mainly against cryptic or SD self-determinants, because T cells directed against them escape tolerance induction

[a]This work was supported by NIH Grant AR40919.

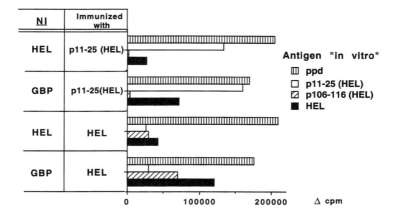

FIGURE 1. NI with HEL diminishes the T-cell proliferative response to a dominant (106-116), but not to a subdominant (11-25), determinant. Immune deviation as an explanation for the tolerance induced after mucosal contact with antigens: the HEL model. BALB/c mice were 8 weeks old when they were given 0.06 mg of HEL (NI). Five days later they were challenged with HEL-CFA. Lymph nodes were taken after 9 days of immunization, and their response to HEL, p106-116, and p11-25 was assayed for proliferation and cytokine production. Note that NI treatment diminishes the (LN) proliferative T-cell response to p106-116 and HEL. On the other hand, the proliferative response to the SD determinant, p11-25, of HEL remains unaffected by the nasal treatment. We tested the pattern of cytokine response to HEL and to p11-25. LN T cells reactive to HEL or p11-25 are present in the LN cells of the pretreated mice.

in the neonatal period.[3] We have been studying oral and nasally induced tolerance to self and nonself proteins. We have found that oral or nasal contact with HEL readily induces Th-1 tolerance to immunodominant, but not SD or cryptic, determinants. In this report we will analyze three experimental situations. In the succeeding paragraphs, 1 and 3, mucosal contacts with HEL and collagen, respectively, reduced the Th-1 and enhanced the Th-2 response. In paragraph 2, nasal installation of myelin basic protein triggered a T-cell proliferative response and accelerated disease in (SJL × B10.PL)F1 mice.

Immune Deviation as an Explanation for the Th-1 Tolerance Induced after Mucosal Contact with Antigens: the HEL Model

As shown in FIGURE 1, NI of HEL in BALB/c mice diminishes the lymph node (LN) proliferative T-cell response to a subsequent immunization with HEL, affecting the dominant response to peptide p106-116. On the other hand, the proliferative response to the SD determinant, p-11-25, of HEL seems to remain unaffected by the nasal treatment (FIG. 1). In this same experiment, we tested the pattern of cytokine response to HEL and to p11-25. Favoring the deviation hypothesis, we found that nine days after immunization with HEL-CFA or p11-25-CFA T cells reactive to HEL or p11-25 are present in the LN cells of mice that had been nasally treated with HEL. These T cells produce much less IFNγ and much more IL-5 in response to immunization with either HEL or p11-25 in CFA, as compared to the cytokine pattern in the control group, which displayed more IFNγ and undetectable levels of IL-5. Inasmuch as we detected an IgG1 response to HEL

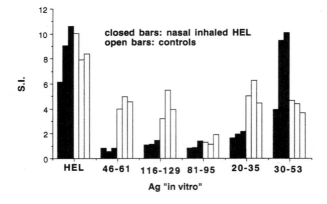

FIGURE 2. Effects of NI with HEL in newborn mice on the hierarchy of determinants in B10.A mice. Mice given 0.06 mg of HEL (NT) in the first week of age do not respond to ID peptides but maintain a response to HEL and SD determinant 30-53.

in the NI animals before any parenteral immunization, we assume that antibody of this isotype, as well as the little proliferation in response to immunization, must result from Th-2 cells primed after mucosal uptake. We are investigating the fine specificity of these T cells arising in the spleen of NI animals before the challenge immunization. Recently we found out that B10.A mice treated neonatally (NI) with HEL do not respond to immunodominant peptides but maintain a response to HEL and SD determinant 30-53 (Fig. 2). From this experiment, we conclude that NI, at least in newborns, diverts the response to SD determinants; in self-proteins, this diversion may account for autoimmunity. These findings in the HEL model provide a basis for the results that we describe in the next two paragraphs in experimental allergic encephalomyelitis (EAE) and collagen-induced arthritis (CIA).

Nasal Installation of Guinea Pig Myelin Basic Protein by (SJL × B10.PL)F1 Mice during the First Week of Age Accelerates the Onset of EAE

Studies in rats had shown that oral administration of guinea pig myelin basic protein (GBP) in neonates (1 week old) enhanced EAE induction when the animals reached adulthood.[4] We have failed to protect (SJL × B10.PL)F1 mice from EAE either by feeding or NI in the neonatal period or in adulthood: in fact, the disease was enhanced by either of these treatments. The following experiment indicates that mucosal contact (NI) with GBP in (SJL × B10.PL)F1 mice primes for a pathogenic immune response. Male F1 mice were six days old when they received a single dose of 60 μg of GBP by NI. The control mice received 60 μg of HEL by NI at the same age. All mice were immunized with GBP-CFA when they reached eight weeks of age. Pertussis toxin was administered ip twice (1 and 2 days after immunization). Surprisingly, instead of being tolerized, disease (EAE) was accelerated (Fig. 3).

Effects of Nasal Installation of Collagen II or a Dominant Collagen II Peptide in the Course of CIA

In the DBA/1 mouse (H-2q), we focused on the response to collagen II (CII) and one prominent determinant, p256-271.[5] NI of bovine CII induced protection from disease;

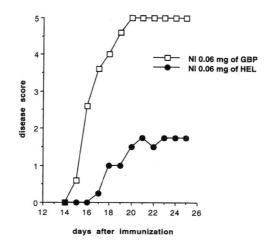

FIGURE 3. Nasal installation of guinea pig myelin basic protein (GBP) to (SJL × B10.PL) F1 mice during the first week of age accelerates the onset of EAE.

strikingly, NI with the immunodominant p256-271 led to a proliferative tolerance, but the disease (CIA) was more severe when the animals were then challenged with bovine CII.

CONCLUSION

Doses 10- to 20-fold lower than needed for oral tolerization are potent in the NI format, and, therefore, as a treatment modality, this offers considerable economy over oral administration. Although untoward responses have been recorded with NI, these may not occur with all peptide tolerogens. It should be possible to determine prospectively the small patient group that is at risk for such a procedure and to then exploit the many devices available for efficiently administrating nasal sprays to humans. It is obviously also of interest to explore those situations in which oral or nasal antigen administration has an effect contrary to expectation. We predict that these situations are ones in which the Th2/antibody response produced exacerbates the disease by enhancing determinant spreading. Alternatively, the mucosal route, per se, might lead to unique processing of the challenge molecule followed by determinant spreading to T cells directed to newly displayed, cryptic, determinant complexes.

REFERENCES

1. WAHDAN, M. H. *et al.* 1982. J. Infect. Dis. **145**(3): 292-295.
2. ROIVAINEN, M. *et al.* 1987. J. Med. Virol. **23**(3): 249-256.
3. SERCARZ, E. *et al.* 1993. Annu. Rev. Immunol. **11**: 729-766.
4. MILLER, A. *et al.* 1994. Eur. J. Immunol. **24**: 1026-1032.
5. ANDERSSON, M. *et al.* 1991. Scand. J. Immunol. **33**(5): 505-510.

Oral Tolerance in Myelin Basic Protein TCR Transgenic Mice[a]

ABBIE MEYER, INGRID GIENAPP, KAREN COX,
JOAN GOVERMAN,[b] LEROY HOOD,[b] AND
CAROLINE WHITACRE

Department of Medical Microbiology and Immunology
Ohio State University College of Medicine
333 West 10th Avenue, Room 2078
Columbus, Ohio 43210
and
[b]*Department of Molecular Biotechnology*
University of Washington School of Medicine
Seattle, Washington 98195

The oral administration of myelin basic protein (MBP) in Lewis rats and some strains of mice results in suppression of clinical signs and histopathologic changes of experimental autoimmune encephalomyelitis (EAE).[1-3] Goverman *et al.*[4] reported the development of TCR double-transgenic mice that expressed the Vα2 and Vβ8.2 αβ TCR that recognizes the immunodominant NAc1-11 epitope of MBP. Cells from these mice, upon transfer into naive recipients, have been reported to undergo a deletion event following the administration of high doses of MBP intravenously.[5] In this study, we examined the effect of oral administration of MBP on the fate and function of MBP-reactive double-transgenic T cells.

A large dose of MBP was administered orally (by gavage), and assessments of transgenic phenotype and proliferative capacity were made in various lymphoid organs 1, 3, 7 or 8, and 10 days later. Flow cytometric analyses showed that the percentage of Vα2/Vβ8.2+ cells was reduced in blood 15-fold compared to pretreatment values on day one. There was an increase in transgenic T cells in the blood compartment on day 3 that reached a maximum on day 7. However, the double-positive cells were again reduced sevenfold over pretreatment values by day 10 after feeding. Similar patterns were observed in lymph node cells (LNC), mesenteric LNC, and spleen (SPL), with marked reductions in double-positive cells at days 1 and 10 after feeding (FIG. 1A).

The MBP proliferative response followed the same pattern as the phenotype assessments. In LNC, mesenteric LNC, and SPL, dramatic reductions in the proliferative response were observed on days 1 and 10, with increases in proliferative capacity on days 3 and 7.

To explore the mechanisms responsible for the biphasic pattern of phenotype and function in the transgenic cells, we first examined the possibility that cells were trafficking into the gut as a result of the oral administration of MBP. Analysis of frozen sections of intestine by immunofluorescence revealed that as early as one day after MBP feeding, there was a large increase in the number of Vα2/Vβ8.2+ cells in the lamina propria of the small intestine (FIG. 1B). The increase was observed throughout the observation period.

We examined the ability of transgenic T cells to secrete cytokines. Frequencies of IL-2 and IL-4-secreting cells were determined by limiting-dilution analysis at various

[a]This work was supported by NIH Grants NS23561 and AI35960.

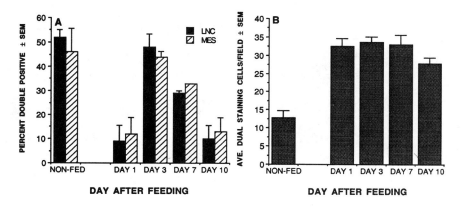

FIGURE 1. Phenotypic assessment of transgenic lymphocytes in peripheral lymphoid organs and the intestine of MBP TCR transgenic mice following oral administration of high-dose MBP. **A:** Flow cytometric detection of $V\alpha2/V\beta8.2$ double-positive cells from peripheral lymph nodes and mesenteric lymph nodes. In both lymph node populations, the transgenic phenotype is dramatically decreased at days 1 and 10 after feeding. **B:** Immunofluorescence detection of $V\alpha2/V\beta8.2$ dual staining cells from 10 high-power 40 × fields of 4 μm frozen sections of upper small intestine, stained with directly labeled monoclonal antibodies. Transgenic lymphocytes are observed to increase at all time points in the small intestine after feeding.

times after oral administration of MBP. At days 1 and 3 following MBP feeding, there was a large increase in the frequency of IL-2-secreting cells in LNC mesenteric LNC, and SPL, which decreased dramatically by days 7-10. By contrast, the frequency of IL-4-secreting cells was low early after feeding but dramatically increased by days 7-10. Thus, there appeared to be a shift from TH1 to TH2 cytokine secretion in multiple lymphoid organs with time after MBP feeding.

In summary, the use of the MBP TCR transgenic mouse for oral tolerance studies permits the tracking of a large population of lymphoid cells with the ultimate capacity for induction of CNS autoimmune disease. Our results suggest that feeding a single large dose of antigen results in an immediate and dramatic decrease in autoreactive lymphocytes in the periphery, perhaps due to trafficking into the gut. A time-dependent decrease in IL-2-secreting cells coupled with a time-dependent increase in IL-4-secreting cells is consistent with a shift from a TH1 to a TH2 type response. By all phenotypic and functional assessments, autoreactive cells are deleted from peripheral lymphoid organs by 10 days after feeding. Therefore, mechanisms of lymphocyte trafficking, changing cytokine secretion patterns, and deletion appear to be involved in high-dose oral tolerance.

REFERENCES

1. WHITACRE, C. C., I. E. GIENAPP, C. G. OROSZ & D. M. BITAR. 1991. J. Immunol. **147:** 2155-2163.
2. BITAR, D. M. & C. C. WHITACRE. 1988. Cell. Immunol. **112:** 364-370.
3. LIDER, O., L. M. B. SANTOS, C. S. Y. LEE, P. J. HIGGINS & H. L. WEINER. 1989. J. Immunol. **142:** 748-752.
4. GOVERMAN, J., A. WOODS, L. LARSON, L. P. WEINER, L. HOOD & D. M. ZALLER. 1993. Cell **72**(4): 551-560.
5. CRITCHFIELD, J. M., M. K. RACKE, J. C. ZUNIGA-PFLUCKER, B. CANNELLA, C. RAINE, J. GOVERMAN & M. J. LENARDO. 1994. Science **263:** 1139-1143.

The Effects of Oral Myelin Basic Protein and Dexamethasone Treatment on Experimental Autoimmune Encephalomyelitis[a]

F. MOKHTARIAN, T. SHIRAZIAN, O. BATUMAN, AND Y. SHI

Division of Immunology
Department of Medicine
Maimonides Medical Center
SUNY Health Science Center
4802 10th Avenue
Brooklyn, New York 11219

INTRODUCTION

Multiple sclerosis (MS) is an autoimmune disease of the central nervous system. Experimental autoimmune encephalomyelitis (EAE) in mice is the best available model, clinically and pathologically, for MS.[1,2] Using this model, attempts have been made to suppress the induction and severity of EAE,[3] in the hope of finding a suitable treatment for MS. Oral administration of myelin basic protein (MBP) is one of the methods used successfully to inhibit EAE and is induced by active immunization with MBP/CFA. The mechanism of this inhibition is either by anergy[4] or by induction of MBP-specific suppressor T cells.[5] The immunosuppressive drug, dexamethasone (DEX), is also used to suppress EAE.[6] In the present investigation, we compared the antigen-specific effect of oral MBP, and the nonspecific suppressive effect of DEX, on the suppression of EAE induced by adoptive transfer of MBP-primed T cells. Both treatments were administered after the transfer of cells.

METHODS

Treatments of Mice

Guinea pig MBP was purified from spinal cords according to standard techniques and used in all studies.[1] SJL mice were adoptively transferred, each with 3×10^7 MBP-primed lymph node cells (LNC), as previously described.[1] These mice were subsequently fed with MBP or OVA (0.5 mg of protein/mouse was given as a control), by an 18-gauge stainless steel feeding needle, on alternate days for 14 days (modified from ref. 5). A third group of mice was injected intraperitoneally with DEX, 280 μg/mouse (16 mg/kg) (Gensia, Pharmaceutical Co. Inc., Irvine, CA), also on alternate days for 14 days, and a fourth group was given both oral MBP and DEX treatments.

[a] This work was supported by a Grant from Maimonides Research and Development Foundation.

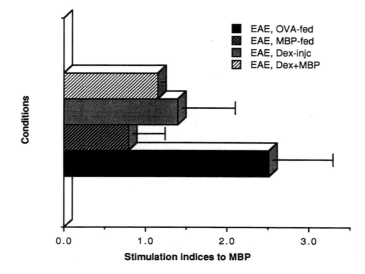

FIGURE 1. Proliferative response of splenocytes (SPL) from mice with EAE to MBP. SPL (2×10^5 cells per well) from OVA-fed, MBP-fed, DEX-injected, and MBP-fed plus DEX-injected mice, 14 days after adoptive transfer of MBP-primed LNC, were cultured with 50 µg/mL of MBP. Experiments were performed in triplicate wells. The results were expressed as mean cpm ± SD of three mice in each group.

Assay for Suppression

For the suppressor T-cell assay, 2×10^5 splenocytes (SPL) from nontreated mice with EAE were added to 2×10^5 mitomycin C-treated SPL from mice treated with oral MBP, DEX, or both, and cultured with or without MBP. After 96 hours in culture, the cells were assayed for proliferation to MBP according to standard techniques. Percent inhibition was expressed as the percent decrease of [^{3}H]TdR incorporation by sample-treated cells when compared to incorporation by untreated cells.

RESULTS AND CONCLUSIONS

The Effect of Treatments with Oral MBP and DEX on the Induction of EAE

Treatment with oral MBP alone, or with DEX plus oral MBP, significantly suppressed proliferation to MBP ($p < 0.05$), whereas treatment with DEX alone did not. The mean stimulation index (SI) to MBP, of MBP-fed mice (0.79), was significantly lower than the control (OVA-fed mice) (2.5). The DEX-treated group proliferated to MBP with a mean SI of 1.4, whereas the group that received both DEX and MBP treatments proliferated with a mean SI of 1.16, which was lower than the OVA-fed and DEX-injected group but higher than the MBP-fed group (FIG. 1). Next, to determine if the lower proliferation of SPL in these mice was due to the presence of suppressor cells, SPL of these treated mice

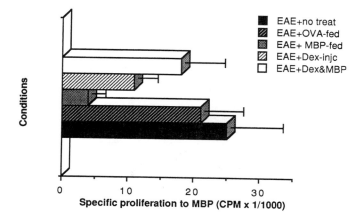

FIGURE 2. *In vitro* suppression of proliferative response to MBP of SPL from mice with EAE. SPL (2×10^5 cells per well) from mice 14 days after adoptive transfer of MBP-primed LNC were cultured with 2×10^5 mitomycin C-treated SPL from nontreated, OVA-fed, MBP-fed, DEX-injected, and MBP-fed plus DEX-injected mice in the presence of 50 μg/mL of MBP. Experiments were performed in triplicate wells. The results were expressed as mean cpm ± SD of three mice in each group.

were added to SPL of mice with EAE. Only the addition of SPL from mice treated with oral MBP, but not DEX, significantly inhibited the proliferation to MBP ($p < 0.05$) (FIG. 2). Treatment with both DEX and oral MBP, however, not only did not improve but reversed the inhibitory effect of oral MBP, probably due to a steroid effect on suppressor cells (FIG. 2). The proliferative response of SPL of mice with EAE to MBP was significantly suppressed at a rate of 81.7% after the addition of SPL from MBP-fed mice. On the other hand, the addition of SPL from mice that were OVA fed to SPL of EAE mice only suppressed the proliferation at the rate of 24.6 percent. SPL from DEX-treated EAE mice inhibited the MBP proliferation at the rate of 60%, whereas mice treated with both DEX and oral MBP only showed 34.8% inhibition (FIG. 2). It was apparent that oral MBP was more effective than DEX in inhibiting the proliferation of recipient mice to MBP.

TABLE 1. The Effect of Oral MBP Treatment, at the Time of Adoptive Transfer, on the Induction of Clinical EAE[a]

	Number of Mice at Different Stages of EAE				
Groups	0	1	2	3	Mean
OVA fed	1	4	4	1	1.45
MBP fed	5	3	0	0	0.38[b]
DEX treated	2	4	2	1	0.80

[a] 0, no abnormality; 1, floppy tail with mild hind-limb weakness; 2, floppy tail with moderate hind-limb weakness; 3, hind-limb paresis but not complete paralysis.
[b] MBP fed < OVA fed, $p < 0.005$.

In Vivo *Suppression of EAE by Oral MBP Feeding and DEX Injection*

MBP feeding and DEX injection both suppressed the development of EAE after the adoptive transfer of MBP-activated LNC (TABLE 1). Only the development of acute EAE in the MBP-fed group (0.38) compared to the OVA-fed group (1.45) was significantly suppressed (p < 0.005). DEX, but not oral MBP treatment, resulted in significant reduction in weight and number of SPL of the treated mice (data not shown). It has been reported that inhibition of EAE is mediated by suppressor T cells through the production of TGF-β.[5] The inhibitory effect of DEX can also be attributed, at least in part, to increased TGF-β production reported to occur in DEX-treated splenic and peripheral T cells.[7]

REFERENCES

1. MOKHTARIAN, F., D. E. MCFARLIN & C. S. RAINE. 1984. Nature (Lond.) **239:** 356-358.
2. RAINE, C. S., F. MOKHTARIAN & D. E. MCFARLIN. 1984. Lab. Invest. **51:** 534-546.
3. MOKHTARIAN, F. 1988. Clin. Immunol. Immunopath. **49:** 308-317.
4. WHITACRE, C. C., I. E. GIENAPP, C. G. OROSZ & D. M. BITAR. 1991. J. Immunol. **147:** 2155-2163.
5. MILLER, A., O. LIDER, A. B. ROBERTS, M. B. SPORN & H. L. WEINER. 1992. Proc. Natl. Acad. Sci. USA **89:** 421-425.
6. REDER, A. T., M. THAPER & M. A. JENSEN. 1994. Neurology **44:** 2289-2294.
7. BATUMAN, O. A., A. P. FERRO, A. DIAZ & S. A. JIMINEZ. 1991. J. Clin. Invest. **88:** 1574-1580.

Oral Insulin Does Not Prevent Insulin-dependent Diabetes Mellitus in BB Rats

JOHN P. MORDES, BRIAN SCHIRF, DAVID ROIPKO,
DALE L. GREINER, HOWARD WEINER,
PATRICIA NELSON, AND ALDO A. ROSSINI

Diabetes Division, Suite 218
University of Massachusetts Medical School
373 Plantation Street
Worcester, Massachusetts 01605
and
Harvard Medical School
Boston, Massachusetts

INTRODUCTION

Oral insulin both delays and reduces the frequency of autoimmune insulin-dependent diabetes mellitus (IDDM) in the NOD mouse,[1] possibly by generating populations of suppressor T cells.[2] The effects of this treatment in the BB rat are unknown. Diabetes-prone (DP) BB rats spontaneously develop pancreatic insulitis followed by selective destruction of beta cells and diabetes between 50-90 days of age.[3] DP-BB rats are severely lymphopenic. Diabetes-resistant (DR) BB rats are coisogenic, nonlymphopenic descendants of DP-BB forebears. Their cumulative incidence of spontaneous diabetes is <1%, but they retain susceptibility to IDDM induction.[3] They become diabetic if depleted of RT6+ T cells and/or treated with the interferon inducer, polyinosinic : polycytidylic acid (poly I : C).[4] Like the NOD mouse, the BB rat is used to model human IDDM. We tested the hypothesis that oral insulin would prevent IDDM in the BB rat.

METHODS

Weanling DR and DP rats of both sexes were obtained with the viral-antibody free colony at our institution and maintained under standard conditions. IDDM was induced in DR rats using two previously described protocols.[4] The first comprised three weekly intraperitoneal injections of poly I : C (5 μg/g in PBS) plus five weekly injections of the DS4.23 cytotoxic anti-RT6.1 monoclonal antibody (mAb). The second protocol comprised only poly I : C, 10 μg/g, three times weekly. Powdered insulin and recombinant rat interferon-α/β (IFN-α/β) were solubilized according to manufacturers' instructions and administered by gavage. Controls and reagent sources are described in the footnotes of each TABLE.

TABLE 1. Frequency of Diabetes and Insulitis in DP Rats Treated with Oral Insulin[a]

Experiment	Treatment	Number	Diabetic (%)	Age at Onset (day)	Insulitis (%)
1	1 mg porcine insulin	11	8 (73%)	98 ± 4	11/11 (100%)
	1 mg albumin	12	10 (83%)	84 ± 12	12/12 (100%)
2	0.5 mg human insulin	6	6 (100%)	74 ± 11	6/6 (100%)
	1.0 mg human insulin	6	6 (100%)	72 ± 9	6/6 (100%)
	2.0 mg human insulin	6	4 (67%)	86 ± 10	6/6 (100%)
	PBS[b]	6	6 (100%)	76 ± 7	6/6 (100%)

[a] Treatments were begun at ≈30 days of age. Experiment 1 summarizes two independent trials using the same protocol. There are no statistically significant differences in the frequency of diabetes or insulitis or in the mean age at diabetes onset among the group in either experiment. Powdered porcine monocomponent insulin was a gift from Eli Lilly, Co., Indianapolis, IN. Recombinant human insulin in powder form was the gift of Novo Nordisk, Copenhagen, Denmark. Oral reagents were given 3 times weekly by gavage. Means are shown ± 1 SD.

[b] PBS = phosphate-buffered saline.

RESULTS

Studies in DP-BB Rats

We first tested oral porcine insulin (1 mg, 3 ×/week) vs. oral albumin (1 mg 3 ×/week) in ≈30-day-old DP rats in two separate trials. Through 120 days of age, spontaneous IDDM occurred with statistically similar frequency and at comparable ages in both groups (TABLE 1, experiment 1). We next tested the combination of human insulin (0.5, 1.0, or 2.0 mg 3 ×/week) plus oral IFN-α/β (5000 U 3 ×/week). IFN was administered on the basis of previous reports for its ability to synergize in oral tolerance protocols, possibly by enhancing the generation of Th2 cells *in vivo*.[2] Spontaneous IDDM occurred with statistically similar frequency and at comparable ages in all groups studied (TABLE 1, experiment 2).

Studies in DR-BB Rats

We first tested the possible tolerizing effect of oral porcine insulin (1.0 mg 3 ×/week) coadministered with the combination of anti-RT6 mAb plus poly I : C, all reagents being started at ≈30 days of age. There was no effect of oral insulin on the development of IDDM (TABLE 2, experiment 1). This protocol was repeated using doses of 0.5, 1.0, and 2.0 mg porcine insulin; 17/18 treated animals and 6/6 controls became diabetic. We next coadministered anti-RT6 mAb plus poly I : C with a combination of IFN-α/β (5000 U 3 ×/week) plus human insulin (0.5, 1.0, or 2.0 mg 3 ×/week). In this experiment, treatment with oral insulin plus IFN was begun at ≈30 days of age, and treatment with mAb and poly I : C was begun one week later. IDDM developed at comparable frequency in all groups with comparable latency after the institution of mAb plus poly I : C (TABLE 2, experiment 2). This protocol was repeated a second time with the single modification of

TABLE 2. Frequency of Diabetes and Insulitis in DR Rats[a]

Experiment	Induction	Treatment	Number	Diabetic (%)	Days to IDDM
1	Poly I:C + anti-RT6 mAb	1 mg porcine insulin	6	6 (100%)	19 ± 1
		1 mg albumin	6	6 (100%)	24 ± 2
2	Poly I:C + anti-RT6 mAb	0.5 mg human insulin + IFN	6	6 (100%)	21 ± 4
		1.0 mg human insulin + IFN	6	5 (83%)	22 ± 5
		2.0 mg human insulin + IFN	6	6 (100%)	19 ± 3
		PBS	6	5 (83%)	21 ± 2
3	Poly I:C + anti-RT6 mAb	0.6 mg insulin β chain + IFN	6	4 (67%)	23 ± 2
		1.2 mg insulin β chain + IFN	6	4 (67%)	24 ± 3
		2.4 mg insulin β chain + IFN	6	6 (100%)	25 ± 6
		No treatment	6	5 (83%)	21 ± 3
4	Poly I:C alone	2.0 mg insulin + IFN	10	7 (70%)	18 ± 6
		IFN alone	10	5 (50%)	20 ± 6

[a] Treatment with oral reagents (3 times weekly by gavage) was begun at ≈30 days of age and continued through 70 days of age. Treatments to induce IDDM were begun 1 week later, except in experiment 1 when they were started at the same time as the oral reagents. The pancreata of all animals demonstrated the presence of insulitis. There are no statistically significant differences in the frequency of diabetes or insulitis or in the mean interval to IDDM onset among groups in any of the experiments. Poly I:C and bovine insulin β chain were purchased from Sigma, St. Louis, MO. Hybridomas producing the DS4.23 anti-RT6.1 mAb are maintained in our laboratory. Recombinant rat interferon-α/β (IFN-α/β) was obtained from Lee Biomolecular Research, San Diego, CA.

using bovine insulin β chain (0.6, 1.2, or 2.4 mg 3 ×/week) in place of intact human insulin.[2] No preventive effects of oral insulin β chain were observed (TABLE 2, experiment 3).

The failure to achieve tolerance in these studies could be attributed to the possible depletion of tolerizing RT6+ T cells. To investigate this possibility, we next tested oral human insulin (2.0 mg 3 ×/week) plus IFN-α/β (5000 U 3 ×/week), both begun one week before the initiation of diabetes induction using high-dose poly I : C alone. Flow cytometric analyses demonstrated that comparable, normal numbers of RT6+ T cells were present in both experimental and control animals during the course of these studies. Nonetheless, IDDM occurred in 70% of insulin-treated rats vs. 50% of controls (TABLE 2, experiment 4).

DISCUSSION

We conclude that oral insulin at these doses does not prevent or delay autoimmune IDDM in BB rats. The basis of the discrepancy with observations in the NOD mouse is not known. Speculatively, it could be argued that the natural lymphopenia of the DP rat and the depletion of RT6+ T cells in the DR rat precludes development of tolerizing suppressor-cell populations. This hypothesis does not readily explain the failure to achieve tolerance in the DR rats treated only with poly I : C to induce IDDM. It is well recognized that NOD mice and BB rats differ substantially with respect to the number and the efficiency of therapies that prevent IDDM.[5] It may be that the immunological mechanisms underlying oral tolerance are dependent on species- or strain-specific characteristics of disease induction that are not well understood.

REFERENCES

1. ZHANG, Z. J., L. DAVIDSON, G. EISENBARTH *et al.* 1991. Proc. Natl. Acad. Sci. USA **88:** 10252-10256.
2. WEINER, H. L., A. FRIEDMAN, A. MILLER *et al.* 1994. Annu. Rev. Immunol. **12:** 809-837.
3. CRISÁ, L., J. P. MORDES & A. A. ROSSINI. 1992. Diabetes Metab. Rev. **8:** 9-37.
4. THOMAS, V. A., B. A. WODA, E. S. HANDLER *et al.* 1991. Diabetes **40:** 255-258.
5. ROSSINI, A. A., J. P. MORDES, E. S. HANDLER *et al.* 1995. Clin. Immunol. Immunopathol. **74:** 2-9.

Mucosal Tolerance to Aflatoxin B₁[a]

A. R. OLIVER,[b] L. K. SILBART,[b] D. F. KEREN,[c]
B. MILLER,[c] AND R. A. McDONALD [c]

[b]Center for Environmental Health
Department of Animal Science
University of Connecticut
CANR, Box U-39
Storrs, Connecticut 06269

[b]Department of Pathology
University of Michigan
Ann Arbor, Michigan 48109

In an attempt to generate a secretory IgA (sIgA) immune response to the dietary carcinogen aflatoxin B_1 (AFB), we coimmunized New Zealand white rabbits through chronically isolated ileal loops[1] with AFB coupled to porcine thyroglobulin (TG) and cholera toxin (CT), a potent mucosal adjuvant.[2] This protocol resulted in a negligible sIgA anti-AFB response (FIG. 1), in contrast to prior studies with conjugates made with the carcinogen 2-acetylaminofluorene.[3,4] The sIgA anti-CT and anti-TG responses of animals immunized

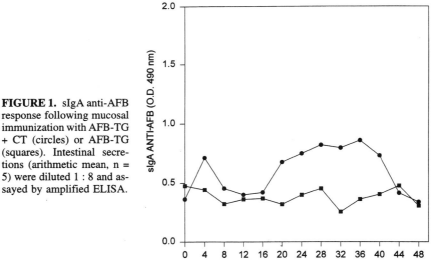

FIGURE 1. sIgA anti-AFB response following mucosal immunization with AFB-TG + CT (circles) or AFB-TG (squares). Intestinal secretions (arithmetic mean, n = 5) were diluted 1 : 8 and assayed by amplified ELISA.

[a]This work was supported in part by USPHS (NCI) Grant CA47132. This is scientific contribution #1623, Storrs Agricultural Experiment Station, University of Connecticut.

TABLE 1. Antibody-secreting cells to AFB and TG following Mitogen Stimulation[a]

Animal	ASC Anti-AFB				ASC Anti-TG			
	MLN	LP	PP	SP	MLN	LP	PP	SP
1	10	<1	10	4	3	<1	4	6
2	ND	<1	12	8	ND	<1	15	8

[a] Lymphocytes from mesenteric lymph nodes (MLN), lamina propria (LP), Peyer's patches (PP), and spleen (SP) of unimmunized rabbits were stimulated with lipopolysaccharide (50 μg/mL) and pokeweed mitogen (2.5 μg/mL), and assayed by ELISPOT for ASC to AFB and TG. Numbers represent ASC per 10^6 lymphocytes. ND = not done.

with AFB-TG plus CT were, however, comparable to those of control animals immunized with TG plus cholera toxin.

Parenteral immunization with AFB-TG emulsified in complete Freund's adjuvant generated a strong serum IgG anti-AFB response, demonstrating the immunogenicity of the conjugate preparation and the presence of appropriate systemic B- and T-cell repertoires to respond to AFB. Mucosal immunization followed by parenteral immunization generated a serum IgG anti-AFB response comparable to that of animals immunized parenterally without prior mucosal immunization. This demonstrates that the tolerance to AFB is specific to the mucosa and that it is not accompanied by systemic suppression (*i.e.,* oral tolerance).

In order to test for the presence of AFB-reactive B-cell precursors in the mucosa, we stimulated lymphocytes from Peyer's patches (PP), spleen (SP), mesenteric lymph nodes (MLN), and lamina propria (LP) of naive animals with lipopolysaccharide and pokeweed mitogen. The stimulated cells were assayed by enzyme-linked immunoadsorbent spot assay (ELISPOT) for the presence of anti-AFB and anti-TG antibody-secreting cells (ASC). As anticipated, ASC were found in SP but also in PP and MLN (TABLE 1), demonstrating that mucosal tolerance to AFB is not a result of B-cell deletion in the gut mucosa.

Taken together, our results demonstrate that rabbits exhibit mucosal but not systemic tolerance to AFB. This tolerance is specific to AFB, is not accompanied by systemic suppression, is not due to deletion of AFB-reactive B cells in the gut, and is not surmountable by CT. This is consistent with the observation that an established mucosal tolerance cannot be broken by coadministration with the heat-labile enterotoxin of *E. coli*,[5] which is structurally and functionally similar to CT. This phenomenon may thus be a result of prior dietary exposure to aflatoxin B_1.

REFERENCES

1. KEREN, D. F., H. L. ELLIOTT, G. D. BROWN & J. H. YARDLEY. 1975. Atrophy of villi with hypertrophy and hyperplasia of Paneth cells in isolated (Thiry-Vella) ileal loops in rabbits. Light-microscopic studies. Gastroenterology **68**: 83-93.
2. HOLMGREN, J., N. LYCKE & C. CZERKINSKY. 1993. Cholera toxin and cholera B subunit as oral-mucosal adjuvant and antigen vector systems. Vaccine **11**: 1179-1184.
3. SILBART, L. K. & D. F. KEREN. 1989. Reduction of intestinal carcinogen absorption by carcinogen-specific secretory immunity. Science **243**: 1462-1464.

4. SILBART, L. K., D. F. KEREN, R. A. McDONALD, P. M. LINCOLN, L. GOSLINOSKI & J. B. SMART. 1992. Characterization of the mucosal immune response to 2-acetylaminofluorene-protein conjugates. Reg. Immunol. **4:** 245-254.
5. CLEMENTS, J. D., N. M. HARTZOG & F. L. LYON. 1988. Adjuvant activity of *Escherichia coli* heat-labile enterotoxin and effect on the induction of oral tolerance in mice to unrelated protein antigens. Vaccine **6:** 269-277.

Tolerance to an Arthritogenic T-cell Epitope of HSP65 and the Regulation of Experimental Arthritis

BERENT J. PRAKKEN, RUURD van der ZEE,
STEPHEN M. ANDERTON, PETER van KOOTEN,
WIETSE KUIS,[a] AND WILLEM van EDEN

Department for Infectious Diseases and Immunology
Faculty of Veterinary Science
PO Box 80165
3508 TD Utrecht, the Netherlands

[a]*University Hospital for Children and Youth*
'Het Wilhelmina Kinderziekenhuis'
Utrecht, the Netherlands

Adjuvant arthritis (AA) is an extensively studied form of experimental arthritis resembling rheumatoid arthritis in a number of pathological aspects. It can be induced in susceptible (Lewis) rats by immunization with mycobacterial antigens. From several experiments it can be concluded that T-cell responses to hsp's play an important immunomodulatory role in the induction AA. First it was shown that AA can be passivily transfered by T cells alone from diseased rats to syngeneic disease-free animals.[1] Furthermore passive transfer of a T-cell clone recognizing the nonconserved 180-188 amino acid sequence in mycobacterial hsp65 was found to induce AA.[2,3] This T-cell clone also responded to cartilage proteoglycan but not to rat hsp60. The clone therefore showed that although self-cross-reactive or ''mimicry'' T cells are able to induce overt autoimmune disease, this was not related to the conserved nature of hsp's.

Several studies have shown that it is possible to induce antigen-specific T-cell tolerance in experimental autoimmune models.[4] Most evidence so far has been collected in the model of experimental allergic encephalomyelitis (EAE).

EAE is a demyelinating autoimmune disease caused by $CD4^+$ T cells specific for myelin basic protein (MBP). It can be induced in susceptible animals by immunization with MBP in CFA. However, oral administration of MBP protects animals from developing EAE. Protection can be established by adoptive transfer of $CD8^+$ T cells, capable of producing TGF-β when stimulated with the relevant antigens.[5] Encephalogenic epitopes of MBP have been characterized, and nasal inhalation of the immunodominant epitope on MBP has also led to protection.

In the present study we investigated whether tolerance could be induced similarly to the AA-related immunodominant epitope and whether this would lead to protection against AA, a disease induced by an antigen as complex as whole mycobacteria.

Two 15-mer peptides containing the individual mycobacterial hsp65 sequences 176-190 (M36) and 211-225 (M43) were used. M36 contains the epitope 180-188 recognized by the arthritogenic T-cell clone, A2b. Furthermore, it is the immunodominant T-cell epitope after induction of arthritis in AA.[6] M43 is a codominant epitope both after induction of arthritis with Mt and after immunization with mycobacterial hsp65.[6] Thus far no role of this epitope has been found in disease induction or in protection from disease.[7]

Lewis rats were tolerized for M36 using the two different protocols (subcutaneous and intranasal). Five to seven days after the last dose, the animals were immunized with mycobacterial hsp65, and 10-14 days later, proliferative responses to M36 and a control peptide (M43) in PLNC were measured in an LST. Control animals received PBS. After tolerization, the proliferative response to M36 was significantly lower in the animals treated with M36 than in the control animals. The proliferative response to M43 and to mycobacterial hsp65 was not affected. Induction of tolerance to M36 followed by induction of AA resulted in a delay in the onset of arthritis, a lower maximum arthritis score, and a weight curve resembling that of normal animals. Induction of tolerance to M36 led to similar effects in a nonbacterial form of experimental arthritis (CP20961 or avridine-induced arthritis): a delay in the onset of arthritis and a much lower maximum arthritis score in the tolerized animals compared to the control animals. These experiments have shown that tolerance for a single specific microbial epitope may cause resistance to various forms of experimental arthritis, including those induced without microbial antigens.

REFERENCES

1. WHITEHOUSE, D. J., M. W. WHITEHOUSE & C. M. PEARSON. 1969. Passive transfer of adjuvant-induced arthritis and allergic encephalomyelitis in rats using thoracic duct lymphocytes. Nature **224:** 1322-26.
2. HOLOSHITZ, J., Y. NAPARSTEK, A. BEN-NUN & I. R. COHEN. 1983. Lines of T lymphocytes induce or vaccinate against autoimmune arthritis. Science **219:** 56-58.
3. VAN EDEN, W., J. E. R. THOLE, R. VAN DER ZEE, A. NOORDZIJ, J. D. A. VAN EMBDEN, E. J. HENSEN & I. R. COHEN. 1988. Cloning of the mycobacterial epitope recognized by T lymphocytes in adjuvant arthritis. Nature **331:** 171-173.
4. HOYNE, G. F., G. O'HEHIR, D. C. WRAITH, W. R. THOMAS & J. R. LAMB. 1992. Inhibition of T cell and antibody responses to house dust mite allergen by inhalation of the immunodominant T cell epitope in naive and sensitized mice. J. Exp. Med. **178:** 1783-8.
5. LIDER, O., L. M. B. SANTOS, C. S. Y. LEE, P. J. HIGGINS & H. L. WEINER. 1989. Suppression of EAE by oral administration of MBP. II. Suppression of disease and *in vitro* immune responses is mediated by antigen specific CD8⁺ cells. J. Immunol. **142:** 748-52.
6. ANDERTON, S. M., R. VAN DER ZEE, A. NOORDZIJ & W. VAN EDEN. 1994. Differential mycobacterial 65kDa hsp T cell epitope recognition after AA inducing or protective immunization protocols. J. Immunol. **152:** 3656-64.
7. ANDERTON, S. M., R. VAN DER ZEE, A. B. J. PRAKKEN, A. NOORDZIJ & W. VAN EDEN. 1995. Activation of T-cells recognizing self 60 kDa heat shock protein can protect against experimental arthritis. J. Exp. Med. **181:** 943-52.

IL-4 Is Not Involved in the Early MLN T-cell Response to Antigen Given Orally with Cholera Toxin, but Those Cells Can Express IL-4R

DENIS P. SNIDER AND MICHAEL SCHAFFELER

Department of Pathology
McMaster University
HSC-3N26H
1200 Main Street West
Hamilton, Ontario, Canada L8N-3Z5

A controversy exists over the precise nature of the T-cell cytokine response to protein antigen that follows intestinal exposure to cholera toxin (CT) and protein antigen. For instance, whereas some research showed a dominant expression of Th2 type cytokines (IL-4, IL-5),[1] other work showed a mixed phenotype of response, including strong IFN-γ responses by Th1 cells.[2,3] We have recently reported production of IgE antibody and allergic sensitization to the antigen hen egg lysozyme (HEL) following oral exposure to CT and admixed HEL.[4] In addition, IL-4 gene knockout mice do not develop a strong mucosal antibody response after oral immunization using CT as an adjuvant.[5] Both observations indicate that the Th2 cytokine, IL-4, is crucial to the adjuvant effect of CT. One problem with interpretation of the cytokine data is that most of the experiments have involved repeated antigen plus CT immunization before detection of T-cell cytokines. More important, the earliest forms of antigen-specific T-helper cells were not examined in these models.

In vitro analysis of the development of antigen-specific Th2 or Th1 cells revealed that a balance of competing cytokines determine the fate of precursor cells to either Th phenotype.[6] IL-4 is the strongest promoter of Th2 development, *in vitro*.[7] The earliest precursors produce and respond to IL-2, but these must then receive an exogenous source of IL-4 to develop into Th2, and thereafter their progeny can secrete IL-4.[8] We have done experiments to examine the earliest HEL-specific production of IL-4 and IL-2, following oral immunization of mice with HEL and CT. This was done to answer two questions. Is there an IL-4-dependent proliferation of these cells, indicative of Th2 development? Is there a source of IL-4 in the MLN that could drive proliferation of these early-arising HEL-specific T cells?

Five days after oral immunization with HEL and CT, whole-cell suspensions of MLN from C3H mice were cultured, and CD4 cells within them proliferated, in the presence of HEL. The proliferating cells expressed CD4 as detected by flow cytometry. Neither the baseline (no HEL) proliferation of these cells nor the HEL-specific proliferation (3-10 × higher) was inhibited by anti-IL-4 antibody. However, anti-IL-2 antibody could inhibit the HEL-specific proliferation completely. Similar observations were made when T cells were purified from the MLN and mixed with irradiated splenic antigen-presenting cells and HEL. None of the cultures (whole MLN or T cell) produced IL-4, as measured by sensitive ELISA (100 pg/mL) or CT-4S bioassay (3 pg/mL). Exogenous recombinant IL-4 synergized with HEL to produce a very large HEL-specific T-cell proliferation. A similar synergistic increase was not observed after addition of recombinant IL-2.

These data indicated that IL-4 was not produced by cells within the MLN, early in the response to immunization with HEL plus CT. However, the HEL-specific CD4 T cells must have expressed IL-4 receptors upon restimulation *in vitro,* because the combination of exogenous IL-4 and HEL generates a synergistic proliferative response. It may be that CT predisposes the generation of mucosal Th2 cells by altering the frequency of cells that can respond to antigen by expressing IL-4R. However, the early responding antigen-specific T cells in the MLN microenvironment have not progressed to an IL-4-producing phenotype (Th2 differentiation).

REFERENCES

1. XU-AMANO, J., H. KIYONO et al. 1993. J. Exp. Med. **178:** 1309-1220.
2. WILSON, A. D., M. BAILEY et al. 1991. Eur. J. Immunol. **21:** 2333-2339.
3. HÖRNQUIST, E. & N. LYCKE. 1993. Eur. J. Immunol. **23:** 2136-2143.
4. SNIDER, D. P., J. S. MARSHALL et al. 1994. J. Immunol. **153:** 647-657.
5. VAJDY, M., M. H. KOSCO-VILBOIS et al. 1995. J. Exp. Med. **181:** 41-53.
6. GAJEWSKI, T. F. & F. W. FITCH. 1988. J. Immunol. **140:** 4245-4252.
7. SWAIN, S. L., A. D. WEINBERG et al. 1990. J. Immunol. **145:** 3796-3806.
8. SAD, S. & T. R. MOSMANN. 1994. J. Immunol. **153:** 3514-3522.

Development of Immune Response to Orally Administered Cow Milk Protein in Young Children

O. VAARALA, J. KASTE, P. KLEMETTI,
T. SAUKKONEN, E. SAVILAHTI, AND
H. K. ÅKERBLOM

Research Laboratory
The Children's Hospital
University of Helsinki
Stenbackinkatu 11
00290 Helsinki, Finland

The development of immune response to oral antigens, particularly cellular immunity, is poorly known in humans. Studies performed in animal models suggest that early exposure to orally administered proteins initiates an immune response to them, whereas in adult animals the same exposure leads to tolerance.[1] Accordingly, antigen feeding has been suggested as a treatment for hypersensitivity disorders and autoimmune diseases.[2]

Twenty newborn infants from mothers with insulin-dependent diabetes mellitus (IDDM) were recruited into the study, which was the pilot stage of a trial for primary prevention of IDDM by elimination of cow milk (CM) proteins during early infancy. In a double-blind trial, 10 infants received an adapted CM-based formula (Enfamil®, Mead Johnson, Evansville, IN; group I), and 10 infants received a casein hydrolysate formula (Nutramigen®, Mead Johnson, Evansville, IN; group II) until the age of 9 months. At the age of 9 months both groups started to get ordinary CM-based formula containing whole CM proteins. Blood samples were obtained at the ages of 6, 9, 12, and 24 months.

Cellular responses to CM proteins were assessed by proliferation assay of peripheral blood mononuclear cells (PBMC) to β-lactoglobulin (BLG), and results were expressed as the stimulation index (SI). Plasma IgG antibodies to BLG were measured by enzyme-linked immunoassay (ELISA). The levels of soluble intercellular adhesion molecule-1 (ICAM-1) were measured by ELISA kits purchased from Bender MedSystems (Vienna, Austria).

No significant antibody levels or proliferation of PBMC to BLG until the age of 9 months was detectable in infants of group II. The difference in the IgG-antibody levels between the groups was significant at the ages of 6 and 9 months ($p = 0.0004$ and $p = 0.001$, respectively; Mann-Whitney test). Similarly, the mean SIs to BLG were higher in group I than in group II, the difference being significant at the age of 9 months ($p < 0.04$, Mann-Whitney test). The SIs to BLG correlated with the level of IgG antibodies to BLG at 9 months of age ($r = 0.577$, $p = 0.02$; Spearman's correlation). The mean SI to BLG and antibody response decreased in group I from 9 to 24 months of age. The mean SIs to BLG were lower in group II than in group I also at the ages of 12 and 24 months when the children in group II were exposed to CM proteins (FIG. 1). The levels of soluble ICAM-1 were significantly higher in group I than in group II during follow-up (FIG. 2) ($p = 0.05$, Friedman test).

We conclude that early exposure to CM proteins induces systemic immune response to CM proteins. The response later declines, supporting the concept of oral tolerization.

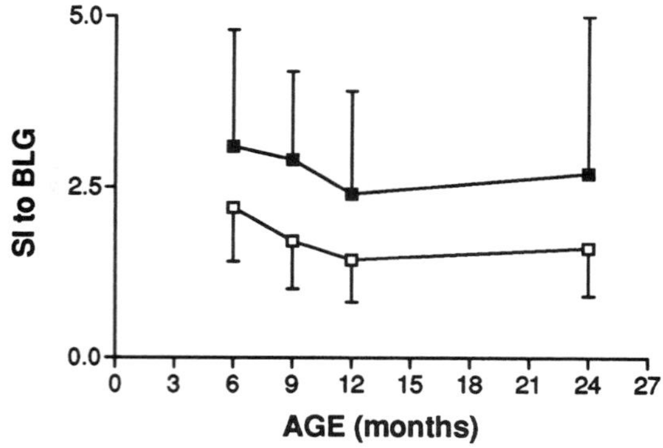

FIGURE 1. Mean levels and standard deviations of stimulation indexes to BLG in children who received cow milk-based formula (■) or casein hydrolysate formula (□) until the age of 9 months.

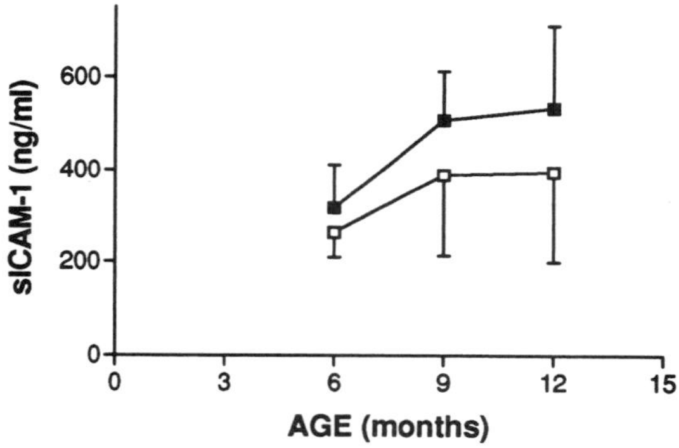

FIGURE 2. Mean levels and standard deviations of soluble ICAM-1 in children who received cow milk-based formula (■) or casein hydrolysate formula (□) until the age of 9 months.

Delayed exposure to CM proteins results in a depressed immune response to these proteins, supporting the view that oral tolerance is an age-dependent phenomenon in humans. Furthermore, the results suggest that orally administered proteins in early infancy induce soluble intercellular adhesion molecules.

REFERENCES

1. STROBEL, S. & A. FERGUSON. 1984. Immune responses to fed antigen in mice. III. Systemic tolerance of priming is related to age at which antigen is first encountered. Pediatr. Res. 18: 588-94.
2. THOMPSON, H. S. G. & N. A. STAINES. 1991. Could specific oral tolerance be a therapy for autoimmune disease? Immunol. Today 11: 396-9.

Intestinal Intraepithelial Lymphocyte Responses to Glucocorticoid Signaling

N. VAN HOUTEN AND G. GASIC

Departments of Pediatrics and Internal Medicine
University of Texas Medical Branch
301 University Boulevard
Galveston, Texas 77555-0366

The immune system associated with the gastrointestinal tract is distinct from the systemic immune system and consists of diverse sequestered compartments. Intestinal intraepithelial lymphocytes (IEL) are incompletely characterized with regard to their functional responses to immunosuppressive agents. These lymphocytes reside between the epithelial cells of the small intestine villi. There is considerable evidence that IEL are derived from progenitor cells independent of direct thymus development, yet the signals that result in development and differentiation of IEL are unknown.[1,2] The signals that determine survival of T cells during selection in the thymus involve ligation of the glucocorticoid receptor in addition to TCR ligation.[3] In normal animals, *in vivo* administration of glucocorticoids results in profound deletion of thymocytes, particularly of the immature population bearing both CD4 and CD8 antigens on their surfaces.[4,5] IEL also contain a subpopulation bearing CD4 and CD8 antigens, yet these CD4[+] CD8[+] IEL are refractory to deletion by glucocorticoids *in vivo*. In fact, no decrease in either yield or cell density of IEL could be identified (FIG. 1). IEL do not respond to the same steroid-mediated signals as their peripheral counterparts. In addition, no major shifts in lymphocyte subpopulations could be seen, as indicated in TABLE 1.

To investigate whether these IEL are, in fact, resistant to the induction of apoptosis, or appear to survive due to a simultaneous influx or proliferation within this compartment, we probed for the appearance of apoptotic nuclei by the terminal deoxynucleotidyl transferase-mediated dUTP nick-end labeling method.[6] Although frequent apoptotic nuclei were identified in the thymus as early as three hours following hydrocortisone administration, no increase in the numbers of apoptotic IEL were identified over the course of 48 hours of treatment. In addition, apoptotic nuclei were also identified in the germinal centers of Peyers's patches of hydrocortisone-treated animals. We have not yet determined whether these are B or T lymphocytes, but we are aware that the toxic effect of steroids reaches the intestinal milieu. The absence of apoptotic nuclei in lymphocytes within the intestinal epithelium indicates that IEL are resistant to apoptotic signals from glucocorticoids.

To determine the mechanism of resistance to the strong deletional signal from hydrocortisone, we investigated Bcl-2 expression in IEL. Bcl-2 has been implicated in the protection of lymphocytes from glucocorticoid-induced apoptosis.[7] Thymocytes express low levels of Bcl-2, consistent with their susceptibility to steroid-induced death, and peripheral lymphocytes express high levels of Bcl-2, consistent with their relative resistance to steroid-induced death. Many, but not all, IEL express high levels of Bcl-2, suggesting alternate mechanisms in their survival. Three populations are observed, of nearly equal proportion, one bearing high levels of Bcl-2, one bearing intermediate levels of Bcl-2, and one with low levels of expression.

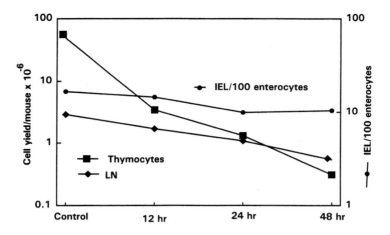

FIGURE 1. Cell yield following hydrocortisone *in vivo*. Resistance of CD4⁺ CD8⁺ IEL to the cytotoxic effect of hydrocortisone. CBA/J mice 8-10 weeks old were injected ip with 4 mg hydrocortisone acetate at 12, 24, or 48 h prior to harvest of thymus and IEL. Total cell yields from thymus and four lymph nodes per mouse were counted. IEL are expressed as number of IEL per 100 enterocytes by hematoxylin-eosin staining of a distal section of the ileum from each mouse. IEL yields by cellular purification paralleled hematoxylin-eosin relative counts; however, due to the extensive protocol for purification of lymphocytes from the epithelium, relative numbers derived by this manner are less meaningful than counts from within the epithelium.

TABLE 1. Lymphocyte Subsets of IEL following Hydrocortisone Administration *in Vivo*[a]

	Control	24 hours	48 hours
TCR α/β	43.7	57.5	46
TCR γ/δ	43.9	33.8	39.2
CD8-β	24.3	41.1	26.7
CD5	15.5	30.1	22.3
CD40L	0.86	0.69	0.86
Thy-1	44.2	58	52.2
CD2	14.1	9.8	17.2

[a] CBA/J mice were injected ip with 4 mg hydrocortisone at 24 or 48 hours prior to tissue harvest. IEL were purified by Percoll gradient, stained with monoclonal antibodies indicated, and analyzed by flow cytometry. Although some variation was seen throughout the experiment, no major population shifts were consistently noted.

Together, these data demonstrate that signaling mechanisms leading to development of IEL differ from peripheral T lymphocytes, as do their responses to immunosuppressive agents. The molecular mechanisms of resistance to apoptotic signals by way of the glucocorticoid receptor remain to be elucidated. Potential pathways include the expression of Bcl-x, a related molecule in function to Bcl-2.[8] Alternately, there may be a direct defect in glucocorticoid receptor signaling, such as is seen in steroid-resistant inflammatory disease.[9]

REFERENCES

1. MOSLEY, R. L., D. STYRE & J. R. KLEIN. 1990. J. Immunol. **145:** 1369-1375.
2. POUSSIER, P., P. EDOUARD, C. LEE, M. BINNIE & M. JULIUS. 1992. J. Exp. Med. **176:** 187-199.
3. ZACHARCHUK, C. M., M. MERCÉP & J. D. ASHWELL. 1991. Ann. N.Y. Acad. Sci. **636:** 52-70.
4. WYLLIE, A. H. 1980. Nature **284:** 555-556.
5. JONDAL, M., S. OKRET & D. MCCONKEY. 1993. Eur. J. Immunol. **23:** 1246-1250.
6. GAVRIELI, Y., Y. SHERMAN & S. A. BEN-SASSON. 1992. J. Cell Biol. **119:** 493-501.
7. STRASSER, A., A. W. HARRIS & S. CORY. 1991. Cell **67:** 889-899.
8. BOISE, L. H., M. GONZALEZ-GARCIA, C. E. POSTEMA, L. DING, T. LINDSTEN, L. A. TURKA, X. MAO, G. NUNEZ & C. B. THOMPSON. 1993. Cell **74:** 597-608.
9. ADCOCK, I. M., S. J. LANE, C. R. BROWN, M. J. PETERS, T. H. LEE & P. J. BARNES. 1995. J. Immunol. **154:** 3500-3505.

Regulation of Chemokine Gene Expression by Contact Hypersensitivity and by Oral Tolerance[a]

YUNN-SHIN YUAN,[b] JENNIFER A. MAJOR,[c] AND
JACK R. BATTISTO [c,d]

[b]Department of Biology
Cleveland State University

[c]Department of Immunology
The Research Institute
Cleveland Clinic Foundation
Cleveland, Ohio 44195

INTRODUCTION

A relatively new group of cytokines, the chemokines, are basic, heparin-binding polypeptides that are locally expressed at inflammatory sites.[1-3] They belong to a superfamily that is divisible into two classes, alpha and beta, on the basis of structure and function. The alpha family members have a C-X-C construct with the two initial cysteines separated by an intervening amino acid, whereas the chemokines of the beta family have no intervening residue. Furthermore, the alpha family members attract and activate neutrophils, whereas those of the beta family are chemoattractants and activators of monocytes. Although other functions for chemokines are rapidly being delineated, their major activity appears to be recruitment of cells to targeted sites.

Certain chemokines have already been shown to be operative in delayed-type hypersensitivity responses in human skin[4] as well as in contact hypersensitivity (CH) in murine skin.[5] In the mouse model the prolonged expression of murine IP-10 (member of the alpha family) and JE/MCP-1 (member of the beta family) genes in the skin during CH to the hapten trinitrochlorobenzene (TNCB) was found attributable to the stimulation emanating from hapten-specific T cells.[5]

In this study we have examined the hypothesis that chemokine gene expression during CH and immunotolerance may be differentially regulated by T lymphocytes.

EXPERIMENTAL DESIGN

The haptens TNCB and oxazalone (OX), that spontaneously couple to self-antigens, were used to initiate CH as well as to induce immunotolerance to CH in mice.

---

[a]Offered in 1994 by Y-S. Yuan in partial fulfillment of the requirements for an advanced degree at CSU.

[d]Address for correspondence: The Cleveland Clinic Foundation, Department of Immunology, 9500 Euclid Avenue, Cleveland, Ohio 44195.

Mice given	Sensitized to TNCB	Challenged TNCB	Tub	IP-10	JE
Nothing	No	Yes			
Nothing	Yes	Yes			
Anti-CD8	Yes	Yes			
Anti-CD4	Yes	Yes			

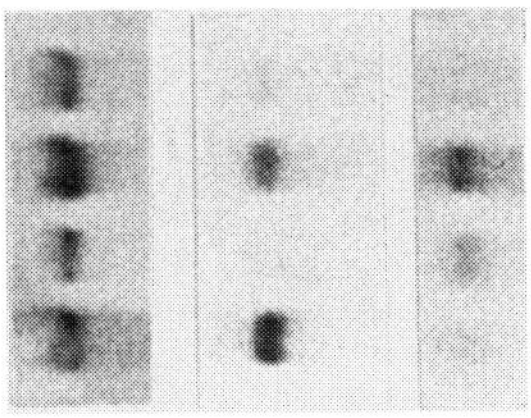

FIGURE 1. Identifying the phenotype of the T cells responsible for mediating chemokine gene activation. Normal mice were given 120 μg of anti-CD4+ or anti-CD8+ antibodies intraperitoneally one day before they, along with normal mice, were painted on abdominal skin with a solution of TNCB in ethanol-acetone. Four to five days later, mice were challenged on both ears with 50 μL of 1% TNCB in olive oil. Extraction of RNA from ear tissue was initiated six hours thereafter. Alpha tubulin (Tub) represents the internal control for the quantity of total mRNA.

CH was induced by painting mice with 0.1 mL of a 5% solution of TNCB or a 3% solution of OX in ethanol/acetone on the fur-clipped abdomen. Thereafter animals were rested for five days before challenging the right ear with 0.05 mL of a 1% solution of TNCB or a 0.5% solution of OX in olive oil, and the left ear with the vehicle alone.

To induce tolerance, the oral administration of haptens preceded the sensitization and challenge protocols. Each lightly etherized mouse was intubated with an olive oil solution of TNCB or OX (7.0 mg/mouse) on two occasions separated by at least one week. They were used a week or more after the final feeding.

Chemokine mRNA levels in the ear skin reaction sites were assayed by Northern hybridization. Extraction of RNA from ear tissue occurred 6 to 18 hours after challenge with either hapten or oil vehicle.

RESULTS AND DISCUSSION

Establishing Which Lymphoid Cells Cause Gene Activation in Contact Hypersensitivity

As the genes for the IP-10 and JE chemokines had been shown to be activated in hypersensitive animals, and as CH is mediated primarily by T lymphocytes of the CD4+ phenotype, it became important to know whether this cell was involved in stimulating each of these genes. To identify the phenotype of responsible T cells, normal mice were given antibodies to the surface molecules that distinguish the two major subsets of T cells (CD4+ and CD8+) in order to inactivate the cells. Thereafter, these mice, along with naive mice, were sensitized to TNCB, challenged on both ears with TNCB in olive oil, and following an appropriate interval, euthanized for extraction of RNA from ear tissue. T cells of the CD8+ phenotype appeared essential for the activation of the IP-10 gene in sensitized mice (FIG. 1). For activating the JE gene, T cells of the CD4+ and CD8+ phenotypes each appeared to be competent (FIG. 1).

Tolerization	Sensitization	GADPH	IP-10	JE
None	OX			
OX Fed	OX			
None	TNCB			
TNCB Fed	TNCB			

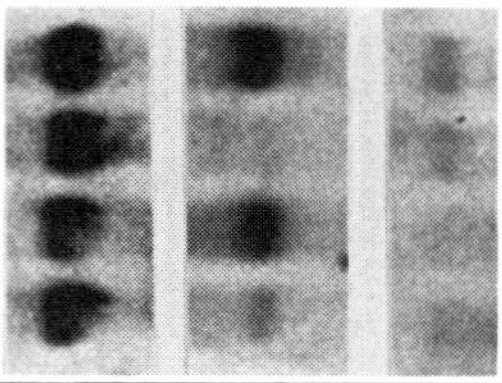

FIGURE 2. Tolerization by feeding haptens down-regulates the activation of the IP-10 gene but not the JE gene. Mice were fed oxazalone (OX, 7 mg) or trinitrochlorobenzene (TNCB, 7 mg) on one occasion and were rested for one week or more. They, along with naive mice, were then treated to induce sensitivity and challenged on the ears four to five days later with the respective hapten. Extraction of RNA was as has been described. The gene that controls synthesis of glyceraldehyde phosphate dehydrogenase (GAPDH) is the internal control for the quantity of total mRNA.

	Condition of Donor	Identity of Splenic Cells	Recipient Sensitized	IP-10
a.	Normal	All	No	
b.	Normal	All	Yes	
c.	Tolerant	All	Yes	
d.	Tolerant	No T cells	Yes	
e.	Tolerant	No CD8$^+$	Yes	
f.	Tolerant	No CD4$^+$	Yes	

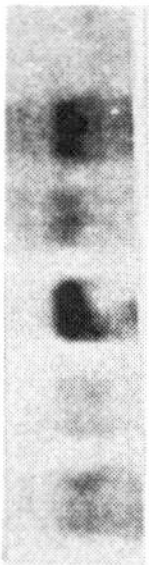

FIGURE 3. T cells of the CD4$^+$ phenotype can control the activation of the IP-10 gene. Equal numbers of splenic cells (50 × 10^6/intended recipient) from mice tolerized by feeding hapten were treated with anti-Thy 1.2, anti-CD8$^+$, anti-CD4$^+$ antibodies and complement, or with complement alone (c). These cells, as well as normal spleen cells, were given iv to naive mice that were then exposed to the five-day sensitization protocol or not. The mice were challenged, and RNA was extracted as has been described.

Effect of Hapten-specific Immunotolerance Achieved by Feeding Hapten on Chemokine Gene Activation

To learn whether tolerance induced toward the hapten would alter the capability to activate the chemokine genes, mice were tolerized before subjecting them to the sensitizing and challenging procedures. One well-known method for inducing immunotolerance is to feed haptens, such as TNCB or OX, by intubation, either once or twice over a three-week interval. Mice that were fed were rested for a week before putting them, along with naive mice, through sensitization and challenging protocols. As may be seen in FIGURE 2, the gene for IP-10 was poorly activated, if at all, in mice that had been tolerized by feeding TNCB or OX. By contrast, the gene for JE appeared not to have been affected in the same way by the tolerization procedure.

To identify the phenotype of the regulatory cells, aliquots of splenic cells of mice tolerized by feeding hapten were treated with anti-Thy 1.2 antibody, anti-CD8⁺ antibody, and anti-CD 4⁺ antibody, as well as complement, or with just complement alone prior to transferring them to naive mice. Examination by FACS of the cells remaining after treatment confirmed that virtually all T cells, CD8⁺ and CD4⁺ cells, had been deleted in the respective groups (data not shown). Thereafter, these mice, along with those given whole populations of normal splenic cells, were exposed to sensitization and/or challenge with TNCB. The T-cell that down-regulated expression of the IP-10 gene was identified as having the CD4⁺ phenotype (FIG. 3).

SUMMARY

In mice with hapten-induced CH, T cells of the CD4⁺ and CD8⁺ phenotypes activated the gene for JE, whereas CD8⁺ T cells alone caused activation of the gene for IP-10. In animals tolerized by feeding either TNCB or OX, hapten-induced expression of IP-10 but not JE mRNA was lost. The down-regulation of IP-10 gene activation was adoptively transferred from tolerized mice to naive mice by CD4⁺ splenic T cells. These findings reflect the differential roles of individual T-cell subsets in both enhancing and diminishing chemokine gene expression in contact hypersensitivity reactions.

REFERENCES

1. OPPENHEIM, J. J., C. O. L. ZACHARIAE, N. MUKAIDA & K. MATSUSHIMA. 1991. Properties of the novel proinflammatory supergene "Intercrine" cytokine family. Annu. Rev. Immunol. **9:** 617.
2. MICHIEL, D. 1993. Chemokines: The missing link. Bio/Technology **11:** 739.
3. LUSTER, A. D. & P. LEDER. 1993. IP-10, a-C-X-C-chemokine, elicits a potent thymus-dependent antitumor response *in vivo.* J. Exp. Med. **178:** 1057.
4. KAPLAN, G., A. D. LUSTER, G. HANCOCK & Z. A. COHN. 1987. The expression of a γ-interferon induced protein (IP-10) in delayed immune responses in human skin. J. Exp. Med. **166:** 1098.
5. GAUTAM, S. C., J. R. BATTISTO, J. A. MAJOR, D. ARMSTRONG, M. STOLER & T. A. HAMILTON. 1994. Chemokine expression in TNCB-mediated contact hypersensitivity. J. Leukocyte Biol. **55:** 452.

Subject Index

Index of Contributors